Thieme

Surgical Ultrasound

René Mantke, MD
Otto von Guericke University
Chairman of the Department
of General and Gastrointestinal
Surgery
City Medical Center
Brandenburg, Germany

Ulrich Peitz, MD
Department of Internal
Medicine Gastroenterology
Raphaelsklinik
Muenster, Germany

With contributions by

Volker Aumann
Thomas Buerger
Christian Goerg
Wolfgang Grechenig
Reinhart Grote
Gerold Kaiper
Juergen Kleinstein
Hardy Krause
Hauke Lang
Hendrik Lehnert
Hans Lippert
Rainer Lueck
Helmut Madjar
Konrad Mahlfeld
Thomas Manger
René Mantke
Johannes Mayr
Harry Rudolf Merk
Géza Pap
Ulrich Peitz
Wolfgang Pichler
Matthias Pross
Kirsten Reschke
Joerg C. Schlegel
Hans Ulrich Schulz
Antje Weimann
Arved Weimann
Hans-Peter Weskott
Uwe Will
Eike Wrenger

957 illustrations

Georg Thieme Verlag
Stuttgart · New York

Library of Congress Cataloging-in-Publication Data
is available from the publisher.

This book is an authorized and revised translation of the German edition published and copyrighted 2001 by Georg Thieme Verlag, Stuttgart, Germany. Title of the German edition: Sonographie für Chirurgen.

Translator: Dietrich Herrmann, Hameln, Germany
Illustrator: Karin Baum, Paphos, Cyprus

Rüdigerstraße 14, 70469 Stuttgart, Germany
http://www.thieme.de
Thieme New York, 333 Seventh Avenue,
New York, NY 10001, USA
http://www.thieme.com

Typesetting by Ziegler + Müller, Kirchentellinsfurt
Printed in Germany by Grammlich, Pliezhausen
10-ISBN 3-13-131871-6 (GTV)
13-ISBN 978-3-13-131871-8 (GTV)
10-ISBN 1-58890-190-4 (TNY)
13-ISBN 978-1-58890-190-3 (TNY)

1 2 3 4 5 6

Dedicated to Hans Lippert
on the occasion of his 60th birthday.

Professor Lippert is Director of the Clinic of General, Visceral, and Vascular Surgery at the Otto von Guericke University Hospital in Magdeburg, Germany.

Foreword

Modern medicine is characterized by a high degree of specialization on the one hand and by problem-oriented multidisciplinary cooperation on the other. In the medical field, this concentration of expertise from different authorities, which applies to diagnostic as well as to therapeutic management, is a rather new way of approaching a problem.

Evaluation of the real-time image by the physician in charge and the possibility of repeating the examination without endangering or straining the patient render ultrasonography a particularly attractive investigation.

Preoperative, intraoperative, postoperative, and interventional application has promoted this universally available method to an integral component of the physical examination in many disciplines in which the ultrasound machine has gained a role equivalent to that of the stethoscope.

Specific qualifications and ongoing training are indispensable in order that experience as well as technical innovations will flow into the diagnostic cycle.

We are accordingly supporting our colleagues in the systematic constitution of ultrasound in our specialty. All physicians should acquire the competence to perform sonographic examinations in the sphere of their specialty so that they can use ultrasound as a basic diagnostic tool.

For many years, Dr Mantke and Dr Peitz have been promulgating excellent knowledge of ultrasound and extensive experience in the teaching of sonographic techniques. With this book they have succeeded in elaborating a systematic presentation of ultrasound applications in surgical disciplines. A wide range of excellent imaging material illustrates the theoretical basic knowledge and certainly benefits the reader.

We hope and expect that this cooperative work will find ready acceptance in medical practice.

Hans Lippert, MD
Professor
Head of the Clinical Department
of General, Visceral, and Vascular Surgery
Otto von Guericke University
Magdeburg, Germany

P. Malfertheiner, MD
Professor
Head of the Clinical Department
of Gastroenterology and Hepatology
Otto von Guericke University
Magdeburg, Germany

Preface

Many readers may ask "Why yet another book on ultrasound?" The answer appears obvious to us: an up-to-date teaching book on ultrasound, comprehensive and yet compact, oriented toward the surgical specialties and focusing on the major topics in surgery is in demand. The ranking of ultrasound among the investigations for surgical diseases has been steadily rising. The reasons are a high diagnostic yield in the first line, combined with availability at almost any time and place, lack of risks, and low cost.

Establishing diagnoses of surgical diseases and deciding on indications for surgical interventions are tasks inherent to the duties of the surgeon, which he or she often fulfills in cooperation with colleagues from related nonsurgical disciplines. The cooperative concept is reflected in the selection of the co-authors for this book. A major part of the text has arisen from interdisciplinary cooperation between surgeons and, for example, endocrinologists, gastroenterologists, gynecologists, orthopedists, and urologists. In most surgical pathologies, sonographic techniques can make substantial contributions along the diagnostic pathway. This applies in particular to surgical emergencies, where ultrasound proves valuable, for example, in the assessment of blunt abdominal trauma and of bowel obstruction, and in the diagnostic confirmation or elimination of cardiac tamponade and of pleural effusions. The debate about which clinical medical disciplines should and may practice diagnostic ultrasound that has been going on for years has in fact long been decided by the reality: the person who is in charge of the patient performs the sonographic examination. Of course that person will ask for guidance and help from the most experienced colleague from his or her institution.

For good reasons, sonographic diagnostic techniques have been incorporated into the logbook of the general surgical trainee and into specialized surgical training programs. In the same way, the formation of a surgical section of the German Society of Ultrasound in Medicine (Deutsche Gesellschaft für Ultraschall in der Medizin [DEGUM]) and the foundation of a Surgical Working Group for Endoscopy and Ultrasound (Chirurgische Arbeitsgemeinschaft Endoskopie und Ultraschall [CAE]) within the German Association of Surgery underline the importance of sonographic examinations in the surgical field.

Ultrasound machines for B-mode and Doppler sonography are nowadays available in every surgical hospital department and in many outpatient clinics and surgeries. Color Doppler ultrasound and its refinements, such as power Doppler ultrasound, are frequently also present or are being shared by members of different disciplines. Miniaturization of ultrasound computers has made possible the construction of portable machines that can be used at the patient's bedside, in the emergency room, or at the site of an accident. Newer technical developments like tissue harmonic imaging and contrast harmonic imaging as well as panoramic and three-dimensional reconstructions are promising to amplify diagnostic possibilities considerably.

The intention of this book is to present surgically relevant knowledge of sonography in a quickly comprehensible and practically oriented form. For this purpose, all sections have been uniformly divided into three units consisting of "Relevant Basic Information," "Sonographic Criteria," and "Consequences for Surgical Treatment." The existing guidelines of the German Association of Surgery have been integrated into the corresponding chapters.

Despite all established surgical standards, every patient requires individual therapeutic decisions. Taking this into account, any book can only be used for basic guidance. The knowledge imparted is founded on numerous publications, the most important of which are listed at the end of the book to enable the reader to gain deeper insight into the matter.

Interpretation of static ultrasound images proves difficult for the unskilled observer. For this reason, each photograph has been accompanied by an explanatory schematic drawing. Sonography does, however, provide and thrive on moving pictures, rendered possible by the process of real-time imaging. The dynamics result on one hand from the examination course itself, with free selection of imaging planes, on the other from the registration of mobile body functions, in particular of the blood flow. Because of these dynamic conditions, the learning of sonography—examination technique as well as image and sound interpretation—requires multiple practical exercises under the guidance of a colleague qualified for training. Practical skills are acquired during daily work as well as from the courses of surgical and radiological colleges. This book has been conceived to provide the necessary theoretical foundation for the resident and fellow in training as much as for the qualified surgeon.

We are particularly indebted to the Directors of our Departments, Professor H. Lippert and Professor P. Malfertheiner, without whose help and generous support the investment of time would not have been tolerable, as much as to our wives Marita Mantke and Lucia Clara Peitz and our children, who had to sacrifice many night and weekend hours with their husbands and fathers. We also express our gratitude to Thomas Scherb MD, Marion Ueckert, Susanne Ristea, and Claudia Güner for the German edition, to Clifford Bergman, Annie Hollins, and Dietrich Herrmann for the English edition, and to the entire team of the Thieme publishing group for their excellent professional support.

Finally, we apologize for any errors that might remain despite the most careful proofreading, and we would sincerely appreciate any constructive critical comment on this book.

René Mantke, Ulrich Peitz

Contributors

Volker Aumann, MD
Department of Pediatrics
University Hospital
Magdeburg, Germany

Thomas Buerger, MD
Associate Professor
Otto von Guericke University
Department of General, Abdominal, and Vascular Surgery
University Hospital
Magdeburg, Germany

Christian Goerg, MD
Professor
Philipps University
Department of Internal Medicine
Marburg, Germany

Wolfgang Grechenig, MD
Professor of Traumatology
University Clinic of Traumatology
Graz, Austria

Reinhard Grote, MD
Professor
Department of Radiology
City Hospital Magdeburg Olvenstedt
Magdeburg, Germany

Gerold Kaiper, MD
Otto von Guericke University
Department of Urology
University Hospital
Magdeburg, Germany

Juergen Kleinstein, MD
Professor
Clinic for Reproductive Medicine and Gynecology Endocrinology
Otto von Guericke University
Magdeburg, Germany

Hardy Krause, MD
Division of Pediatric Surgery
Department of General, Abdominal, and Vascular Surgery
University Hospital
Magdeburg, Germany

Hauke Lang, MD, FACS
Department of General and Transplantation Surgery
University of Essen
Essen, Germany

Hendrik Lehnert, MD, FRCP
Professor
Chair of Medicine
Warwick Medical School
Coventry University Hospital
Coventry, United Kingdom

Hans Lippert, MD
Professor of Surgery
Head of Department of General, Abdominal, and Vascular Surgery
University Hospital
Magdeburg, Germany

Rainer Lueck, MD
Department of Abdominal and Transplantation Surgery
Hanover Medical School
Hanover, Germany

Helmut Madjar, MD
Department of Gynecology
Professor and Chairman
German Diagnostic Clinic
Wiesbaden, Germany

Konrad Mahlfeld, MD
Department of Orthopedics
Otto von Guericke University
Magdeburg, Germany

Thomas Manger, MD
Professor
Department of General, Visceral, and Pediatric Surgery
SRH Wald Hospital Gera GmbH
Academic Hospital of the Friedrich Schiller University Jena
Gera, Germany

René Mantke, MD
Associate Professor
Otto von Guericke University
Magdeburg, Germany
Chairman of the Department of General and Gastrointestinal Surgery
City Medical Center Brandenburg
Brandenburg, Germany

Johannes Mayr, MD
Professor
Department of Pediatric Surgery
University of Basel
Basel, Switzerland

Harry Rudolf Merk, MD, MSc
Department of Orthopedics
Ernst Moritz Arndt University
Greifswald, Germany

Géza Pap, MD
Department of Orthopedics
Otto von Guericke University
Magdeburg, Germany

Ulrich Peitz, MD
Associate Professor
Department of Internal Medicine
Gastroenterology
Raphaelsklinik
Muenster, Germany

Wolfgang Pichler, MD
University Clinic of Traumatology
Graz, Austria

Matthias Pross, MD
Associate Professor
Department of Surgery
DRK Kliniken Berlin/Koepenick
Berlin, Germany

Kirsten Reschke, MD
Otto von Guericke University
Department of Endocrinology and Metabolism
Magdeburg, Germany

Joerg C. Schlegel, PhD
Marketing Manager
Ultrasound Business Group
Toshiba Medical Systems Europe BV
Head Office
Zoetermeer, Netherlands

Hans Ulrich Schulz, MD
Professor of Surgery
Department of General, Abdominal, and Vascular Surgery
University Hospital
Magdeburg, Germany

Antje Weimann, MD
Transplantation Outpatient Clinic
Department of Abdominal, Transplantation, Vascular, and Chest Surgery
University of Leipzig
Leipzig, Germany

Arved Weimann, MD
Head of Department of General and Abdominal Surgery
St. George Hospital
Affiliated Hospital of the University of Leipzig
Leipzig, Germany

Hans-Peter Weskott, MD
Department of Ultrasound
Klinikum Region Hannover
Siloah General Hospital
Hanover, Germany

Uwe Will, MD
Department of Internal Medicine III
Municipal Hospital
Gera, Germany

Eike Wrenger, MD
Center for Nephrology and Dialysis
Langenhagen (Hanover), Germany

List of Abbreviations

β-HCG beta-human chorion gonadotropin
AAA abdominal aortic aneurysm
ABC airways, breathing, circulation
ABI ankle-brachial pressure index
ADF advanced dynamic flow
AFP alpha-fetoprotein
ALT alanine aminotransferase
AP alkaline phosphatase
A-P anteroposterior
APACHE acute physiology and chronic health evaluation
APC argon plasma coagulation
ASA acetylsalicylic acid
ASIC application-specific integrated circuit
AST aspartate aminotransferase
AV ateriovenous
bFGF basic fibroblast growth factor
BPH basic prostatic hyperplasia
CBC complete blood count
CBD common bile duct
CCA common carotid artery
CCK cholecystokinin
CEA carcinoembryonic antigen
CEUS contrast-enhanced ultrasonography
CFA common femoral artery
CFDI color flow Doppler imaging
CFV common femoral vein
CHD common hepatic duct
CIA common iliac artery
CIV common iliac vein
CNS central nervous system
CRP C-reactive protein
CT computed tomography
CUP cancer of unknown primary
CVI chronic venous insufficiency
CVP central venous pressure
CW continuous wave
D dimension(al)
DD differential diagnosis
DEGUM Deutsche Gesellschaft für Ultraschall in der Medizin (German Association of Ultrasound in Medicine)
DFA deep femoral artery
DFV deep femoral vein
DGOT Deutsche Gesellschaft für Orthopädie und Traumatologie (German Society of Orthopedics and Traumatology)
DI damping index
DICOM digital imaging and communication in medicine
DSA digital subtraction angiography
DSO Deutsche Stiftung Organtransplantation (German Foundation of Organ Transplantation)
DVT deep venous thrombosis
EBV Epstein–Barr virus
ECA external carotid artery
ECG electrocardiogram
EDV, V_{ed} end-diastolic (blood flow) velocity
EGF epidermal growth factor
EIA external iliac artery
EIV external iliac vein
EMG exomphalos, macroglossia, gigantism (syndrome)
ERC endoscopic retrograde cholangiography
ERCP endoscopic retrograde cholangio-pancreatography
ESR erythrocyte sedimentation rate
ESWL extracorporal shock wave lithotripsy
ET embryo transfer
EUS endoscopic ultrasound, endosonography
FAP familial adenomatous polyposis
FAST focused assessment by sonography for trauma
FNA fine-needle aspiration
FNAB fine-needle aspiration biopsy
FNH focal nodular hyperplasia
FPV femoropopliteal vein
fT_3 free triiodothyronine
fT_4 free tetraiodothyronine (thyroxine)
FV femoral vein
GGT gamma-glutamyl transpeptidase
GI gastrointestinal
GIST gastrointestinal stromal tumor(s)
GLDH glutamate dehydrogenase
GnRH gonadotropin releasing hormone
GSaV greater saphenous vein
H&H hemoglobin and hematocrit
H. pylori Helicobacter pylori
Hb hemoglobin
HCC hepatocellular carcinoma
HCT hematocrit
HELLP hemolysis, elevated liver enzyme, low platelet count
HIDA hepatobiliary iminodiacetic acid
HIS Hospital Information System
HNPCC hereditary nonpolyposis colorectal cancer
HU Hounsfield unit
i.v. intravenous(ly)
IBD inflammatory bowel disease
ICA internal carotid artery
ICU intensive care unit
IDDM insulin-dependent diabetes mellitus
IDUS intraductal ultrasound
IGF insulin-like growth factor
IHPS infantile hypertrophic pyloric stenosis
IIA internal iliac artery
IIV internal iliac vein
IJV internal jugular vein

IMA inferior mesenteric artery
INR international normalized ratio
INSS International Neuroblastoma Staging System
IOS intraoperative ultrasound
IPMT intraductal papillary mucinous tumor
IVC inferior vena cava
IVF in vitro fertilization
IVUS intravascular ultrasonography
KUB kidneys, ureters, bladder
LDH lactate dehydrogenase
LHV left hepatic vein
LMWH low molecular weight heparin
LN lymph node
LSaV lesser saphenous vein
L–T_4 l-thyroxine
LTx liver transplant(ation)
MALT mucosa-associated lymphoid tissue
MBO mechanical bowel obstruction
MCL mid-clavicular line
MCS microscopy, culture, and sensitivity
MEN multiple endocrine neoplasia
MHV middle hepatic vein
MI mechanical index
MIBI methoxyisobutylisonitrile
MPR multiplanar reslicing
MRA magnetic resonance angiography
MRC magnet resonance cholangiography
MRCP magnetic resonance cholangio-pancreatography
MRI magnet resonance imaging
Nd:YAG Neodymium:yttrium-aluminum-garnet
NSAID nonsteroidal anti-inflammatory drug
PA popliteal artery
PAOD peripheral occlusiver arterial disease
PCN percutaneous nephrostomy
PCNL percutaneous nephrolithotomy
PCR polymerase chain reaction
PDT photodynamic therapy
PET positron emission tomography
PI pulsatility index
PID pelvic inflammatory disease
PoV portal vein
PPS post-phlebitic syndrome
PRF pulse repetition frequency
PRIND prolonged reversible ischemic neurological deficit
PSA prostate-specific antigen
PSV peak systolic velocity
PT prothrombin time
PTA percutaneous transluminal angioplasty
PTC percutaneous transhepatic cholangiography
PTCD percutaneous transhepatic cholangiography and drainage
PTFE poly(tetrafluoroethylene)
PTT partial thromboplastin time
PV popliteal vein
PW pulsed wave
PTX pancreas transplant
RBC red blood count
RES reticuloenothelial system
RFA radiofrequency ablation
RHV right hepatic vein
RI resistance index
ROI region of interest
RR (blood pressure measured with the method described by) Riva-Rocci
RT/CT radiochemotherapy
SFA superficial femoral artery
SFJ sapheno-femoral junction
SFV superficial femoral vein
SLAP superior labrum anterior–posterior
SLE systemic lupus erythematosus
SLT split liver transplant
SMA superior mesenteric artery
SMV superior mesenteric vein
SPECT single-photon emission computed tomography
SPJ sapheno-popliteal junction
SPV systolic peak (flow) velocity
SV splenic vein
T_3 triiodothyronine
T_4 thyroxine = tetraiodothyronine
TA tibial artery
TAUS transabdominal ultrasound
TEA thrombendarterectomy
TEE transesophageal echocardiography
TEM transanal endoscopic microsurgery
TGC time gain compensation
TIA transient ischemic attack
TIPSS transjugular intrahepatic portosystemic stent shunt
TPO-Ab thyrocyte peroxidase antibody
TRAb TSH receptor antibodies
TRUS transrectal ultrasound
TSH thyroid-stimulating hormone
TSH-R-Ab TSH-receptor antibody
TURP transurethral resection of the prostate
TV tibial vein
Tx transplantation
UCA ultrasonic contrast agent
US ultrasound/ultrasonography
VA vertebral artery
VIP vasoactive intestinal (poly)peptide
VV vertebral vein
WBC white blood count
WHO World Health Organization

Contents

1 Acute Abdomen

U. Peitz, R. Mantke, J. Kleinstein

Appendicitis

Basic Facts

- Appendicitis is primarily a clinical diagnosis. The typical patient presents with initial visceral or referred pain in the periumbilical or epigastric region, possibly compounded later by the physical signs of the beginning of peritonitis. Depending on the location of the inflamed appendix, the pain will shift to the right or left lower quadrant and even the right hypochondrium. Acute appendicitis in children and the elderly, as well as in the pregnant patient, may be particularly difficult to confirm.
- The lifetime incidence of appendicitis averages 10%. Inflammation of the appendix may occur at any age, though it most commonly arises in the second and third decades of life.
- Sonography of a patient with suspected appendicitis is guided by these objectives: keeping the negative laparotomy rate below 20% and the perforation rate at surgery below 10%.
- The diagnostic sensitivity of sonography in appendicitis is very much operator dependent, even though in experienced hands it may reach 90%. Thus, while a nonvisualized appendix does not exclude the possibility of inflammation, the specificity of this imaging modality is generally high–approaching 95% in several studies (Puylaert, 1990; Schwerk et al., 1989).
- Sonography helps to differentiate acute appendicitis from other diseases, in particular bacterial or viral infections in the ileocecal region, Crohn disease, gynecological conditions, ureteral obstruction, etc. (Puylaert, 1990).
- *Additional workup:* laparoscopy, in cases of significant diagnostic ambiguity perhaps preceded by CT of the abdomen.

Sonographic Criteria

- Usually, the normal appendix is too small and not echogenic enough for distinction from the surrounding structures. It may be demonstrated in the presence of ascites (Fig. 1.**1**).
- **Appendicitis:** The inflamed appendix appears as a tender, aperistaltic tube > 6 mm in diameter (Figs. 1.**2**–1.**5**). Less frequently it assumes the shape of a sausage ring. Differential diagnosis must include concomitant appendiceal swelling in IBD.
- The muscle layer of the appendix is usually preserved in acute appendicitis (Figs. 1.**1**–1.**5**). Owing to edematous swelling, wall layering may become more pronounced, in which case on cross-sections the appendix will look like a small target sign (Figs. 1.**1**, 1.**3**).
- For ease of orientation, trace the cecum to its base where the appendix originates. Frequently, the cecum will also be swollen by edema (Figs. 1.**2**, 1.**4**).
- Demonstration of the ileocecal valve will help to differentiate between the terminal ileum and appendix.
- Ectopic locations of the appendix include the retrocecal and true pelvic as well right upper quadrant positions. The retrocecal region is best assessed by scanning from the midaxillary line to behind the cecum (Fig. 1.**5**).
- Inflamed perienteric fatty tissue and/or omentum surrounding the distended appendix may induce cap-shaped enhancement ("echogenic halo" or "omental cap," although omentum and mesentery cannot be differentiated) (Figs. 1.**3**–1.**5**).
- Fluid collection around the appendix may be due to suppuration or may signal beginning perforation.
- In free perforation with diffuse peritonitis, the appendix can frequently no longer be delineated,
- A pericecal abscess is characterized by fluid around the base of the cecum, walled off by mesentery or omentum. Enlarged lymph nodes may be demonstrated, and sometimes the remains of the appendix are seen in the abscess cavity (Fig. 1.**6**).
- Differential diagnosis of ileocecal inflammation and/or mesenteric lymphadenitis:
  - Extended uniform thickening of the wall of the ileum, possibly extending into the cecum and ascending colon, affecting mainly the mucosa and the submucosal layer (Fig. 1.**7**).
  - Active, possibly heightened, peristalsis.
  - Demonstration of a distended ileocecal valve (Fig. 1.**8**).
  - Mesenteric lymphadenitis: enlarged (diameter > 5 mm) hypoechoic mesenteric lymph nodes (Fig. 1.**7**).

Consequences for Surgical Treatment

Diagnosis	Characteristic Findings	Management
Acute appendicitis	Distended appendix, cap-shaped hyperechoic perienteric fat ("omental cap"), typical clinical signs	Laparoscopic or open appendectomy
Pericecal abscess	Hypoechoic or anechoic mass in the right lower quadrant, possibly with gas collections	Drainage

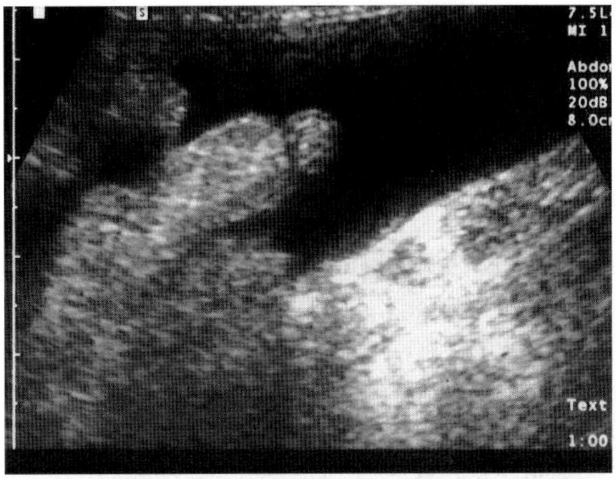

Fig. 1.1 **a** Cross-sectional image showing the normal appendix and mesoappendix in a patient with ascites in liver disease. The appendix displays the typical five-layered gut signature.

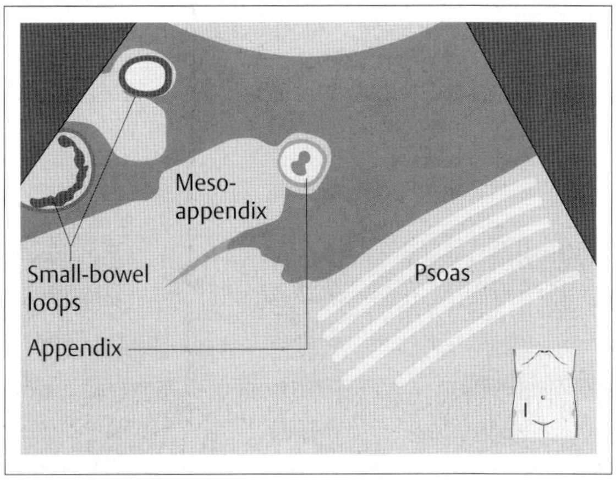

Fig. 1.1 **b** Line drawing.

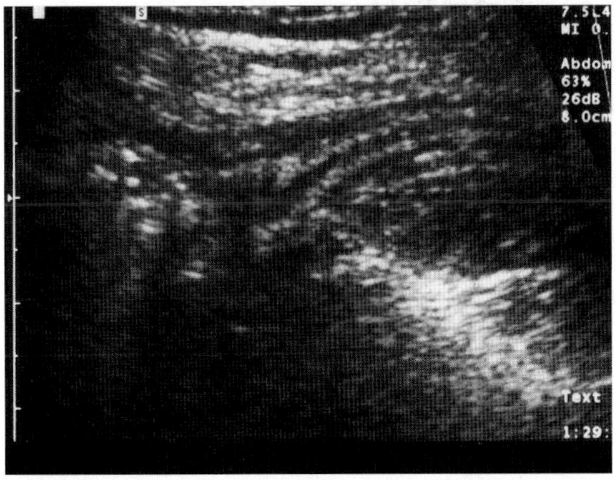

Fig. 1.2 **a** Acute appendicitis with phlegmon on histopathology. In the long axis the distended appendix measures 15 mm in diameter. The five-layered gut signature is preserved.

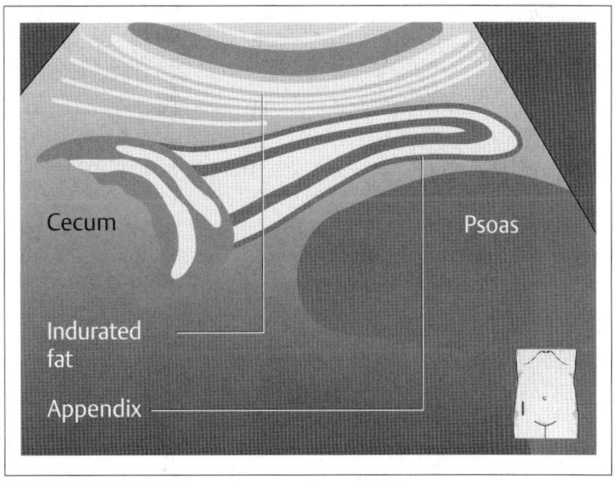

Fig. 1.2 **b** Line drawing.

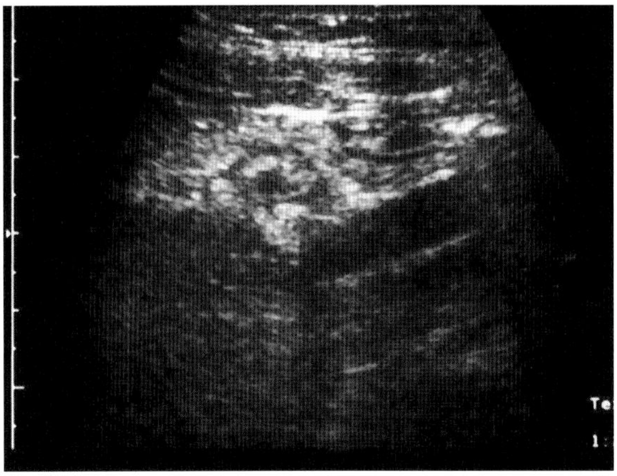

Fig. 1.**3a** Same patient as in Fig. 1.**2**. Transverse view of the distended appendix with preserved gut signature, encased by hyperechoic fat.

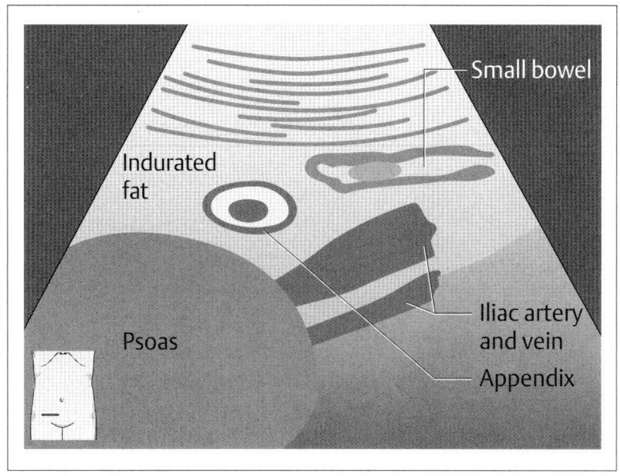

Fig. 1.**3b** Line drawing.

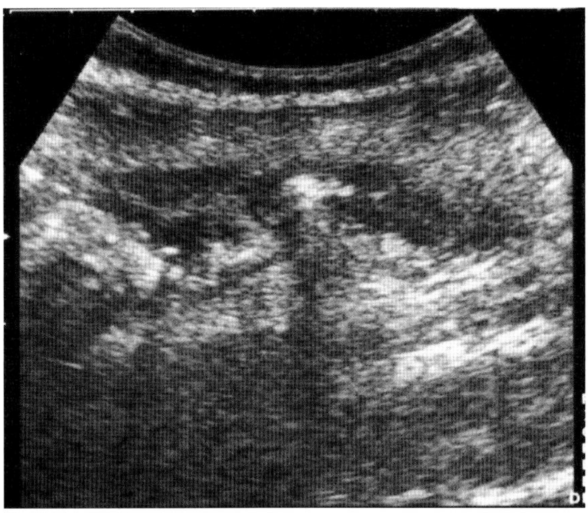

Fig. 1.**4a** Acute suppurative appendicitis. Long-axis view of the distended appendix (maximum diameter 12 mm) with its origin at the also swollen cecum. Either appendicolith or intraluminal gas with characteristic posterior shadowing. The appendix is encased by hyperechoic fat.

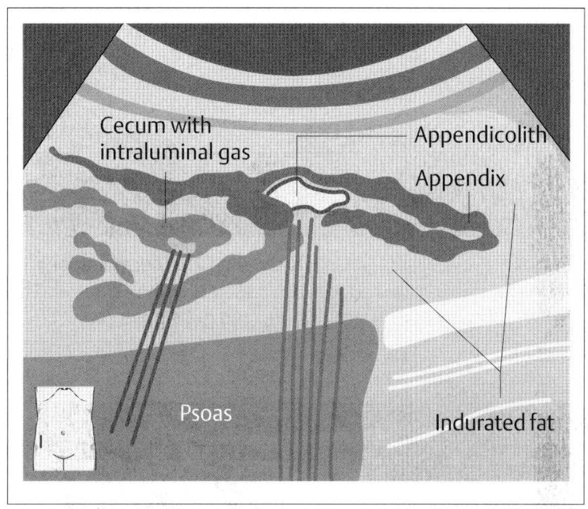

Fig. 1.**4b** Line drawing.

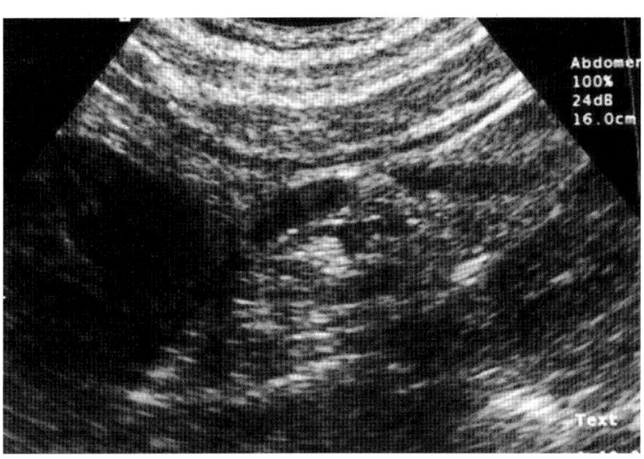

Fig. 1.**5a** Retrocecal appendicitis. Long-axis view of the distended appendix (maximum diameter 11 mm) in its retrocecal position dorsolateral to the ascending colon and reaching cephalad to the lower pole of the right kidney. There is less hyperechoic fat, as this area primarily contains little fat. Small intraluminal gas echo.

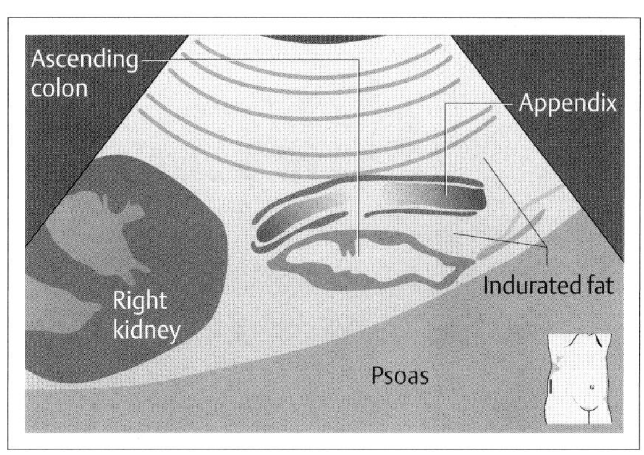

Fig. 1.**5b** Line drawing.

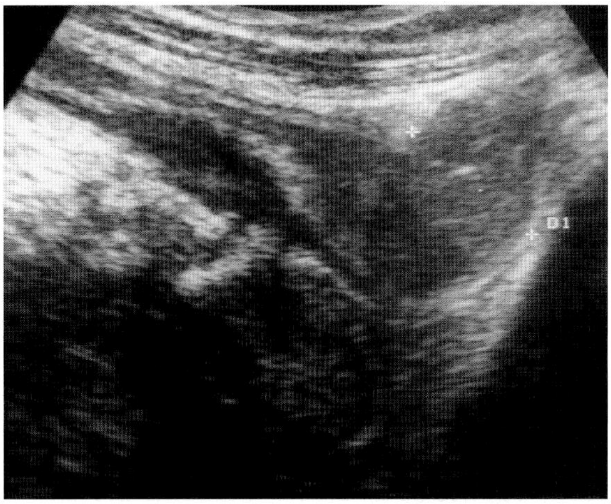

Fig. 1.**6 a** Small periappendiceal abscess. The appendix can only be identified by its hyperechoic lumen. Its wall is indistinguishable from a small hypoechoic mass, which in turn blends in with the muscle layer of the terminal ileum. The latter appears stenosed, owing to compression from outside. Caveat: misdiagnosis of Crohn disease.

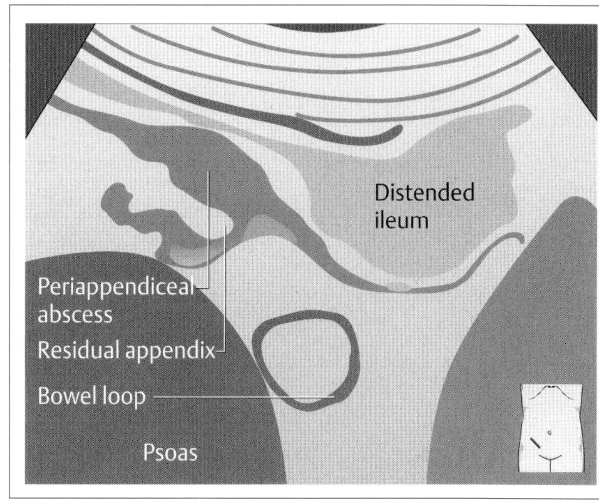

Fig. 1.**6 b** Line drawing.

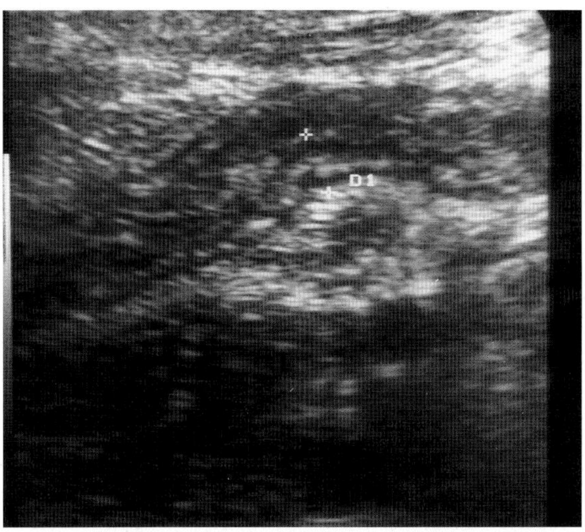

Fig. 1.**7 a** Ileocecal inflammation due to bacterial infection with Yersinia. The wall of the terminal ileum is thickened, primarily its mucosal and submucosal layers. There is a mildly enlarged mesenteric lymph node (8 mm).

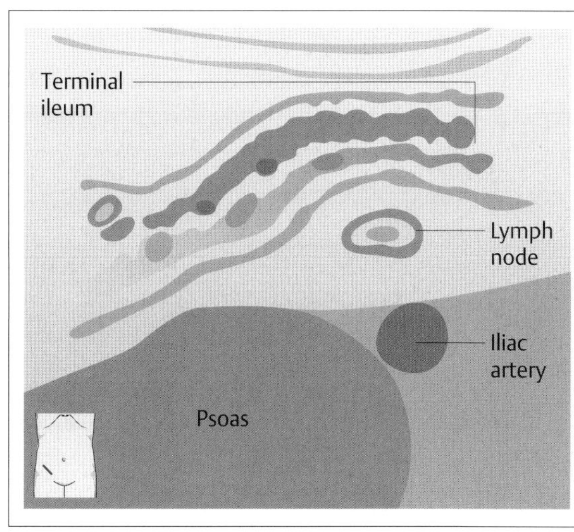

Fig. 1.**7 b** Line drawing.

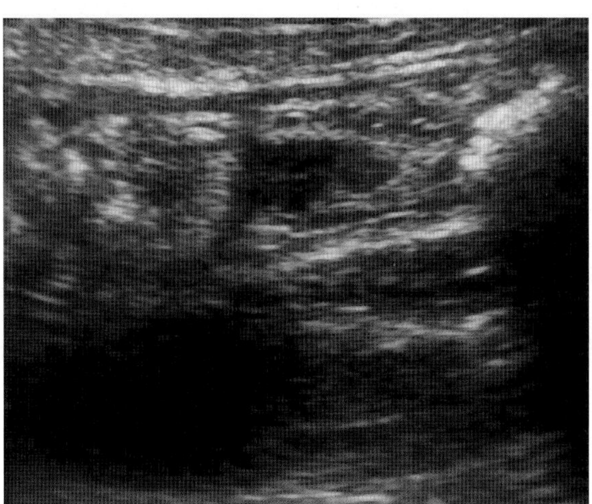

Fig. 1.**8 a** Same patient as in Fig. 1.**7**. Long-axis view of the cecum and ascending colon. Inside the lumen, on cross-section the ileocecal valve is discerned as a hypoechoic orifice-like structure.

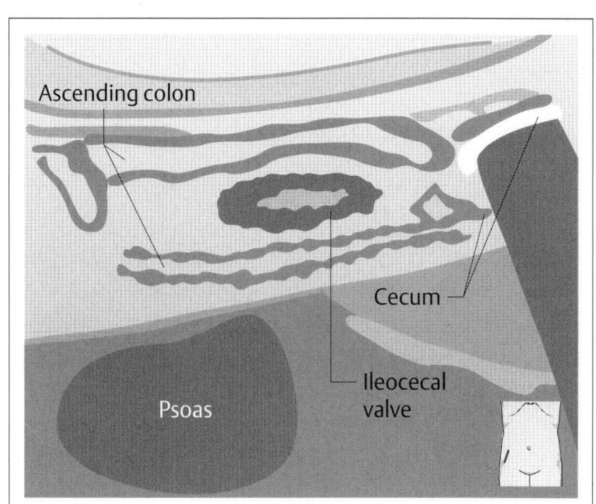

Fig. 1.**8 b** Line drawing.

Acute Cholecystitis

Basic Facts

Causes and Pathophysiology

- Cholelithiasis in 95% of cases (see Chapter 7, p. 159).
  Pathogenesis: usually due to calculous obstruction of the cystic duct, less frequently obstruction by bile duct stones or tumor.
  Sequelae:
  - Bacterial infection (in about 80% of cases).
  - Chemical irritation by lysolecithin and other bile components.
  - Ischemia secondary to increased wall tension.
- Nonobstructive acalculous cholecystitis in the remaining 5% of cases.
  Pathogenesis:
  - Stress, especially in critically ill patients (see Chapter 4, Ultrasound in the Intensive Care Unit, p. 70).
  - Primary infection (e.g., with streptococci, salmonella, leptospira, Vibrio cholerae, parasites; in patients with AIDS, cytomegalovirus infections are of particular relevance).
  - Diabetes.
  - Toxic effects from local chemoembolization.

Clinical Presentation

- There may be a history of biliary colic. Patients typically complain of continuous pain in the right upper quadrant and epigastrium, worsened by deep inspiration, with referral to the back and right shoulder. Tenderness in the right upper quadrant, sometimes with guarding, is found on physical examination. In one-third of the patients, a tender gallbladder may be palpated ("Murphy's sign").
- Pathological laboratory parameters of inflammation: elevated WBC, CRP, ESR.

Complications

- Empyema of the gallbladder or intramural abscess formation.
- Localized or diffuse peritonitis, possibly without frank perforation.
- Perforation and viscus penetration. In hyperacute cholecystitis, free perforation into the peritoneal cavity commonly results in diffuse biliary or purulent peritonitis. More protracted courses tend to result in perforations walled off by omentum and/or adjacent viscus. Progression to a pericholecystic abscess can ensue, with penetration into neighboring organs, in particular into the liver (Bakalakos et al., 1996). In even more protracted cases, the gallbladder may perforate into the stomach, or more frequently into the duodenum or more distal bowel, with passage of stones into the gastrointestinal lumen, sometimes resulting in intestinal obstruction (gallstone ileus) due to impaction of a calculus (pp. 14–17, Intestinal Obstruction).
- Sonography is the diagnostic imaging modality of choice and is frequently sufficient on its own. It has proved superior to CT and MRI in acute gallbladder disease (Harvey and Miller, 1999; Park et al., 1998).
- *Additional workup:* plain abdominal films (mainly for differential diagnosis), ERCP. Rarely required: MRCP, PTC, CT, HIDA scan, EUS.

Sonographic Criteria

Hydropic Gallbladder

- Large, tense, and tender gallbladder ("sonographic Murphy's sign").
- Gallbladder size is variable, its typical maximum dimensions being: length 10 cm, diameter 4 cm. Long-term chronic inflammation quite often results in a shrunken gallbladder. In the elderly with cholecystolithiasis the gallbladder may be significantly distended, reaching into the pelvis in extreme cases, yet causing only mild clinical symptoms, if any.
- More important than size is the presence of tense filling characterized by an ovoid shape (Figs. 1.**9**–1.**11**), lack of compressibility with the ultrasound probe or on digital palpation, local tenderness over the gallbladder, and indentation of adjacent structures including the abdominal wall (Fig. 1.**9**).
- For ectopic locations see Chapter 7, Biliary System, p. 158.

Acute Cholecystitis

- Evidence of a hydropic gallbladder.
- Gallbladder wall thickness of more than 3 mm. This is a nonspecific sign (Wegener et al., 1987)–for differential diagnosis see Table 1.**1.** The thickness of the gallbladder wall is inversely proportional to the wall tension, i.e., wall thickness decreases with increasing intraluminal pressure. Thus, normal wall thickness does not rule out cholecystitis, and the diameter of the wall does not correlate with the severity of inflammation (Figs. 1.**9**–1.**11**).
- Stratification of the gallbladder wall into three (Fig. 1.**9**) or more (Fig. 1.**10**) layers is frequently cited as clear evidence of acute cholecystitis, but its specificity has been found to be poor (Teefey et al., 1991).
- Asymmetric thickening of the gallbladder wall, detachment of its innermost layer, or intraluminal membrane formation are often manifestations of an intramural abscess (Figs. 1.**10,** 1.**11**).
- Sludge within the gallbladder. If the entire lumen is filled with floating echoes, an empyema is highly likely (Fig. 1.**11**), but sonomorphological differentiation from sludge is impossible. Sludge is a sign of low specificity (Chapter 7, Biliary System, p. 158), but one of several criteria in acalculous cholecystitis.

- A gallbladder encased by a hypoechoic rim, revealing pericholecystic edema especially when it is in contact with the liver, is another nonspecific sign. Its other causes are identical to those of gallbladder wall thickening (Table 1.**1**).
- Walling off of the inflammatory process by hyperechoic fatty tissue (Figs. 1.**9**, 1.**10**) is usually less pronounced in cholecystitis than in acute appendicitis or diverticulitis.
- Inflammatory reaction of neighboring bowel segments is seen on ultrasound as hypoechoic edematous distension of the bowel wall (Fig. 1.**10**).
- *Complications:*
  - Perforation: fluid collections around the gallbladder, in most cases walled off by omentum or adjacent viscus (Fig. 1.**9**). Sonography cannot discriminate the nature of the fluid; e.g., bile cannot be differentiated from pus.
  - Formation of a hepatic abscess: liquid intrahepatic mass contiguous with the inflamed gallbladder. Simple edema of liver parenchyma may yield a similar image.
  - Emphysematous cholecystitis: gas collections within the gallbladder wall, visualized by ring-down (comet-tail) artifacts and posterior shadowing, may be difficult to differentiate from a gallbladder full of stones, porcelain gallbladder (calcified wall), and cholesterolosis of the gallbladder (see Chapter 7, Biliary System, p. 164).
  - Uncommon: dilated bile ducts due to CBD obstruction (for differential diagnosis see Chapter 7, Biliary System, p. 167). Most such cases are associated with ascending cholangitis.

Consequences for Surgical Treatment

Diagnosis	Characteristic Findings	Management
Uncomplicated acute cholecystitis	Typical clinical presentation and laboratory parameters; tense, tender gallbladder with thickened wall and pericholecystic edema	Symptom duration < 72 hours: laparoscopic (or open) cholecystectomy; symptom duration > 72 hours: nonoperative attempt with antibiotics, cholecystectomy when acute inflammation has subsided
Acute cholecystitis with complications	As above plus: signs of intramural or pericholecystic abscess formation	Laparoscopic (if the surgeon is sufficiently experienced), otherwise open cholecystectomy
Acute cholecystitis with complications	Possible malignancy or Diffuse peritonitis or Decompensated hepatic cirrhosis or Prior major surgery in the same area	Open cholecystectomy
Acute cholecystitis with bile duct obstruction	Signs of acute cholecystitis complemented by jaundice, elevated bilirubin, AP and GGT levels, and dilated bile ducts on sonography	If possible, ERCP and endoscopic management of the obstruction followed by elective cholecystectomy; alternatively, cholecystectomy with intraoperative cholangiography and possibly bile duct exploration

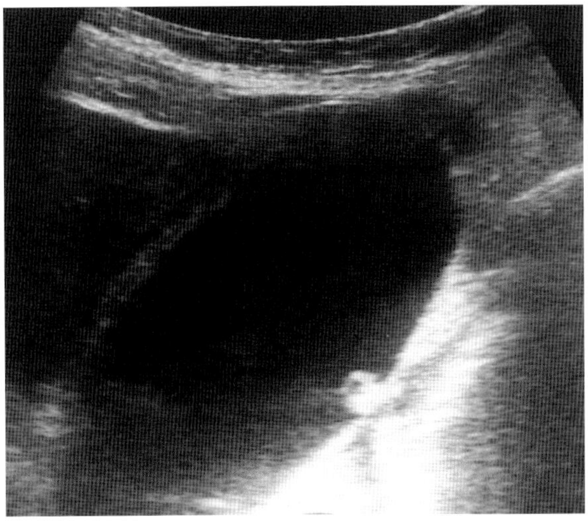

Fig. 1.9 a Acute cholecystitis with walled-off perforation at the fundus. The bulging gallbladder encroaches on the abdominal wall. Only mild thickening (5 mm), owing to severe tension in the triple-layered gallbladder wall. The hypoechoic pericholecystic rim correlates with edema. The hyperechoic fatty tissue around the fundus cannot be differentiated from the gallbladder wall. The small fluid collection within the fat corresponds to the walled-off perforation. Intraluminal gallstone with posterior shadowing and sludge.

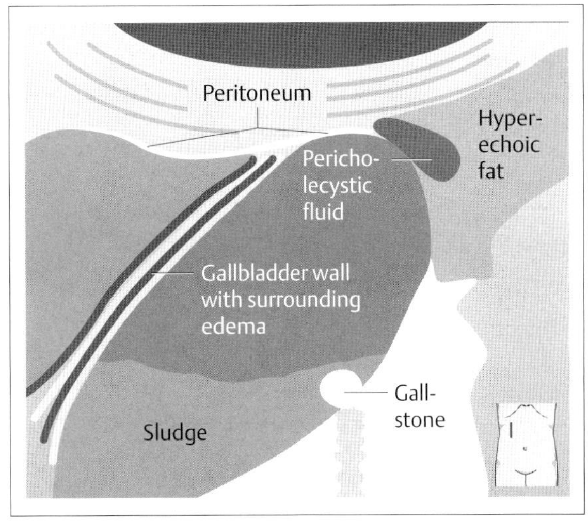

Fig. 1.9 b Line drawing.

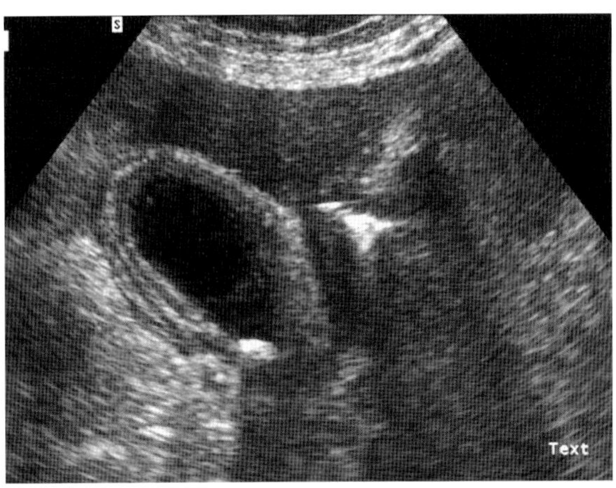

Fig. 1.10 a Acute cholecystitis. Bulging gallbladder with grossly thickened (11 mm) multilayered wall. Surrounding reactions: pericholecystic and duodenal wall edema, encasement by hyperechoic fatty tissue. Intraluminal gallstone with posterior shadowing and sludge.

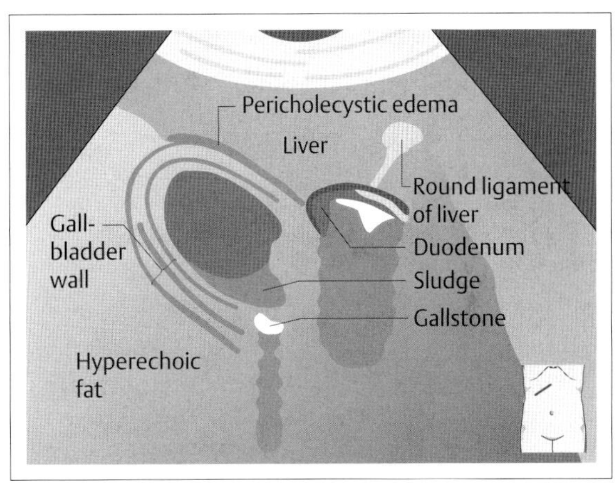

Fig. 1.10 b Line drawing.

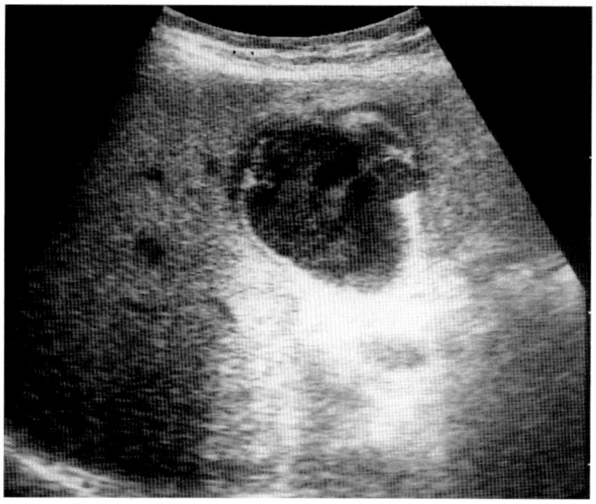

Fig. 1.**11 a** Acute cholecystitis with gallbladder empyema and multiple intramural abscess formations. Bulging gallbladder with thickened triple-layered wall and multiple hypoechoic intramural foci. Numerous intense intraluminal echoes, finely dispersed.

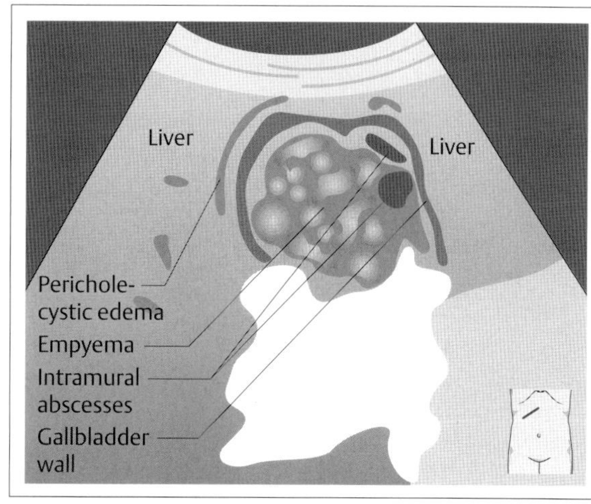

Fig. 1.**11 b** Line drawing.

Table 1.**1** Etiology of diffuse thickening of the gallbladder wall

Primarily Diseased Organ	Pathology	Sonographic Characteristics of the Gallbladder Wall
Gallbladder	Acute cholecystitis	Usually hypoechoic; multilayered; possibly with intramural foci; bulging gallbladder
	Chronic cholecystitis:	Hyperechoic
	Gallbladder carcinoma, lymphoma, or other rare neoplasm	Mostly focal, rarely diffuse; loss of wall layering; usually hypoechoic
	Adenomyomatosis	See section Chapter 7, Biliary Tree
	Gallbladder varices	Intramural tubular structures with venous flow pattern on Doppler US
Liver	Acute hepatitis	Triple- or multi-layered, hypoechoic; usually poorly filled gallbladder (applies to all entries from Acute hepatitis to Hypoproteinemia)
	Portal hypertension	
	Malignancy or inflammation near the gallbladder	
Other abdominal organs	Ascites	
	Peritoneal carcinomatosis	
	Penetrating GI ulcer	
	Pancreatitis	
Diseases with global edema formation	Right heart failure	
	Liver failure	
	Renal failure	
	Hypoproteinemia	

Acute Pancreatitis

Basic Facts

- *Pathophysiology:* Premature intracellular or intraductal activation of pancreatic enzymes triggers autodigestion of the pancreas. Manifests with local inflammation characterized by increased capillary permeability and exudation of fluid with subsequent local edema, and possibly necrosis, of pancreatic parenchyma and surrounding fatty tissue. In severe cases, circulation of toxic products from cell death results in systemic capillary leakage. This leads to intravascular volume depletion and, in combination with the simultaneously induced vasodilatation, to hypovolemic shock.

Causes

- Common: alcohol, cholelithiasis. Patients with regular excessive alcohol consumption often present with recurrent acute episodes of an underlying chronic pancreatitis.
- Uncommon: drugs, infection (viral, parasitic), autoimmune disorders, ischemia (shock, cardiopulmonary surgery, vasculitis), local factors (trauma, perforating ulcer, ERCP), metabolic disorders (hypercalcemia, hyperlipidemia), among others.

Incidence

- Around 40 cases per 100 000 inhabitants every year.

Clinical Presentation

- Severe constant epigastric or midabdominal pain radiating to the back, flanks, and/or the lower abdomen. Bloated, moderately tense to rigid abdomen due to decreased peristalsis and chemical peritonitis. Circulatory failure may ensue.
- Two stages of severity are predictive of outcome:
  - Edematous pancreatitis (about 85%) carries a favorable prognosis.
  - Necrotizing pancreatitis (about 15%); frequently associated with multiorgan failure and a mortality of around 30%. Fatal outcome most often is related to superinfection of the necrotic tissue, occurring in 40–70% of cases, most frequently during the third week of illness.

Diagnostic Criteria

- Typical clinical manifestations and elevation of serum amylase and lipase levels to > 3× upper normal level. Enzyme levels in the blood do not correlate with severity. The two courses are differentiated by clinical and laboratory scores (among others, Ranson's criteria, APACHE II score, CRP > 120 mg/l) and by cross-sectional imaging modalities (sonography being the gold standard, CT with i.v. contrast bolus injection to identify necrosis, presenting as a nonperfused region within the pancreas) (Block et al., 1985; United Kingdom Guidelines, 1998).
- The sensitivity of sonography is limited, since in 30% of patients with purely edematous pancreatitis no pathology is discerned (Habscheid, 1987). In particular, in severe cases the pancreas is often hidden behind gas-filled bloated loops of bowel (Schölmerich et al., 1989). If the pancreas is easily identified, sonographic findings have a high specificity and a strong positive predictive value (Hollerbach et al., 1994).
- Sonography is particularly valuable for recognition of complications and follow-up. Superinfected necrosis may have a bearing on possible indication for surgery; specimens can be collected by sonographically guided FNA of necrotic areas and/or fluid collections (Rau et al., 1998).
- *Additional workup:* laboratory panel (pancreatic enzymes, parameters of inflammation, CBC, electrolytes, blood sugar, liver and renal parameters, blood gas analysis), CT, ERCP in cases of biliary etiology, EUS, MRCP.

Sonographic Criteria

- **Edematous Pancreatitis**
  - Swelling of part of or the entire pancreas, recognized by volume increase with concomitant hypoechoic texture (Fig. 1.**12**). (For normal values of pancreatic size, see Chapter 7, Pancreas, p. 146). The extent of hypoechogenicity depends on the pancreatic texture to date, and is less pronounced in preexisting chronic pancreatitis, old age, or pancreatic lipomatosis.
  - Acute focal pancreatitis is often localized in the head of the pancreas (Loren et al., 1999). Differential diagnosis: somewhat hypoechoic anterior pancreas anlage, in most cases probably due to a maldistribution of fat (Matsumoto et al., 1995), pancreatic malignancy.
  - In particular, acute-on-chronic pancreatitis is characterized by spotty hypoechogenicity or adjacent hyper- and hypoechoic zones (Figs. 1.**13**, 1.**16**).
  - Hypoechoic peripancreatic rim (Fig. 1.**12**).
  - Fluid-filled lesser sac, with possibly a small amount of fluid in the remainder of the peritoneal cavity.
  - Edematous, i.e., hypoechoic, posterior gastric wall, which may be hard to differentiate from the fluid within the lesser sac (Fig. 1.**12**). Thickening of the gallbladder wall (Nyberg and Laing, 1983).
  - Compressed by edema, the pancreatic duct usually cannot be discerned. Exception: prevailing pancreatic duct dilatation in chronic pancreatitis (Fig. 1.**16**) or pancreatic duct obstruction.

- **Necrotizing Pancreatitis**
  - Findings as in edematous pancreatitis, plus:
  - Liquefaction of pancreatic parenchyma, i.e., areas of rather hypoechoic to almost anechoic sonotexture (Figs. 1.**13,** 1.**16**). Better differentiation between edema and necrosis of the pancreas by i. v. contrast-enhanced CT rather than sonography.
  - Frayed contour of the pancreas (Figs. 1.**13,** 1.**16**).
  - Bands of fat necrosis visualized as hypo- to anechoic structures bilaterally in the anterior perirenal space (Fig. 1.**15**), as well as in the mesocolon, mesentery (Fig. 1.**17**), and greater and lesser omentum. Extension into the lower abdomen is possible, and fat necrosis may also occur at distant (extraperitoneal) sites, such as the mediastinum, the subperitoneal region of the pelvis, or the scrotum. The perirenal fat is usually spared, well protected by Gerota's fascia (Fig. 1.**15**).
  - Ascites may develop exclusively within the lesser sac (Figs. 1.**13,** 1.**16**), and/or anywhere else in the peritoneal cavity, where it may concentrate in the subhepatic, subphrenic, or lower abdomen. Such fluid is usually inflammatory in nature. However, sonographic differentiation from frank blood or hemorrhagic exudate is impossible. The mixture of exudate, blood, and fat necrosis results in a semisolid mass of reticular, spider web–like texture and resembles the sonograms of intra-abdominal hemorrhage (Fig. 1.**17**).
  - Bowel wall edema (Figs. 1.**15,** 1.**17**) secondary to chemical peritonitis and/or impaired perfusion (systemic capillary damage, involvement of the mesentery).
  - Fluid may also collect inside the bowel wall, especially in the descending part of the duodenum, as well as in the liver and spleen, in most cases beneath the capsule (Fig. 1.**17**).
- **Contribution of US in the Elucidation of Etiology:**
  - Gallbladder stones may point to biliary pathogenesis. Very high likelihood in case of dilated bile ducts (Fig. 1.**12**), biochemical parameters of cholestasis, or if calculi are found within the bile ducts (see Chapter 7, Biliary System, p. 162). However, bile duct dilatation in acute pancreatitis may also be caused by stenosis of the CBD due to edema of the head of the pancreas, or by tubular stenosis secondary to chronic pancreatitis.
  - In alcoholic pancreatitis, frequently there are signs of acute-on-chronic inflammation (Fig. 1.**16**) and fatty infiltration of the liver or cirrhosis.
- **Complications That May Be Demonstrated Sonographically**
  - Pleural effusion, more often on the left than on the right.
  - Bowel distension progressing to paralytic ileus (see Mechanical Bowel Obstruction and Paralytic Ileus later in this chapter).
  - Delayed gastric emptying in paralytic ileus or stenosis of the duodenum, the latter resulting from swelling of or pseudocyst formation in the head of the pancreas (see Chapter 7, Chronic Pancreatitis, p. 147). Edema of the duodenal wall may also contribute to gastric outlet obstruction (Fig. 1.**17**).
  - Obstruction of the CBD with subsequent dilatation.
  - Pseudocyst formation by fibrous walling off of fluid collections within the pancreas (Fig. 1.**14**) or along the noted bands of necrosis. As defined in the 1998 United Kingdom guidelines, at least 4 weeks must have elapsed since the acute episode of pancreatitis before a peripancreatic fluid collection may be regarded as being a pseudocyst; otherwise it should simply be referred to as a "fluid collection."
  - Sonography can demonstrate superinfection of a fluid collection or pseudocyst only by indirect means, i.e., the gas formed by anaerobic bacteria. Superinfection is confirmed via US-guided FNA (Fig. 1.**14**).
  - Venous thrombosis, most often in the splenic vein and less commonly in the portal vein and/or superior mesenteric vein.
  - Erosion of the arterial wall may be demonstrated by color-flow Doppler imaging (see Chapter 7, Chronic Pancreatitis, p. 149).

Consequences for Surgical Treatment

Diagnosis	Characteristic Findings	Management
Acute edematous pancreatitis	Typical symptoms with upper quadrant pain, pancreatic enzymes elevated to > 3 × upper normal level, hypoechoic swelling of the pancreas, peripancreatic edema, effusion in the lesser sac	Conservative treatment; no preventive administration of antibiotics
Acute necrotizing pancreatitis	The above findings plus: liquefaction of pancreatic parenchyma, frayed pancreatic contour, bands of necrosis, CRP > 120 mg/l	Conservative treatment in the ICU, preventive antibiotics; in case of deterioration/infection, laparotomy with necrectomy, irrigation, and drainage
Biliary pancreatitis	Choledocholithiasis and/or dilated CBD accompanied by the elevated enzyme levels of biliary obstruction	ERC ± papillotomy and stone extraction or nasobiliary tube drainage; alternatively, open cholecystectomy with bile duct exploration
Pancreatic abscess	Clinical signs of infection; fluid collections (± gas) within the pancreas or along the bands of necroses, walled off by a membrane; FNA positive for pus	Drainage: in localized, easily accessible fluid collections endoscopic drainage through the stomach or duodenum is preferred, otherwise percutaneously; alternatively, laparotomy with abscess evacuation and external drainage

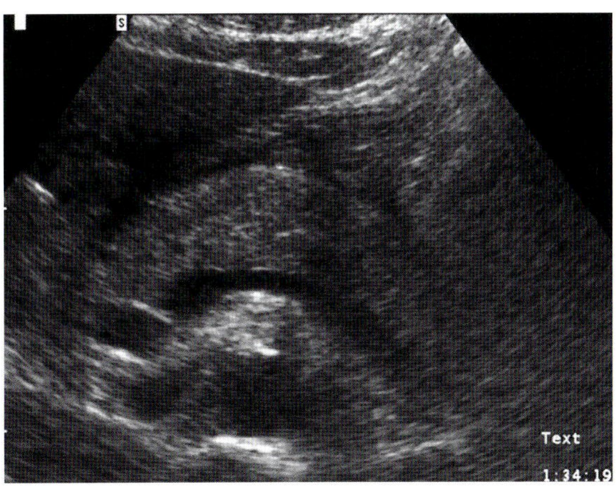

Fig. 1.**12 a** Acute edematous pancreatitis. Engorged pancreas (diameter of the body 23 mm) with speckled hypoechoic texture, the peripancreatic edema blending in with the hypoechoic posterior gastric wall. Distended CBD (11 mm), suggestive of biliary etiology.

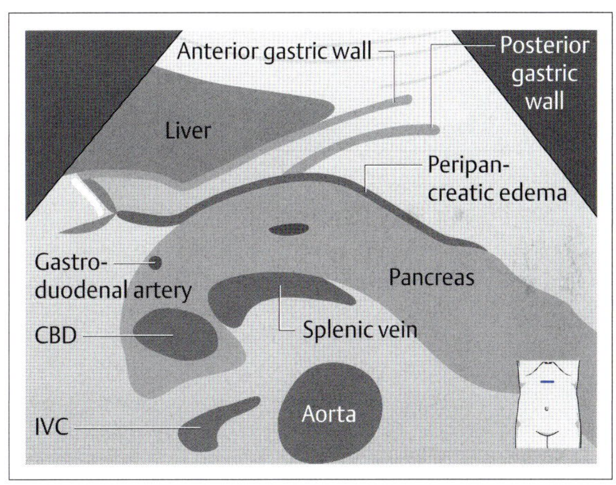

Fig. 1.**12 b** Line drawing.

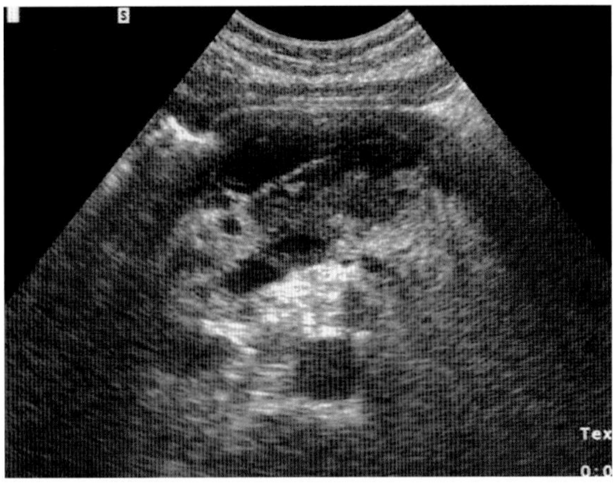

Fig. 1.**13a** Acute necrotizing pancreatitis. Edema in the body of the pancreas, which is hypoechoic compared with the echotexture of the head and tail. The anechoic area with frayed contour in the anterior part of the body correlates with parenchymal necrosis. Fluid-filled lesser sac.

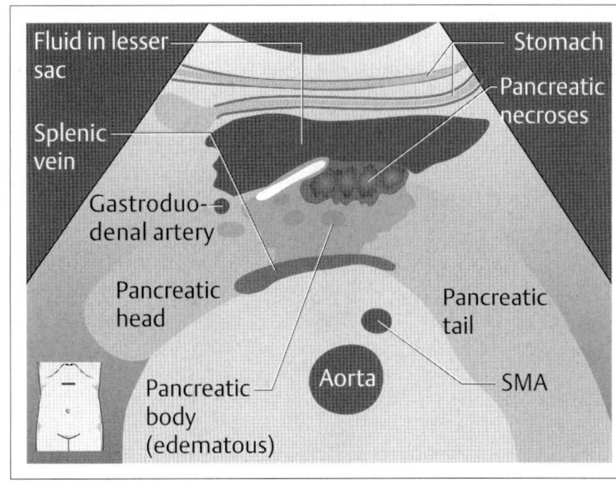

Fig. 1.**13b** Line drawing.

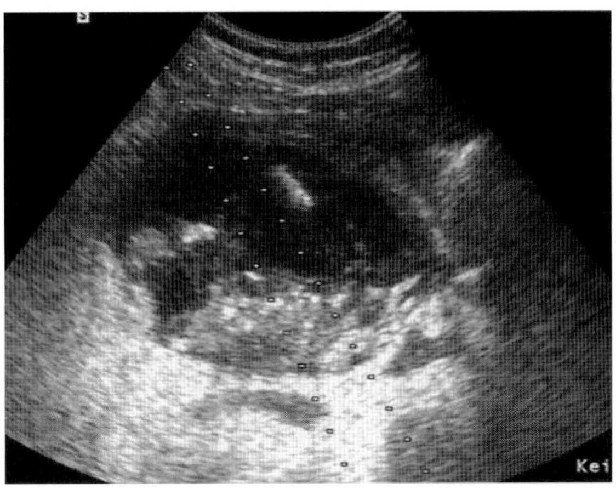

Fig. 1.**14a** Same patient as in Fig. 1.**13**, 11 days later. An encapsulated fluid collection (maximum diameter 9.5 cm) has formed, originating from the pancreatic body and containing particulate matter. US guided (dotted lines) FNA for microbiology and drainage.

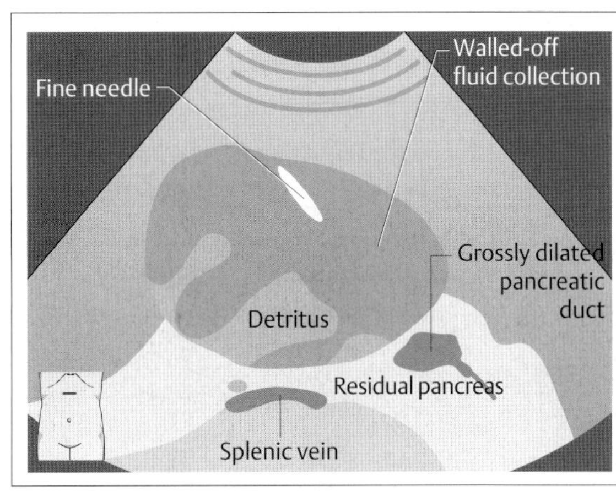

Fig. 1.**14b** Line drawing.

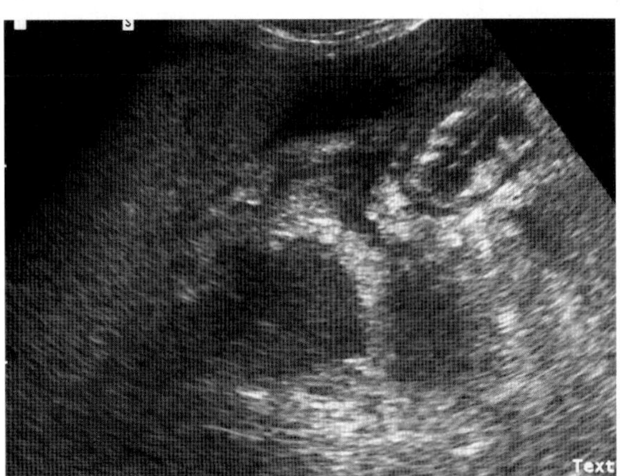

Fig. 1.**15a** Fatty-tissue necrosis in the right anterior pararenal gutter, easily identified by the hypoechoic bands running through the untouched hyperechoic fat. Also edema of the colon and ascites.

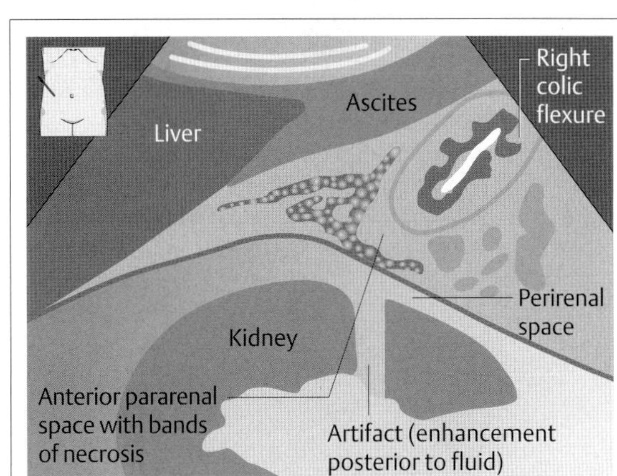

Fig. 1.**15b** Line drawing.

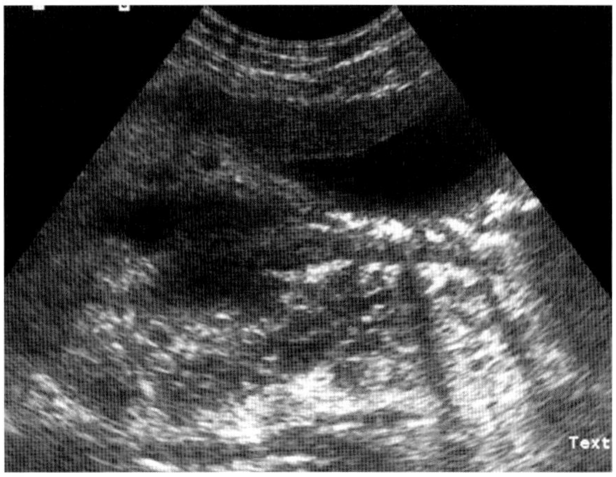

Fig. 1.**16a** Acute-on-chronic pancreatitis. Atrophic pancreas with reticular hyperechoic texture, calcification, and an irregularly dilated duct (5 mm). Interspersed between the hyperechoic parts and calcifications are blotchy hypoechoic areas, and in the transition zone between head and body there is focal necrosis with loss of the anterior contour of the organ. There is fluid in the lesser sac, both posterior and anterior to the stomach. Any air between the gastric folds must not be confused with calcification of the pancreatic parenchyma.

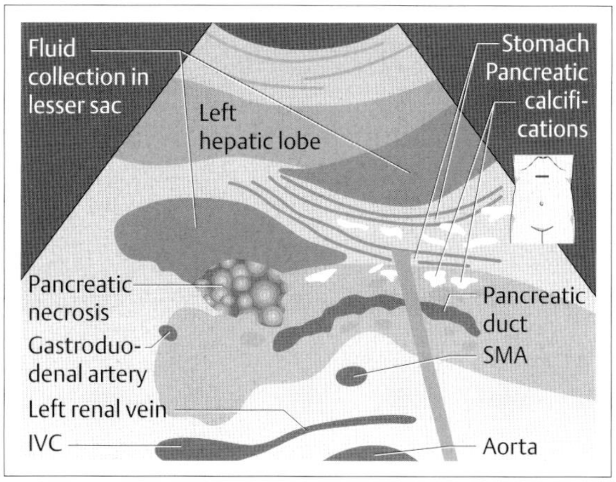

Fig. 1.**16b** Line drawing.

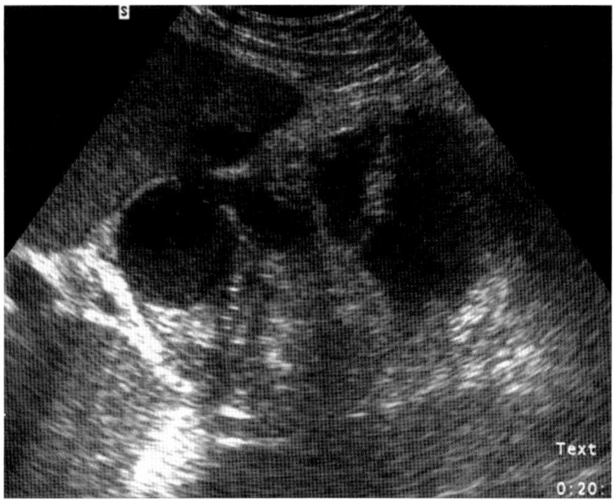

Fig. 1.**17a** Same patient as in Fig. 1.**16**, 2 weeks after onset of symptoms. Beginning encasement of the fluid collections within the mesentery, below the splanchnic surface of the liver, and in the edematous wall of the descending part of the duodenum, the lumen of which is narrowed.

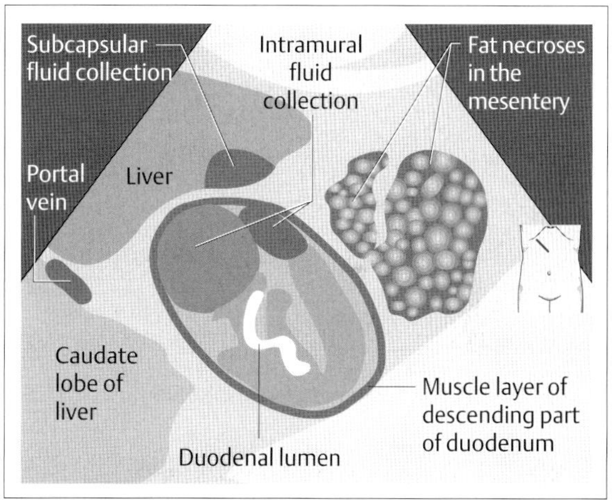

Fig. 1.**17b** Line drawing.

Mechanical Bowel Obstruction and Paralytic Ileus

Basic Facts

- Sonographic diagnosis of intestinal obstruction is based on gastric and intestinal distension (Figs. 1.**18**, 1.**19**, 1.**22**, 1.**23**) (Ko et al., 1993; Seitz and Merz, 1998).
- If they are filled with fluid the size of the intestinal loops is easily determined, but measurement is difficult or impossible in the presence of gas. Thus, sonography is particularly helpful in early-phase mechanical bowel obstruction (MBO) or ileus (Seitz and Merz, 1998).
- While peristalsis is present in MBO, it is lacking in paralytic ileus. Once peristalsis is sluggish, differentiation between advanced MBO and incomplete paralytic ileus may prove impossible.
- Although the level of obstruction may frequently be visualized, this is less often true for its cause (Ko et al., 1993), e.g., hernia, inflammatory or neoplastic mass, strangulation (Fig. 1.**20**), intussusception, gallstone (Fig. 1.**22**), bezoar, etc.
- The etiology of paralytic ileus may be inferred from signs of intestinal ischemia (see p. 21), or from evidence of a concomitant or underlying disease, e.g., acute pancreatitis, cardiac or renal failure, etc.
- Free intraperitoneal fluid may be encountered in advanced ileus or as a sequela of the associated or underlying disorder.
- *Additional workup:*
  radiographic series consisting of plain chest and upright abdominal films, abdominal CT study.

Sonographic Criteria

- Although a **dilated gastric antrum** can be visualized in the epigastrium, in supine position it is usually seen to be filled with gas. A fluid-filled body and fundus may be demonstrated from the left midaxillary line, anterior to the left kidney and inferior to the spleen.
- Partial obstruction/ileus typically goes along with small-bowel diameter of 2–3 cm, diameters above 3 cm usually imply complete obstruction/ileus (Figs. 1.**18**, 1.**19**, 1.**22**).
- Increased **fluid-filling of the jejunal loops** will facilitate visualization of the circular folds with their "keyboard" or "step-ladder"-like appearance (Figs. 1.**18**, 1.**19**, 1.**22**).
- The **diameter of the large bowel** is frequently more difficult to assess due to its inherently higher gas content. This measure is of low validity in any case, as it varies quite strongly under physiological conditions. Usually, the cecum is widest, while in the left colon a diameter of more than 5 cm should be regarded as abnormal (Fig. 1.**23**).
- **Peristalsis** can be assessed by fluctuation of chyme and gas echoes within the intraluminal fluid and by contraction of the intestinal wall. Such active motility is to be differentiated from passive fluid shifts and bowel movement with respiration.
- **Paralytic ileus** is characterized by sluggish peristalsis, while in MBO motility is usually heightened proximal to the obstruction and there may be pendulating peristalsis. The level of obstruction may be identified, since the loops upstream of the obstruction will be distended while those distal to it are collapsed (Fig. 1.**19**), and/or if the cause of obstruction shows up directly–e.g., tumor (see Chapter 7, Gastrointestinal Tract, Tumors, p. 113), inflammation (see Chapter 7, Chronic Inflammatory Bowel Disease, p. 116), or intussusception (see Chapter 18, Pediatric Sonography, p. 372) Sometimes the strangulated (edematous, aperistaltic) bowel segment itself can be demonstrated, e.g., as contents in a hernia sac or in closed-loop obstruction due to adhesive bands (Fig. 1.**20**).
- **Gallstone obstruction:** gas within the gallbladder lumen (Fig. 1.**21**) is regularly observed along with evidence of MBO (Fig. 1.**22**). The gallstone within the intestinal lumen may (Fig. 1.**22**) or may not be visualized. (Caveat: differential diagnosis includes calcified mesenteric lymph nodes.)

Consequences for Surgical Treatment

Diagnosis	Characteristic Findings	Management
MBO	Clinical signs of acute abdomen, vomiting, on US dilated prestenotic bowel loops (small intestine caliber > 3 cm), pendulating peristalsis, and empty bowel distal to the obstruction	Plain abdominal film, surgery (e.g., tumor resection, division of adhesions or bands, hernia repair, etc.)
Incomplete MBO	In comparison with above, less severe clinical symptoms and less pronounced sonographic signs (small-bowel caliber distended to 2–3 cm)	Nonoperative reestablishment of the GI passage by "drip and suck" possibly, contrast studies with water-soluble contrast medium; diagnostic endoscopy; reduction of a hernia
Paralytic ileus	Distension of the entire small and large bowel, absence of peristalsis (e.g., after surgery, in inflammation, mesenteric ischemia, electrolyte imbalance, etc.)	Treatment of the underlying disease; may be combined with medical or mechanical GI stimulation

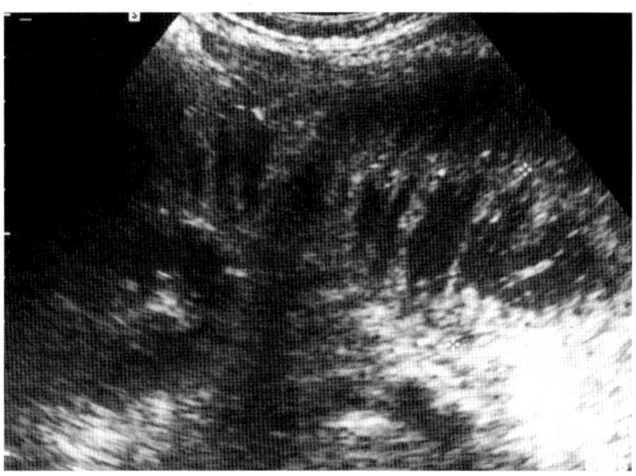

Fig. 1.**18a** Small-bowel obstruction. Distended jejunum (42 mm) with "keyboard" and "step-ladder"-like appearance.

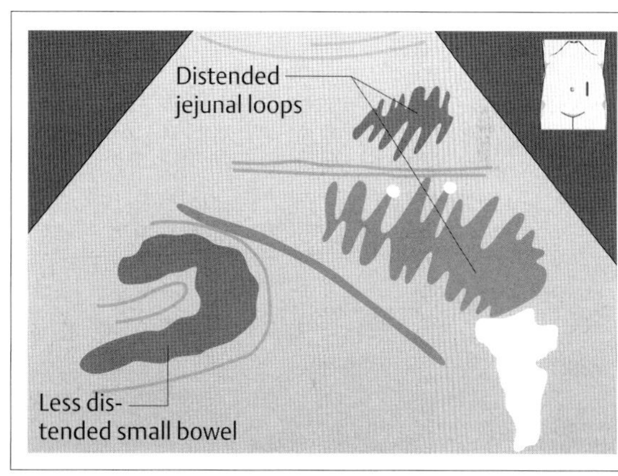

Fig. 1.**18b** Line drawing.

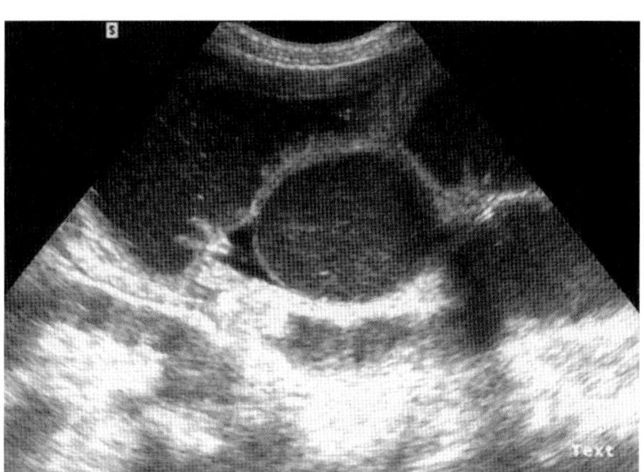

Fig. 1.**19a** Small-bowel obstruction by band. Massive distension of the small intestine (up to 5 cm), while the ascending colon –delineated anterior to the right kidney–is empty and collapsed; the level of obstruction may be inferred to be in the lower small bowel. The small amount of ascites signifies advanced ileus.

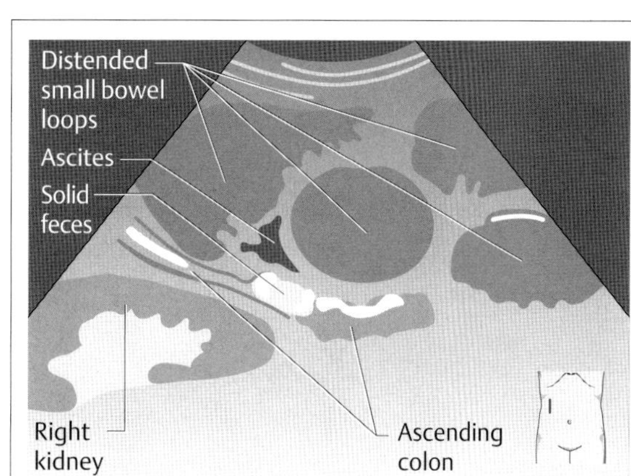

Fig. 1.**19b** Line drawing.

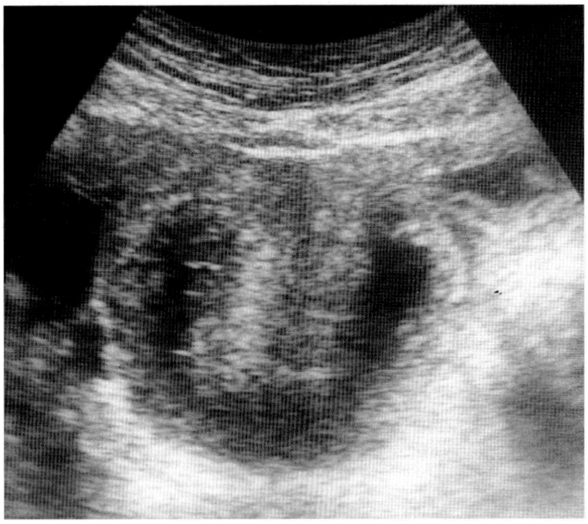

Fig. 1.**20 a** Closed-loop obstruction with subsequent gangrene due to strangulation of a small-bowel segment by an adhesive band. The distended aperistaltic segment is shaped like a "sausage ring" and is further characterized by a thickened wall and loss of wall layering. Intermixing of distended and normal small-bowel segments.

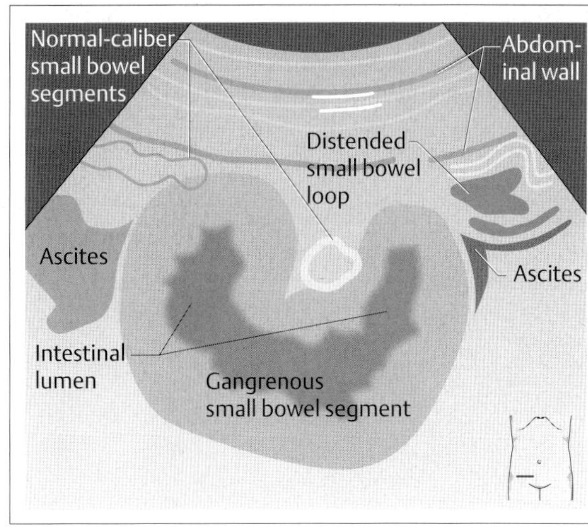

Fig. 1.**20 b** Line drawing.

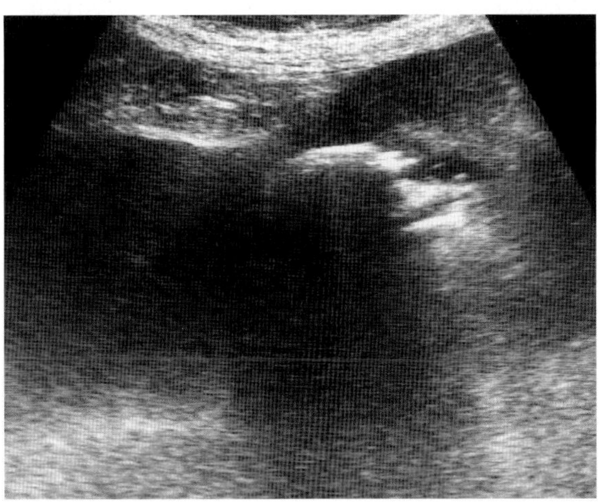

Fig. 1.**21 a** MBO due to gallstone. As the gallbladder contains gas and demonstrates irregular thickening of its wall, reflecting chronic inflammation, this is almost pathognomonic of a fistula between the gallbladder and the lumen of the GI tract.

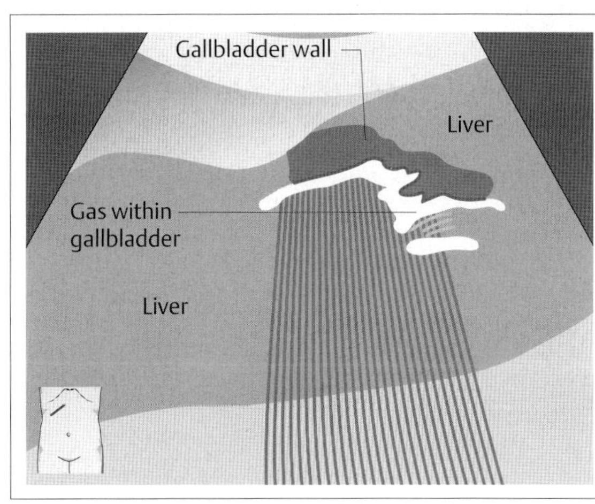

Fig. 1.**21 b** Line drawing.

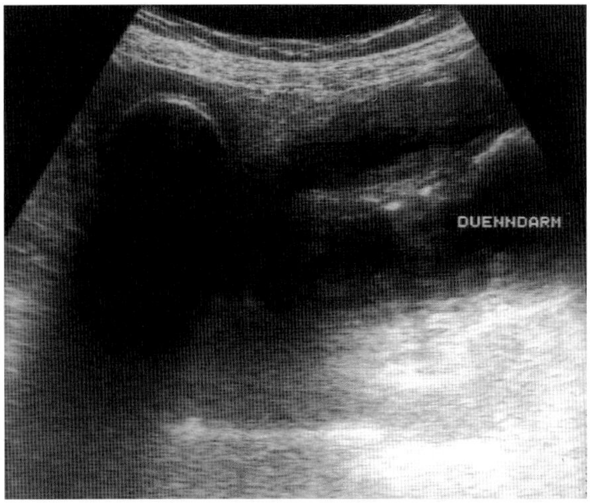

Fig. 1.22 a Same patient as in Fig. 1.21: Dilated small bowel, gallstone within the intestinal lumen, identified by the sickle-shaped, almost total echo reflection by the calculus with posterior shadowing. The calculus is encased by the hypoechoic bowel wall.

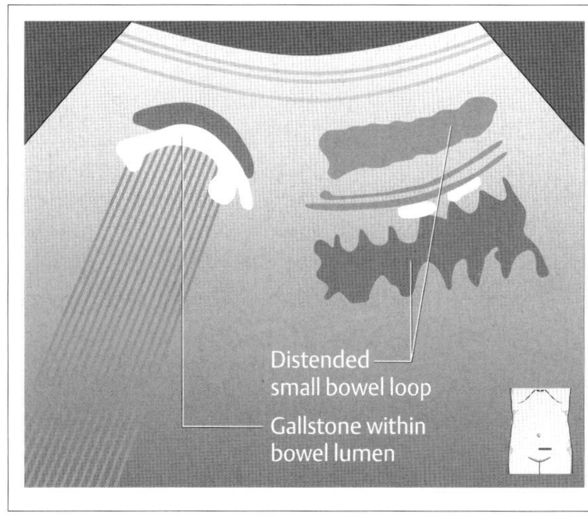

Fig. 1.22 b Line drawing.

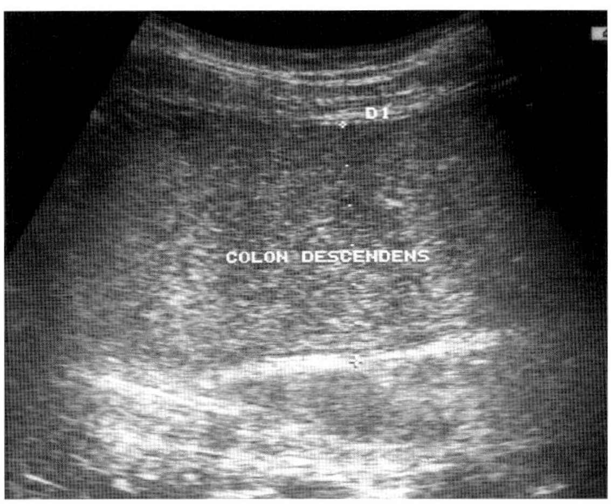

Fig. 1.23 a Large bowel obstruction. Descending colon filled with liquid feces and distended to a diameter of 6 cm.

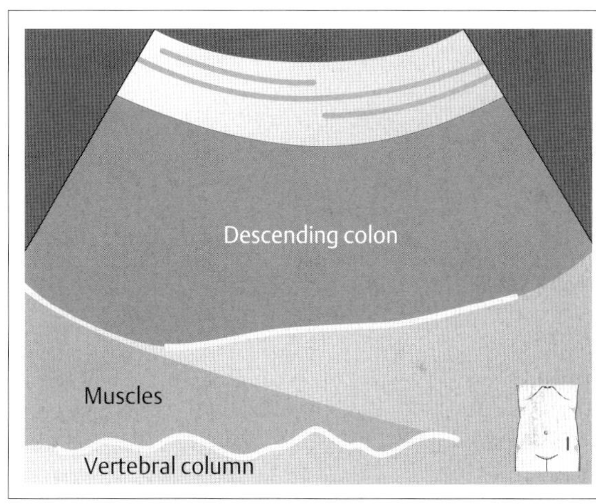

Fig. 1.23 b Line drawing.

Perforation of the Gastrointestinal Tract

Basic Facts

- GI perforations are most frequently due to peptic ulcers in the stomach or duodenum. Less common causes include diverticulitis, trauma, iatrogenic perforation (e.g., during endoscopy), Crohn disease, bowel ischemia, or malignancy.
- Diagnosis is based on the clinical signs of peritonitis and evidence of free intraperitoneal gas, "pneumoperitoneum."
- In experimental settings, as little as 1 ml of air could be demonstrated by sonography (Seitz and Reising, 1982). Knowledge and experience in sonographic detection of free air have so far remained even more elusive than with other imaging modalities. However, sonography is highly sensitive in experienced hands and represents an important complement to radiography (Chang-Chien et al., 1989; Meiser and Meissner, 1986; Seitz and Reising, 1982). It can sometimes provide information on the site of perforation (Fig. 1.**26**) (Patel and Gopichandran, 1999; Tsai et al., 1998; Yamamoto et al., 1997; Yang et al., 1999).
- *Additional workup:* radiological confirmation of the pneumoperitoneum–upright chest film and plain abdominal film erect or in left lateral decubitus, or CT of the abdomen (which may also depict inflammatory wall thickening).
- In at least one-third of patients with GI perforations, the pneumoperitoneum cannot be demonstrated initially and will not be seen until several hours after the onset of clinical symptoms. In such cases, repeated radiographic and US examinations may be valuable, especially after upper GI endoscopy.
- The incidental finding of asymptomatic free air in the peritoneal cavity does not necessarily warrant surgery (Hoover et al., 1992; Kirchner et al., 1996; Patel and Gopichandran, 1999). This may be present after laparotomy, transvaginal gynecological interventions, or GI endoscopy (especially colonoscopy), in a variety of forms of intestinal pneumatosis, etc.

Sonographic Criteria

- **Free air** is identified by its bright echo along the parietal peritoneum with ring-down, reverberation, and shadowing artifacts (Figs. 1.**24**–1.**26**).
- Differentiation of free air from intraluminal gas: free air is not surrounded by gastric or bowel wall, and changes in location are independent of the GI structures. Intraluminal gas shifts in parallel with the diaphragm, while free air does not. In contrast, when posture is changed, free air always accumulates in the topmost part of the peritoneal cavity (Fig. 1.**25**).
- The patient should therefore be positioned such that the anterior surface of the liver represents the highest point of the abdomen; to this end, turn the supine patient somewhat to the left and slightly elevate the upper body. Free air will then be discerned along the anterior surface of the liver (Fig. 1.**24**). Possible misdiagnosis includes air within the basal segments of the lungs or colonic gas anterior to the liver in patients with Chilaiditi syndrome.
- **Gas echoes** between omentum and abdominal wall or within the omental layers (Fig. 1.**25**).
- If there is little air, the presumed site of perforation may be identified by its inflammatory thickening of the intestinal wall and by adjacent hyperechoic fatty tissue (see Chapter 7, Gastroduodenal Ulcer, Appendicitis, Diverticulitis, p. 111, 120). Occasionally, gas bubbles may pearl from such an area (Fig. 1.**26**) (Patel and Gopichandran, 1999)
- In addition, **free intra-abdominal fluid** with floating echoes due to mixing of gas, residual food, or inflammatory cells can frequently be seen. Look for the interface between free fluid and free air, corresponding to the air–fluid levels on upright abdominal films (Fig. 1.**24**).
- In advanced stages, the intestinal wall–and possibly the gallbladder wall–becomes diffusely thickened and hypoechoic, secondary to the development of generalized peritonitis.

Consequences for Surgical Treatment

Diagnosis	Characteristic Findings	Management
Frank perforation with peritonitis	Tender rigid abdominal wall; on US, intra-abdominal gas echoes; free air confirmed by plain abdominal film	Emergency laparotomy
Suspected upper GI tract perforation	Clinical signs suspicious of perforation, but no free gas on sonography or radiography	EGD, repeat imaging may be indicated; when in doubt, laparoscopy
Incidental finding of free air	Sonographic or radiological evidence of free intraperitoneal air in an asymptomatic patient	Inpatient observation, workup of cause

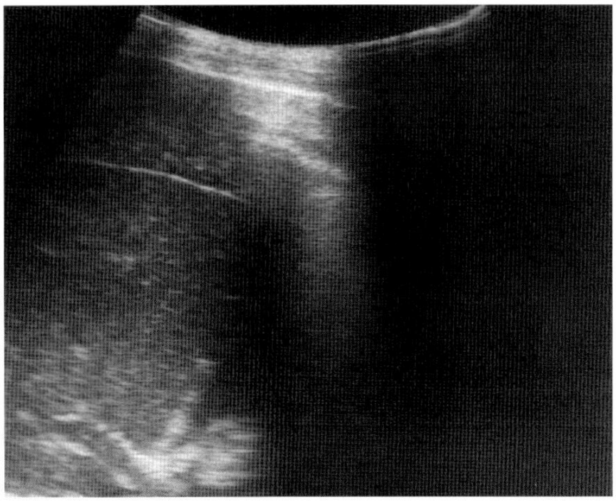

Fig. 1.**24a** Free intraperitoneal air and perihepatic fluid. The floating echoes within the fluid are due to gastric contents oozing from a perforated gastric ulcer.

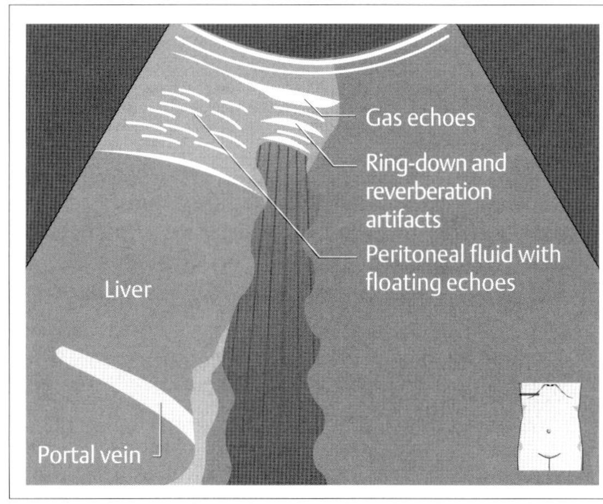

Fig. 1.**24b** Line drawing.

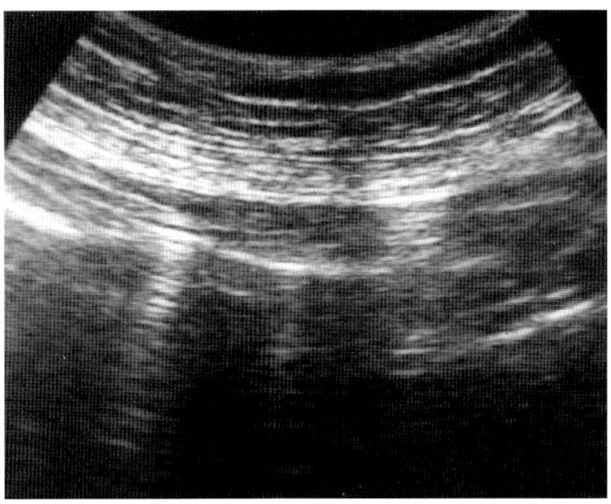

Fig. 1.**25a** Free air between omentum and anterior abdominal wall, shifting position when the patient changes posture. In contrast, intraintestinal gas echoes will shift in parallel with respiration.

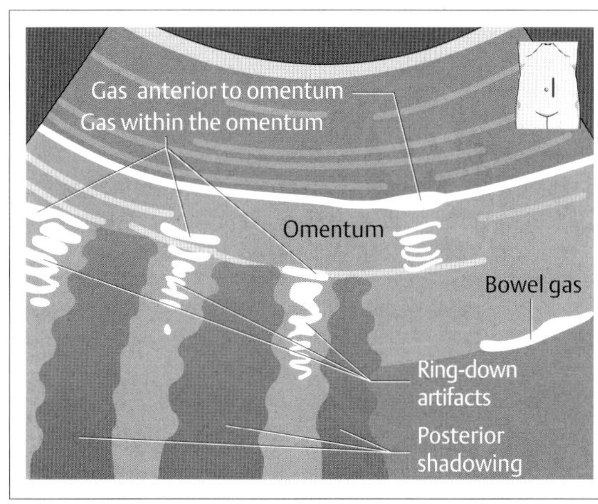

Fig. 1.**25b** Line drawing.

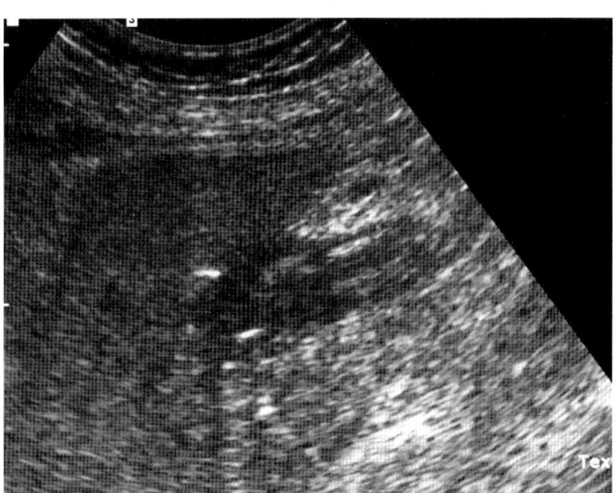

Fig. 1.**26a** Gastric ulcer in a thickened hypoechoic stomach wall, the gas echo marking the lesion. In addition, extraluminal free air between stomach and liver. Hyperechoic fat of the lesser omentum and mesentery capping the ulcer.

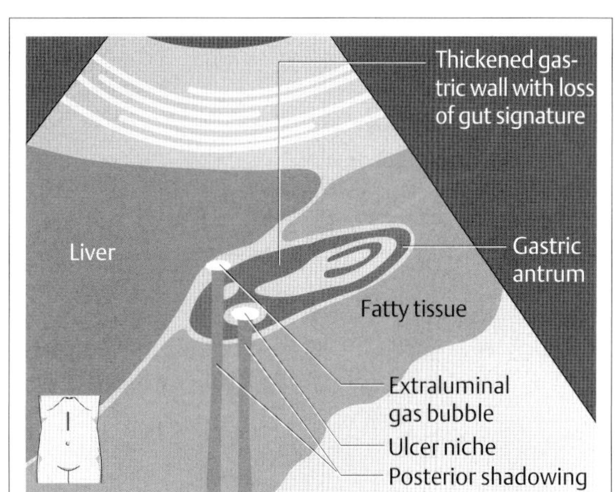

Fig. 1.**26b** Line drawing.

Abdominal Aortic Aneurysm

Basic Facts

- "Abdominal aortic aneurysm" (AAA) is defined as a pathological dilatation of the abdominal aorta.
- According to customary definitions, in AAA the caliber of the aorta must be > 3 cm.
- AAAs are frequently spindle-shaped with elongation of the original aorta. Sonographic measurement of the maximum caliber, quite often the antero–posterior diameter, is vital for treatment planning.
- 95 % of all AAAs are restricted to the infrarenal aorta.
- In patients aged 65 years and older the incidence of AAA is between 4.4 % and 8.4 %, with a male preponderance of 9 : 1.
- There is an exponential relationship between aneurysm size, rate of growth, and risk of rupture.
- The probability of rupture leaps from a maximum of 3 % per year for aneurysms with a diameter < 6 cm to 15 % per year for diameters ≥ 6 cm.
- The role of arteriosclerosis in the pathogenesis is still being debated, while mycosis, Marfan syndrome, or inflammation are rare causes.
- Small aneurysms not yet ruptured tend to be asymptomatic (80 % of all patients with AAA) but may become an important source of distal emboli.
- If sonography cannot confirm the diagnosis or if assessment is hampered in ruptured AAAs, spiral CT is markedly superior to ultrasound and should always be performed.
- **Symptomatic AAA:** Back pain and diffuse abdominal pain are typical of expanding aneurysms. Penetration into neighboring organs is possible.
- **Aortic rupture:** Sudden expansion of the aortic wall is reflected by violent abdominal pain (acute abdomen) and back pain, which may radiate into pelvis or left flank, typically followed by hemorrhagic shock.

Sonographic Criteria

- On transverse view, AAAs have a hyperechoic wall, frequently with a mural thrombus of somewhat irregular outline and lesser echogenicity.
- Sonography may miss involvement of the iliac artery.
- Rupture initially results in retroperitoneal hematoma (Fig. 1.**27**). In frank intra-abdominal rupture, free fluid can be demonstrated.
- In dissected aneurysms, the detached part of the intima may appear as a thin hyperechoic band floating within the lumen.

- **Important issues to be addressed by sonography:**
  - Rupture, free intra-abdominal fluid
  - Size and caliber
  - Involvement of the mesenteric and/or renal arteries (which branch off about 2 cm inferior to the origin of the superior mesenteric artery)
  - Involvement of the iliac arteries
  - Presence of mural thrombus
- *Additional workup:* contrast enhanced angio-CT, MRI, DSA.

Consequences for Surgical Treatment

Diagnosis	Characteristic Findings	Management
AAA	Ruptured AAA with retroperitoneal hematoma or free intra-abdominal fluid	Emergency surgery (mortality 60–80 %, if in hypovolemic shock)
AAA	No rupture, but symptomatic	Diagnosis confirmed by spiral CT, followed by urgent surgery
AAA	Incidental finding	Spiral CT; if transverse diameter exceeds 5.0–5.5 cm, elective aneurysm surgery is recommended

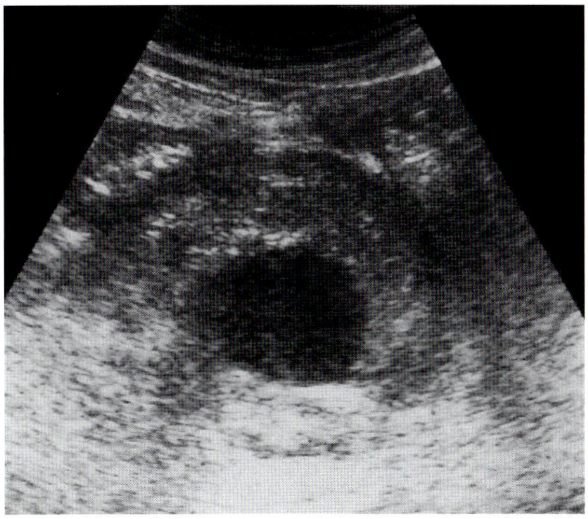

Fig. 1.**27a** Abdominal aortic aneurysm with walled-off perforation into the right retroperitoneum. On this transverse view, the A–P diameter measures 8 cm.

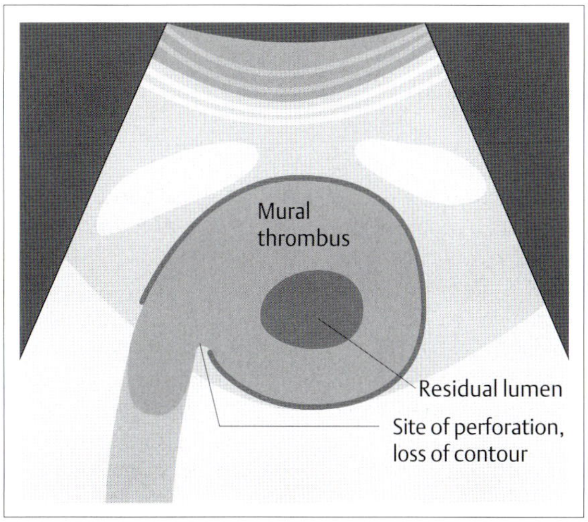

Fig. 1.**27b** Line drawing.

Intestinal Ischemia

Basic Facts

- The occlusive and nonocclusive forms of intestinal ischemia differ in their pathophysiology. Nonocclusive intestinal ischemia is found mainly as a sequela to severe general illness with low cardiac output and/or mesenteric vascular spasms. The usual cause of occlusive intestinal ischemia is arterial embolism or thrombosis, less commonly venous thrombosis. Intestinal ischemia accounts for 0.5–2% of cases of acute abdomen.

Clinical Presentation

- A triphasic course is typical:
  - Acute colicky abdominal pain with normal to heightened peristalsis.
  - Symptomatic relief with sluggish bowel motility.
  - Development of bacterial peritonitis due to transmural migration.
- Incomplete ischemia of the bowel wall, whether induced by arterial hypoperfusion or impaired venous outflow, results in edema or necrosis of the mucosa. Only in case of complete ischemia will transmural involvement ensue.
- Arterial embolism prevails in the vascular bed of the superior mesenteric artery, whereas the splenic flexure is the most common site in nonocclusive intestinal ischemia.
- Under favorable imaging conditions, Doppler ultrasound may reveal signs of arterial stenosis or venous thrombosis (Klein et al., 1995; Teefey et al., 1996).

Sonographic Criteria

- Extensive circular hypoechoic thickening of the bowel wall (Figs. 1.**28**, 1.**29**).
- Segmental involvement is common.
- The early stage is limited to the mucous membrane and submucosal layer, with thickening of the circular folds or of the semilunar folds of the colon, respectively (producing the "thumbprint" sign on radiographs) (Figs. 1.**28**, 1.**29**).
- In the intermediate and later phase, the affected segment becomes aperistaltic.
- In late stages, ascites is present in addition to paralytic ileus (Fig. 1.**30**).
- Intramural gas, indicative of a gangrenous intestinal wall (Fig. 1.**31**), and possible gas embolism of the intrahepatic portal vein branches (Figs. 1.**32**, 1.**33**) signify a poor prognosis.

- However, the view is frequently obstructed by gaseous distension of the bowel. Bowel wall thickness strongly depends on the wall tension, i.e., on the caliber of the intestine (Figs. 1.**28**–1.**31**).
- *Additional workup:* Arterial angiography of the celiac trunk and mesenteric arteries. In peritonitis, standard workup for bowel perforation or exploratory laparoscopy is called for.

Consequences for Surgical Treatment

Diagnosis	Characteristic Findings	Management
Suspected acute arterial ischemia or acute mesenteric vein thrombosis	Acute abdomen; extended circular thickening of the hypoechoic bowel wall; segmental aperistalsis; possibly Doppler-US confirmation of mesenteric vascular occlusion	Based on angiographic findings: in cases of nonocclusive disease, medical/radiological management; possibly thrombectomy or embolectomy; In suspected transmural ischemia, laparoscopy/laparotomy and bowel resection is warranted

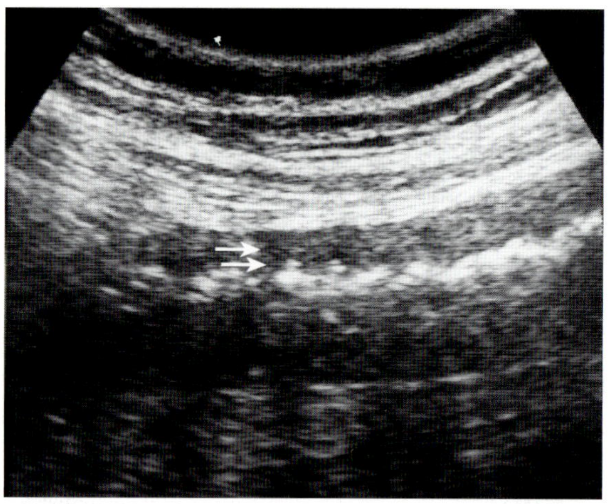

Fig. 1.**28 a** Nontransmural ischemia of the jejunal wall in a longitudinal view: hypoechoic swelling of the mucosa and submucosal layer (arrows). The circular folds can be discerned; peristalsis is diminished.

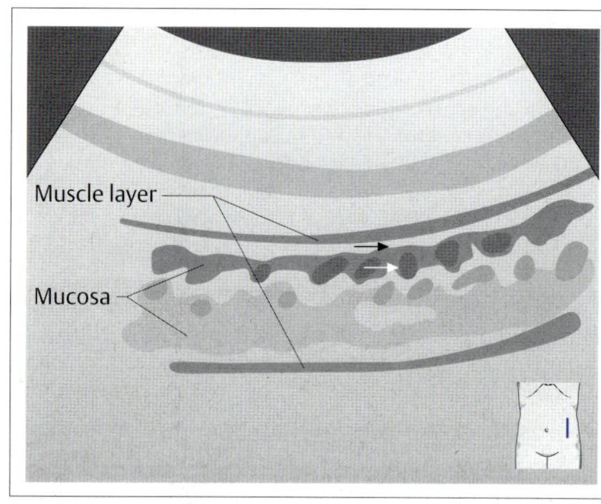

Fig. 1.**28 b** Line drawing.

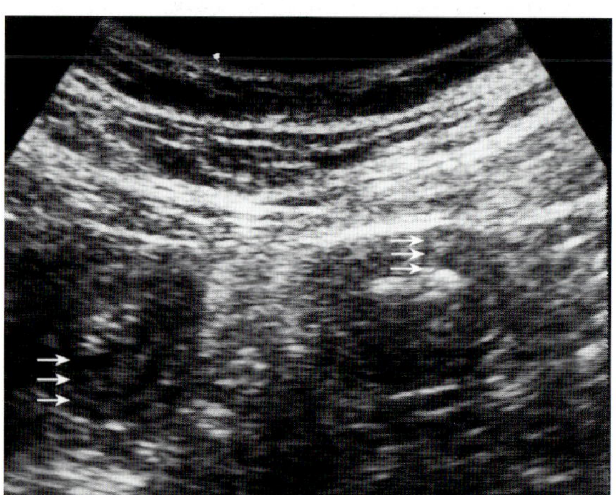

Fig. 1.**29 a** Same patient as in Fig. 1.**28**. Cross-sectional view of two distended jejunal loops. The three arrows mark the mucous membrane, submucosa, and muscle layer.

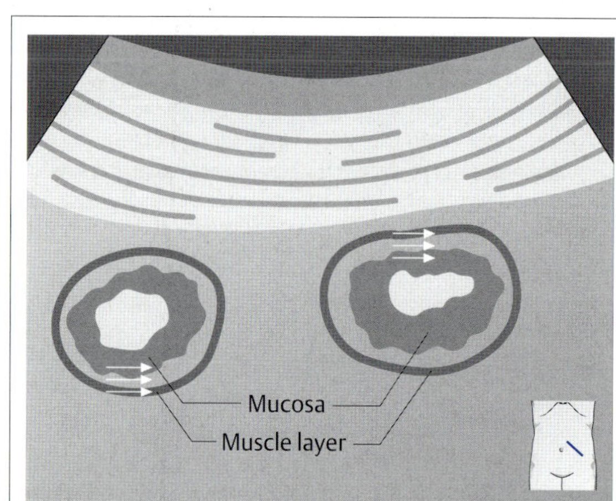

Fig. 1.**29 b** Line drawing.

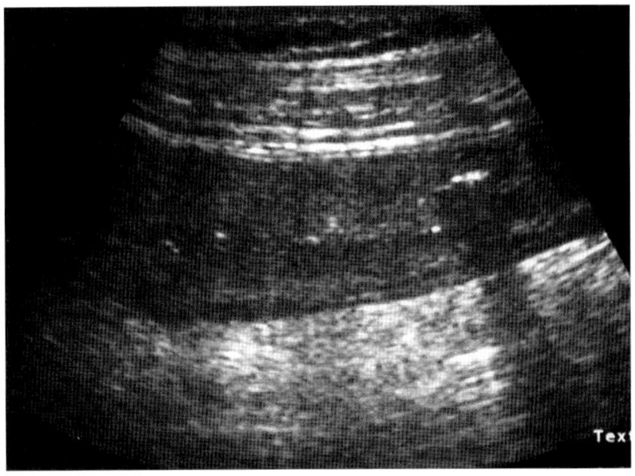

Fig. 1.**30 a** Nontransmural ischemic colitis of the descending and sigmoid colon. Long-axis view of the descending colon with swollen, diffusely delineated mucosal and submucosal layers. In contrast, the muscle layer is clearly defined–composed of two hypoechoic bands corresponding with the inner circular and outer longitudinal layers. The narrowed lumen is identified by the sparse intraluminal gas echoes. A sessile gas echo within the wall is suspicious for an ulcer. On colonoscopy, several ulcers were encountered.

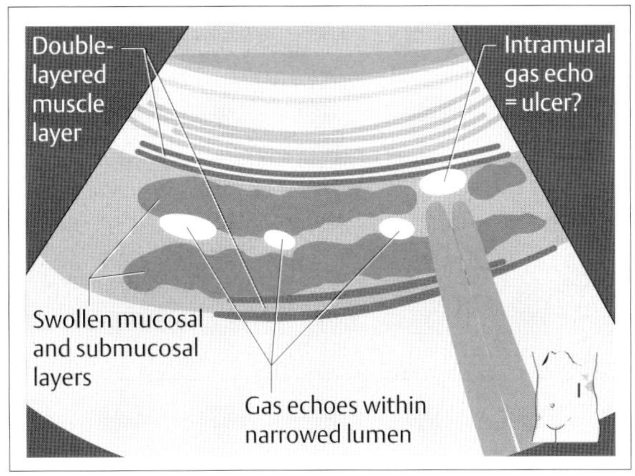

Fig. 1.**30 b** Line drawing.

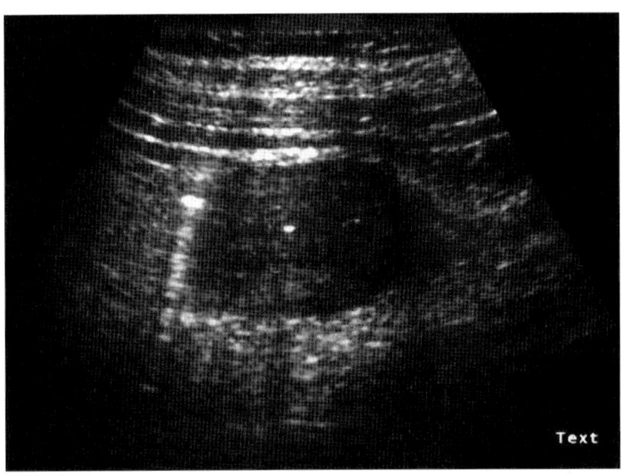

Fig. 1.**31 a** Same patient as in Fig. 1.**30**. Transverse view of the descending colon with swollen, diffusely delineated mucosal and submucosal layers. In contrast, the muscle layer is clearly defined–composed of two hypoechoic bands corresponding with the inner circular and outer longitudinal layers. The narrowed lumen is identified by the central intraluminal gas echoes. Incidental finding of a sessile gas echo on the colonic wall corresponding with a diverticulum.

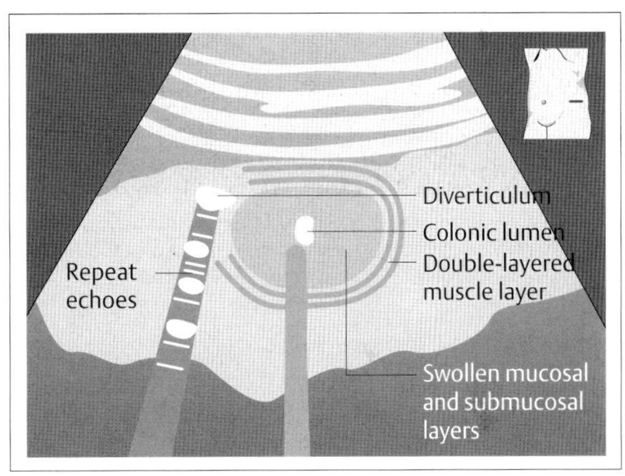

Fig. 1.**31 b** Line drawing.

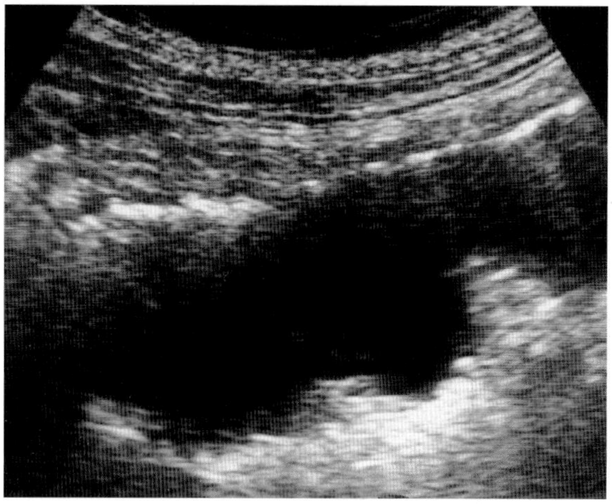

Fig. 1.32 a Ischemic bowel wall necrosis. Dilated bowel with intramural gas collection, demonstrated by the bright echoes with reverberation artifacts. They are localized within the wall and not the lumen, since the gas echoes collect along both discernible gut walls and do not float to the topmost position.

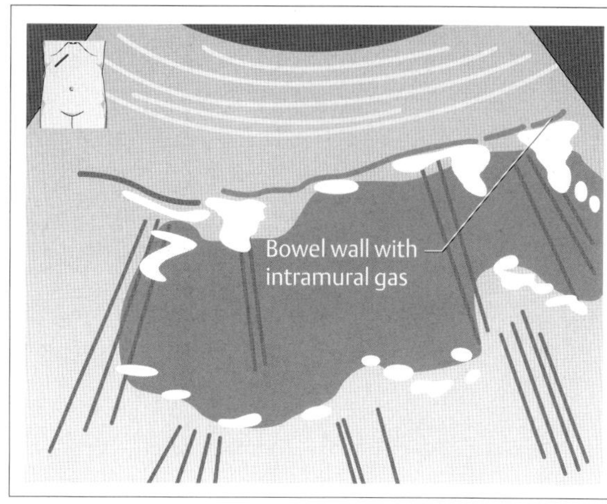

Fig. 1.32 b Line drawing.

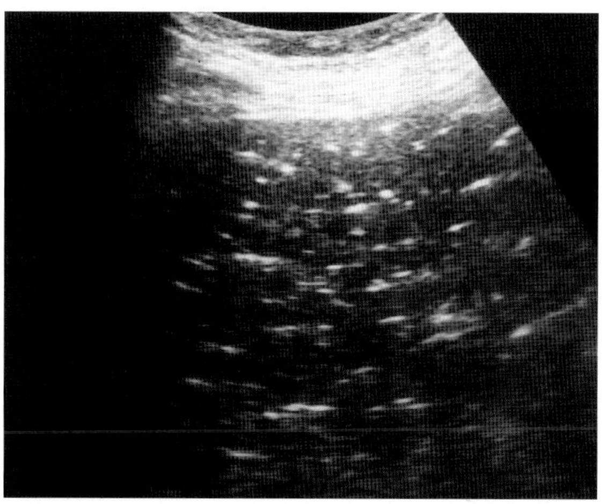

Fig. 1.33 a Same patient as in Fig. 1.32. Gas embolism of the portal vein due to intestinal gangrene. Finely dispersed gas echoes throughout the liver. The patient succumbed to septic shock within two hours after admission.

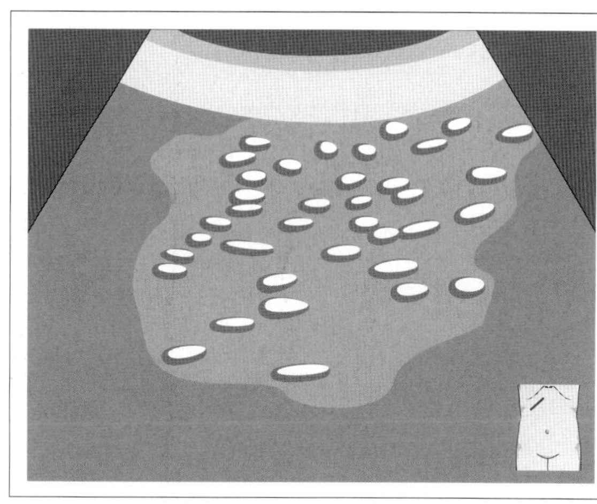

Fig. 1.33 b Line drawing.

Bowel Wall Hematoma

Basic Facts

Causes

- The etiology of bowel wall hematoma is divided almost evenly between the following (Lorente-Ramos et al., 1999; Rupprecht et al., 1984):
  - Coagulation disorders, mainly induced by anticoagulant medication. The most common site is the jejunum.
  - Trauma, predominantly affecting the duodenum, with children being at greater risk than adults.
  - Various other pathologies, including acute pancreatitis, vasculitis (especially Henoch-Schönlein purpura), vascular anomalies.
- The hematoma encompasses all layers, in particular the submucosa, leading to incomplete or complete obstruction.
- Accordingly, most clinical cases present as MBO, while GI bleeding is observed in only 30% of patients.
- *Additional workup:* CT of the abdomen (typically, the hematoma has an initial density > 50 HU). Most difficult differential diagnosis: intestinal ischemia. When in doubt, angiography or laparoscopy is warranted.

Sonographic Criteria

- Traumatic **duodenal hematoma** frequently assumes the aspect of a fusiform mass in the duodenal wall.
- Bowel wall hematomas due to coagulation disorders present as extended circular hypoechoic wall swelling, similar to that in bowel ischemia, with thickened circular (Fig. 1.**34**) or semilunar folds (Fig. 1.**36**), respectively. Typically, the swelling of the wall is even more pronounced than in intestinal ischemia (> 10 mm), and is associated with obstruction (Figs. 1.**34**–1.**36**).
- This **thickening of the gut wall** primarily affects the submucosa, which can be differentiated from the less echogenic muscle layer, especially on transverse views (Fig. 1.**35**).
- Signs of MBO may be evident upstream of the site of obstruction (Fig. 1.**34**).
- Additional hematomas may be found in the mesentery and retroperitoneum.

Consequences for Surgical Treatment

Diagnosis	Characteristic Findings	Management
Suspected hematoma of the intestinal wall	Clinical picture: coagulation disorder, trauma, acute pancreatitis, or vascular pathology; Sonography: extended symmetric circular thickening of the gut wall, particularly so of the submucosa, with intestinal obstruction; possible signs of MBO upstream of the site of obstruction.	Diagnosis confirmed by another modality (CT or laparoscopy): conservative management; correction of coagulation disorder. Segmental resection is indicated in cases of persistent GI bleeding or peritonitis; in suspected intestinal ischemia, splanchnic angiography may be indicated.

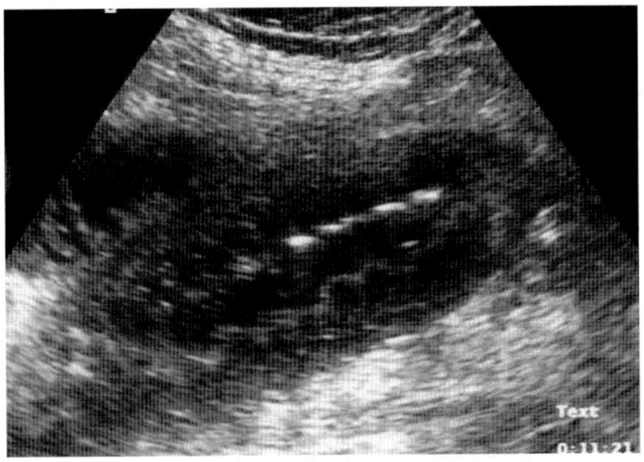

Fig. 1.**34 a** Intramural hematoma of the jejunum. A 71 year-old man with mechanical bowel obstruction secondary to warfarin overdose. Over a length of about 50 cm, the bowel wall is thickened, hypoechoic, and rigid. This is particularly so for the submucosal layer, with swollen, closely adjacent circular folds. The wall thickness between the folds cannot be measured. Including the folds, the thickness of the bowel wall measures 20 mm. The lumen is almost completely obstructed, as implied by the central intraluminal gas echoes. Adjacent dilated small-bowel loop with heightened motility but no thickened wall, corresponding to mechanical obstruction.

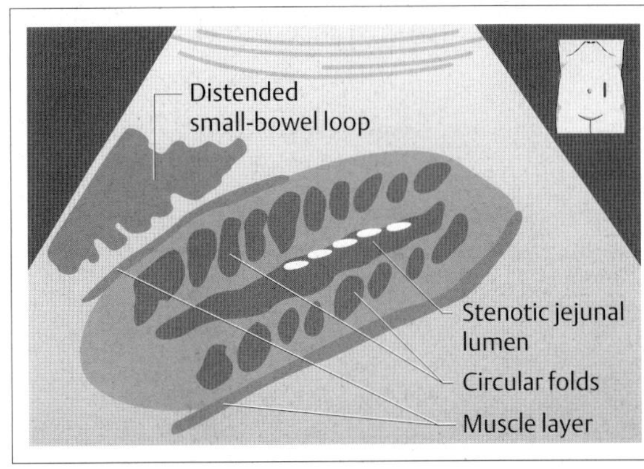

Fig. 1.**34 b** Line drawing.

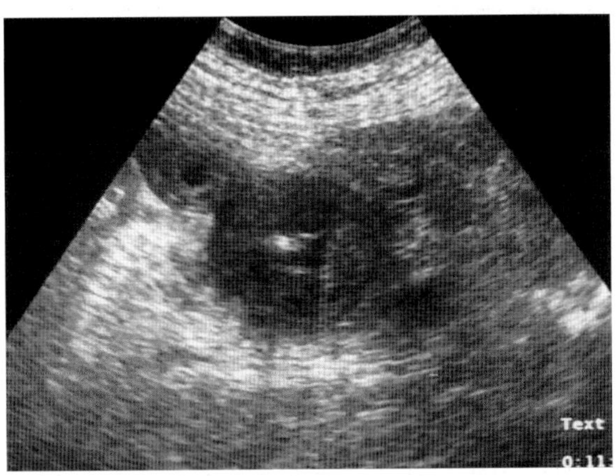

Fig. 1.**35 a** Transverse view of the jejunal wall hematoma depicted in Fig. 1.**34** with the totally symmetric circular bowel wall thickening; this affects predominantly the submucosa, which is hyperechoic to the muscle layer. Narrowed lumen outlined by the gas echoes. Overall diameter of the jejunum is 41 mm. The adjacent mildly dilated and normal small bowel loops are indicative of mechanical obstruction.

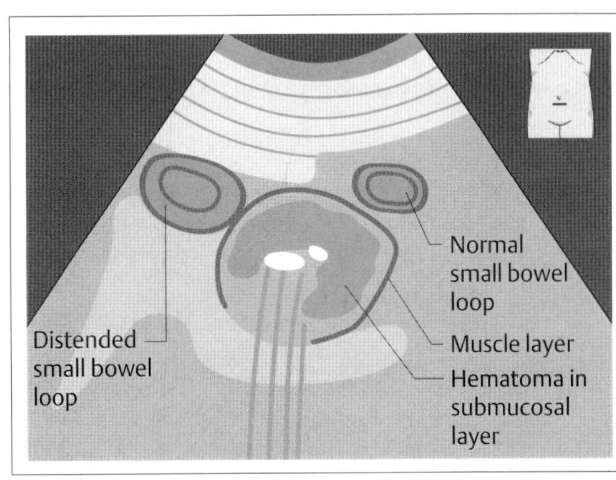

Fig. 1.**35 b** Line drawing.

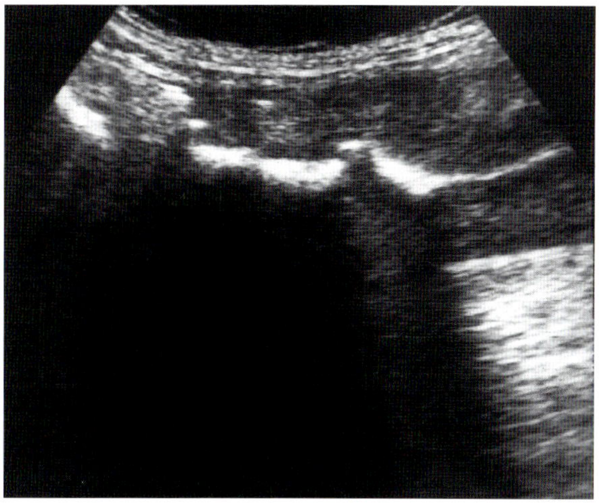

Fig. 1.**36 a** Intramural hematoma of the colon. A 71 year-old woman with left lower quadrant pain secondary to warfarin overdose. Descending colon with transition between normal wall with five-layered gut signature and wall thickening of up to 20 mm, extending over a length of 15 cm. Severe swelling of the semilunar folds.

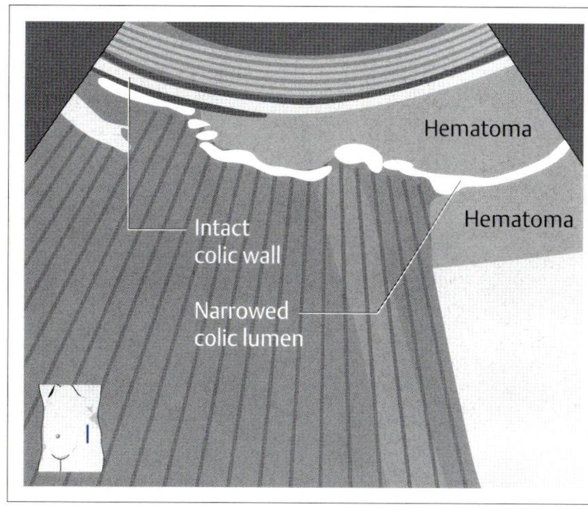

Fig. 1.**36 b** Line drawing.

Gynecological Disorders

Pelvic Inflammatory Disease (PID)

Basic Facts

- Peak incidence in young, sexually active women between 16 and 24 years.
- PID may mimic acute abdomen due to localized or generalized peritonitis.
- Important differential diagnoses include ovarian cyst torsion, ectopic pregnancy, appendicitis, and urinary tract infection.
- Differentiation may be facilitated by CBC, ESR, CRP, and pregnancy testing as well as urinalysis.
- Acute infections as well as their sequelae may yield important sonographic findings.
- *Additional workup:* vaginal, cervical, and urethral cultures. Optional: exploratory laparoscopy.

Sonographic Criteria

- Transvaginal sonography is superior to abdominal ultrasound in the assessment of gynecological pathology.
- Normal fallopian tubes are almost impossible to identify by sonography.
- Acute PID may produce increased fluid collections in the pouch of Douglas.
- Adnexal mass with loss of normal ovarian texture secondary to multicystic ovarian enlargement (Fig. 1.**37**).
- One complication of previous PID may be distal occlusion of the fallopian tube, giving rise to the typical hydrosalpinx (sactosalpinx) and correlating clinically with tubal sterility (Fig. 1.**38**).
- Hydrometra following fluid discharge from a hydrosalpinx into the uterine cavity is rare (Fig. 1.**39**).

Consequences for Surgical Treatment

Diagnosis	Characteristic Findings	Management
Acute PID	Pelvic complaints, fever	I. v. antibiotics, anti-inflammatory drugs
Tubo-ovarian abscess	Persisting fever and pain	Surgical evacuation (via laparotomy or laparoscopy)
Hydrosalpinx	Sterility, chronic pain	Microsurgical salpingostomy; alternatively, IVF-ET

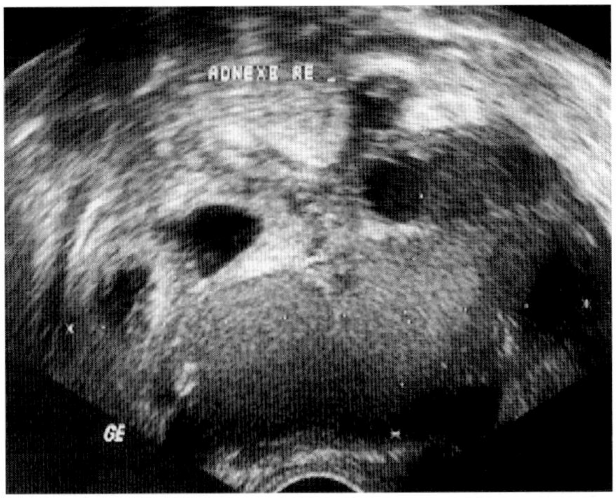

Fig. 1.**37 a** Ovarian abscess. Transvaginal sonography of the right ovary with central abscess formation and peripheral follicles.

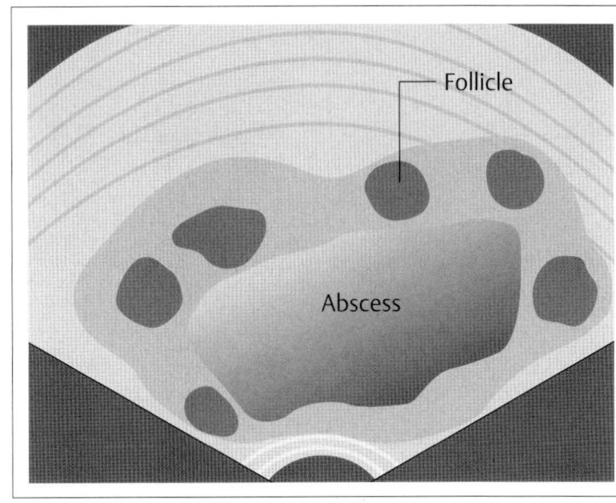

Fig. 1.**37 b** Line drawing.

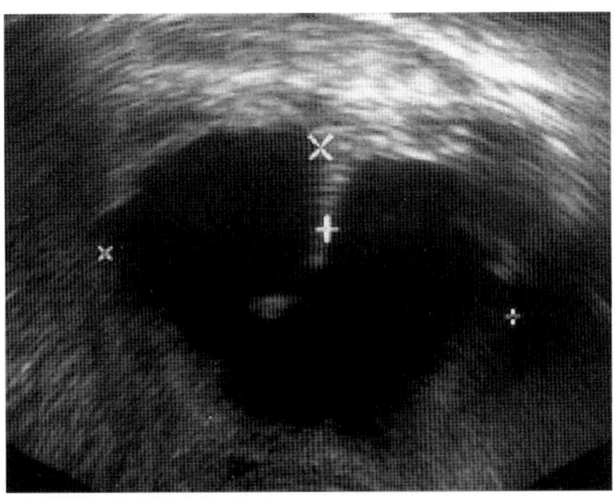

Fig. 1.**38 a** Tortuous hydrosalpinx shaped like a post horn (transvaginal sonogram).

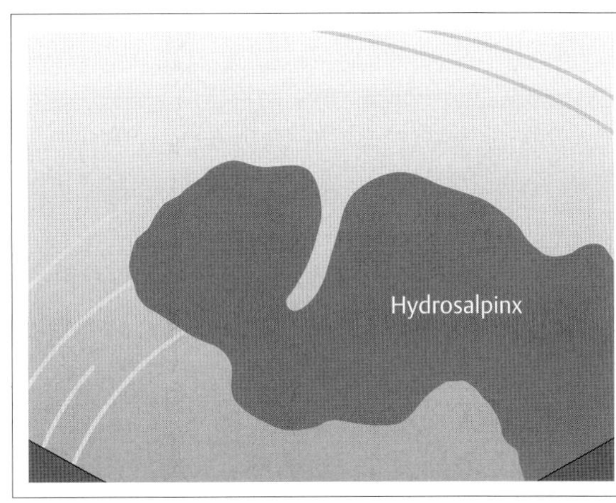

Fig. 1.**38 b** Line drawing.

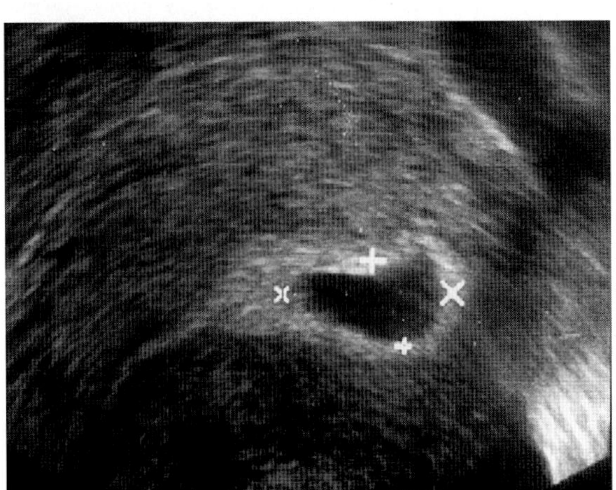

Fig. 1.**39 a** Hydrometra demonstrated on transvaginal sonogram.

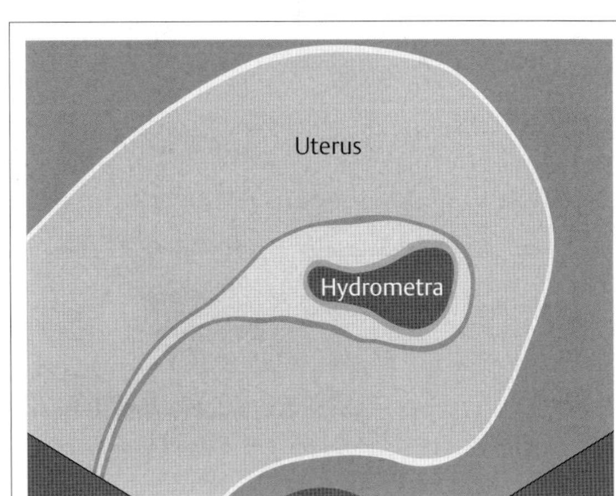

Fig. 1.**39 b** Line drawing.

■ Ovarian Neoplasms

Basic Facts

- Ovarian neoplasms may be found at any age.
- The incidence of functional ovarian neoplasms peaks during the reproductive phase.
- Due of the high incidence of functional cysts in ovarian neoplasms, "watchful waiting" with serial sonography, possibly under hormone medication, is preferable to precipitate surgery.
- Ovarian tumors may cause acute pain, owing to their size, position, and torsion (pedicle).
- Sonomorphology can differentiate between cystic (anechoic), solid (hyperechoic), and mixed (hypo- and hyperechoic) forms.
- *Additional workup:* tumor marker CA 125; color flow Doppler imaging; since CT and MRI are of limited diagnostic value, laparoscopy is preferred.

Sonographic Criteria

- Normal ovaries are identified more easily by tracing the ipsilateral external iliac vessels to which they relate (Fig. 1.**40**).
- **Smaller tumors** are better delineated by transvaginal sonography, while larger masses are depicted in toto by additional transabdominal sonogram.
- The more irregular the shape of an ovarian mass and the more pronounced its texture of cystic and solid areas, the higher the likelihood of malignancy.
- Ovarian tumors with papillary proliferation, ascites, and/or focal hepatic lesions are highly likely to be malignant.

Consequences for Surgical Treatment

Diagnosis	Characteristic Findings	Management
Unilocular ovarian cyst	Incidental finding, little tenderness	Nonoperative; follow-up with serial sonography; possibly, endocrine blockage of ovarian function (oral contraceptive)
Suspected ovarian cyst torsion	Acute pain, vomiting, localized peritonitis	Exploratory laparoscopy
Suspected ovarian malignancy	Heterogeneous mass and ascites	Preoperative workup: chest radiograph, barium enema, cystoscopy; followed by laparotomy

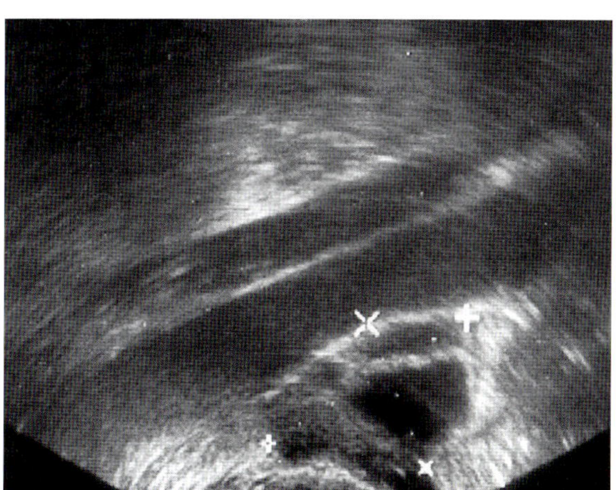

Fig. 1.**40 a** Topographic relationship between ovary and external iliac vessels. Typical transvaginal sonographic image of the functioning ovary.

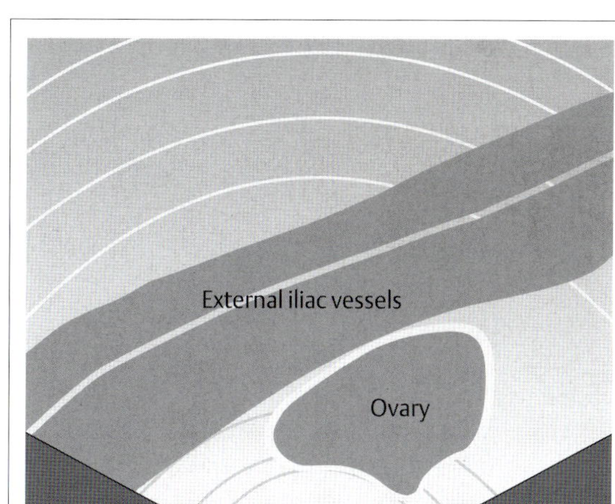

Fig. 1.**40 b** Line drawing.

Ectopic Pregnancy

Basic Facts

- According to WHO data, the incidence of ectopic pregnancy is around 2% of all pregnancies.
- Population at risk: women with episodes of PID or previous pelvic surgery.
- Early diagnosis (in the 5th to 7th week) helps to prevent complications.
- Pelvic complaints culminating in peritonitis are the possible cardinal symptom.
- Tubal abortion and tubal rupture are potential complications.
- (Suspected) Diagnosis is usually based on history, bimanual palpatory findings, pregnancy testing, and transvaginal sonography.
- *Additional workup:* cardiovascular parameters, pregnancy test, CBC; broad indication for exploratory laparoscopy.

Sonographic Criteria

- Transvaginal sonography is the prime modality.
- If β-HCG testing is positive and normal intrauterine pregnancy cannot be visualized, ectopic or otherwise abnormal pregnancy must be suspected.
- A "pseudogestation sac" may mimic intrauterine pregnancy.
- Intact ectopic pregnancy is rare.
- Frequently, a heterogeneous mass or a ring is seen at one of the fallopian tubes (Fig. 1.**41**).
- Excessive free fluid in the pouch of Douglas or elsewhere within the abdomen is suggestive of tubal abortion or rupture.

Consequences for Surgical Treatment

Diagnosis	Characteristic Findings	Management
Suspected ectopic pregnancy	Uterine bleeding, pain	Pregnancy test; gynecological assessment; transvaginal sonography; laparoscopy
Tubal abortion, tubal rupture	Pain, circulatory failure, signs of hypovolemic shock	Circulatory support; emergency laparoscopy/laparotomy

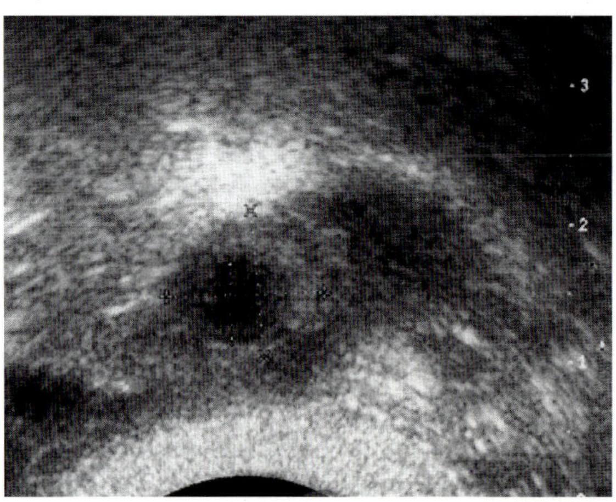

Fig. 1.**41 a** Transvaginal sonography of ectopic pregnancy presenting as a ring-shaped structure in the isthmoampullary section of the fallopian tube.

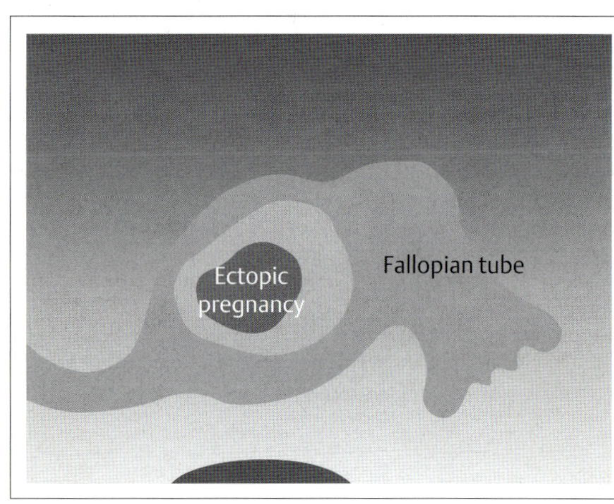

Fig. 1.**41 b** Line drawing.

Bibliography

Bakalakos EA, Melvin WS, Kirkpatrick R. Liver abscess secondary to intrahepatic perforation of the gallbladder, presenting as a liver mass. Am J Gastroenterol. 1996; 91: 1644–6.

Block S, Maier W, Clausen C, Büchler M, Malfertheiner P, Beger HG. Diagnostik der nekrotisierenden Pankreatitis. Vergleich von Kontrastmittel-CT und Ultraschall in einer klinischen Studie. Dtsch Med Wochenschr. 1985; 110: 826–32.

Chang-Chien CS, Lin HH, Yen CL, Lee CM, Lin SM. Sonographic demonstration of free air in perforated peptic ulcers: comparison of sonography with radiography. J Clin Ultrasound. 1989; 17: 95–100.

Habscheid W. Sonomorphologie der akuten Pankreatitis unter Berücksichtigung des Schweregrades. Ultraschall Med. 1987; 8: 134–7.

Harvey RT, Miller WT Jr. Acute biliary disease: initial CT and follow-up US versus initial US and follow-up CT. Radiology. 1999; 213: 831–6.

Hollerbach S, Ruser J, Ochs A, Frick E, Schölmerich J. Aktueller Stellenwert der abdominellen Pankreassonographie. Eine retrospektive Analyse von 585 sonographischen Pankreasuntersuchungen. Med Klin. 1994; 89: 7–13.

Hoover EL, Cole GD, Mitchell LS, Adams CZ Jr., Hassett J. Avoiding laparotomy in nonsurgical pneumoperitoneum. Am J Surg. 1992; 164: 99–103.

Kirchner J, Lorenz M, Heyd R, Gute P, Jacobi V. Pneumoperitoneum und Pneumoretroperitoneum ohne Perforation. Zentralbl Chir. 1996; 121: 861–5.

Klein HM, Lensing R, Klosterhalfen B, Tons C, Gunther RW. Diagnostic imaging of mesenteric infarction. Radiology. 1995; 197: 79–82.

Ko YT, Lim JH, Lee DH, Lee HW, Lim JW. Small bowel obstruction: sonographic evaluation. Radiology. 1993; 188: 649–53.

Limberg B. Sonographie des Gastrointestinaltraktes. Berlin, Heidelberg: Springer; 1998.

Lippert H. Praxis der Chirurgie. Stuttgart: Thieme; 1998.

Loren I, Lasson A, Fork T, et al. New sonographic imaging observations in focal pancreatitis. Eur Radiol. 1999; 9: 862–7.

Lorente-Ramos RM, Santiago-Hernando A, Del Valle-Sanz Y, Arjonilla-Lopez A. Sonographic diagnosis of intramural duodenal hematomas. J Clin Ultrasound. 1999; 27: 213–6.

Matsumoto S, Mori H, Miyake H, et al. Uneven fatty replacement of the pancreas: evaluation with CT. Radiology. 1995; 194: 453–8.

McGagan JP, Goldberg BB. Diagnostic Ultrasound. Philadelphia, New York: Lipincott-Raven; 1997.

Meinel K, Issel EP, Watzek H. Geburtshilfliche und gynäkologische Ultraschalldiagnostik. Stuttgart: Thieme; 1991.

Meiser G, Meissner K. Sonographische Diagnostik beim komplizierten peptischen Ulkus. Ultraschall Med. 1986; 7: 268–74.

Merz E. Sonographische Diagnostik in Gynäkologie und Geburtshilfe. Stuttgart: Thieme; 1997.

Nyberg DA, Laing FC. Ultrasonographic findings in peptic ulcer disease and pancreatitis that simulate primary gallbladder disease. J Ultrasound Med. 1983; 2: 303–7.

Park MS, Yu JS, Kim YH, et al. Acute cholecystitis: comparison of MR cholangiography and US. Radiology. 1998; 209: 781–5.

Patel SV, Gopichandran TD. Ultrasound evidence of gas in the fissure for ligamentum teres: a sign of perforated duodenal ulcer. Br J Radiol. 1999; 72: 901–2.

Puylaert JBCM. Ultrasound of Appendicitis and its Differential Diagnosis. Berlin, Heidelberg: Springer; 1990.

Rau B, Pralle U, Mayer JM, Beger HG. Role of ultrasonographically guided fine-needle aspiration cytology in the diagnosis of infected pancreatic necrosis. Br J Surg. 1998; 85: 179–84.

Rupprecht HJ, Braun B, Neher M, Schweden F. Darmwandeinblutung während Antikoagulantientherapie. Diagnose durch Sonographie und Computertomographie. Dtsch Med Wochenschr. 1984; 109: 1686–8.

Schölmerich J, Johannesson T, Brobmann G, et al. Die Sonographie bei der akuten Pankreatitis – Diagnose, Ätiologieklärung und Prognoseabschätzung. Ultraschall Med. 1989; 10: 290–4.

Schwerk WB, Wichtrup B, Rothmund M, Ruschoff J. Ultrasonography in the diagnosis of acute appendicitis: a prospective study. Gastroenterology. 1989; 97: 630–9.

Seitz K, Merz M. Sonographische Ileusdiagnostik. Ultraschall Med. 1998; 19: 242–9.

Seitz K, Reising KD. Sonographischer Nachweis freier Luft in der Bauchhöhle. Ultraschall Med. 1982; 3: 4–6.

Sohn C, Holzgreve W. Ultraschall in Gynäkologie und Geburtshilfe. Stuttgart: Thieme; 1995.

Teefey SA, Baron RL, Bigler SA. Sonography of the gallbladder: significance of striated (layered) thickening of the gallbladder wall. Am J Roentgenol. 1991; 156: 945–7.

Teefey SA, Roarke MC, Brink JA, et al. Bowel wall thickening: differentiation of inflammation from ischemia with color Doppler and duplex US. Radiology. 1996; 198: 547–51.

Tsai KC, Wang HP, Huang GT, Wang SM. Preoperative sonographic diagnosis of sealed-off perforated gastric ulcer. J Clin Ultrasound. 1998; 26: 269–71.

United Kingdom Guidelines for the Management of Acute Pancreatitis. British Society of Gastroenterology. Gut. 1998; 42, Suppl 2: S1–13.

Wegener M, Börsch G, Schneider J, Wedmann B, Winter R, Zacharias J. Gallbladder wall thickening: a frequent finding in various nonbiliary disorders – a prospective ultrasonographic study. J Clin Ultrasound. 1987; 15: 307–12.

Yamamoto M, Okamura T, Tomikawa M, et al. Perforated diverticulum of the transverse colon. Am J Gastroenterol. 1997; 92: 1567–9.

Yang CS, Wang HP, Huang GT, et al. Perforation of jejunal lymphoma – ultrasonographic diagnosis of free air over left flank area. Hepatogastroenterology. 1999; 46: 2436–8.

2 Thoracic and Abdominal Trauma

R. Mantke

Indications for Sonography

The focused assessment by sonography for trauma, or FAST, is a routine component of the initial workup in thoracic and abdominal trauma. FAST is performed by the surgeon as an extension of the physical examination immediately after arrival of the patient in the emergency room. Thus, every surgeon must master this technique and its interpretation. Even if the trauma obviously does not affect the chest and abdomen, thoracic and abdominal sonography should still be an integral part of the basic assessment.

At present, the primary goal of FAST is to identify fluid, presumably blood, as a surrogate in blunt-injury patients with lesions of solid organs (liver, spleen, kidneys, pancreas), hollow viscera (gastrointestinal tract, bladder), heart, and the great vessels. Sonography should be preferred to diagnostic peritoneal lavage.

The algorithm in Fig. 2.**1** outlines the primary management of major trauma.

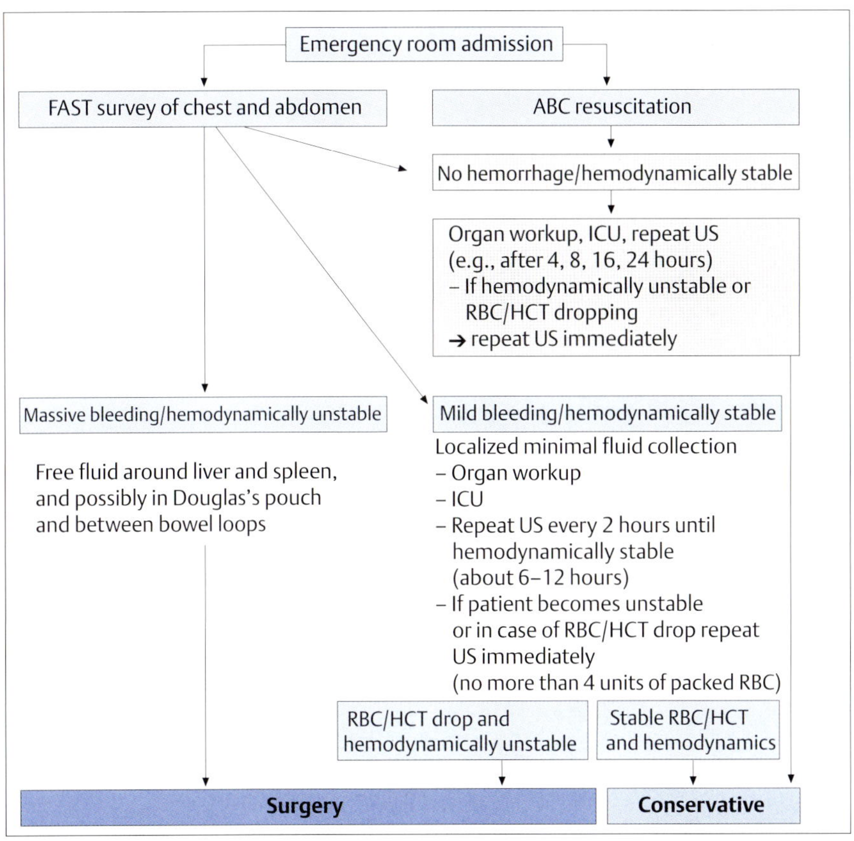

Fig. 2.**1** Algorithm for sonography in trauma management.

Specific Technique and Diagnostic Evaluation

- Patient in standard (supine) position.
- Convex 3.5–5.0 MHz transducer.
- Choice of viewing plane: → Fig. 2.**2**.
- Assessment of individual organs: see corresponding chapters.
- Douglas's pouch is most reliably assessed through a full bladder.
- The most common sites of free fluid must be evaluated with particular care:
  - Hepatorenal recess (Morrison's pouch)
  - Splenorenal recess and perisplenic space
  - Costodiaphragmatic recess
  - Douglas's pouch
- Detailed search for subtle parenchymal lesions is permissible only in hemodynamically stable patients.
- Circulatory failure associated with demonstration of free intraperitoneal fluid mandates immediate laparotomy.

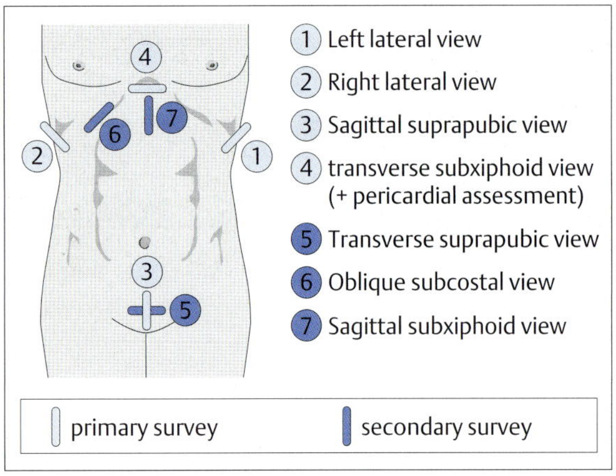

Fig. 2.**2** Recommended viewing planes (primary and secondary survey) in the sonographic evaluation of abdominal trauma.

Table 2.**1** Incidence of specific injuries in a series of 356 patients with severe blunt abdominal trauma (data from 1991, Department of Surgery, University of Mannheim Medical Center, [Lippert, 1997])

	n	%
Spleen	167	46.9
Liver	131	36.7
Kidneys	53	148
Mesentery	46	12.9
Small bowel	34	9.5
Pancreas	27	7.5
Major vessels	25	7.0
Diaphragm	20	5.6
Urinary bladder	16	4.4
Colon	13	3.6
Stomach	9	2.5

Free Intra-abdominal Fluid

- The distribution of injuries giving rise to free intraperitoneal fluid is shown in Table 2.**1**.
- In > 90% of cases, any free intra-abdominal fluid seen subsequent to thoracic and abdominal trauma will correspond to blood from parenchymal injuries.
- Free fluid will usually be found at the sites specified above.
- Free fluid between the bowel loops or in Douglas's pouch signifies severe bleeding.
- The intra-abdominal location of the free fluid, however, should not lead to premature conclusions about the organ injured, because active and passive changes in patient posture (during transport!) may cause fluid shifts. If in doubt about the nature/etiology of the fluid, ultrasound-guided diagnostic aspiration can be performed without losing time (Fig. 2.**3**).
- Sonography may reliably reveal as little as 50 ml of free perihepatic or perisplenic fluid.

Sonographic Criteria

- Free fluid is seen as an anechoic region outside any organ, vessel, or other defined structure.
- With changes in posture, fluid will shift to the most dependent location. Fluid will also react to external compression.
- Free fluid collects primarily in the perihepatic or perisplenic space (Figs. 2.**4** to 2.**8**).
- Differentiation between blood and ascites: sonographically, ascites is less homogeneous as it is rich in protein, contains bands of fibrin, and may correlate with the signs of cirrhosis of the liver (Fig. 2.**9**).

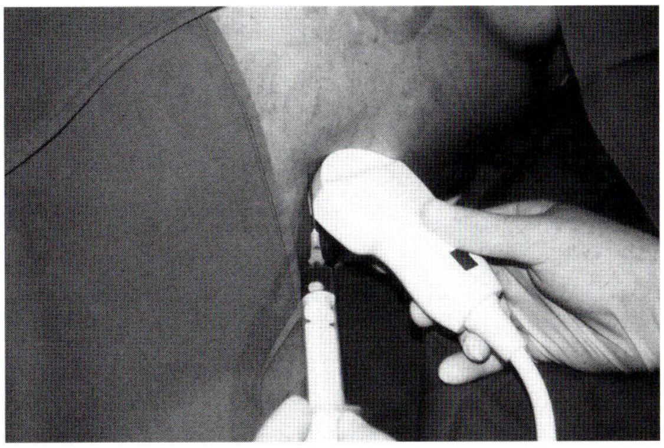

Fig. 2.**3** Freehand ultrasound-guided aspiration of free intra-abdominal fluid.

Consequences for Surgical Treatment

Diagnosis	Characteristic Findings	Management
Free intra-abdominal fluid: Hemodynamically stable, steady H&H	Small localized amount of free fluid (< 5 mm)	Watchful waiting with serial sonography, initially every two hours
Free intra-abdominal fluid: Hemodynamically unstable, H&H drop	Massive amount of free fluid (> 10 mm), either localized or spread diffusely throughout the abdomen	Emergency laparotomy; no further investigations, since this would only result in potentially fatal time loss

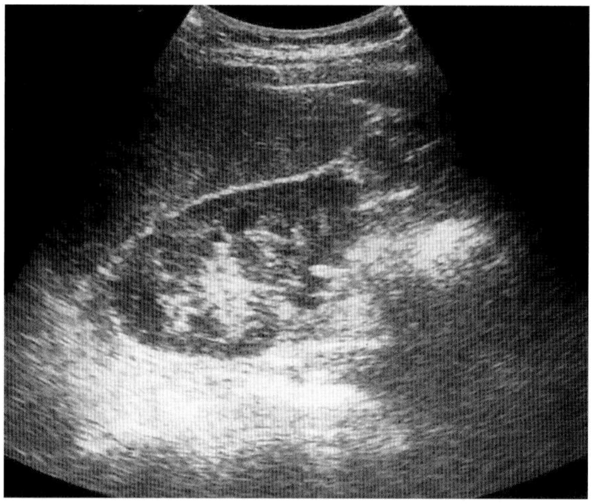

Fig. 2.**4a** Normal view of spleen and left kidney (splenorenal recess).

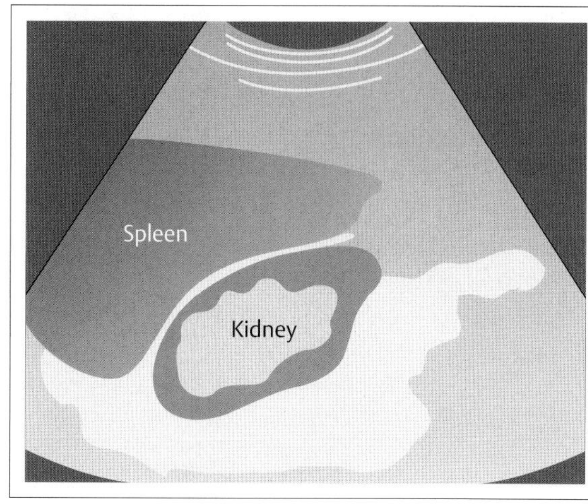

Fig. 2.**4b** Line drawing.

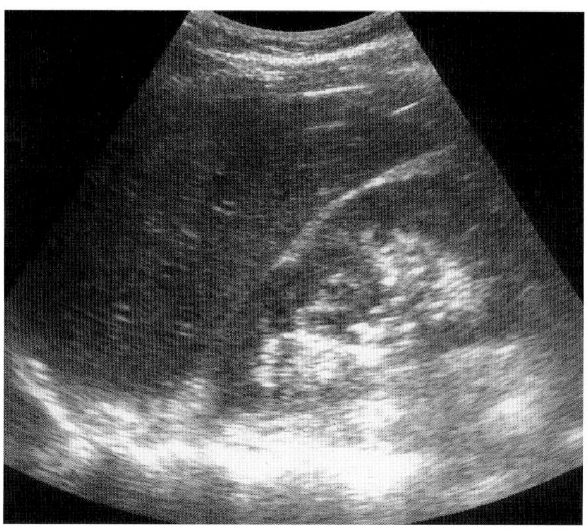

Fig. 2.**5a** Normal view of liver and right kidney (Morrison's pouch).

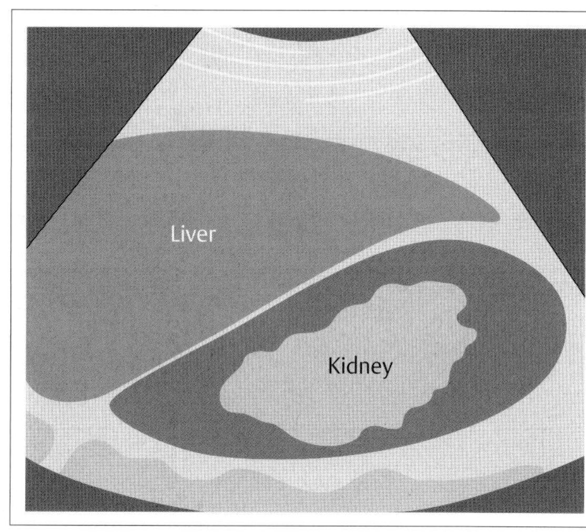

Fig. 2.**5b** Line drawing.

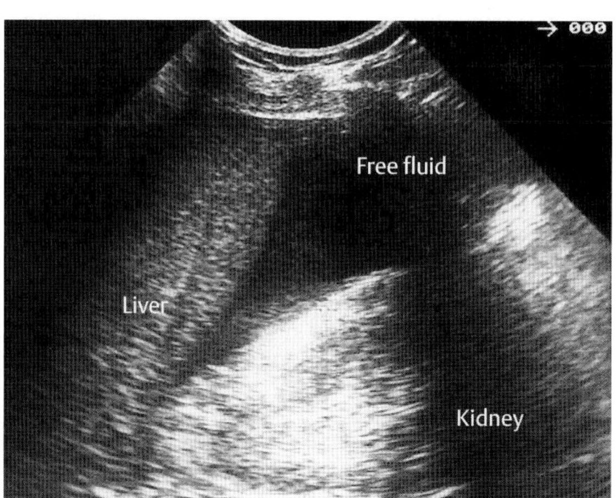

Fig. 2.**6a** Free fluid in Morrison's pouch after blunt abdominal trauma with splenic rupture.

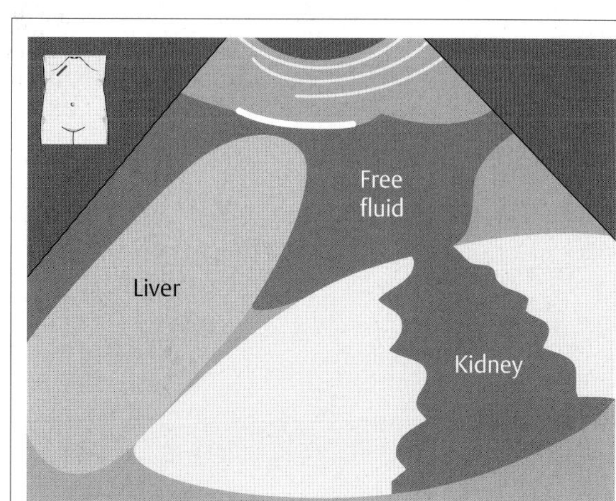

Fig. 2.**6b** Line drawing.

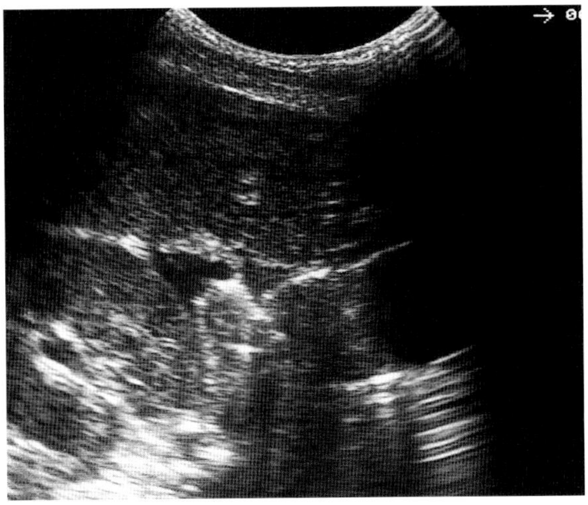

Fig. 2.7 **a** Small amount of free fluid in the hepatorenal recess following abdominal trauma.

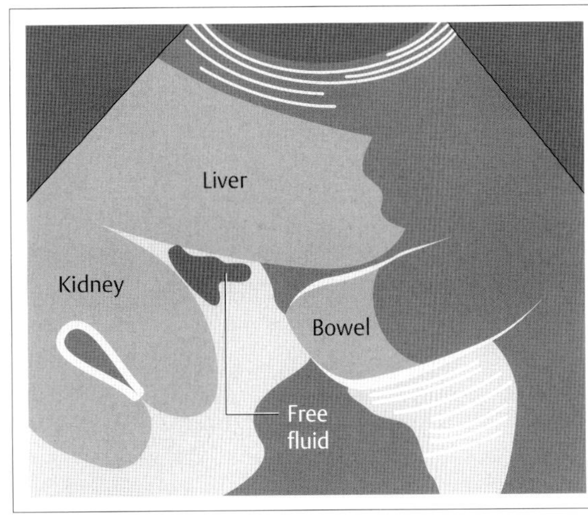

Fig. 2.7 **b** Line drawing.

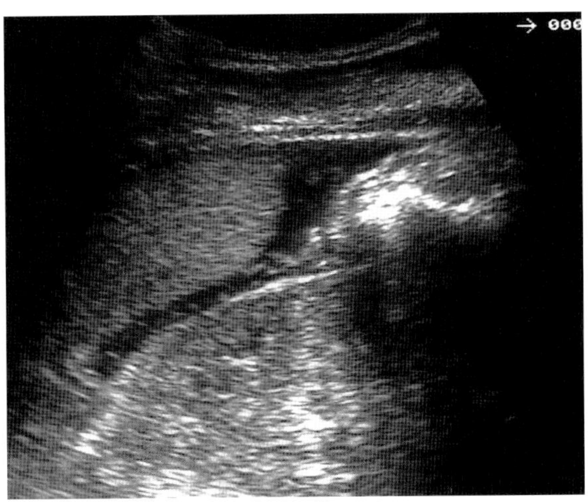

Fig. 2.8 **a** Free fluid around a ruptured spleen. The parenchymal lesion cannot be demonstrated.

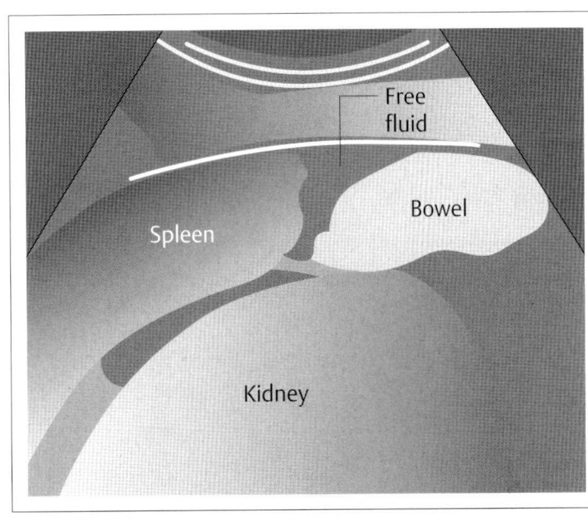

Fig. 2.8 **b** Line drawing.

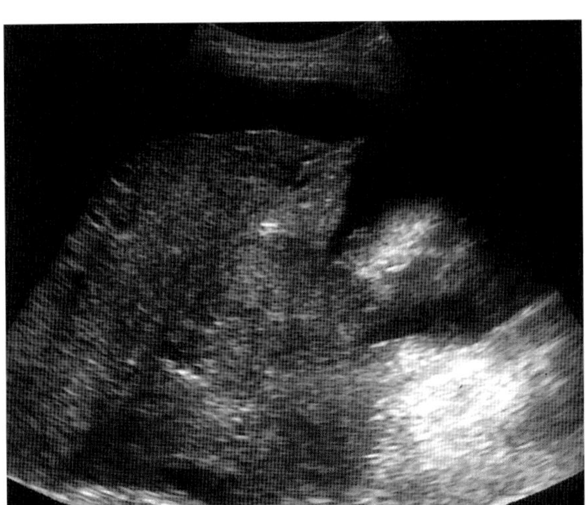

Fig. 2.9 **a** Ascites in a patient with a cirrhotic liver, characterized by inhomogeneous echotexture and irregular contour.

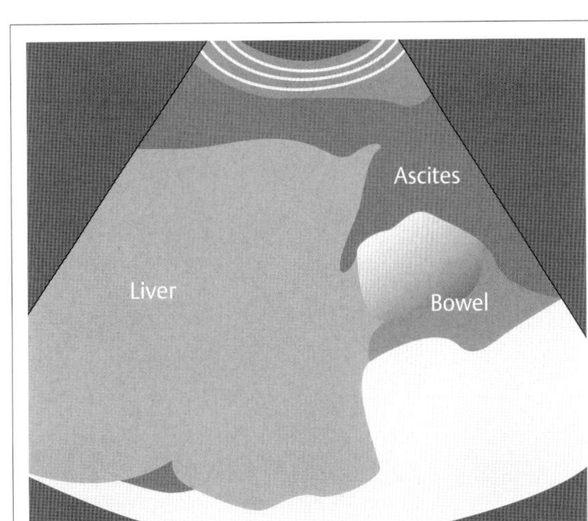

Fig. 2.9 **b** Line drawing.

Splenic Trauma

Basic Facts

- The spleen is the most frequently injured intra-abdominal organ (in 25–60% of all severe abdominal trauma cases).
- In 25%, splenic trauma is combined with fractured ribs or other intra-abdominal organ injuries. Concomitant injury of the left diaphragm is encountered in 2% of abdominal trauma.
- *Type of injury:* subcapsular and intrasplenic hematoma, partial or complete rupture, avulsion of the splenic pedicle (rare).
- Delayed rupture is possible days, even weeks, after splenic trauma. Therefore, close sonographic follow-up (in case of abnormal findings, at least daily during the first week) and inpatient observation are mandatory.

Sonographic Criteria

- Acute intraparenchymal hemorrhage presents as a hyperechoic zone within the spleen. With time it may take on a hypoechoic aspect, owing to liquefaction.
- A strictly subcapsular blood collection may appear hypoechoic from the onset.
- With progressive organization, hematomas become more heterogeneous and are then more easily identified.
- A heterogeneous irregular contour is characteristic of parenchymal injury (Fig. 2.**10**).

- Small fresh intraparenchymal hematoma and small ruptures frequently escape initial detection.
- *Additional workup:* contrast enhanced angio-CT, angiography; laparoscopy.

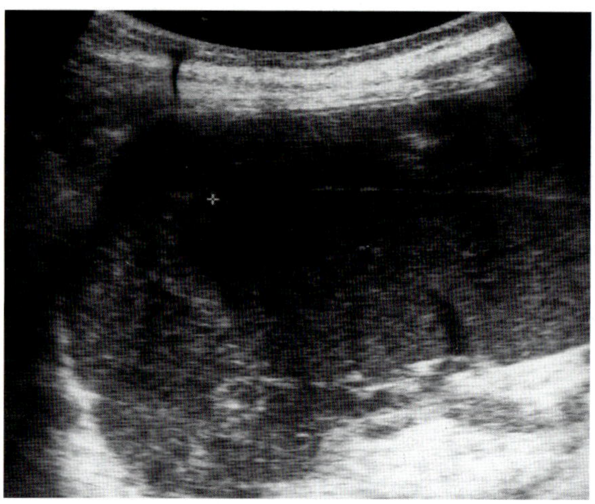

Fig. 2.**10 a** Inhomogeneous, somewhat hyperechoic lesion in the upper pole of the spleen with perisplenic hematoma after abdominal trauma.

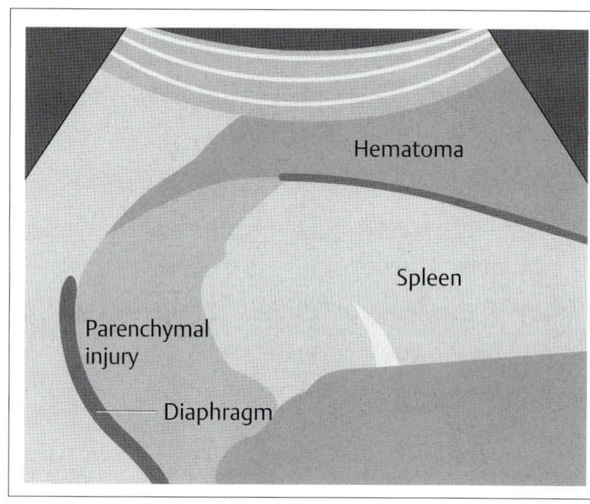

Fig. 2.**10 b** Line drawing.

Consequences for Surgical Treatment

Diagnosis	Characteristic Findings	Management
Subcapsular hematoma, in hemodynamically stable patient	No free fluid	Watchful waiting with repeat sonography; if necessary, transfusion until self-tamponade sets in
Splenic rupture: hemodynamically stable, steady H&H	Small localized amount of free fluid (< 5 mm), parenchymal lesion not seen sonographically	Close observation with repeat sonography
Splenic rupture: Hemodynamically unstable, H&H drop	Massive amount of free fluid (> 10 mm), either localized or spread diffusely throughout the abdomen; obvious parenchymal lesion	Surgical exploration attempting splenic preservation (topical fibrin adhesive, Vicryl mesh, infrared coagulation), splenectomy

Liver Trauma

Basic Facts

- Injuries of the liver are seen in 5–12% of all severe abdominal trauma cases.
- Up to 30% are accompanied by right-sided rib fractures.
- The liver is the second most often injured abdominal organ, with predominant involvement of the larger right lobe.
- **Type of injury:** intrahepatic or subcapsular hematoma, capsular or parenchymal tear (small/large), lobar rupture, extensive bilateral lobar rupture, avulsion of the hepatoduodenal ligament (extremely rare). Clinical staging according to Moore (Moore et al., 1989) (Table 2.**2**).
- *Additional workup:* contrast enhanced angio-CT, angiography (possibly combined with definitive embolization).

Sonographic Criteria

- Intrahepatic hematomas demonstrate irregular outlines and are in most cases hypoechoic (Figs. 2.**11**, 2.**12**).
- Small parenchymal tears may be missed on sonography.
- In massive parenchymal injury, free intraperitoneal fluid dominates the sonogram; the liver may no longer be homogeneous and may be distanced from the abdominal wall.

Table 2.**2** Moore's liver injury scale (AAST 2005)

Grade		
I	Hematoma	Subcapsular, < 10% surface area
	Laceration	Capsular tear, < 1 cm parenchymal depth
II	Hematoma	Subcapsular, 10–50% surface area: intraparenchymal < 10 cm in diameter
	Laceration	Capsular tear, 1–3 cm parenchymal depth, < 10 cm length
III	Hematoma	Subcapsular, > 50% surface area of ruptured subcapsular or parenchymal hematoma; intraparenchymal hematoma > 10 cm or expanding
	Laceration	> 3 cm parenchymal depth
IV	Laceration	Parenchymal disruption involving 25–75% of hepatic lobe or 1–3 Couinaud's segments within a single lobe
V	Laceration	Parenchymal disruption involving > 75% of hepatic lobe or >3 Couinaud's segments within single lobe
	Vascular	Juxtahepatic venous injuries; i. e., retrohepatic venacava/central major hepatic veins
	Vascular	Hepatic avulsion

Consequences for Surgical Treatment

Diagnosis	Characteristic Findings	Management
Subcapsular hematoma, in hemodynamically stable patient	No free fluid	Watchful waiting with repeat sonography; if necessary, transfusion until self-tamponade sets in
Liver rupture: hemodynamically stable, steady H&H	Small localized amount of free fluid (< 5 mm), parenchymal lesion frequently not seen sonographically	Watchful waiting with repeat sonography
Liver rupture: Hemodynamically unstable, H&H drop	Massive amount of free fluid (> 10 mm), either localized or spread diffusely throughout the abdomen	Immediate laparotomy with repair by suture, beamer, packing; resection/explantation of the liver only as last resort

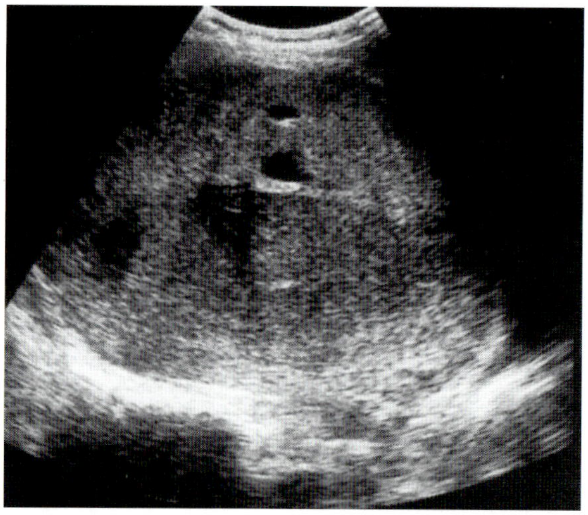

Fig. 2.11 a Large hypoechoic hemorrhage into the right lobe of the liver after abdominal trauma (size 14 cm × 7 cm).

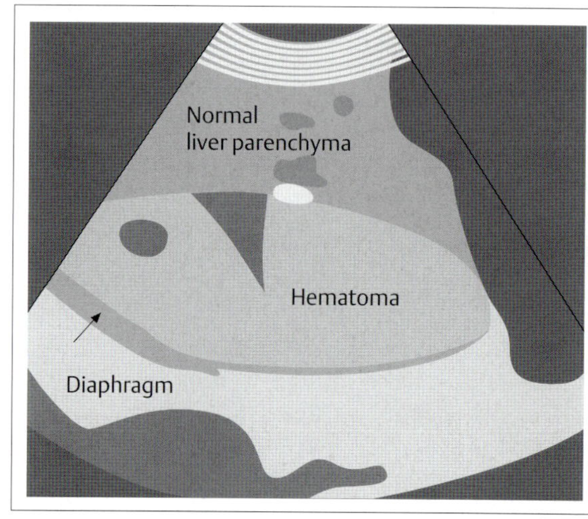

Fig. 2.11 b Line drawing.

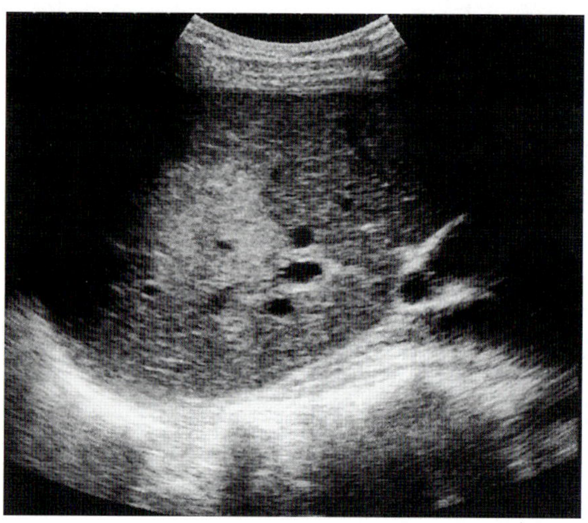

Fig. 2.12 a Two day-old hyperechoic hematoma in the right lobe of the liver with irregular outline (51 mm × 56 mm).

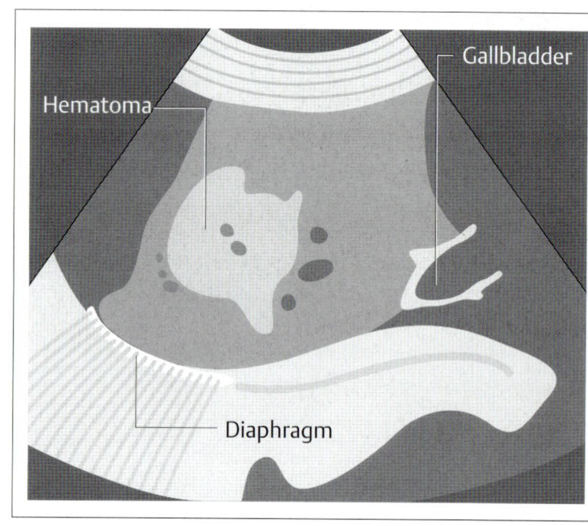

Fig. 2.12 b Line drawing.

Pancreatic Trauma

Basic Facts

- Pancreatic injury is a rare event, occurring in 2% of major blunt abdominal trauma cases.
- It may accompany multiple organ injury, but may just as likely represent isolated trauma, e.g., handlebar injury (more frequent in children).
- Because of its position anterior to the spine, the transition zone between head and body of the pancreas is at particular risk.
- **Type of injury:** Contusion, hematoma, rupture (Table 2.**3**)
- Frequently accompanied by duodenal tearing.
- Pancreatic injury may escape initial detection.

Table 2.**3** AAST Pancreas Injury Scale (2005)

Grade*		
I	Hematoma	Minor contusion without duct injury
	Laceration	Superficial laceration without duct injury
II	Laceration	Major contusion without duct injury or tissue loss
	Hematoma	Major laceration without duct injury or tissue loss
III	Laceration	Distal transection or parenchymal injury with duct injury
IV	Laceration	Proximal transection or parenchymal injury involving ampulla
V	Laceration	Massive disruption of pancreatic head

- Late-onset pancreatitis is possible (violent epigastric pain; peritonitis; guarding; procalcitonin, amylase, and lipase levels, WBC, and CRP elevated).
- *Additional workup:* contrast-enhanced CT, ERCP.

Sonographic Criteria

- Usually, sonography cannot identify **pancreatic rupture**.
- Under favorable viewing conditions–unlikely in the emergency setting–**pancreatic edema** (engorged hypoechoic echotexture) or intraparenchymal **hematoma** (hypoechoic mass) may be demonstrated.
- Over the course, a **posttraumatic pseudocyst** may arise (Fig. 2.**13**).
- In most cases, emergency sonography will not yield further details.
- In case of pancreatic pathology on sonography further workup is mandatory!

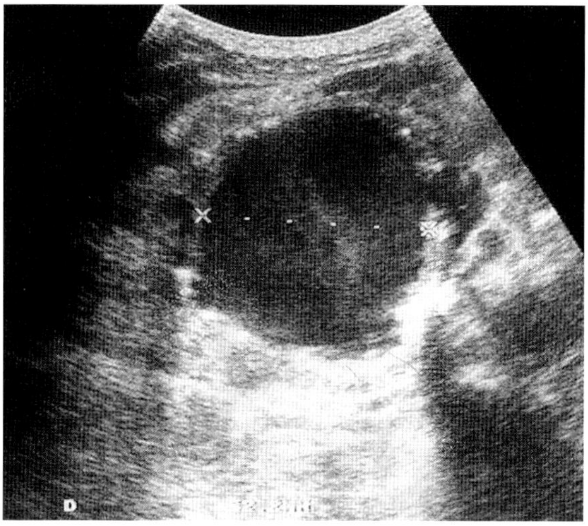

Fig. 2.**13 a** Pancreatic pseudocyst at the head/body (diameter 3.2 cm) six months after multiple organ injury.

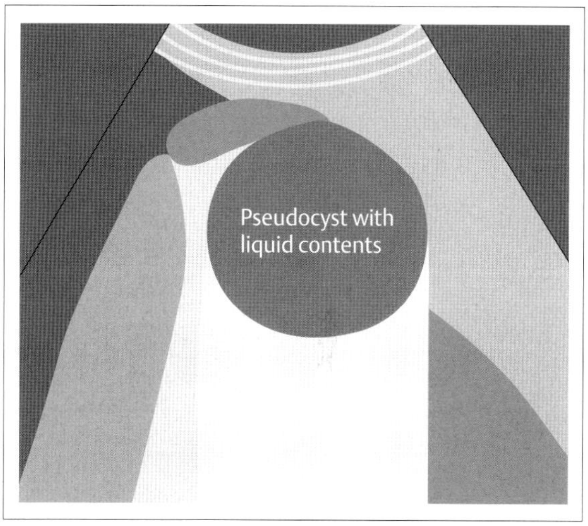

Fig. 2.**13 b** Line drawing.

Consequences for Surgical Treatment

Diagnosis	Characteristic Findings	Management
Contusion with hematoma or minor parenchymal tear	Possibly hematoma appearing as a hypoechoic mass	Expectant management, initially as in acute pancreatitis
Major parenchymal disruption without duct injury	Possibly hematoma and/or free intraperitoneal fluid	Exploratory laparotomy, selective debridement of destroyed pancreatic tissue, external drainage
Extensive (> 50 %) parenchymal disruption to the left of the mesenteric vessels, or duct injury	Possibly hematoma and/or free intraperitoneal fluid	Debridement, possibly partial pancreatectomy
Massive disruption of the pancreatic head injury with possible duct injury	Possibly hematoma and/or free intraperitoneal fluid	Debridement and external drainage
Injury of the pancreatic head with transaction of the duct	Possibly hematoma and/or free intraperitoneal fluid	Organ preservation should be attempted (debridement followed by internal or external drainage), e. g., Roux-en-Y pancreaticojejunostomy
Combined pancreatic and duodenal injury	Possibly hematoma and/or free intraperitoneal fluid	Whipple's operation only as last resort due to high mortality (30–40 %), possibly Berne diverticulization or pyloric exclusion (Vaughn)

Gallbladder Trauma

Basic Facts

- Direct injury to the gallbladder in abdominal trauma is rare (incidence < 2%).
- *Type of injury:* hematoma, rupture, perforation.
- The clinical picture is characterized by somewhat late-onset acute abdomen.
- *Additional workup:* contrast enhanced angio-CT, ERCP; laparoscopy.

Sonographic Criteria

- Gallbladder injuries can rarely be directly visualized.
- Intracholecystic blood increases the echogenicity of the gallbladder (DD: sludge).
- Nonvisualization of the gallbladder associated with subhepatic free fluid is highly suggestive of gallbladder rupture.

Consequences for Surgical Treatment

Diagnosis	Characteristic Findings	Management
Intraluminal hematoma, possibly hemobilia, stable circulation and H&H	Increased intraluminal echogenicity	Watchful waiting; possibly cholecystectomy after the acute phase
Gallbladder perforation	Nonvisualized gallbladder, subhepatic free fluid	Immediate cholecystectomy/laparoscopy

Renal Trauma

Basic Facts

- Incidence: in 6–10% of all severe abdominal trauma cases.
- Kidneys with preexisting pathology (e.g., cystic kidney disease or horseshoe kidney) are more susceptible to traumatic injury.
- *Type of injury:* parenchymal lesions, injury to the renal calices and pelvis, avulsion of the ureter and the renal pedicle, embolism/thrombosis (Table 2.**4**).
- Gross hematuria is the cardinal symptom, usually accompanied by flank pain and possibly hypovolemic shock.
- In microscopic hematuria, sonography or other imaging modalities frequently cannot demonstrate a parenchymal lesion.
- If renal trauma is strongly suspected, the role of sonography is but part of the overall diagnostic workup.
- *Additional workup:* contrast enhanced angio-CT; iv urogram; color flow Doppler imaging; and angiography.

Sonographic Criteria

- Fresh subcapsular hematomas are hypoechoic, while intraparenchymal hematomas may also be hyperechoic (Figs. 2.**14**, 2.**15**).
- Tiered parenchyma may indicate a possible rupture.
- Smaller parenchymal lacerations may be missed on ultrasound.

Table 2.**4** AAST Kidney Injury Scale (2005)

Grade*		
I	Contusion	Microscopic or gross hematuria, urological studies normal
	Hematoma	Subcapsular, nonexpanding without parenchymal laceration
II	Hematoma	Nonexpanding perirenal hematoma confirmed to renal retroperitoneum
	Laceration	< 1.0 cm parenchymal depth of renal cortex without urinary extravasation
III	Laceration	< 1.0 cm parenchymal depth of renal cortex without collecting system rupture or urinary extravasation
IV	Laceration	Parenchymal laceration extending through renal cortex, medulla, and collecting system
	Vascular	Main renal artery or vein injury with contained hemorrhage
V	Laceration	Completely shattered kidney
	Vascular	Avulsion of renal hilum which devascularizes kidney

- If a kidney cannot be completely visualized or displays a washed out echotexture, a contrast-enhanced CT scan should always be performed, the general condition of the patient permitting.

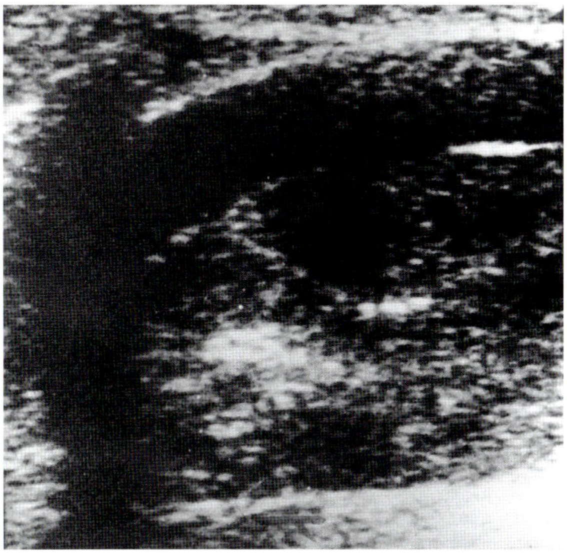

Fig. 2.**14 a** Posttraumatic subcapsular hematoma of the left kidney (by kind permission of Dr. Kaiper, Department of Urology, University of Magdeburg Medical Center).

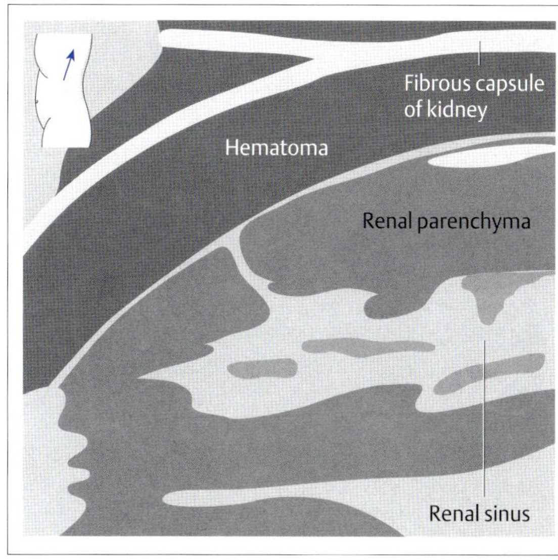

Fig. 2.**14 b** Line drawing.

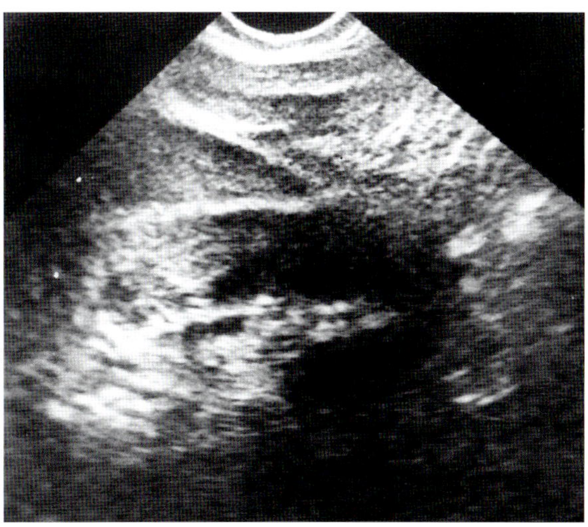

Fig. 2.**15 a** Rupture in the upper third of the right kidney with mostly intrarenal hematoma (by kind permission of Dr. Kaiper, Department of Urology, University of Magdeburg Medical Center).

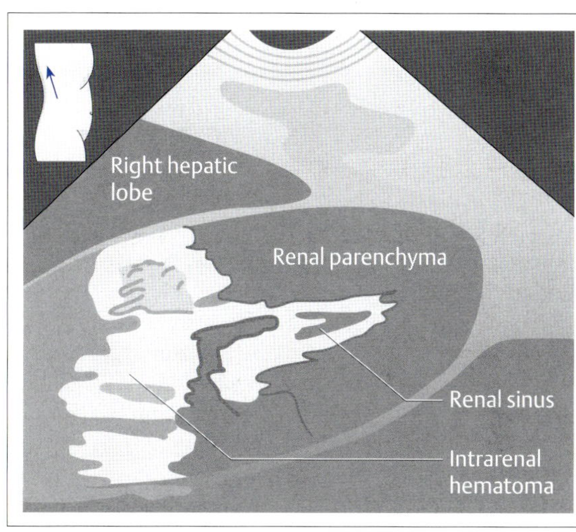

Fig. 2.**15 b** Line drawing.

Consequences for Surgical Treatment

Diagnosis	Characteristic Findings	Management
Contusion, minor parenchymal tear	Possibly renal hematoma	Watchful waiting
Deep parenchymal laceration communicating with the renal pelvis	Loss of normal organ contour, hematoma	Exploratory surgery; if possible organ preservation and repair, otherwise nephrectomy
Crush injury	Large lateral retroperitoneal hematoma, nonvisualized kidney	Nephrectomy
Ureter injury	Nonvisualization	Reconstruction, nephrostomy, or ileum interposition

Bowel and/or Mesentery Trauma

Basic Facts

- The small bowel is more susceptible to injury (about 5%) in major abdominal trauma than is the colon.
- Apart from intramural hematoma, there may be subtotal or total disruption of the bowel.
- Mesenteric injury is more common than bowel lesions themselves.
- Neither can be reliably identified on sonography, and their clinical picture is that of acute abdomen.
- Guarding and induced paralytic ileus impair the sonographic examination enormously.
- Localized free fluid collections may indicate bowel injury.
- Such free fluid corresponds either with blood or bowel contents.

Sonographic Criteria

- Free bowel contents display a heterogeneous echotexture and contain particulate matter.
- If a localized leak is demonstrated, its nature can be verified by US-guided FNA.
- Thickening of the bowel wall due to edema or hematoma displays as a hypoechoic lesion.

- *Additional workup:* Plain upright abdominal film (looking for free air), contrast-enhanced CT, small or large bowel enema with water-soluble contrast medium; exploratory surgery in case of acute abdomen.

Consequences for Surgical Treatment

Diagnosis	Characteristic Findings	Management
Mural or mesenteric hematoma, possibly associated with paralytic ileus	Sonographic assessment is rarely possible	Primarily nonoperative; stimulation of peristalsis
Bowel perforation	Ileus, possibly localized free fluid (with particulate matter), free gas on sonography or radiogram	Possibly laparoscopy for diagnostic confirmation; exploratory surgery, segmental bowel resection

Rupture of the Diaphragm

Basic Facts

- The incidence of diaphragmatic injuries is higher in blunt abdominal trauma (about 3%) than in thoracic trauma.
- Over 90% of all tears affect the left diaphragm as the right side is protected by the liver.
- The injury is frequently missed on initial examination.
- *Additional workup:* chest film, contrast-enhanced CT, standard GI contrast studies (using water-soluble contrast agents).

Sonographic Criteria

- Direct contact of usually intra-abdominal hollow viscera and lung tissue, both being displaced cranially.
- Sometimes, the discontinuity in the diaphragm can be demonstrated.

Consequences for Surgical Treatment

Diagnosis	Characteristic Findings	Management
Left-sided diaphragmatic rupture	Direct intrathoracic contact of lungs and abdominal organs, diaphragmatic continuity is interrupted	Surgical exploration and repair, chest tube

Retroperitoneal Hematoma

Basic Facts

- Retroperitoneal hematoma may originate from retroperitoneal vascular injuries (vena cava, aorta, renal and suprarenal vessels, lumbar arteries, numerous smaller branches).
- Basic anatomy facilitates contralateral spread.
- Intraperitoneal blood collection is possible by diapedesis.

Sonographic Criteria

- Large heterogeneous, primarily hypoechoic masses with diffuse contour (Fig. 2.**16**)

- Localization: lateral (flank), caudal (pelvis), or medial (central) region.
- *Additional workup:* contrast-enhanced CT; angiography.

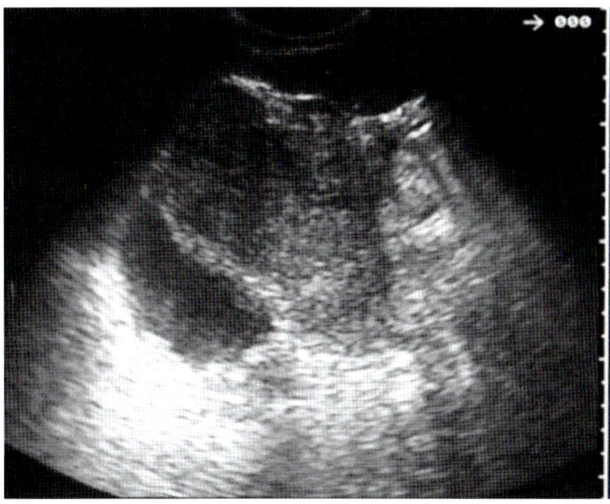

Fig. 2.**16 a** Extensive retroperitoneal hematoma in a patient with a pelvic fracture, reaching into the lesser pelvis and displacing the bladder.

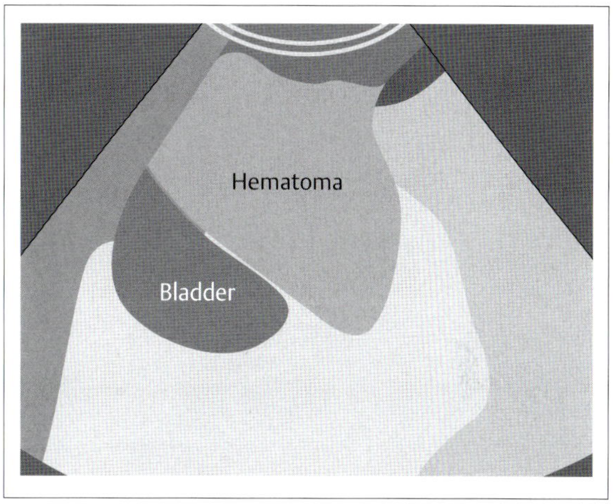

Fig. 2.**16 b** Line drawing.

Consequences for Surgical Treatment

Diagnosis	Characteristic Findings	Management
Retroperitoneal hematoma: hemodynamically stable patient	Localized hematoma without perforation into the abdominal cavity	Watchful waiting with repeat sonography; if necessary, transfusion until self-tamponade sets in (treatment of choice)
Retroperitoneal hematoma without evidence of self-tamponade: Hemodynamically unstable, H&H drop	Massive, mostly central hematoma	Surgical intervention indicated only in case of uncontrolled hemorrhage, implying injury to major vessels (renal veins, inferior vena cava, less so arteries)

Thoracic Trauma

Basic Facts

- Pneumothorax can easily be diagnosed on physical examination (resonant hemithorax with absent breath sounds and tactile fremitus).
- The most common cause is rib fractures, in which case the clinical signs are pain enhanced on movement and respiration, local tenderness, and possibly crepitation.
- In up to 10% of cases, fractures of the 1st to 3rd ribs are accompanied by trauma to the major vessels.
- Sonography can easily demonstrate free fluid in the costodiaphragmatic recess.
- *Additional workup:* chest film, contrast-enhanced CT, or angiography if vascular injury is suspected.

Sonographic Criteria

- Anechoic mass in the costodiaphragmatic recess displacing the lung (Fig. 2.**17**).
- With time, hematoma organization leads to increased heterogeneous echogenicity, possibly with septation.

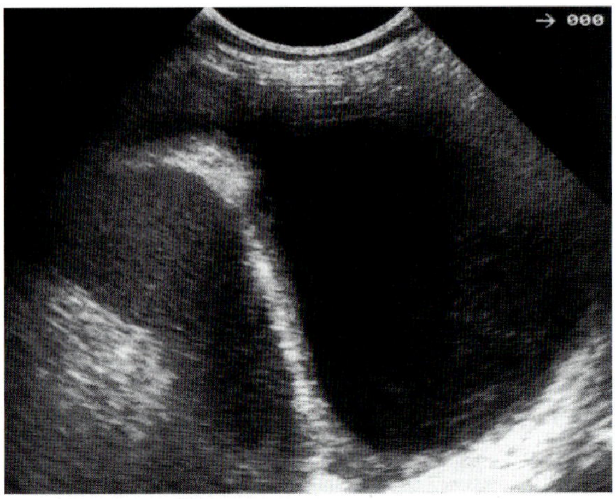

Fig. 2.**17 a** Left-sided hemothorax in a patient with fractures of the 4th to 6th ribs. Sonogram on admission.

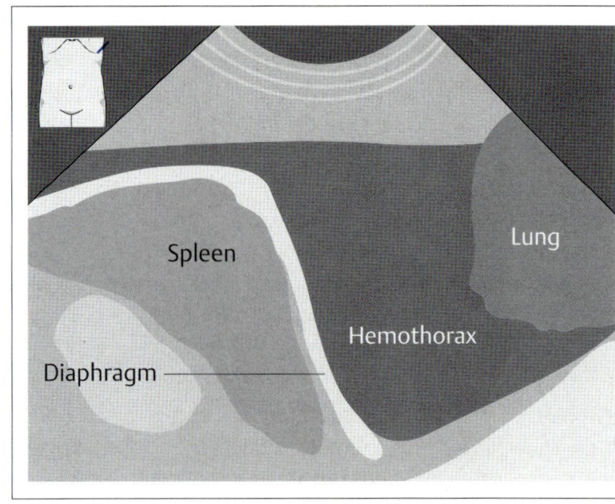

Fig. 2.**17 b** Line drawing.

Consequences for Surgical Treatment

Diagnosis	Characteristic Findings	Management
Free intrathoracic fluid: patient hemodynamically stable, breathing spontaneously, no flail chest	Small amount of free fluid in the costodiaphragmatic recess (1–2 cm)	Watchful waiting with repeat sonography
Free intrathoracic fluid: hemodynamically unstable or ventilated patient with flail chest	Larger amount of free fluid in the costodiaphragmatic recess (> 2 cm)	Chest tube drainage, thoracotomy in case of uncontrolled bleeding (> 200 ml/h or transfusion requirements exceeding 6 units of packed red cells)

Bibliography

AAST (American Association for the Surgery of Trauma). www.aast.org/injury/injury.html; 2005.

Blaivas M, Brannam L, Hawkins M, Lyon M, Sriram K. Bedside emergency ultrasonographic diagnosis of diaphragmatic rupture in blunt abdominal trauma. Am J Emerg Med 2004; 22: 601–4.

Krestin GP. Akutes Abdomen. Stuttgart: Thieme; 1994.

Lippert H. Praxis der Chirurgie. Stuttgart: Thieme; 1997.

Moore EE, Shackford SR, Pachter HL et al. Organ injury scaling: Spleen, liver and kidney. J. Trauma 1989; 12: 1664–6.

Moylan A. Principles of Trauma Surgery. New York: Gower Medical Publishing; 1992.

Poletti PA, Platon A, Becker CD et al. Blunt abdominal trauma: does the use of a second-generation sonographic contrast agent help to detect solid organ injuries? AJR Am J Roentgenol 2004; 183: 1293–301.

Sato M, Yoshii H. Reevaluation of ultrasonography for solid-organ injury in blunt abdominal trauma. J Ultrasound Med 2004; 23: 1583–96.

Schmidt G. Ultraschall-Kursbuch. Stuttgart: Thieme; 1996.

3 Intraoperative Sonography (IOS) of the Hepatobiliary System and Pancreas and for Staging

R. Mantke, T. Manger

Indications for Sonography

Intraoperative sonography (IOS) has been making continuous inroads in the operating theater and is increasingly being integrated into the surgical concepts of standardized patient management (Fig. 3.**1**).

Within the last two decades IOS has come into its own, especially in hepatobiliary and pancreatic surgery, and is becoming increasingly more important in operative decision making in other areas.

Precise staging of esophageal, gastric, hepatic, and pancreatic malignancies becomes possible by the combined application of laparoscopy and IOS. Depending on the stage determined, multimodal treatment strategies can be initiated (e.g., neoadjuvant chemotherapy). In case of peritoneal carcinomatosis identified during such a staging procedure, this will spare the patient a needless laparotomy.

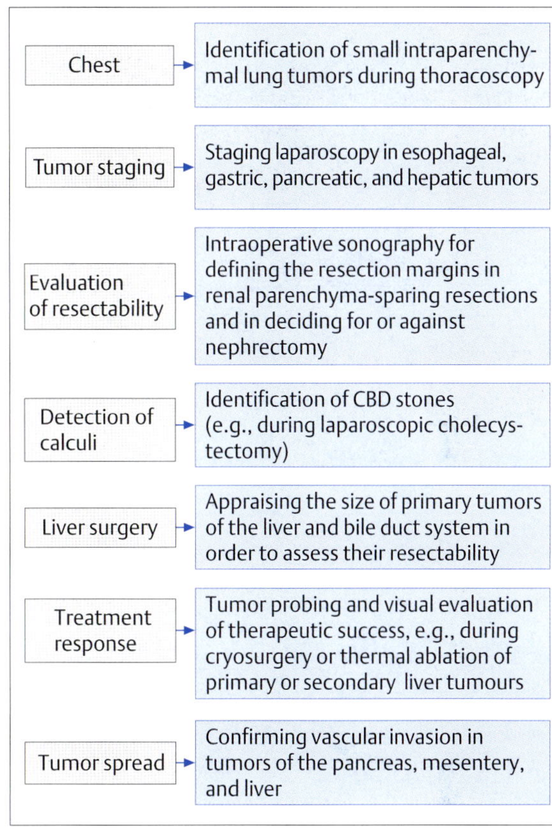

Fig. 3.**1** Accepted applications of intraoperative sonography.

IOS–General Facts

- A standard ultrasound system is used.
- However, good performance and ease of handling call for dedicated probes with frequencies of 5–10 MHz.
- 7.5 MHz transducers with a sound penetration of 6–8 cm have generally been employed.
- Since in IOS there is direct contact between the probe and the organ under investigation, this prevents bothersome artifacts from other organs and the abdominal wall.
- When combined with the current powerful ultrasound units, 7.5 MHz probes can detect even small pathologies, such as calculi down to a size of 1 mm, cysts from 1–2 mm, and tumors from 3–4 mm diameter upward.
- Sterility of probes for intraoperative use is achieved by cold gas sterilization or use of a plastic sterile cover (Fig. 3.**2**).
- Most surgeons prefer small T- or I-shaped probes for easy handling even in tight areas, like the dome of the liver.
- In contact scanning, the probe is placed directly on the tissue or organ surface, e.g. liver or pancreas; due to the near-field problem, this will not permit assessment of the immediate surface.
- Examination of relatively small structures such as the extrahepatic bile ducts, or the surface/superficial area of organs such as the liver or pancreas, might require probe-standoff scanning where the operative field is somewhat flooded with normal saline for acoustic coupling.
- The less preceding surgical dissection, the better the image quality of IOS and the higher its positive predictive value and specificity.

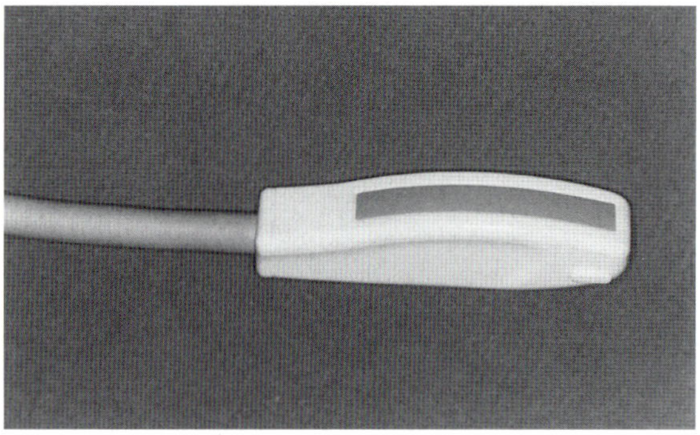

Fig. 3.2a Finger-tip probe from Toshiba.

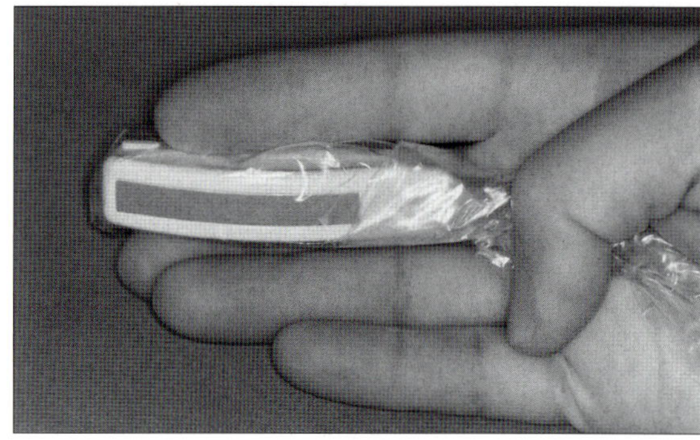

Fig. 3.2b Finger-tip probe from Toshiba with sterile plastic cover.

Staging Laparoscopy and Laparoscopic IOS in Esophageal, Gastric, and Pancreatic Carcinoma

Basic Facts

- The patient is place in anti-Trendelenburg position with the legs spread, and at least three trocars are needed for a meaningful exploration (Fig. 3.**3**).
- Laparoscopic sonography of parenchymal organs tries to overcome the lack of tactile feedback provided by digital palpation in open surgery, thus eliminating a major drawback of laparoscopy, particularly when dealing with hepatic surgery.
- Given normal anatomy, laparoscopic sonography will obviate the need for mobilizing of the liver, as modern probes feature excellent handling in three-dimensional space (Fig. 3.**4**).
- In up to 23% of laparoscopies performed for staging of gastric carcinomas, the combination of direct vision and IOS identified intrahepatic metastases not detected during preoperative imaging, including contrast-enhanced CT (Lowy et al., 1996).
- The technique of laparoscopic IOS is more demanding than that of open IOS, since the examiner has to gaze at both the video monitor and the sonogram.
- Currently, staging laparoscopy benefits the patient in cancer of the esophagus, stomach, and pancreas; in addition to the usual staging criteria, IOS can help detect previously nonvisualized hepatic metastases and tumor invasion into other organs.
- While previously assessment of the liver via rigid laparoscopic ultrasound probes necessitated frequent probe change-over from one trocar to the other, the current line of flexible probes has simplified and speeded up this examination significantly.
- The steps of laparoscopic IOS of the liver and pancreas are depicted in Figs. 3.**5**–3.**7**.
- Laparoscopic IOS of the pancreas is preceded by evacuation of gastric contents (by the anesthesiologist via a nasogastric tube) and introduction of 100–300 ml of saline into the upper abdomen. Level the table to avoid fluid run-off into the pelvis!

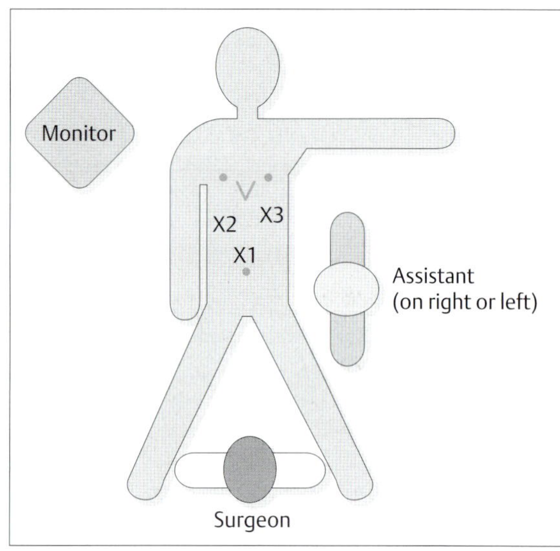

Fig. 3.3 Suitable placement of trocars in staging laparoscopy with laparoscopic IOS for tumors in the upper abdomen.

- The pancreas may be scanned through the structures covering it anteriorly (stomach, duodenum, gastrocolic ligament, and lesser sac).
- Artifacts generated by gastric or duodenal gas may be suppressed by slight compression with the probe; at times, filling the stomach with lactated Ringer's or normal saline solution will improve acoustic conditions considerably.
- Figure 3.**8** depicts one option for laparoscopic IOS in gastric carcinoma.
- *Additional workup:* Any mass identified on IOS should be biopsied for histopathological workup (mandatory in known malignancy), e.g., by introperative aspiration or excision.

Sonographic Criteria

- See IOS of the liver (p. 53–54)

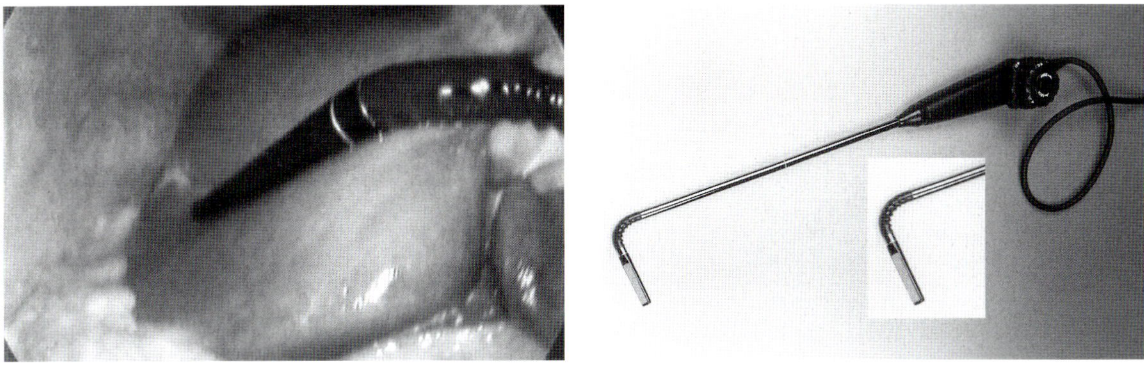

Fig. 3.**4 a and b** Flexible ultrasound probe from Toshiba for laparoscopy; cold gas sterilization.

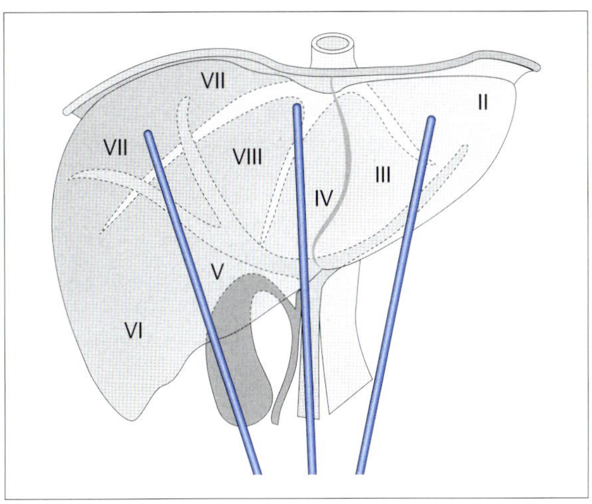

Fig. 3.**5** Orientation is facilitated by tracing the hepatic veins and portal vein branches–schematic line drawing of the liver segments. Ultrasound probe introduced through the umbilical trocar.

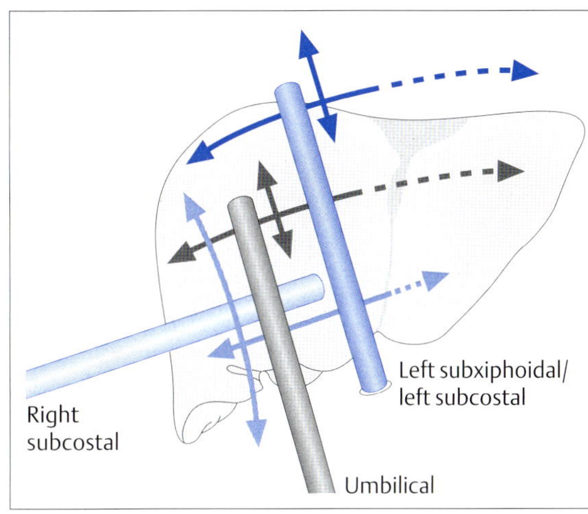

Fig. 3.**6** Possible positions of the laparoscopic probe and corresponding views of the liver.

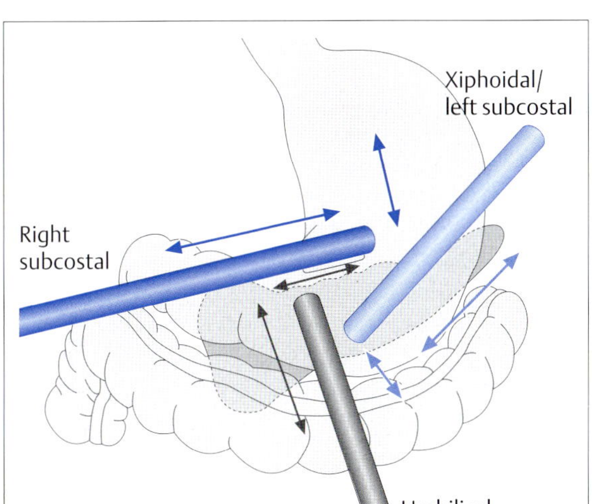

Fig. 3.**7** Possible positions of the laparoscopic probe and corresponding views of the pancreas.

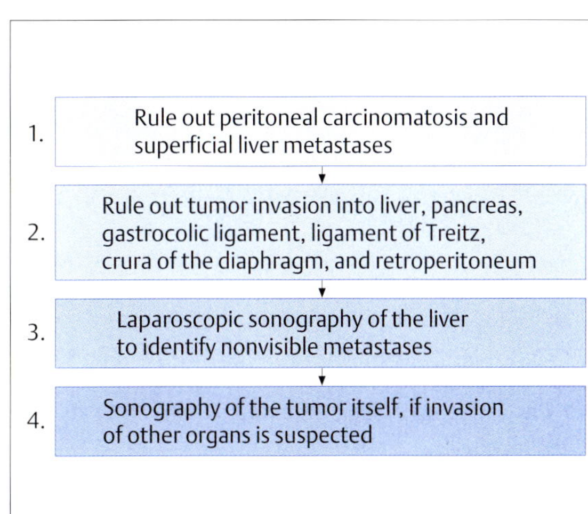

Fig. 3.**8** One option for laparoscopic staging of gastric carcinoma.

Consequences for Surgical Treatment

Diagnosis	Characteristic Findings	Management
Hepatic metastasis in gastric carcinoma	Solitary hepatic metastasis	a) Confirmation by histology, followed if possible by palliative gastrectomy (survival longer than after exploration alone [8 vs. 2.8 months; Becker, in Lippert 1998]), possibly with immediate excision of the metastasis b) Confirmation by histology; gastric bypass only if necessary, e.g., in gastric outlet obstruction; palliative chemotherapy
Hepatic infiltration in gastric carcinoma	In continuity	Gastrectomy together with resection
Hepatic metastasis in gastric carcinoma	Diffuse hepatic spread	Confirmation by histology; gastric bypass only if necessary, e.g., in gastric outlet obstruction; palliative chemotherapy
Hepatic metastasis in esophageal carcinoma	Solitary or diffuse spread	– Confirmation by histology Resection of tumor not indicated, but rather palliative management (irradiation, chemotherapy, laser treatment, stenting)
Hepatic metastasis in pancreatic carcinoma	Solitary or diffuse spread	– Confirmation by histology – Resection of tumor not indicated Possibly bypass surgery for bile duct or duodenal obstruction

Laparoscopic IOS of the Biliary Tree

Basic Facts

- Screening of the extrahepatic bile ducts by IOS during laparoscopic cholecystectomy will detect CBD stones with a sensitivity of 87.5% and a specificity of 100% (Goletti et al., 1995).
- Once mastered, laparoscopic IOS will be quicker than laparoscopic cholangiography and may be employed without risk in pregnant women and patients allergic to contrast agents (Soyer et al. 1997).
- In contrast to cholangiography, no dissection is required; irrigation with saline will improve acoustic coupling.
- The issue is not yet settled whether routine laparoscopic IOS would always prevent unwanted laparoscopic cholecystectomy in gallbladder carcinoma.
- Scanning of the extrahepatic biliary tree proceeds in transverse views from the hepatic portal caudad to the duodenal papilla (Fig. 3.**9**).
- The laparoscopic ultrasound probe is introduced via a left or right epigastric trocar (in the latter case, once the probe is advanced through the foramen of Winslow into the lesser sac the hepatoduodenal ligament may also be scanned from its posterior aspect).
- Laparoscopic IOS is less effective than intraoperative cholangiography in the detection of small stones in the intrapancreatic bile duct as well as in the identification of ductal pathology.
- *Additional workup:* In ambiguous IOS findings of the CBD, laparoscopic cholangiography should be performed.

Sonographic Criteria

- The classic appearance of choledocholithiais is that of a rounded, bright echogenic lesion with posterior acoustic shadowing (Fig. 3.**10**).

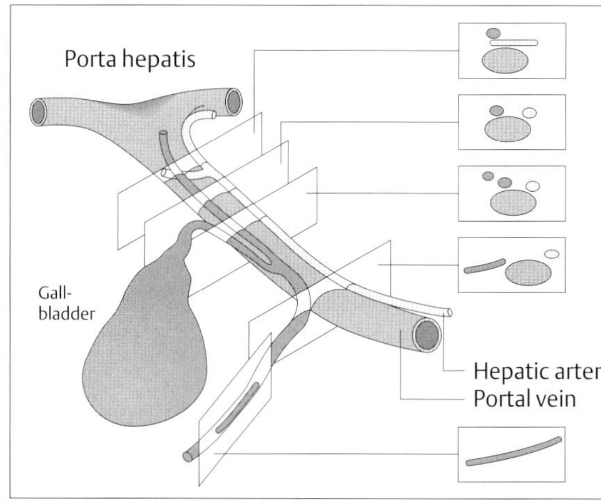

Fig. 3.**9** Transverse views in laparoscopic IOS of the extrahepatic biliary tree (modified from Kolecki and Schirmer, 1998).

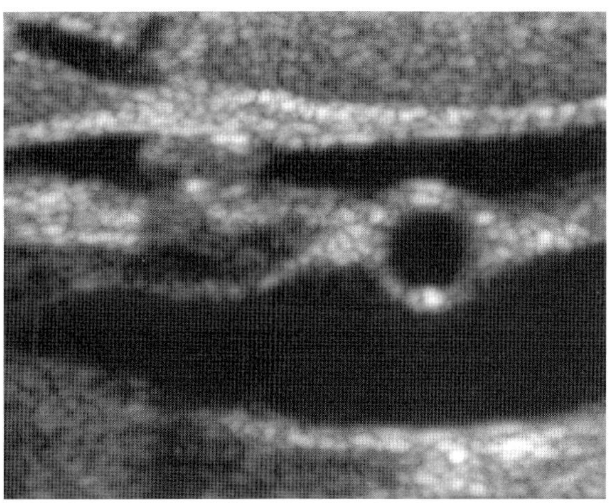

Fig. 3.**10 a** Choledocholithiasis; calculus with posterior shadowing.

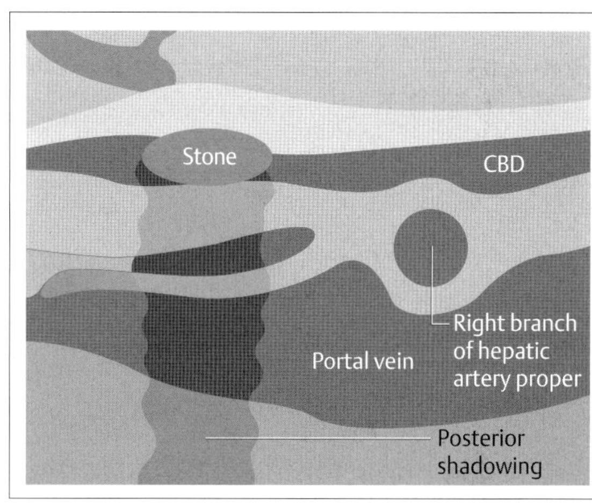

Fig. 3.**10 b** Line drawing.

Consequences for Surgical Treatment

Diagnosis	Characteristic Findings	Management
Choledocholithiasis	Confirmed or suspected preoperatively	Preoperative ERCP and sphincterotomy plus stone extraction
Choledocholithiasis	Incidental finding during operation	Two-stage procedure: Postperative ERCP and sphincterotomy plus stone extraction
Choledocholithiasis	Incidental finding during operation, huge or impacted calculus	Laparoscopic or open CBD exploration

Intraoperative Sonography of the Liver in Primary Hepatic Malignancy and Colorectal Metastasis

Basic Facts

- Use of 5–7.5 MHz transducers and the lack of rib-induced artifacts in IOS result in a far superior quality when compared with transabdominal sonography.
- IOS of the liver can help identify segmental boundaries (Fig. 3.11).
- Even IOS may miss hepatic metastases < 5 mm (depending on their echogenicity)
- For IOS of the entire convexity of the liver, the organ should be mobilized first by transecting the left and right triangular as well as the falciform ligaments.
- Because of its large dimensions, the right lobe of the liver should also be scanned from its posterior aspect.
- IOS of the liver is particularly well suited in the identification of small lesions seated deep within the parenchyma.
- Pre- and intraoperative sonographic findings will differ in up to 29% of cases (Alanen et al., 1995).
- Depending on the study, 5–14% of previously undetected metastases of colorectal cancer are identified only by IOS of the liver.
- In up to 21% of cases results of intraoperative palpation of the liver will differ from those of IOS.
- Palpation has proved more sensitive than IOS for lesions on the hepatic surface itself.
- The localization and extent of additional liver metastases detected by IOS will affect surgical management in 4–42% of cases (Alanen et al., 1995; Goletti et al., 1995; Kolecki and Schirmer, 1998).
- In up to 54% of primary malignancies of the liver IOS may have a decisive impact on the intraoperative management (Röthlin et al. 1996).
- Compared with metastasis of colorectal cancer, the sensitivity in hepatocellular carcinoma (HCC) is lower because it has proved difficult to differentiate regeneration masses from HCC.
- The sensitivity and specificity of detecting hepatic metastases of colorectal cancer are 93.8% and 94.4%, respectively (Table 3.**1**).
- Dynamic biphasic contrast-enhanced CT of the liver has a lower sensitivity than IOS combined with palpation (Haider et al. 1995, Kolecki et al. 1998).
- Bimanual palpation is followed by transverse and longitudinal sonography of the liver, most often by contact scanning; when combined with palpation IOS will yield the highest degree of diagnostic certainty.
- A standardized IOS protocol and use of uniform nomenclature are extremely valuable (Table 3.**2**).
- Suspicious hepatic foci should always undergo US-guided FNA and be submitted for frozen section.

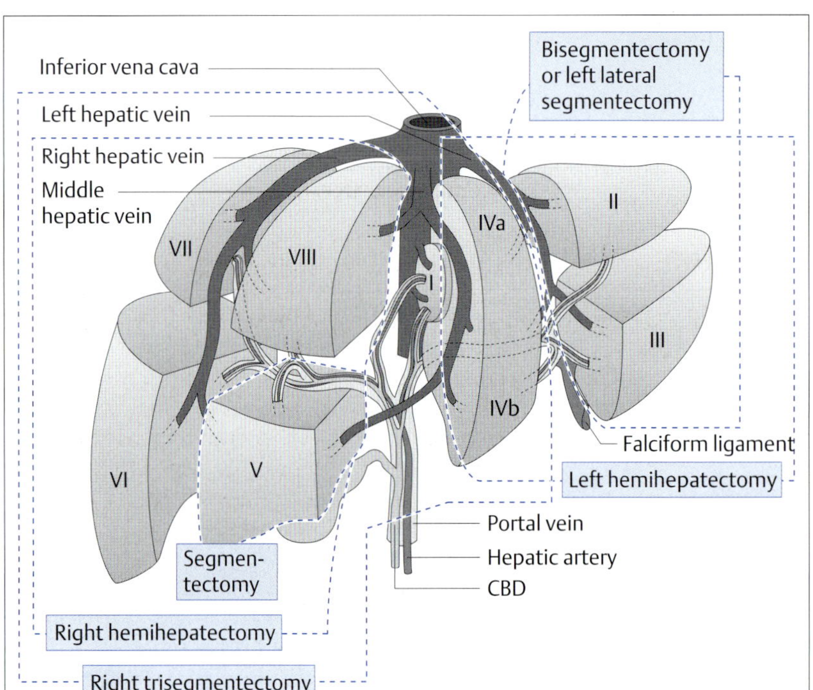

Fig. 3.**11** Couinaud's functional segmental anatomy of the liver (modified from Durst and Rohen, 1996).

Table 3.1 Sensitivity and specificity of IOS compared with preoperative transabdominal sonography, contrast-enhanced CT, and exploratory surgery. (Modified from Machi and Siegel, in Gandolfi and Fukuda, 1997)

	Preoperative Sonography %	**CT** %	**Surgical Exploration** %	**IOS** %
Sensitivity	40.8	49.0	66.0	93.3
Specificity	95.8	94.4	89.3	94.4
Overall accuracy	73.4	75.9	79.8	94.2

Table 3.2 Standardized protocol for IOS of the liver (modified)

- Start with the left lobe (segments II–III).
- The probe is moved craniocaudad along the anterior surface of the liver.
- The scanning parameters are continuously adapted to the change in organ size.
- Next, the left lobe is scanned in the transverse plane.
- The portal branches are checked along their course for thrombosis and obstruction.
- Normal segments and any abnormal findings should always be documented by one image each.
- Segment IV is scanned in the same fashion; this segment is ideally suited for assessing the confluence of the hepatic vein with the IVC regarding possible thrombosis or tumor.
- Usually, segment IV also offers the best viewing window for segment I (caudate lobe) and the portal trunk as well as the CBD.
- Scanning of the right hepatic lobe also starts with the medial segment of the left lobe (segment IV), once again first craniocaudad to the right side and then in the transverse plane.
- When examining the right lobe, particular attention must be paid to the possibility that intrahepatic lesions might be registered twice, once from the frontal aspect and once more from the posterior aspect of the dome of the liver.
- Here, the middle hepatic vein must be identified, as it constitutes the boundary between segment IV and the right hepatic lobe.
- Since the right lobe is bigger, the scanning parameters on the ultrasound unit must be updated continuously in order to attain the same echo strength from the surface to the full depth.
- Segmental assessment of the right lobe, including documentation, follows the same rules as on the left, with the hepatic veins and portal branches once again serving as landmarks for correct segmental identification and looking for focal lesions, thrombosis, or obstruction by a tumor.

- The examiner may get his or her bearings by tracing the hepatic veins and the portal vein branches (Couinaud's anatomy of the liver–Fig. 3.**11**)
- The criteria for malignancy of hepatic masses are:
  - Infiltrating growth
  - Tumor invasion into the hepatic veins or branches of the portal vein
  - Hypoechoic rim ("halo" sign)
  - Confluent lesions
  - Presence of multiple tumor generations
  - Signs of displacement
  - Central necrosis or calcification
- Definitive differentiation between benign and malignant hepatic lesions is not possible based on IOS alone–thus, frozen section is mandatory.
- *Additional workup:* Any mass identified on IOS should be biopsied for histopathological workup (mandatory in known malignancy), e.g., by introperative aspiration or excision.

Sonographic Criteria

- **A cyst** presents as an anechoic mass with relative posterior enhancement, and the shape of its wall can be deformed by pressure (hematoma, abscess, and bilioma may mimic a cyst). Differentiation is possible by FNA (Fig. 3.**12**)
- **Focal fatty infiltration** appears as hyperechoic islands and focal fatty sparing presents as hypoechoic islands within normal liver parenchyma; these are usually are triangular, ovoid or flame-like in shape, and involve the periportal region, the gallbladder fossa, or the dome of the right lobe; the intrahepatic vascular bed remains untouched.
- The sonographic appearance of typical **hemangiomas** is round or oval; they are distinctly hyperechoic and display an echogenic texture (Fig. 3.**13**).

- **Liver metastases** may be anechoic (resembling cysts, e.g., in sarcoma or ovarian cancer–rather rare overall), hypoechoic (more common in lung and breast cancer), isoechoic (with hypoechoic halo), or hyperechoic (more common in colorectal cancer); regressive changes may result in hypoechoic necrosis or calcification (Figs. 3.**14**–3.**19**).
- **Focal nodular hyperplasia** (FNH) appears as a hypoechoic or isoechoic mass of sometimes cloudy echotexture, and at times displaying tortuous feeding arteries or microcalcification (Fig. 3.**20**).
- Since **hepatic adenomas** consist only of hepatocytes (in contrast to FNH), they are isoechoic or hypoechoic with the normal adjacent liver parenchyma and display a hypoechoic halo (pseudocapsule).
- **Primary hepatic malignancy** cannot be differentiated from liver metastasis on the basis of sonography alone (Figs. 3.**21**–**23**).

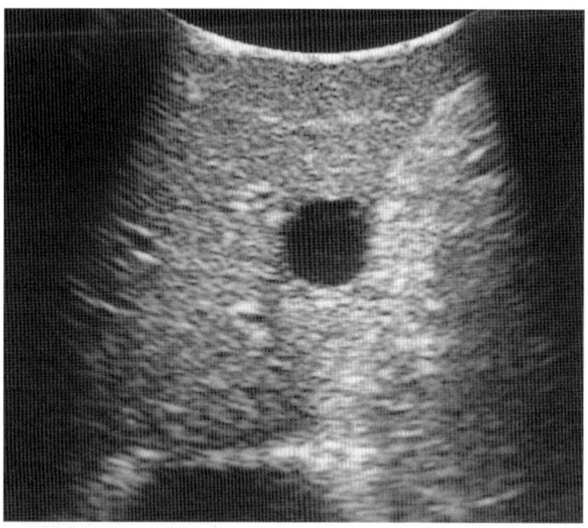

Fig. 3.**12 a** IOS of the liver with small (1 cm) anechoic cyst near the surface of the left lobe.

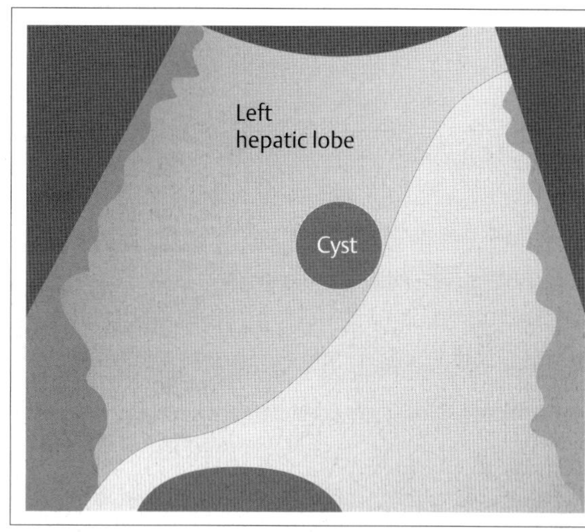

Fig. 3.**12 b** Line drawing.

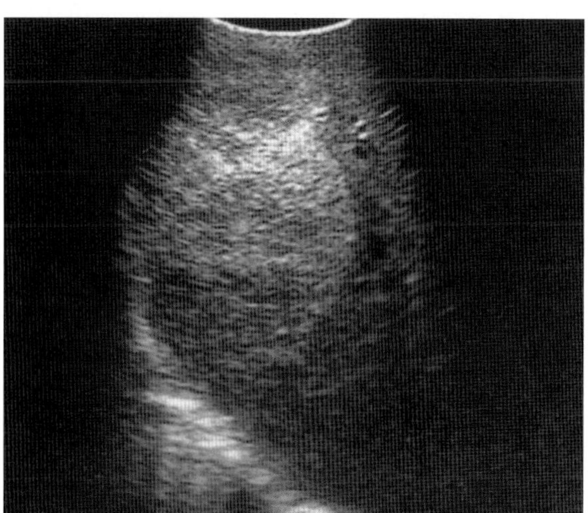

Fig. 3.**13 a** IOS of the liver with typical hyperechoic hemangioma in the right lobe, with echogenicity and in close relation with the diaphragm (cavernous hemangioma on histology).

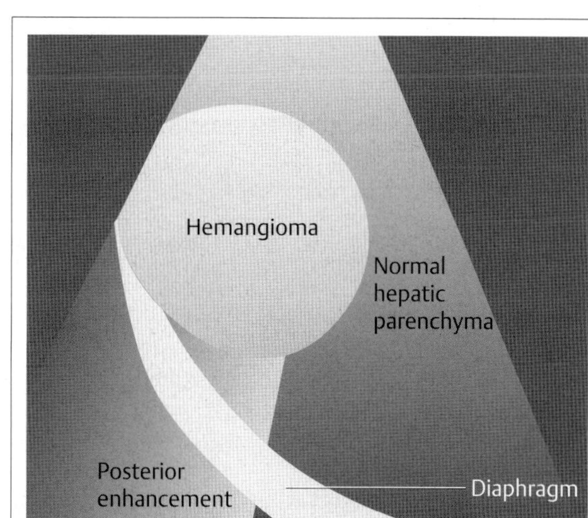

Fig. 3.**13 b** Line drawing.

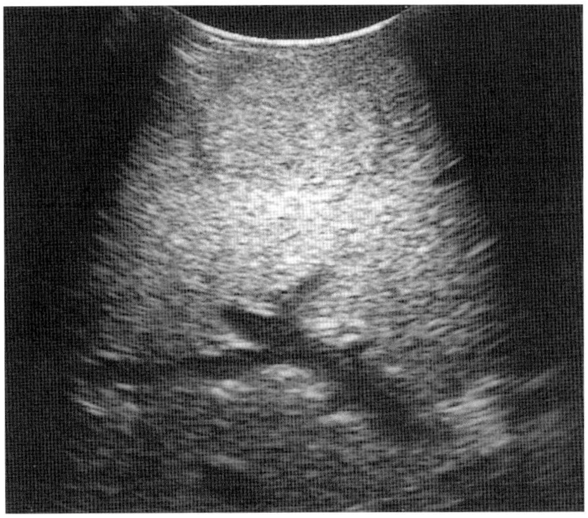

Fig. 3.**14a** IOS of the liver with a somewhat isoechoic metastasis of pancreatic cancer. Appearance of a hypoechoic halo.

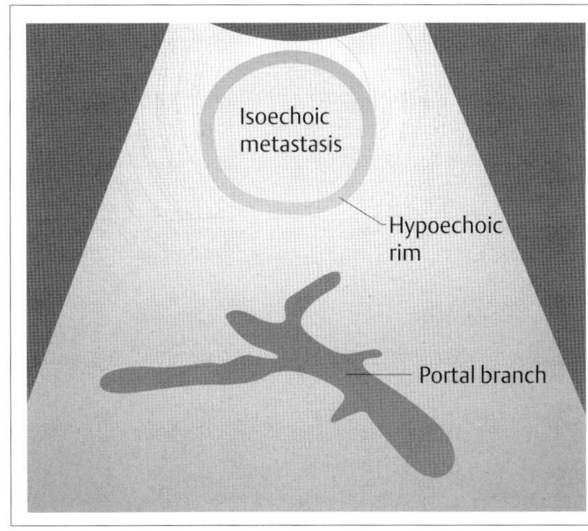

Fig. 3.**14b** Line drawing.

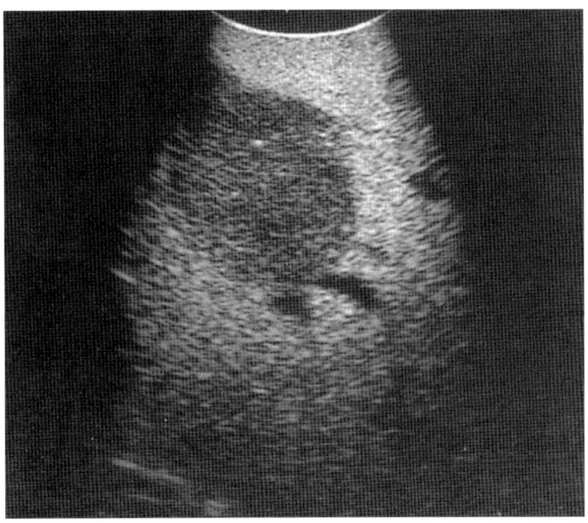

Fig. 3.**15a** IOS of the liver with a hypoechoic metastasis of choroidal melanoma in segment VII.

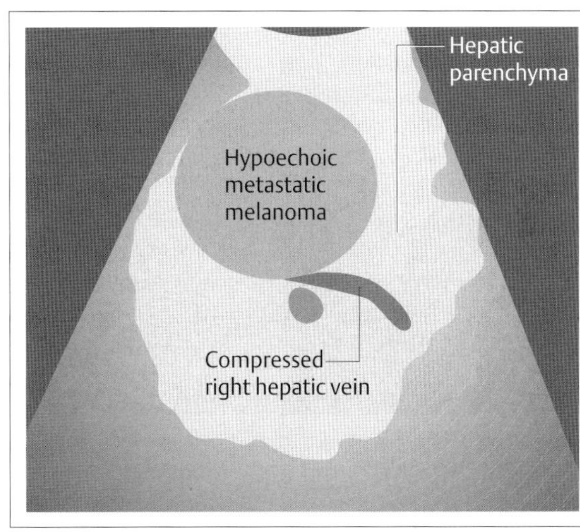

Fig. 3.**15b** Line drawing.

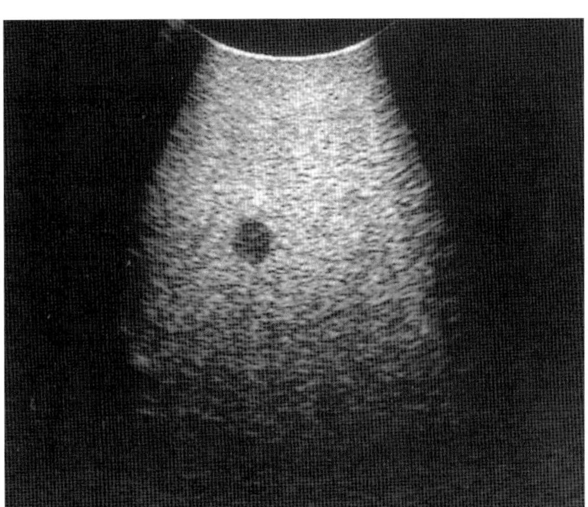

Fig. 3.**16a** IOS of the liver with a nonpalpable 8 mm small metastasis of choroidal melanoma in segment VI.

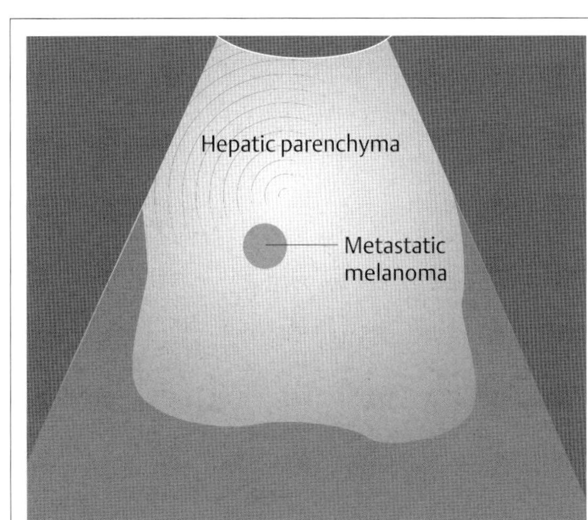

Fig. 3.**16b** Line drawing.

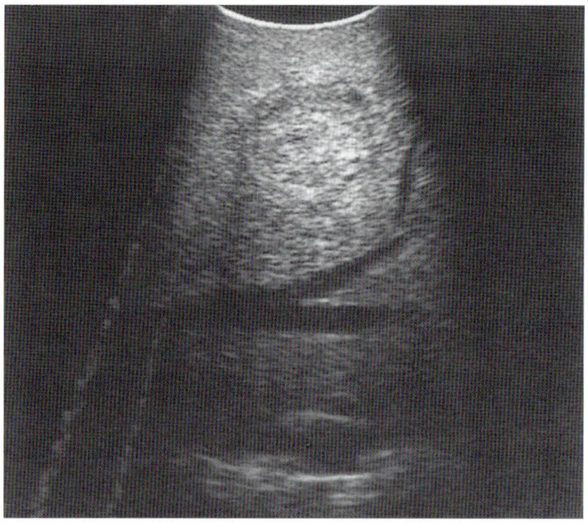

Fig. 3.17 a IOS of the liver with a 1.5 cm large nonpalpable hyperechoic metastasis of colorectal carcinoma, delineating its relation with the right hepatic vein (post-chemotherapy changes in the consistency of the normal parenchyma).

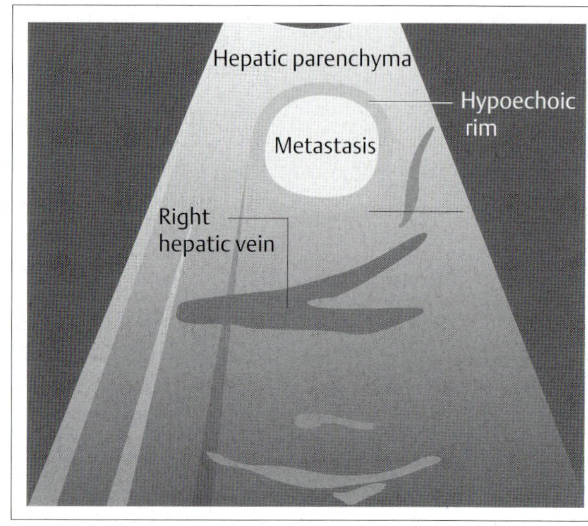

Fig. 3.17 b Line drawing.

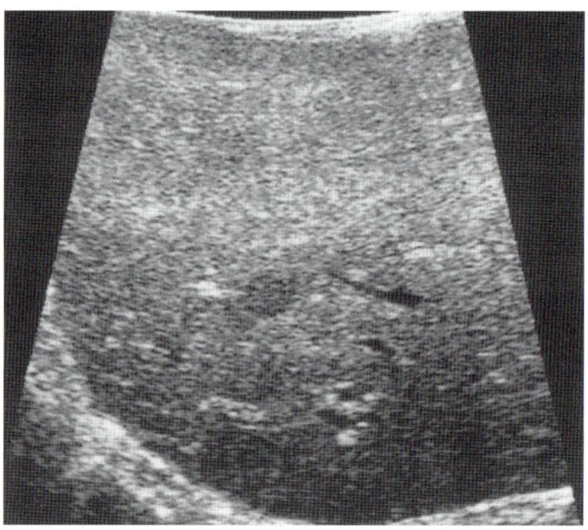

Fig. 3.18 a IOS of the liver with a nonpalpable 5 mm small hypoechoic metastasis of liposarcoma in the right lobe.

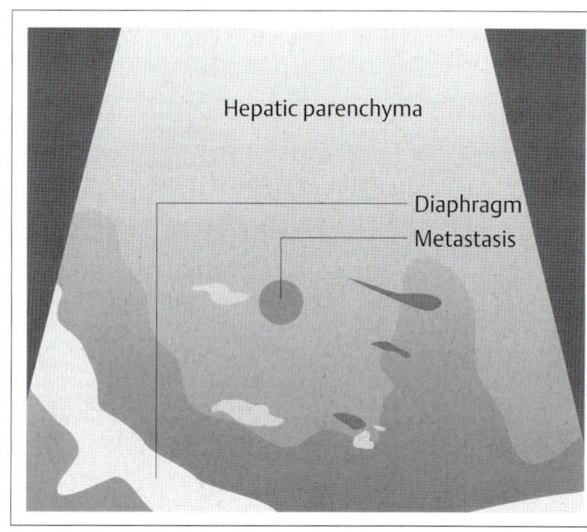

Fig. 3.18 b Line drawing.

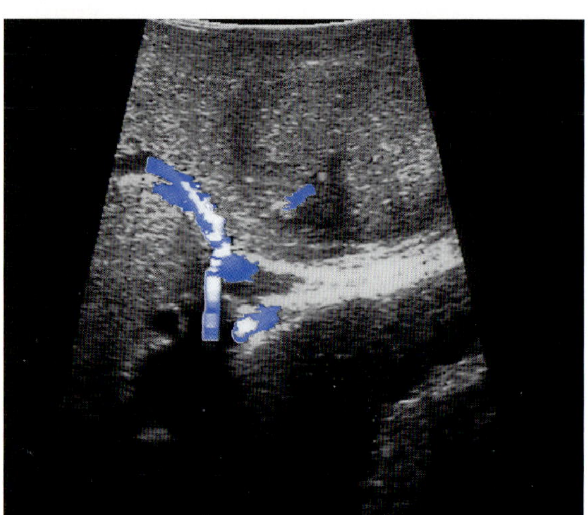

Fig. 3.19 a IOS of the liver with a large central metastasis of colorectal carcinoma, encroaching on the trunk of the portal vein to within 5 mm; resection would be possible, but with dubious safety margin.

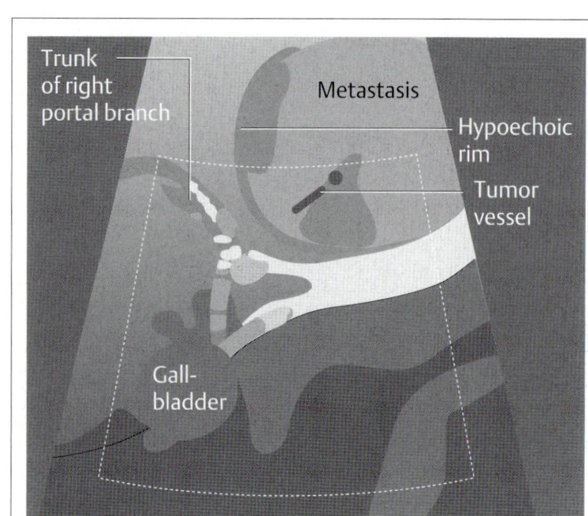

Fig. 3.19 b Line drawing.

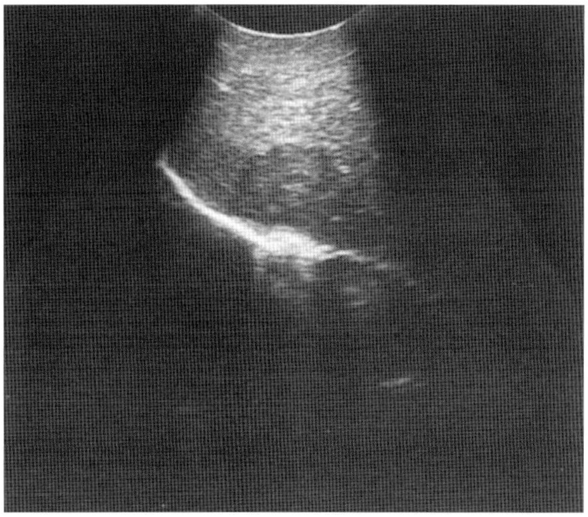

Fig. 3.**20 a** IOS of the liver with a hypoechoic, somewhat cloudy mass in segment VII (FNH on histopathology).

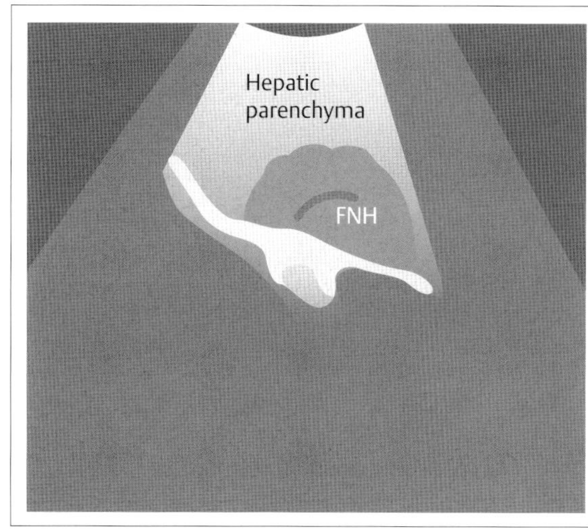

Fig. 3.**20 b** Line drawing.

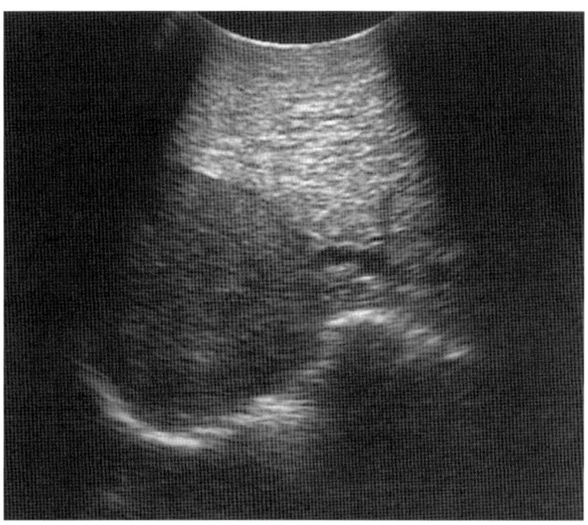

Fig. 3.**21 a** IOS of the liver with a hypoechoic mass in segment VIII in a noncirrhotic liver (HCC on histopathology).

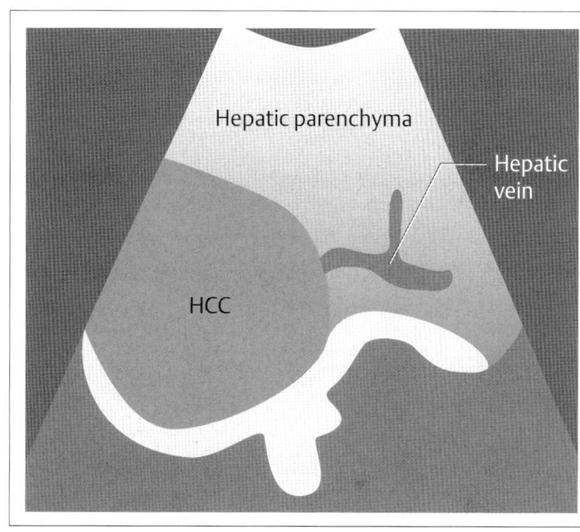

Fig. 3.**21 b** Line drawing.

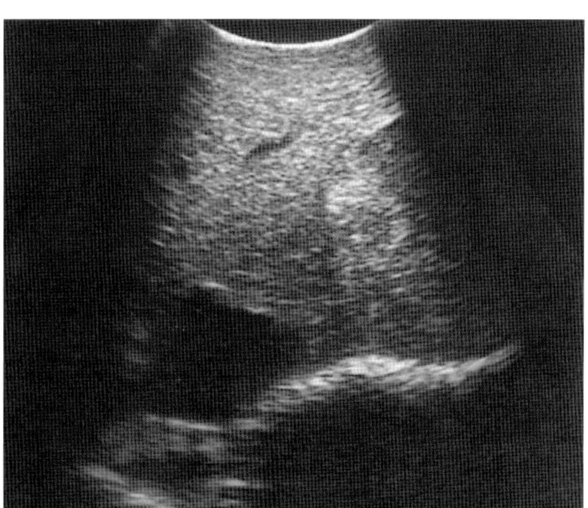

Fig. 3.**22 a** IOS of the liver with a mass in segment VIII, depicting its relation with the inferior vena cava (HCC on histopathology).

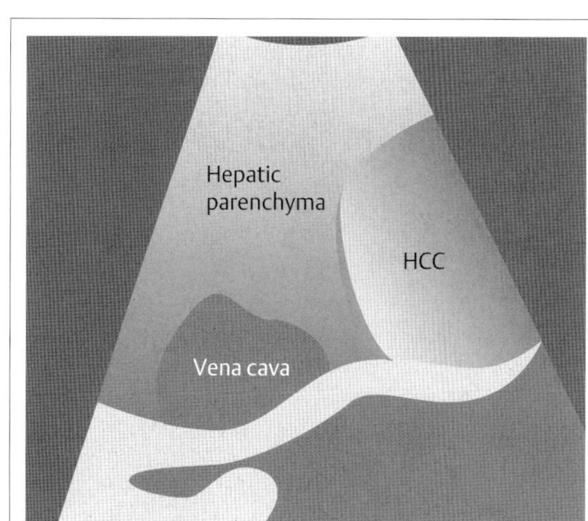

Fig. 3.**22 b** Line drawing.

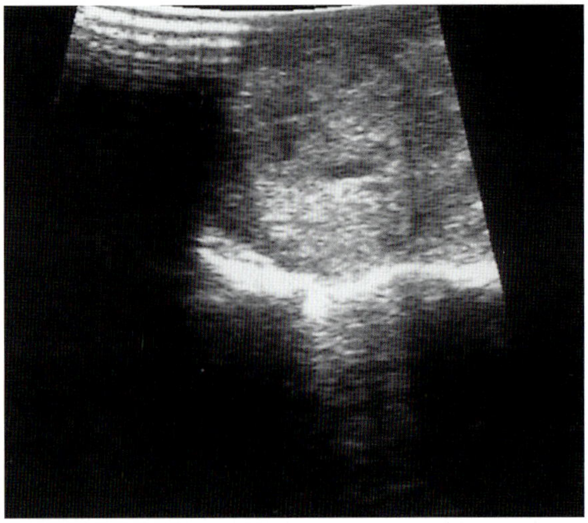

Fig. 3.**23 a** Histologically confirmed HCC in segment VI of a cirrhotic liver, with focal regression changes and heterogeneous texture.

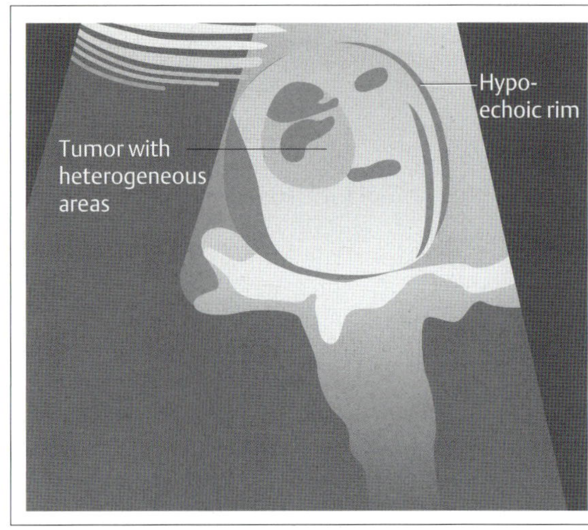

Fig. 3.**23 b** Line drawing.

Consequences for Surgical Treatment

Diagnosis	Characteristic Findings	Management
Hepatic metastasis of colorectal cancer	Solitary or multiple, usually unilateral, no extrahepatic spread	– Resection with curative intent – Determining factor in liver resection is the amount of healthy liver remaining, and not the hepatic involvement per se
Hepatic metastasis of colorectal cancer	Diffuse spread in all segments	– Confirmation by histology – Palliative systemic chemotherapy
Cholangiocarcinoma	Unilateral without extrahepatic spread	Resection
Cholangiocarcinoma	Involving both lobes or metastasized	No resection; possibly bile duct drainage, palliative chemoembolization/chemotherapy
FNH	Asymptomatic, small	No resection in case of nonoperative diagnosis; observation; diagnosis should be confirmed by histopathology. If diagnosed intraoperatively possible resection will depend on the situation.
FNH	Symptomatic, size > 10 cm, with bleeding	Relative indication for resection
Hepatic adenoma	Inherent risk of rupture/ malignant transformation regardless of size	Resection indicated
HCC	< 5 cm, solitary, unilateral; remaining parenchyma (usually with cirrhotic transformation) sufficient for liver function?	Resection will depend on the extent of the cirrhosis, residual liver function, and portal hypertension. (possible assessment for liver transplantation)
HCC	> 5 cm, metastatic, in severe cirrhosis	No resection; possibly chemoembolization, cryosurgery, thermal ablation, ethanol injection, palliative systemic chemotherapy

Intraoperative Sonography of the Pancreas

Basic Facts

- Indications for IOS in pancreatic surgery:
  - Differentiation between chronic pancreatitis and malignant mass.
  - In confirmed pancreatic malignancy, assessment of the spatial relation (invasion?) of the tumor to the portal vein and the superior mesenteric artery.
  - Localization of small endocrine tumors within the parenchyma.
  - After transection of the gastrocolic ligament and the Kocher maneuver, the pancreas can be assessed both by palpation and by IOS.
  - Acoustic coupling is improved by immersing the lesser sac in normal saline.
- The head of the pancreas sits to the right of the left border of the superior mesenteric vein; the pancreatic body extends from the left border of the superior mesenteric vein to the left border of the aorta; and the tail of the pancreas courses from the left border of the aorta to the splenic hilum.

Chronic Pancreatitis

- Figure 3.**24** depicts the morphological findings seen in chronic pancreatitis.
- IOS will localize the following complications of chronic pancreatitis or rule them out, especially if palpation is impaired by the indurated, inflamed tissue:
  - Pancreatic fibrosis
  - Poststenotic ductal dilatation > 2 mm
  - Scarring
  - Pseudocyst formation
  - Bile duct narrowing
  - Small abscesses
  - Splenic and/or portal vein thrombosis
- Pronounced chronic pancreatitis frequently gives rise to postprandial pain and endocrine/exocrine pancreatic insufficiency.
- Postnecrotic cysts as sequelae of acute inflammatory episodes often contain brownish hemorrhagic secretions.
- Retention cysts (following ductal dilatation) are filled with clear to slightly turbid viscous fluid.
- Pseudocysts (no inner epithelial lining) resulting from acute pancreatitis may become much larger than retention cysts.
- Distal CBD stenosis, symptomatic duodenal stenosis, and severe chronic pain in chronic pancreatitis are indications for surgery.
- Severe pancreatitis may induce thrombosis of the portal vein. Take care with resection procedures!
- All pancreatic pseudocysts with hyperechoic mural structures should be suspected of cystadenoma, especially if their contents are mucinous.
- Pancreatic duct calculi may be beaded like a string of pearls and may be found in the main duct as well as its branches.
- IOS may facilitate duct localization in side-to-side drainage procedures.

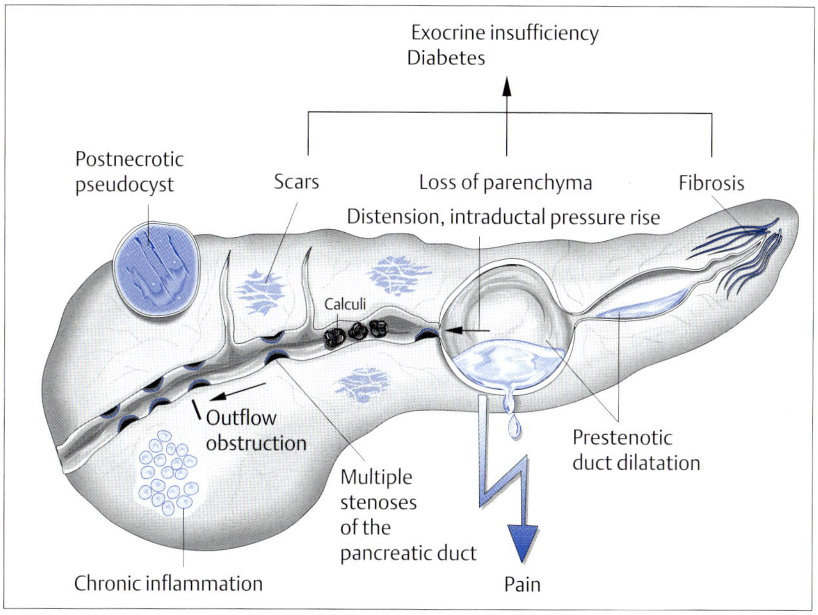

Fig. 3.**24** Important morphological findings in chronic pancreatitis (from Lippert, 1998).

Endocrine Tumors of the Pancreas

- Most endocrine tumors of the pancreas measure 0.2–4 cm (mean 0.8 cm); they comprise insulinomas (60%), gastrinomas (18%), and less often glucagonomas, VIPomas, somatostatinomas, and nonsecretory islet cell tumors.
- Even IOS cannot identify with certainty endocrine tumors below 0.3 cm.
- In endocrine tumors of the pancreas, IOS with its sensitivity of about 85% is far superior to all other imaging modalities (the sensitivity of bimanual palpation is about 45%).
- 99% of all insulinomas are intrapancreatic, about 90% are solitary; there is no predisposition of any segment, and their rate of malignancy is < 10%.
- Only about 30% of gastrinomas are intrapancreatic, primarily in the head of the pancreas, and their rate of malignancy is > 50%.
- Gastrinomas are often multiple and give rise to the Zollinger–Ellinson syndrome.
- Most gastrinomas are found in a triangle bordered by the following structures:
  - Junction of the cystic duct and the CBD
  - Inferior section of the third part of the duodenum
  - Border between head and body of the pancreas
- About 70% of all gastrinomas are found in the duodenal wall–here, palpation is superior to IOS.

Cancer of the Pancreatic Head

- In cancer of the pancreatic head, IOS and exploration help establish the criteria of inoperability in:
  - Peritoneal carcinomatosis
  - Hepatic metastasis (including IOS)
  - Extraregional lymphatic spread
  - Invasion of the portal vein or superior mesenteric artery (relative indication because of possible graft interposition)
- Quite often, tumor invasion into the distal CBD, resulting in jaundice, will be the initial symptom leading to the diagnosis.
- Adenocarcinomas originating from the ductal epithelium are by far the most common tumors of the pancreas, with about 75% arising in the head of the pancreas.
- Only 40% of those patients undergoing surgery will be resected with curative intent (5-year survival rate about 5–10%).
- *Additional workup:* Intraoperative needle biopsy for histological confirmation by frozen section.

Sonographic Criteria

- Fibrosis is characterized by finely granular induration of the parenchyma.
- The typical cyst is anechoic (Fig. 3.**25**).
- The pancreatic duct may be distended and anechoic (Fig. 3.**26**).
- Calcifications are strongly hyperechoic and produce posterior shadowing.
- Most endocrine tumors are hypoechoic (Figs. 3.**27**–3.**29**).
- Cystadenomas comprise cystic anechoic and solid hyperechoic regions.
- Most pancreatic carcinomas are circumscribed hypoechoic (less often isoechoic) lesions, bulging the normal contour of the organ and possibly invading the portal vein, superior mesenteric artery, celiac trunk, distal CBD, and local lymph nodes (Fig. 3.**30**).

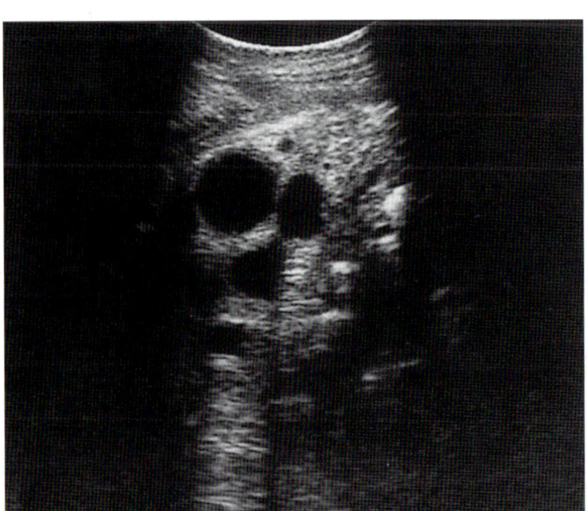

Fig. 3.**25a** IOS of the pancreas in chronic pancreatitis with typical anechoic pseudocysts in the pancreatic head; transgastric view.

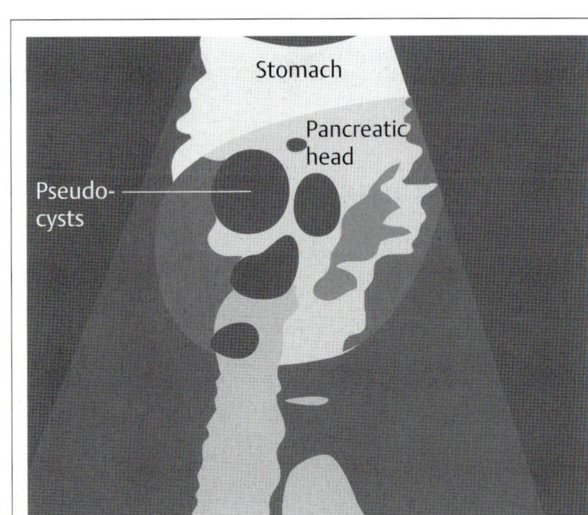

Fig. 3.**25b** Line drawing.

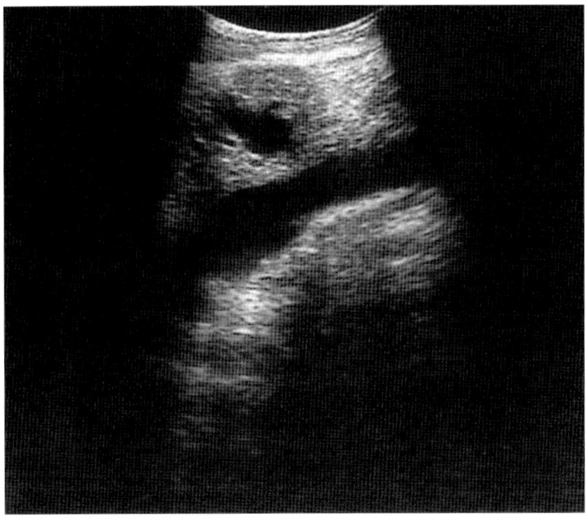

Fig. 3.**26 a** Transgastric IOS of the pancreas in chronic pancreatitis with enlarged anechoic head and duct distended to 9 mm.

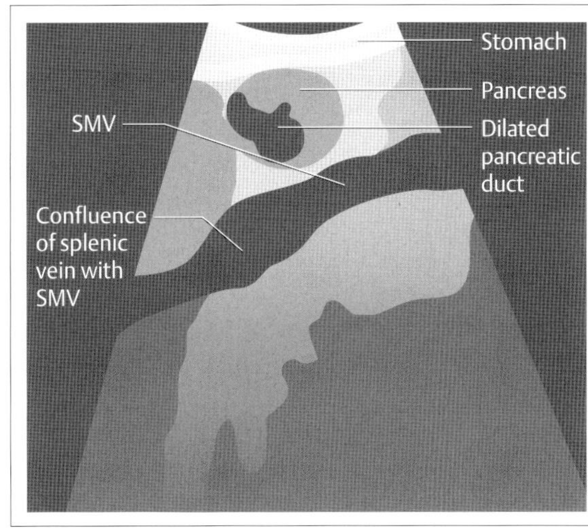

Fig. 3.**26 b** Line drawing.

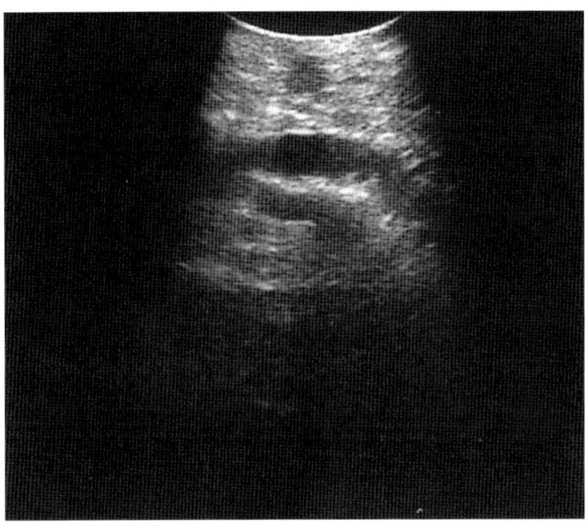

Fig. 3.**27 a** Insulinoma of about 9 mm in the pancreatic head, palpable, with typical hypoechoic texture.

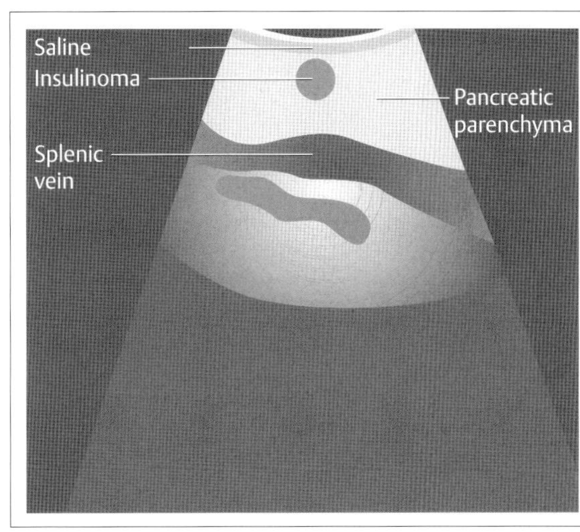

Fig. 3.**27 b** Line drawing.

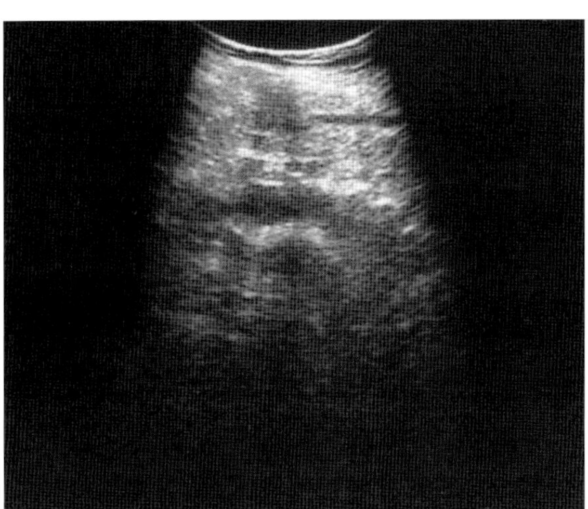

Fig. 3.**28 a** Insulinoma in the pancreatic body, directly related to the pancreatic duct. Resection is safely possible only with drainage via pancreaticojejunostomy.

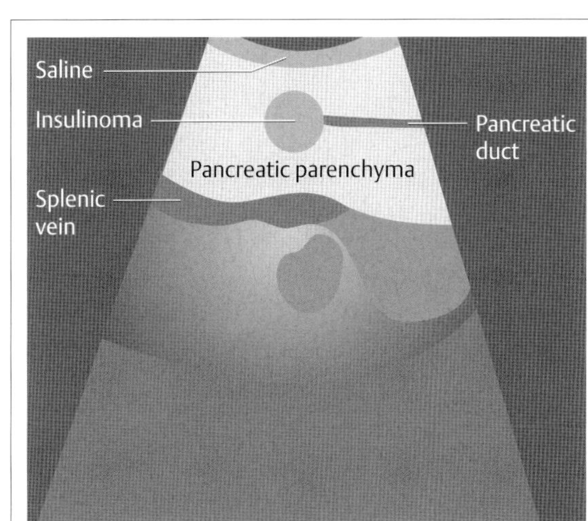

Fig. 3.**28 b** Line drawing.

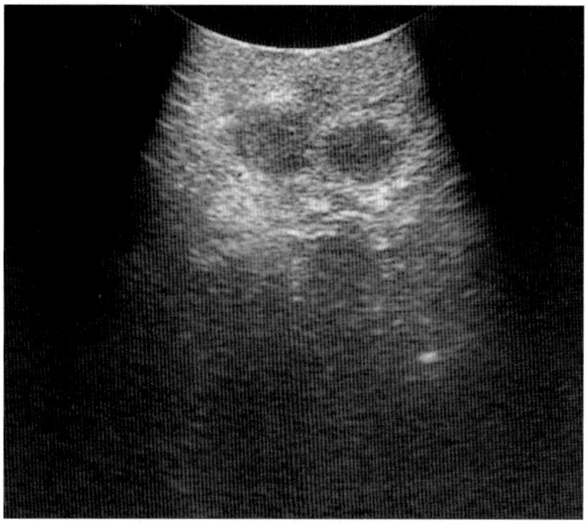

Fig. 3.**29 a** On direct IOS of the pancreas two hypoechoic gastrinomas of about 8 mm each in the pancreatic body, with hepatic metastasis.

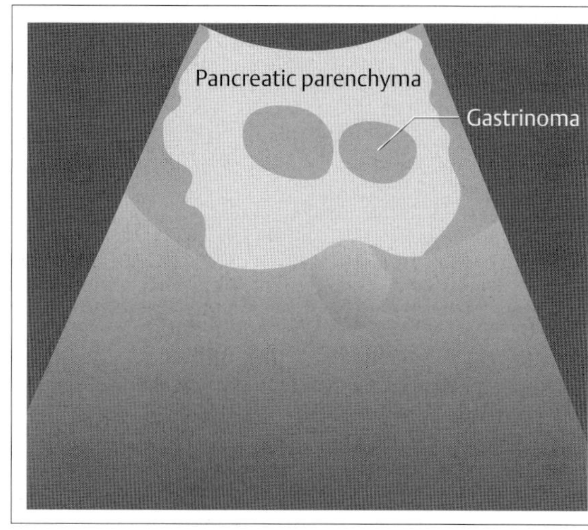

Fig. 3.**29 b** Line drawing.

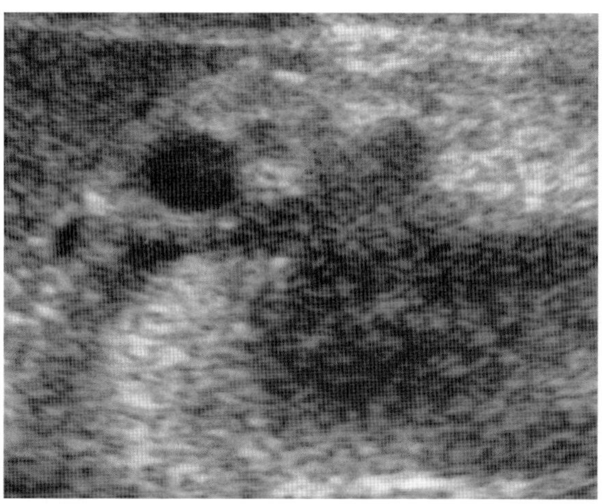

Fig. 3.**30 a** IOS of the pancreas in pancreatic carcinoma of the uncinate process, growing toward the root of the mesentery and reaching the superior mesenteric vein.

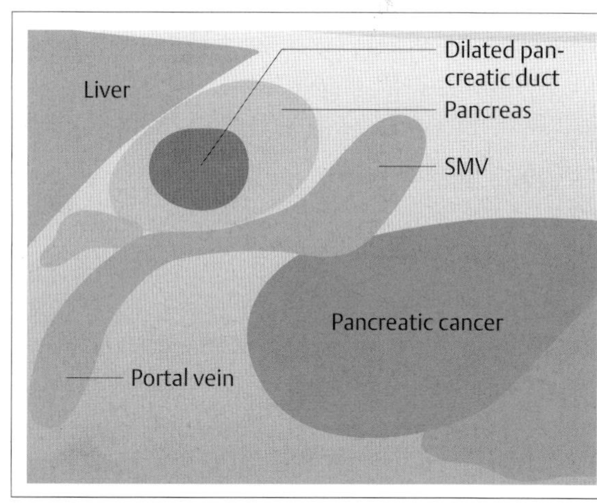

Fig. 3.**30 b** Line drawing.

Consequences for Surgical Treatment

Diagnosis	Characteristic Findings	Management
Cancer of the pancreatic head	No invasion of portal vein or superior mesenteric artery No distant lymph node or organ metastasis	Pancreaticoduodenectomy (Whipple–Kausch procedure or Traverso–Longmire procedure)
Cancer of the pancreatic head	With invasion of portal vein or superior mesenteric artery	In some cases (only if R0!) extended pancreaticoduodenectomy with vascular grafting may be indicated
Cancer of the pancreatic head	Extraregional lymph node or organ metastasis	Resection of tumor not indicated In symptomatic cases bypass surgery, possibly palliative postoperative chemotherapy
Chronic pancreatitis with mass in pancreatic head	No retention cysts of ductal stenosis in body and tail of pancreas	Duodenum-preserving resection of the pancreatic head (Beger procedure)
Chronic pancreatitis	Entire organ compromised by retention cysts, ductal distension, ductal calculi	Duodenum-preserving resection of the pancreatic head and side-to-side pancreatico-jejunostomy (Frey procedure)
Endocrine tumor	Localized in the head/body of the pancreas No malignancy	Excision or "coring out" (in case of tight relation to the pancreatic duct system internal drainage via Roux-en-Y may be indicated) Whipple procedure, if complete excision is impossible.
Endocrine tumor	Localized in the head/body of the pancreas With malignancy	Whipple procedure (following oncological principles)
Endocrine tumor	Localized in the pancreatic tail No malignancy	Spleen-preserving resection of the pancreatic tail
Endocrine tumor	Localized in the pancreatic tail With malignancy	Distal pancreatectomy with splenectomy and lymphadenectomy following oncological principles

Cryosurgery and Thermal Ablation of Primary Liver Tumors and Hepatic Metastases

Basic Facts

- In cryosurgery of nonresectable primary liver tumors and hepatic metastases, placement of the cryosurgery probes and assessment of freezing is guided by IOS.
- Depending on the model, a maximum of 5 probes can be inserted, using liquid nitrogen for freezing (– 196 °C).
- Cell death is by extra- and intracellular as well as microvascular ice crystallization during the freezing process, and by fusion of individual ice crystals as well as by microvascular thrombosis and ischemia during thawing (Baust et al., 1997).
- Successful cryoablation depends on fast freezing and slow thawing, and possible refreezing.
- The treatment of choice for primary and secondary malignancies of the liver is resection; however, for a variety of reasons, in the majority of patients the tumors are nonresectable (only about 20% of hepatic metastases in colorectal cancer and patients with HCC are amenable to curative resection).
  - If curative resection is not an option, cryoablation or thermal ablation may be a viable alternative
- Preoperative workup should include transabdominal sonography and contrast-enhanced CT or MRT of the liver (images not older than 4 weeks); in primary liver tumors and hepatic metastases of colorectal cancer, extrahepatic spread must be excluded, and in the latter case local recurrence must also be ruled out.
- All hepatic masses must undergo needle biopsy for histopathological confirmation.
- After hepatic cryoablation, complete remission was seen in up to 25% of nonresectable patients (Baust et al., 1997).
- The IOS must be performed and assessed by a physician member of the surgical team.
- The liver must be mobilized by transection of its supporting ligaments (see IOS of the Liver in this chapter).
- Performing the IOS (see IOS of the Liver in this chapter).
- The extrahepatic parts of the cryoprobe must be insulated to prevent damage outside the target region.
- With modern cryosurgery equipment employing "supercooled" nitrogen (– 209 °C) a volume of roughly 180 cm^3 and a diameter of about 7 cm will be frozen within 20 minutes; as the temperature rises rapidly with the distance from the probe, overlapping freezing regions will increase effectiveness.
- In small nonpalpable tumors, probe placement under simultaneous IOS is preceded by placement of a thinner guide needle in order to keep the trauma to the tumor as low as possible.
- Once the correct localization has been ascertained, the cryoprobe is placed parallel to the needle.
- Special "guide wire" systems with dilators have also been used successfully in nonpalpable tumors; here, monitored by IOS, dilators with increasing diameter are passed over the guide wire thus dilating the parenchymal channel.
- Larger, easily palpated tumors are steadied with one hand while inserting the probe with the other, after which probe placement is checked and corrected by IOS, if necessary.
- The first cryoprobe should be advanced to the deepest point of the tumor.
- Depending on the freezing radius specified for the probes, further probes are then placed around this central probe; the freezing zones should encroach on the normal parenchyma of the liver for at least 1 cm.
- In cryotherapy, cellular death results from freezing, dehydration during thawing, and the ischemia due to vascular injury.
- IOS is also suitable for monitoring, since frozen liver tissue displays increased acoustic impedance, which in turn results in increased echogenicity and distinctive total posterior shadowing.
- The temperature within the resultant hyperechoic rim is about 0 °C.
- Depending on the probe employed, the – 40 °C isothermals so important for cellular death are located 5–8 mm within the sonographically visualized interface.
- The visualized acoustic shadowing should therefore exceed the tumor margins by at least 1 cm in all directions and should be monitored during freezing by IOS.
- If the freezing zone appears insufficient, a further cryoprobe may be placed near the margin to complete cryoablation.
- There is a close correlation between the extent of freezing and the visualized shadowing (Gilbert et al., 1985).
- Larger vessels may interfere with uniform spreading of the freezing zone because the circulating blood is at body temperature and will prevent freezing of the vascular wall and the tissue in the immediate vicinity.
- The deepest point of the frozen volume is best scanned from the inferior aspect of the liver, since there is no interference by posterior shadowing.
- If probe placement had been correct, the thawing process will not have to be monitored continuously.
- Some authors favor double freezing of the tumor (Baust et al., 1997).
- In cryoablation close to larger bile duct branches, perfusion with warm saline will prevent unwarranted freezing of the ducts (Silverstein et al., 1997).
- In principle, laparoscopic cryoablation is also possible if the tumors are suitably localized.
- Repeat postoperative sonography and an abdominal CT scan are mandatory after cryosurgery.
- The following complications are possible:
  - Bleeding from the cryoprobe channels (one may fill up the channels with small particles of collagen fleece)
  - Subcapsular hematoma
  - Abscess
  - Right-sided pleural effusion
  - Bilioma (Caveat: compared with larger blood vessels bile ducts freeze earlier)
  - Thrombosis and formation of arteriovenous shunts

- Thermal ablation is much more common because of the much easier handling of the equipment and less intraoperative bleeding complications. IOS is used for the placement of the laser probes or radiofrequency ablation (RFA) probes, but sonography cannot monitor tissue injury here quite as well as in cryoablation.
- Indications for RFA:
  - Not more than 5 liver lesions
  - Diameter of metastases < 3.5–4 cm (depends on the equipment)
- Contraindications for RFA:
  - Tumor outside the liver
  - Liver failure
  - Infections
  - Metastases too large(> 3.5–4 cm in diameter), or too numerous (more than 5)
- Thrombosis of the portal vein is a relative contraindication

Sonographic Criteria

- On transverse views the inserted probes are identified as hyperechoic structures with comet-tail artifacts directed into the depth (Fig. 3.**31**).
- Frozen liver tissue reflects the ultrasound beam at the boundary layer and there is distinct posterior shadowing (Fig. 3.**32**).
- After thawing, the normal adjacent liver tissue will be seen as a hypoechoic border around the tumor, while the latter will keep its original echogenicity.

- *Additional workup:*
  During surgery: temperature measurement
  After surgery: transabdominal sonography, MRT, contrast-enhanced CT

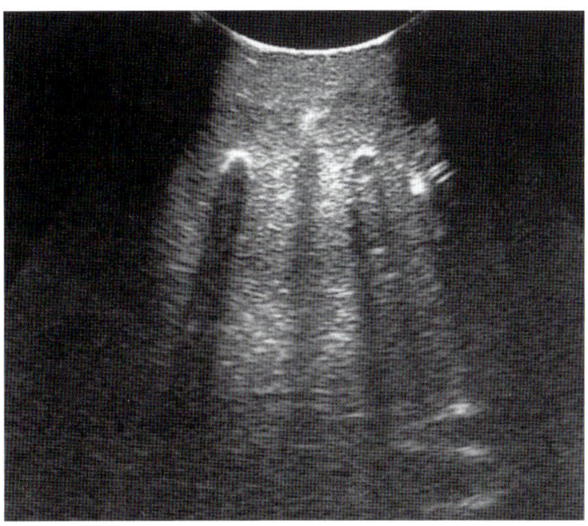

Fig. 3.**31 a** Transverse view of a hepatic metastasis, 4 cm in diameter, of colorectal cancer in segment VIII during cryoablation. Two probes are placed on the outside, while the guide wire in the center has not yet been replaced by a probe and produces posterior acoustic shadowing.

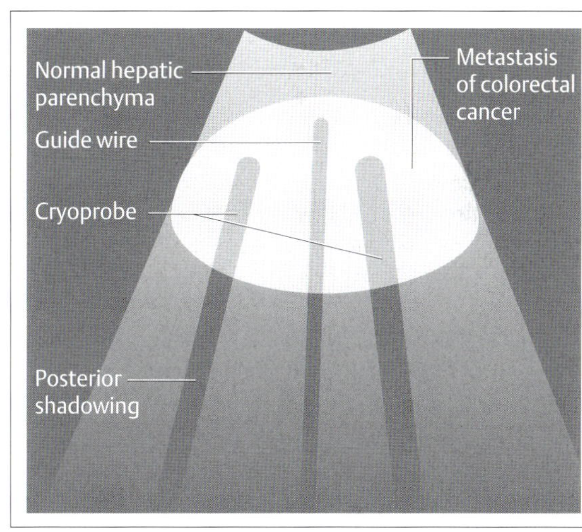

Fig. 3.**31 b** Line drawing.

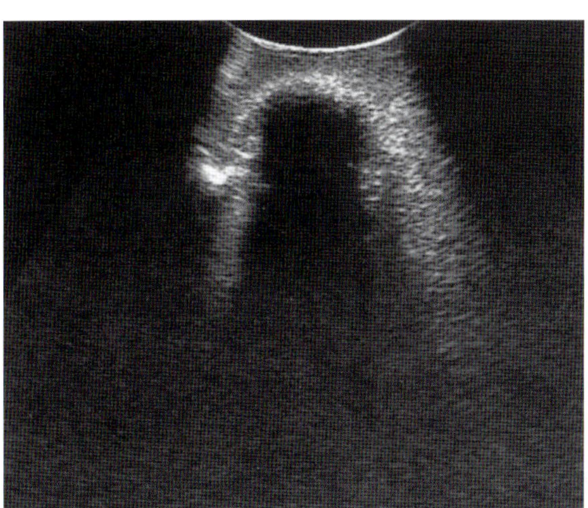

Fig. 3.**32 a** IOS in ongoing freezing, demonstrating distinctive posterior shadowing in the frozen region.

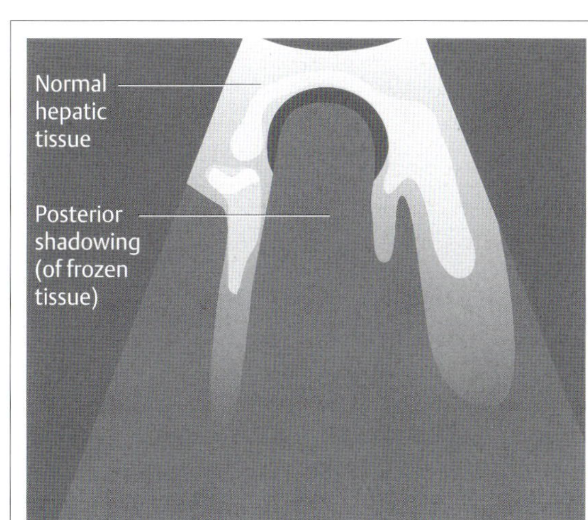

Fig. 3.**32 b** Line drawing.

Consequences for Surgical Treatment

Diagnosis	Characteristic Findings	Management
Colorectal metastasis	Total cryoablation/thermal ablation	Follow-up with CT or MRT and tumor markers
Colorectal metastasis	Subtotal cryoablation/thermal ablation	In addition, palliative systemic chemotherapy; follow-up with CT or MRT and tumor markers
Primary liver tumors	Total cryoablation/thermal ablation	Follow-up with CT or MRT and tumor markers
In primary liver tumors	Subtotal cryoablation	Possibly intra-arterial chemoembolization, palliative chemotherapy, ethanol injection; follow-up with CT or MRT and tumor markers

Bibliography

Baust J, Gage AA, Ma H, Zhang CM. Minimally invasive cryosurgery-technological advances. Cryobiology. 1997; 34: 373–84.

Buscarini E, Savoia A, Brambilla G, et al. Radiofrequency thermal ablation of liver tumors. Eur Radiol. 2005; 15(5): 884–94.

Ferrai FS, Stella A, Gambacorta D, et al. Treatment of large hepatocelluar carcinoma: comparison between techniques and long term results. Radiol Med 2004; 108(4): 356–71.

Gandolfi L, Fukuda M. Current Trends in Digestive Ultrasonography. Basel: Karger; 1997.

Gilbert JC, Onik GM, Hoddick WK, Rubinsky B. Realtime ultrasonic monitoring for hepatic cryosurgery. Cryobiology. 1985; 22: 319–30.

Haider MA, Leonhardt C, Hanna SS. The role of intraoperative ultrasonography in planning the resection of hepatic neoplasms. Can Assoc Radiol J. 1995; 46: 98–104.

John TG, Greig JD, Carter DC, Garden OJ. Carcinoma of the pancreatic head and periampullary region. Tumor staging with laparoscopy and laparoscopic ultrasonography. Ann Surg. 1995; 221(2): 156–64.

Kolecki R, Schirmer B. Intraoperative and laparoscopic ultrasound. Surg Clin North Am. 1998; 78: 251–71.

Lin LW, Ye Z, Xue ES, Gao SD, He YM. Intraoperative ultrasonography in hepatobiliary surgery. Hepatobiliary Pancreat Dis Int. 2002; 1(3): 425–8.

Lippert H. Praxis der Chirurgie. Stuttgart: Thieme; 1998.

Siewert JR, Harder F, Allgöwer M, et al. Chirurgische Gastroenterologie. Berlin, Heidelberg: Springer; 1990.

Silverstein JC, Staren E, Velasco J. Thermal bile duct protection during liver cryoablation. J Surg Oncol. 1997; 64: 163–4.

Skogseid B, Grama D, Rastad J, et al. Operative tumor yield obviates preoperative pancreatic tumor localization in multiple endocrine neoplasia type 1. J Intern Med. 1995; 238(3): 281–8.

Soyer Ph, Mosnier H, Choti MA, Rymer R. Intraoperative and laparoscopic sonography of the liver. Eur Radiol. 1997; 7: 1296–302.

Torzili G. Contrast-enhanced intraoperative ultrasonography in surgery for liver tumors. Eur J Radiol. 2004; 51 (Suppl): S25–9. Review.

Torzili G, Makuuchi M. Intraoperative ultrasonography in liver cancer. Surg Oncol Clin N Am. 2003; 12(1): 91–103. Review.

Torzili G, Makuuchi M. Tricks for ultrasound-guided resection of colorectal liver metastases. Hepatogastroenterology. 2003; 50(49): 1–3. Review.

Torzili G, Olivari N, Moroni E, et al. Contrast-enhanced intraoperative ultrasonography in surgery for hepatocellular carcinoma in cirrhosis. Liver Transpl. 2004; 10(2 Suppl 1): S34–8.

Vogl TJ, Schwarz W, Blume S, et al. Preoperative evaluation of malignant liver tumors: comparison of unenhanced and SPIO (Resovist)-enhanced MR imaging with biphasic CTAP and intraoperative US. Eur Radiol. 2003; 13(2): 262–72; Epub 2002 Sep. 10.

4 Sonography in the Intensive Care Unit

M. Pross, R. Mantke

Evaluation of the critically ill patient in the intensive care unit (ICU) is often very difficult. The clinical presentation of postoperative complications may be masked by general systemic reactions to (surgical) trauma. Thus, bedside sonography enables the intensivist to garner important objective information rapidly and repetitively for postoperative decision making. Little discomfort for the patient, portability, and round-the-clock availability are the most important advantages of this diagnostic tool.

Indications for Sonography

The indication for sonography should be rather broad and arrived at without delay–for differential diagnosis of ambiguous findings and assessment of the postoperative course, including US-guided interventions resulting therefrom.

Examination Technique

- Bedside sonography is performed with the patient in standard (supine) position; for evaluation of possible pleural effusion, the patient is positioned with the upper body moderately elevated.
- For selection of the pertinent probe position and view, see the chapters on specific organs.
- Use 3.5–7.5 MHz transducers.
- In the immediate postoperative period (up to 48 hours), the surgical incision should be draped with a sterile adhesive sheet and sterile acoustic coupling gel (or K–Y jelly) or povidone-iodine (Betadine) should be used.
- For evaluation of the lower abdomen in patients with an indwelling/suprapubic catheter, the bladder is filled retrogradely with 200–300 ml of sterile normal saline.
- After the examination has been completed, both probe and ultrasound unit must be cleaned according to current infection control guidelines.

Pleural Effusion

Basic Facts

- Pleural effusion is a collection of (usually serous) fluid in the pleural space between the visceral and the parietal pleura.
- Other kinds of fluid (hemothorax, chylothorax, and empyema) may also be encountered.
- **Clinical symptoms:** Dyspnea, absent basal breath sound, and dullness on percussion.
- Multifactorial etiology: heart failure, pericarditis, pleural carcinomatosis, mediastinal organ injury, renal failure, liver cirrhosis with portal hypertension, and nephrotic syndrome; postoperatively, inflammatory processes prevail (subphrenic abscesses, pancreatitis, pneumonia, pleural effusions secondary to abdominal surgery, and severe intra-abdominal inflammation).
- The largest diameter of the effusion is noted together with its localization, e.g., in mid-axillary line when supine; the patient is best examined in semi-reclining position or at least with the upper body slightly elevated.
- *Additional workup:* plain chest radiography, fluoroscopy, thoracic CT.

Sonographic Criteria

- Crescent-shaped anechoic mass in the basal parts of the pleural cavity (Fig. 4.**1**).
- The presence of numerous hyperechoic internal reflections is indicative of pleural empyema.

Consequences for Surgical Treatment

Diagnosis	Characteristic Findings	Management
Minor pleural effusion	Anechoic basal mass measuring 1–2 cm from chest wall to lung surface	No intervention; treatment of underlying disease (possibly with diuretics); serial sonograms
Major pleural effusion	Extensive anechoic basal mass > 2 cm	US-guided sterile thoracentesis at the most dependent point
Simple pleural empyema	Mixed anechoic and hyperechoic reflections; signs of inflammation	Thoracentesis, chest tube drainage; MCS
Septated pleural empyema	Mixed anechoic and hyperechoic reflections; signs of inflammation; multi-chambering visualized	Attempt thoracentesis and drainage; if unsuccessful, attempt evacuation by thoracoscopy.

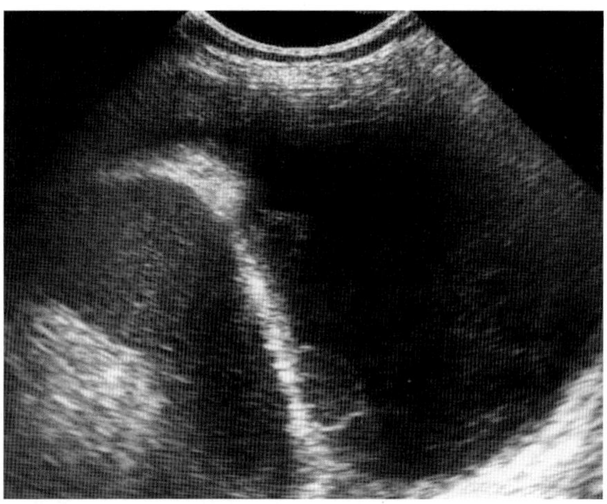

Fig. 4.**1 a** Large left-sided anechoic pleural effusion secondary to pancreatitis.

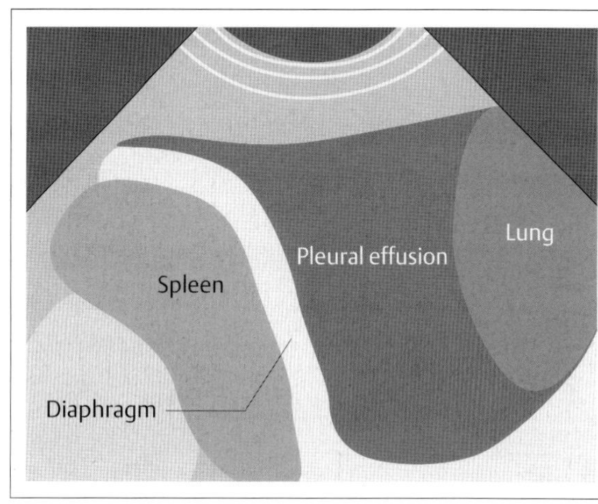

Fig. 4.**1 b** Line drawing.

Pericardial Effusion

Basic Facts

- Etiology: trauma, handling during surgery (pericardial irritation), other underlying disease (pericarditis, renal failure, and others), tumor, and infection.
- Hemodynamically relevant pericardial effusion mandates rapid action. Clinical symptoms: low-output cardiac failure, neck vein distension, and elevated CVP.
- Sonography is the diagnostic modality of choice; the effusion is visualized either by transesophageal echocardiography or from the subxiphoid position via the hepatic window.
- *Additional workup* (none necessary, if only pericardial effusion needs to be confirmed/ruled out): Plain A–P chest radiography: broadened cardiac silhouette.

Sonographic Criteria

- Subxiphoid view through the left lobe of the liver: anechoic pericardial mass (Fig. 4.**2**).
- The presence of numerous hyperechoic internal reflections is indicative of hemopericardium.

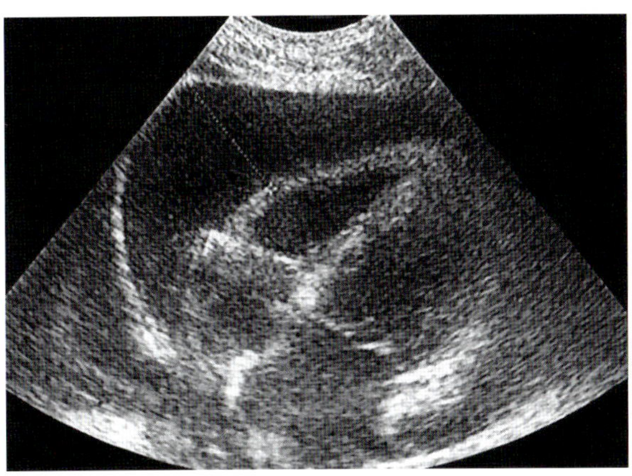

Fig. 4.**2a** Extensive pericardial effusion in a patient with systemic lupus erythematosus (subcostal view).

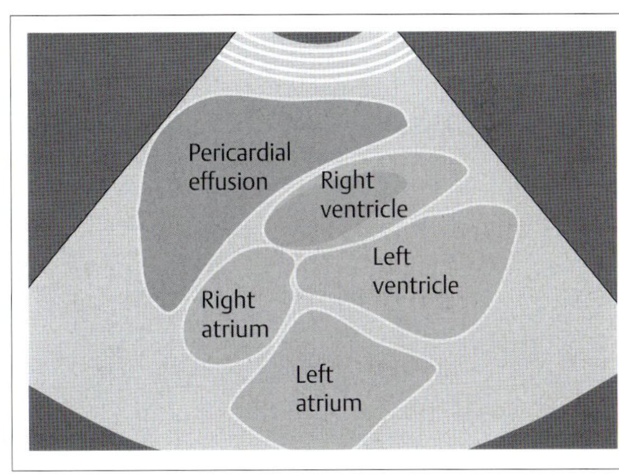

Fig. 4.**2b** Line drawing.

Consequences for Surgical Treatment

Diagnosis	Characteristic Findings	Management
Minor effusion	Anechoic precardial mass < 1.5 cm, no effect on circulation	Cardiac monitoring; diuretics
Major effusion	Anechoic precardial mass > 1.5 cm, usually with hypotension	US-guided pericardiocentesis
Cardiac tamponade	Usually posttraumatic; severe hypotension, distended neck veins	Immediate pericardiocentesis, possibly followed by surgical revision

Cholecystitis in the ICU Setting

Basic Facts

- Acute acalculous cholecystitis ("stress-related cholecystitis") is one complication after major surgery and in polytrauma patients and carries an incidence of 5%.
- Decreased bile flow secondary to postoperative or posttraumatic starvation and aperistalsis of the upper abdomen induce functional obstruction, aggravated by tissue hypoxia with successive cell damage, in turn secondary to disease-related circulatory centralization, or intensive care measures.
- Conditions in the surgical ICU impair evaluation of clinical and laboratory parameters and confound establishment of the diagnosis.
- Co-morbidity, the ambiguous course with difficult assessment, and the frequently fulminating development during the postoperative phase contribute to a high mortality.

Sonographic Criteria

- Enlarged round gallbladder with indistinctly contoured margin.
- Triple layered thickened wall of more than 3–4 mm (Fig. 4.**3**).
- Hypoechoic rim correlating with perifocal edema.
- Pericholecystic fluid.

- Caveat: Postoperative enlargement of the gallbladder is quite common.
- Sensitivity and specificity of sonography are increased by dynamic ultrasound techniques (ceruloplasmin test, CCK test).
- *Additional workup:* abdominal CT.

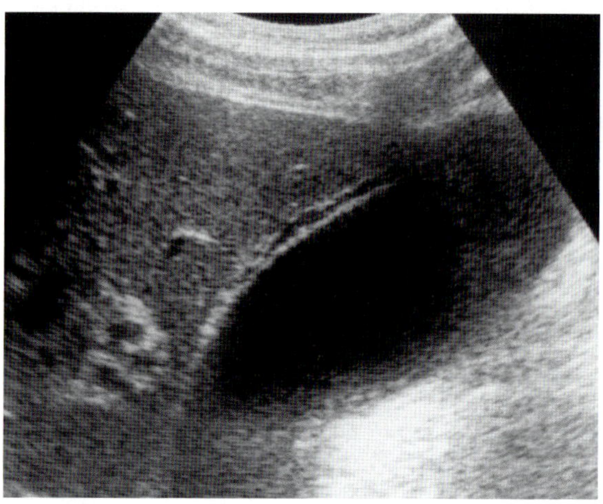

Fig. 4.**3 a** Acute acalculous cholecystitis with wall thickening.

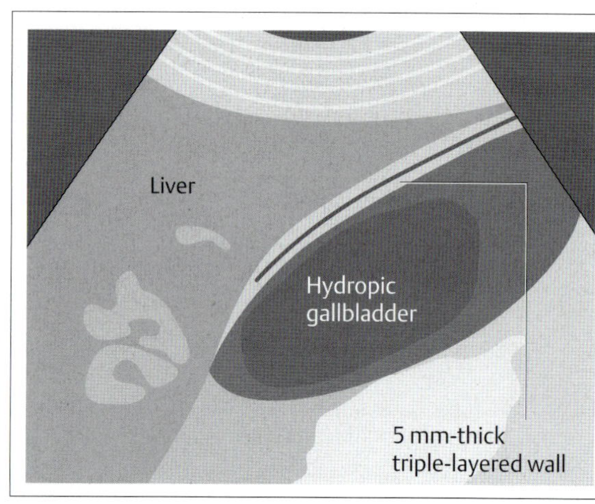

Fig. 4.**3 b** Line drawing.

Consequences for Surgical Treatment

Diagnosis	Characteristic Findings	Management
Inflammation	Typical sonographic signs of inflammation; pericholecystic fluid; general signs of infection, and fever; elevated WBC; no acute abdomen	Antibiotics; observation; serial sonography
Inflammation	Typical sonographic signs of inflammation; pericholecystic fluid; general signs of infection and fever; elevated WBC; acute abdomen	Cholecystectomy

Postoperative Bleeding and Hematoma

Basic Facts

- The incidence of postoperative bleeding in the general surgical population averages 3.5–4.3%, depending on the procedure: 0.1–0.5% after appendectomy, up to 8% after partial liver resection, and up to 12% in necrotizing pancreatitis.
- 90% of all bleeding is seen within 48 hours of surgery.
- Caveat: Surgeons often tend to regard coagulation disorders as the sole reason for the bleeding. Dry drainage tubes do not rule out postoperative hemorrhage.
- The situation requires unbiased objective assessment, taking into account: amount/type of fluid drained, kind and complexity of the procedure/trauma, hemodynamic status, volume depletion, transfusion requirements, coagulation and liver panel, urinary output; serial sonography.
- Early reoperation is warranted since morbidity and mortality rise with prolonged hypovolemic shock.
- *Additional workup:* CT or angiography only in exceptional cases.

Sonographic Criteria

- Hypoechoic/anechoic mass primarily at/near the operative field; in case of massive hemorrhage, there may be diffuse intra-abdominal spread (Figs. 4.**4**–4.**7**).
- Heterogeneous echoes within the mass are the result of coagulation (Fig. 4.**8**).

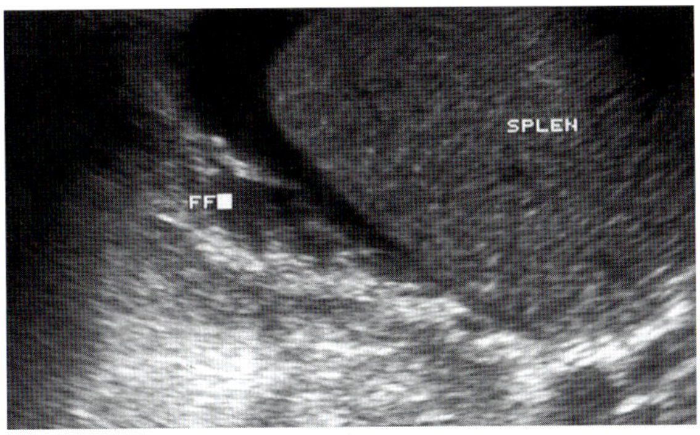

Fig. 4.**4 a** Free intra-abdominal fluid (FF) after a 6-hour segmental liver resection, with perisplenic blood and around the lower pole of the spleen.

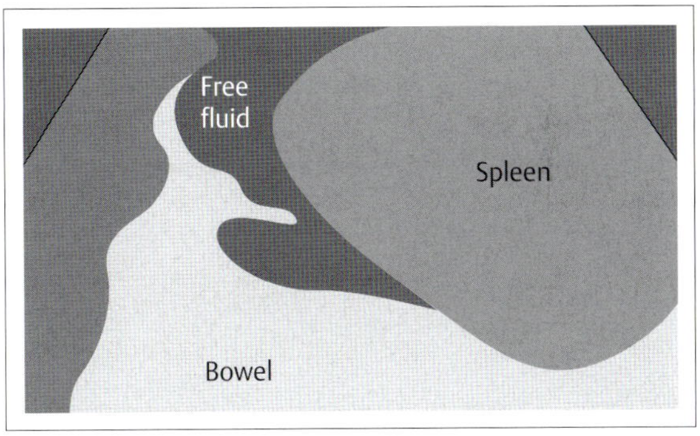

Fig. 4.**4 b** Line drawing.

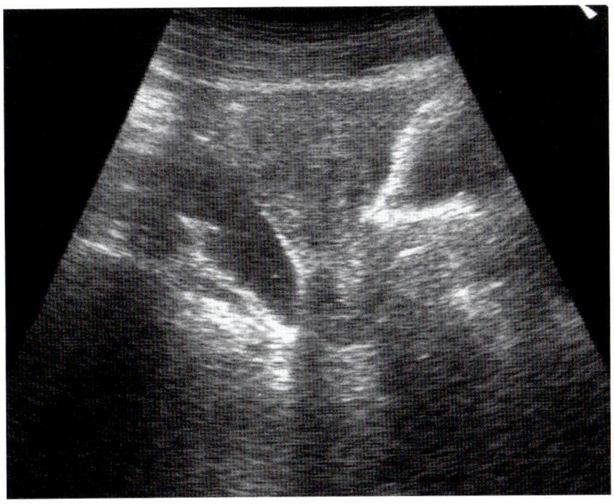

Fig. 4.**5 a** Free fluid in the pouch of Douglas after laparoscopic cholecystectomy. Paracentesis may help differentiate between blood and irrigation fluid.

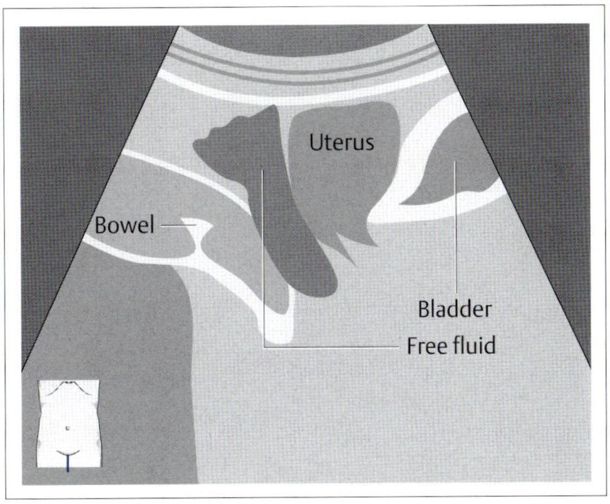

Fig. 4.**5 b** Line drawing.

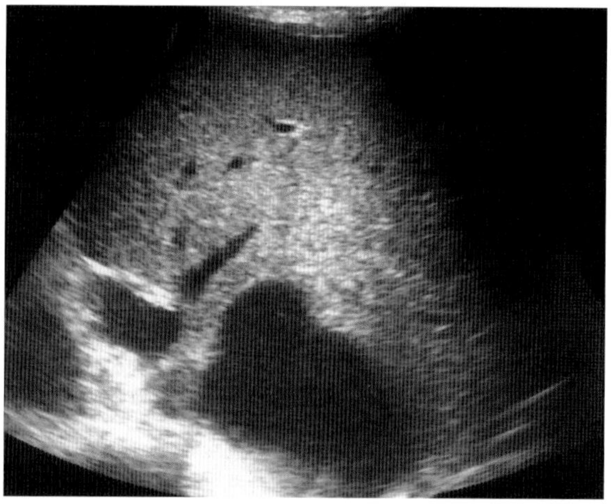

Fig. 4.6 a Circumscribed paracaval hematoma three days after liver transplantation, not requiring revision.

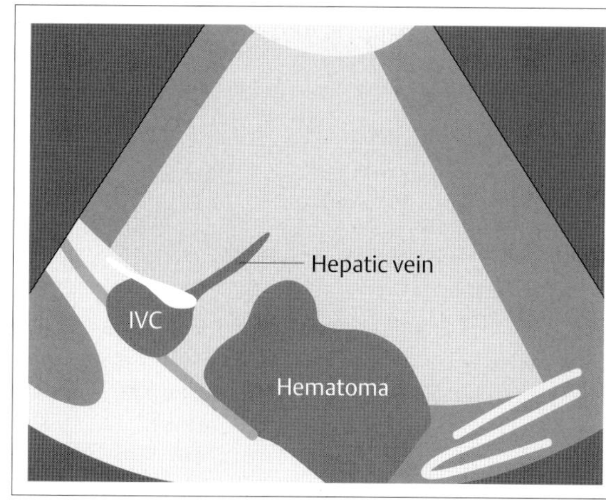

Fig. 4.6 b Line drawing.

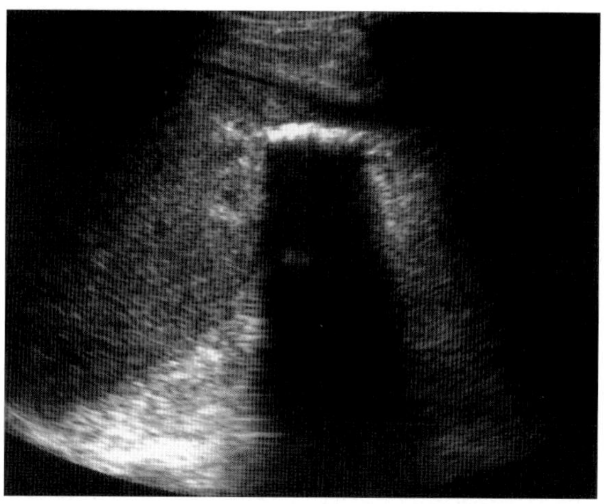

Fig. 4.7 a Repeat sonography for postoperative hemorrhage after liver transplantation. Hemostasis was achieved by packing with iodoform gauze, visualized as textile foreign body.

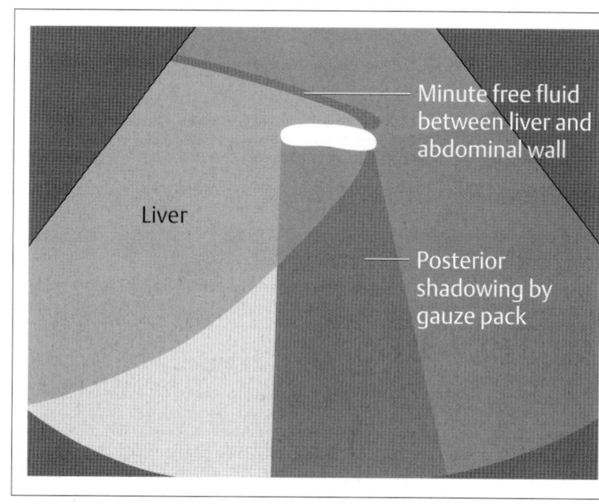

Fig. 4.7 b Line drawing.

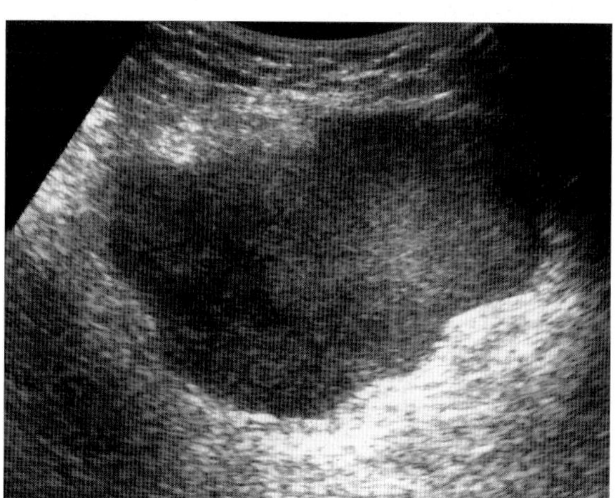

Fig. 4.8 a Heterogeneous hematoma, measuring 8 × 5 cm, along the left iliac axis after vascular surgery.

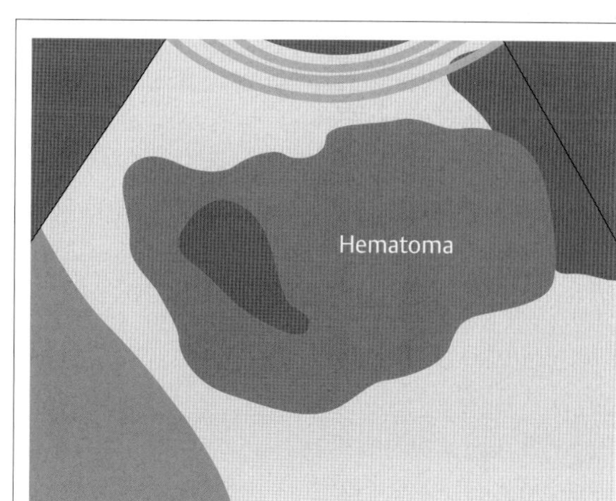

Fig. 4.8 b Line drawing.

Consequences for Surgical Treatment

Diagnosis	Characteristic Findings	Management
Circumscribed intra-abdominal collection of fluid	Hypo-/anechoic mass at/near the operative field; stable H&H; stable circulation	Serial sonography, watchful waiting; rapid reoperation in case of H&H drop
Massive intra-abdominal collection of fluid	Large hypo-/anechoic mass at/near the operative field and possibly in the pouch of Douglas; H&H drop; hemodynamic instability	Reoperation, preferably while the general condition is still reasonably stable
Abdominal wall hematoma	Hypoechoic mass within the abdominal wall	Serial sonography; wait for self-tamponade; reoperation in case of massive hematoma or arterial bleeding

Biloma

Basic Facts

- Incidence: up to 6% in hepatic resection, up to 3% in extrahepatic bile duct surgery.
- Drainage should always be attempted to avoid biliary peritonitis and superinfection.
- *Additional workup:* ERCP, abdominal CT.

Sonographic Criteria

- Circumscribed, usually subhepatic anechoic mass at/near the operative field (Fig. 4.**9**).
- In case of infection, quite often internal echoes and possibly small pockets of gas may be present.

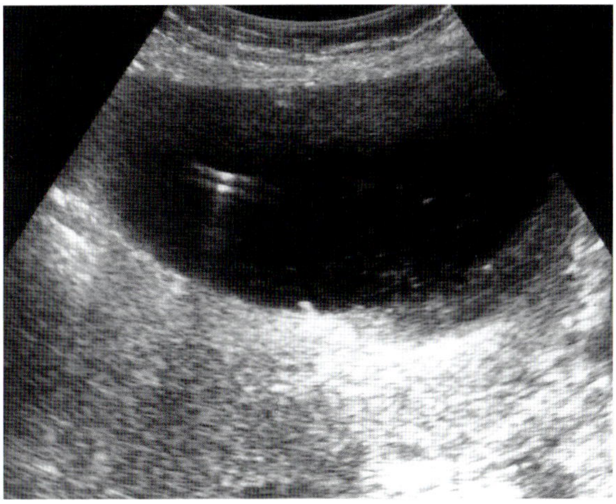

Fig. 4.**9 a** Biloma anterior to the liver after liver transplant. Longitudinal view with pigtail catheter already inserted.

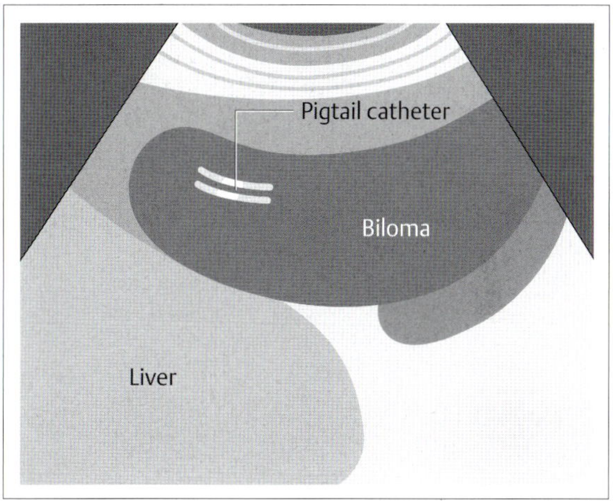

Fig. 4.**9 b** Line drawing.

Consequences for Surgical Treatment

Diagnosis	Characteristic Findings	Management
Biloma	Sharply circumscribed anechoic mass	Paracentesis, interventional drainage; once bile flow has subsided initiate further diagnostic workup (ERC and stenting)
Biloma	Multiple anechoic masses, free intra-abdominal fluid, beginning peritonitis	Reoperation and drainage

Abscess

Basic Facts

- The incidence of postoperative intra-abdominal abscess formation varies (3–6%) with the procedure, with GI tract surgery being at particular risk.
- If the clinical picture points to postoperative infection, abscess formation must always be ruled out.
- The most common sites for the collection of inflammatory fluid are the operative field, both subdiaphragmatic recesses, between the bowel loops, both paracolic gutters, and/or the pouch of Douglas.
- Conditions favoring abscess formation include hematoma, necrosis, foreign body, and an immunocompromised patient.
- Diagnostic workup must be prompted by the clinical picture of inflammation (undulating temperature spikes; elevated nonspecific parameters of inflammation; nonspecific abdominal symptoms; aperistalsis). Meticulous physical examination always precedes sonography.
- *Additional workup:* contrast-enhanced CT, MRI, paracentesis.

Sonographic Criteria

- Hypo-/hyperechoic masses with ill-defined margins containing small pockets of gas (Fig. 4.**10**).
- Sometimes a hyperechoic pyogenic rim is visualized.

Consequences for Surgical Treatment

Diagnosis	Characteristic Findings	Management
Intra-abdominal abscess	Classic sonographic signs visible; elevated laboratory parameters of inflammation; fever	Preferably drainage by radiological intervention; otherwise: surgical evacuation
Subcutaneous/subfascial abscess	Collection of hypo-/hyperechoic fluid	Removal of stitches/sutures, drainage, irrigation

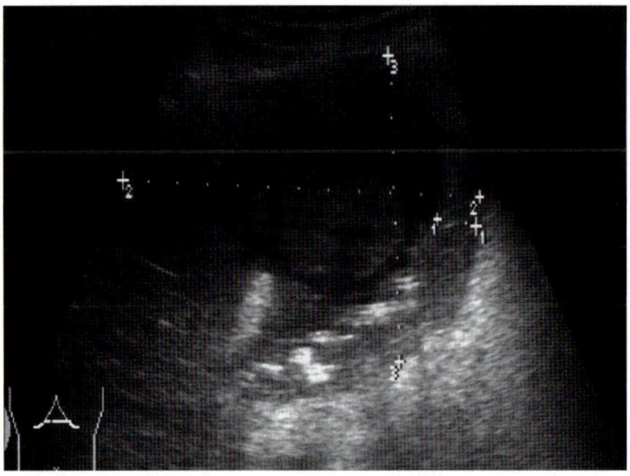

Fig. 4.**10a** Tender hypoechoic mass, measuring 8 × 5 cm, encased by indurated hyperechoic fatty tissue. This is the sonogram of an intra-abdominal abscess.

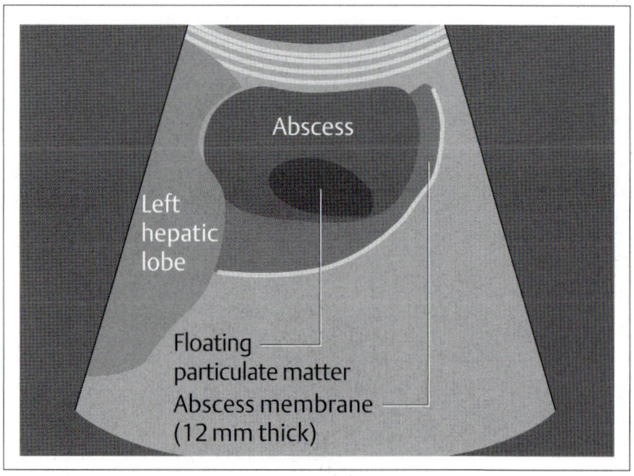

Fig. 4.**10b** Line drawing.

Ultrasound-Guided Central Venous Cannulation and Placement of Suprapubic Catheters

Basic Facts

- Most patients in the ICU require a central venous line for adequate fluid replacement and CVP monitoring, possibly also for parenteral nutrition or as temporary access for hemodialysis.
- Preferred location (low complication rate): right external or internal jugular vein; only if conditions warrant it (e.g., injury to the cervical spine, jugular vein thrombosis) should other vessels be cannulated.
- Indication for suprapubic catheter placement in the ICU: need for prolonged urinary diversion after surgery or trauma.
- Contraindications: hemorrhagic diathesis, contracted bladder, bladder tumors, nondistensible bladder. Relative contraindications: previous lower abdominal surgery.
- Cannulation has been standardized and generally does not require ultrasound-guidance; however, US-guidance may prove helpful in anatomically challenging situations; sonography before catheter placement will improve the safety of the procedure.

Sonographic Criteria

- Normal anechoic internal jugular vein with complete loss of lumen on compression (Fig. 4.**11**).
- For suprapubic catheter placement: the bladder will be visualized as anechoic retropubic mass (Fig. 4.**12**), particularly after retrograde filling with normal saline via a Foley catheter.

Consequences for Surgical Treatment

Diagnosis	Characteristic Findings	Management
Full bladder	Anechoic retropubic fluid collection	Suprapubic catheter placement
Nondistensible bladder	No increase in the anechoic retropubic fluid collection	No cannulation
Normal neck	No thrombosis of the internal jugular vein	Classic cannulation of the right jugular vein
Abnormal cervical anatomy	Thrombosis of the internal jugular vein in external compression	No cannulation at this site; alternative access via the left jugular or subclavian vein

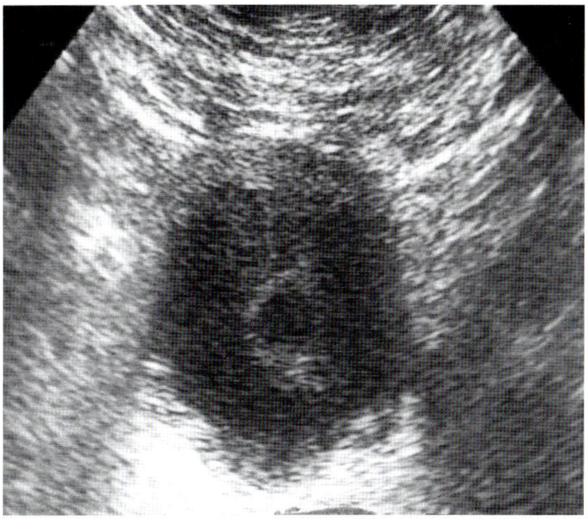

Fig. 4.**11 a** Transverse view of the normal anatomy of the left neck.

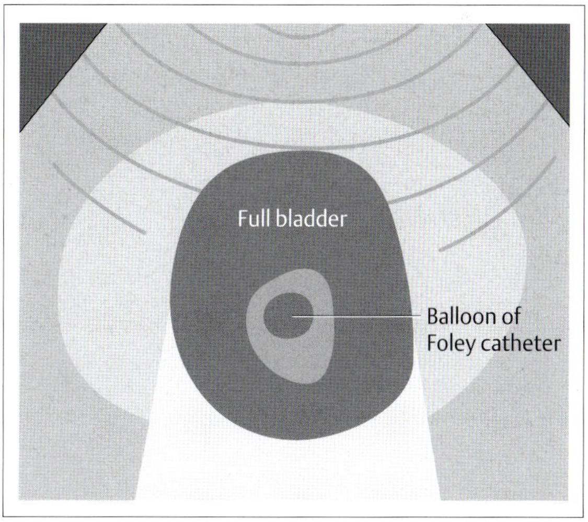

Fig. 4.**11 b** Line drawing.

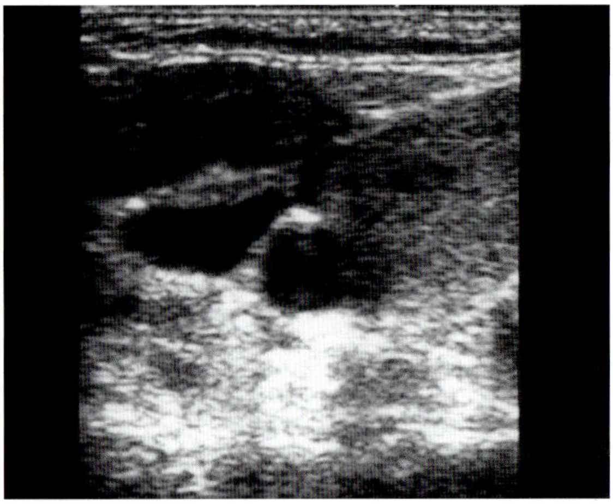

Fig. 4.**12 a** View of the full bladder, safe for suprapubic catheter placement.

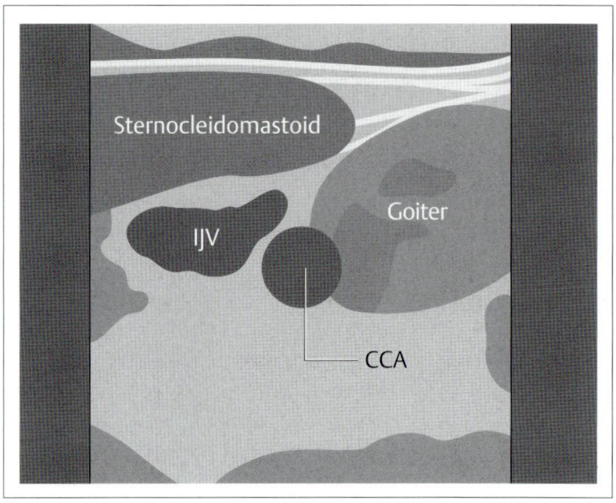

Fig. 4.**12 b** Line drawing.

Bibliography

Imhof M, Ohmann C, Röher HD. Die Intensivgallenblase-passageres Phänomen oder therapiebedürftiges Problem? Chirurg. 1995; 66: 360–5.

Lippert H, Ed. Praxis der Chirurgie, Allgemein- und Viszeralchirurgie. Stuttgart: Thieme; 1998.

Mazziotti A, Cavallari A, Eds. Techniques in Liver Surgery. London: Greenwich Medical Media; 1997.

McGahan JP, Goldberg BB. Diagnostic ultrasound–a logical approach. Washington, New York: Lippincott Raven; 1998.

Töns C, Schumpelick V, Eds. Chirurgische Notfall- und Intensivmedizin. Stuttgart: Enke; 1997.

5 Interventional Sonography

U. Peitz, R. Mantke, R. Grote

■ General Considerations

Introduction

Cross-sectional imaging modalities such as sonography and computed tomography (CT) have significantly extended the scope of diagnostic and therapeutic aspiration and biopsy. Most importantly, aspirations that were previously performed blind have become safer. Examples include Menghini aspiration biopsy of the liver (Caturelli et al., 1996; Greiner and Franken, 1983; Lindor et al., 1996), thoracentesis, and central venous access (Teichgräber et al., 2000). In addition, biopsy of small lesions and aspiration of fluid collections, which otherwise escape palpation and standard fluoroscopy, have become possible. The following discussion of aspiration techniques relates to diagnostic as well as therapeutic procedures, since the first step for both is always insertion of a needle.

Choosing the Imaging Modality

Whether the intervention is best supported by sonography or X-ray tomography, in particular computed tomography, primarily depends on which method best depicts the target lesion and needle track and allows for safe guided needle placement (Table 5.**1**). Studies comparing these competing modalities have found sonography to be best suited overall for guided procedures (Dameron et al., 1999; Sheafor et al., 1998).

Visualization of the Needle

Both the shaft and the tip of the needle can be visualized on the monitor. However, the tip is much brighter and more echogenic, in most cases giving rise to a double reflection (Fig. 5.**1**). Visualization of the tip generally does not depend on the angle between the needle and the ultrasound beam. Even if the needle and beam run parallel, the tip can still be identified. Conversely, the shaft of the needle is visualized more easily the less obtuse the angle between the needle and the plane of the transducer, the optimum being a right angle. For teaching and training purposes, it helps to demonstrate the delineation of a needle by placing it in a water bath (Fig. 5.**1**).

The tip of the needle may be harder to identify within hyperechoic tissue of heterogeneous texture, due to the smaller difference in echogenicity with the surroundings. Obviously, the larger their diameter the easier needles are to depict. Visualization may be facilitated by rotating the needle or slightly withdrawing any stylet used. Various types of tip bevel have been designed in order to improve sonographic visualization, but practical aspects are, of course, much more likely to dictate needle selection. Injection of a small amount of air will help delineate the region of the tip by multiple gas reflections around it, but at the same time this will impair precise tip localization.

Table 5.**1** Advantages and disadvantages of sonography over computed tomography for guided aspiration/biopsy

Availability		⊕ Inexpensive ⊕ Portability
Radiation exposure		⊕ None
Visualization of target volume and needle track	Resolution	⊕ Resolution superior to CT for near targets (e.g., thyroid) ⊕ Resolution inferior to CT for probe-target separation > 10 cm
	Artifacts	⊕ Fewer artifacts from metal ⊕ Total reflection of beam by intestinal gas and bone
Visualization of the entire needle insertion		⊕ Freely and rapidly interchangeable views ⊕ Real-time monitoring of the needle insertion

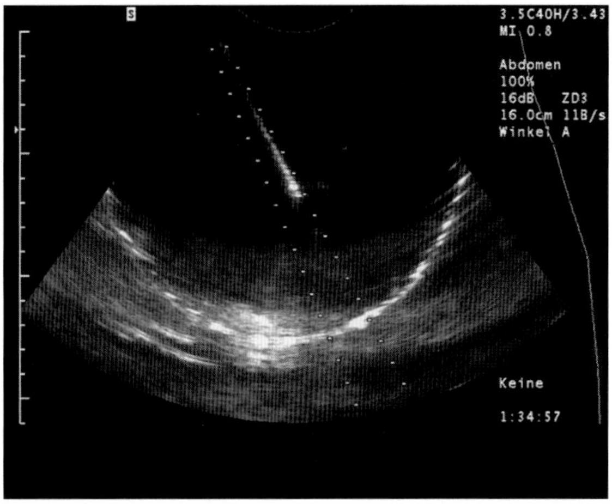

Fig. 5.**1 a** Sonogram of a fine needle in a water bath. Two virtual needle guide lines can be seen on the monitor. The access route has been adjusted to the upper line. The needle enters the sonogram from the side through the removable needle guide.

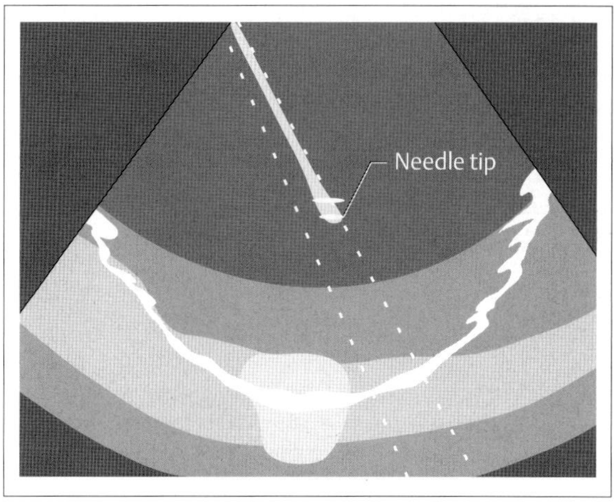

Fig. 5.**1 b** Line drawing.

Sonographic Guidance Techniques

Depending on the type of sonographic guidance employed in targeting, there are two basic techniques: freehand needle placement and the use of needle guides.

Freehand Needle Placement

The freehand technique again encompasses two variants:

- In indirect ultrasound guidance (Fig. 5.**2 a**), first the direction and depth of needle insertion are determined by sonography. The needle is then inserted from the predetermined site without real-time sonographic visualization. Superficial anatomical landmarks and markings on the skin of the patient facilitate orientation. This technique lends itself only to large lesions or to assessment of diffuse changes in parenchymal organs.
- In the freehand technique with real-time needle placement (Fig. 5.**2 b**), the needle is placed either adjacent to or remote from the probe ("off-probe aspiration") and followed sonographically until the tip enters the target. By placing the needle just to the side of the ultrasound plane, but at a slight angle, and by subtly sweeping the probe back and forth, the operator images the entire length of the needle.

Needle Guides

The use of needle guides involves a fixed attachment to the ultrasound transducer. This allows the needle to be passed at a given angle in relation to the viewing plane, i.e., the tip and shaft of the needle remain in constant view. The guides are either removable (Figs. 5.**2 c**, 5.**3 a**) or are an integral part of the probe (Fig. 5.**2 d, e,** Fig. 5.**3 b–c**). In the latter case, the needle will pass along a central canal within the ultrasound probe. Because a canal attenuates the imaging quality somewhat, aspiration-dedicated probes do not lend themselves to routine imaging. Moreover, aspiration-dedicated probes with a central canal are configured as linear arrays, lacking the advantages offered by the smaller curved-array and sector probes (see Chapter 6, Technical Principles). Ultrasound probes with built-in needle guides fall into either of these two basic categories:

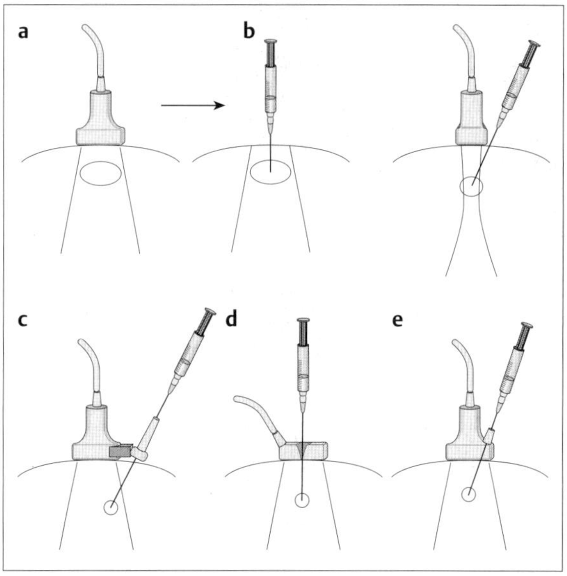

Fig. 5.**2** Techniques of ultrasound-guided aspiration
a Two-stage freehand aspiration
b Freehand aspiration under real-time ultrasound guidance
c Aspiration with a removable needle guide sleeve
d Aspiration using dedicated probe with central canal
e Aspiration using dedicated probe with built-in needle guide sleeve

a
b
c
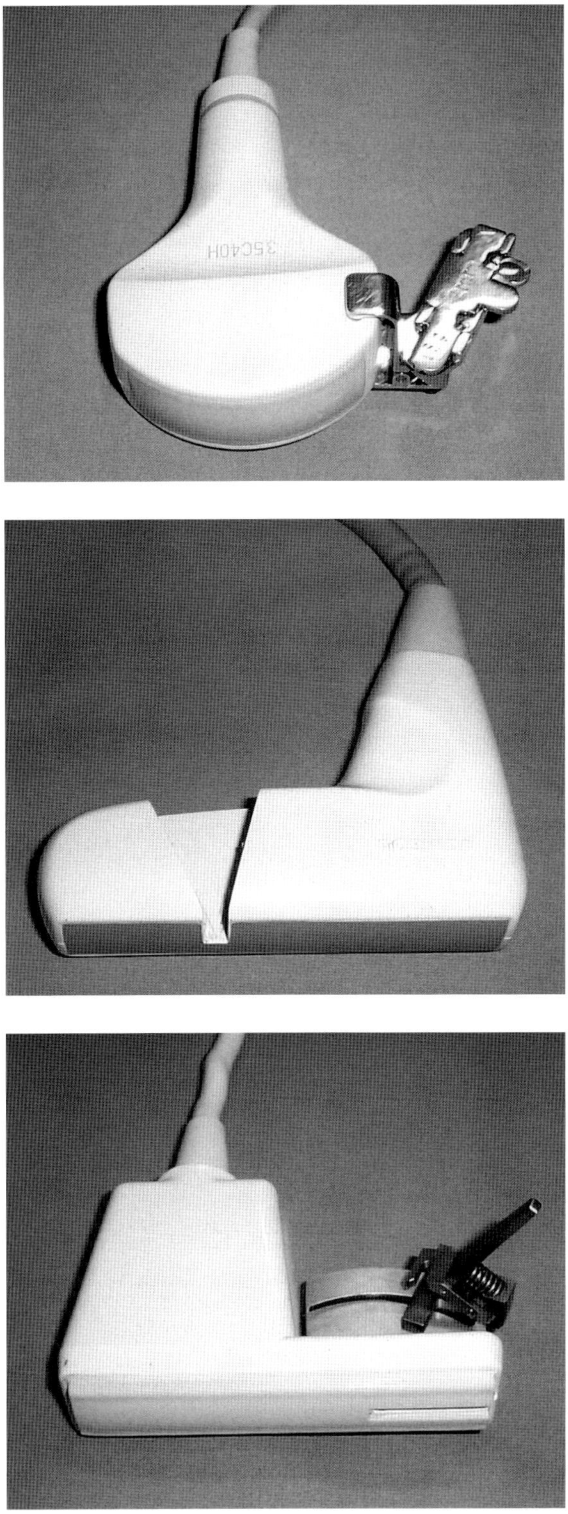

Fig. 5.3 Aspiration-dedicated probes.
a Aspiration-dedicated probe with removable needle guide sleeve
b Aspiration-dedicated probe with central canal
c Aspiration-dedicated probe with built-in needle guide sleeve

- Needle guide with a canal fixing the needle parallel to the direction of the beam, but still leaving some leeway for motion (Figs. 5.**2d**, 5.**3b**).
- Probe with built-in needle guide sleeve tightly fitting around the needle, thus permitting aspiration at precise angles (Figs. 5.**2e**, 5.**3c**). Usually, the examiner is free to set the angle between the needle and the probe. The sleeves come in a variety of diameters and therefore can be matched precisely with the needle selected.

Recently, both principles have been combined. The aspiration-dedicated probe with central canal depicted in Fig. 5.**3b** may be supplemented by an adapter sleeve for the canal. The advantage of having some leeway of needle motion within the central canal compared with the sleeve is a lower risk of injury, e.g., with respiratory motion; the disadvantage is that of somewhat less precise targeting.

Needle guide sleeves also come with an adapter frame for mounting on standard probes (Figs. 5.**2c**, 5.**3a**). Such needle guides are inexpensive and are available for almost all types of probes. Compared with aspiration-dedicated probes incorporating a central canal, they suffer from two minor drawbacks: firstly, the needle track cannot be visualized in the upper near field but only when it enters the image somewhat deeper from the side (Fig. 5.**1**); and secondly, the range of permissible angles is narrower. However, for most practical purposes the removable needle guides are perfectly adequate.

The planned route for the needle to follow must be depicted on the monitor as a dotted virtual guide line. The software of the ultrasound unit allows the user to match the guide line with the needle guide. This calibration should be done in a water bath (Fig. 5.**1**).

Choice of Aspiration Technique

Aspiration-dedicated probes will yield the most precise targeting of small masses. For the great majority of cases, the results do differ between removable and built-in needle guides. Sleeves offer the additional advantage that fine needles will not bend quite as easily outside the body. In particular, long fine needles will tend to bend when passing through firm tissue such as the skin.

Nevertheless, freehand aspiration in one form or another may still have its use in certain situations. It is less cumbersome, especially when it comes to maintaining sterile conditions, and a shorter needle can be used with more freedom of motion. This gives the examiner a better feeling for the consistency of the organ aspirated as well as movement of the patient, in particular any respiratory excursions. As the operator feels such unintentional needle movements, he or she can give way to them and thereby prevent bending of the needle inside the body, avoiding potential injury. Skill and personal experience of the examiner will also contribute to the choice of aspiration technique.

Usually, ultrasound-guided aspiration by just one individual appears preferable to having both probe and needle guided by two people, as coordination is clearly facilitated when the same person handles the probe with one hand and advances the needle with the other.

Asepsis

Liberal skin disinfection and formal (fenestrated) draping are mandatory, and perhaps also a sterile gown for the operator. Regarding sterility of the probe, there are three options:

- Freehand technique: the disinfected probe is placed remote from the site of needle insertion.
- Freehand needle placement and the use of needle guides: placing the probe within a sterile glove or dedicated cover (do not forget the acoustic coupling gel inside the glove/cover).
- Fundamental to all techniques, in particular for probes with needle guide sleeves: cold gas sterilization of the probe according to the manufacturer's instructions, or at least sterilization of the needle guide sleeve and disinfection of the transducer.

Best results are obtained with prepackaged commercial sterile ultrasound gel for acoustic coupling. Skin disinfectants may also be employed for acoustic coupling, although compared with ultrasound gel they somewhat degrade imaging quality.

Patient Preparation

- Informed, and if possible written, consent at least one day before the procedure.
- Ability of the patient to cooperate.
- No coagulation disorder:
  - Routine background information with attention to a history of bleeding disorders, liver disease, and medications is more important than the laboratory studies listed below. Standard coagulation laboratory panels reveal neither the vascular component of the coagulation cascade nor thrombocytopathy.
  - Limits for needle diameter ≥ 1 mm: Quick's PT assay > 60%, PTT < 45 s, platelet count > 100 000/μl.
  - Limits for needle diameter < 1 mm; by definition these are the so-called "fine needles": Quick's PT assay > 60%, PTT < 45 s, platelet count > 80 000/μl (Weiss and Duntsch, 1996).
  - Other authors have advanced lower limits for FNA: Quick's PT assay > 50%, PTT < 45 s, platelet count > 50 000/μl (Nolsoe et al., 1990). However, in present-day surgery the preoperative bleeding time test is no longer regarded as being meaningful when assessing the risk of hemorrhagic complications (Peterson et al., 1998; Wagner, 1998).
  - Apart from the coagulation status, the risk of hemorrhage will also depend on the gauge of the needle used (see below) and the characteristics of the tissue, i.e., on the organ in question and the (pathological) texture of the tissue. Thus, the risk will be higher in cirrhotic patients than in those with noncirrhotic diffuse liver disease. Focal lesions are more prone to hemorrhage than diffuse pathologies (Glaser and Pausch, 1995). The compressibility of the needle insertion site also plays a substantial role. Consequently, breast lesions may even be biopsied with the patient under anticoagulant medication (Melotti and Berg, 2000).
  - Low-dose heparin or platelet aggregation inhibitors are not contraindications per se. The risk of possible bleeding is difficult to assess in patients on multidrug regimens. Data on the bleeding risk in patients on acetylsalicylic acid (ASA) or nonsteroidal anti-inflammatory drugs (NSAIDs) are scant. ASA did not increase the risk of bleeding after FNA and biopsy of the prostate (Herget et al., 1999). Just as in operations (Schafer, 1999) and endoscopic GI polypectomies (Shiffman et al., 1994), low-dose ASA (100 mg/day) and NSAIDs are considered safe in procedures without an inherently high risk of hemorrhage. However, if ASA and NSAIDs are deemed a risk, they have to be discontinued at least four days beforehand, or even better one week.
- A fasting period of six hours is only called for in paracentesis, which otherwise would be impaired by gas in the GI tract, or for procedures requiring surgical standby.

Analgesia and Sedation

Local or systemic analgesia is not required for fine-needle aspirations, which actually can be more uncomfortable with local anesthesia than without (Daltrey and Kissin, 2000). Large-caliber needles with a diameter ≥ 1.0 mm usually require a skin incision and thus local anesthesia as well. The injection of a local anesthetic slightly impairs visualization as the solution will always be intermixed with tiny air bubbles. Special attention should be paid to drawing up the anesthetic without bubbles.

When aspirating and draining organs not amenable to local anesthesia, such as the peritoneum and pleura, and in patients sensitive to pain, a systemic opioid analgesic may be administered (beware of the side effects!).

Sedation would, however, reduce cooperation and entail the risk of respiratory depression. All organs that move with respiration are best punctured in deep inspiration, as pain tends to trigger involuntary inspiration that might result in bending of the needle.

Diagnostic Aspiration and Biopsy

Most diagnostic aspirations and biopsies are performed to obtain tissue specimens, but US-guidance may also be employed in the instillation of contrast agents before radiological studies, e.g., in PTC or percutaneous pancreatography.

Needles

Typing needles by their diameter into large-caliber (14–19 gauge; diameter > 1 mm) and small-caliber (20–25 gauge; diameter < 1 mm) needles is based on the observation that the risk of complications depends primarily on the size of the needle (Menghini, 1970; Piccinino et al., 1986; Weiss and Duntsch, 1996).

Large-caliber needles, usually with a diameter of 1.4–1.6 mm, are mostly employed in the biopsy of parenchymal organs, such as the liver and the kidneys, for histological examination of diffuse changes. Fine-needles lend themselves to aspiration of fluids as well as biopsy of pathological masses.

Based on the type of collection, the needles can be grouped into the injection-aspiration or the cutting-core biopsy type. Needle terminology is inconsistent and quite often varies with the manufacturer. Injection-aspiration needles are employed in the collection of fluid and cytological specimens as well as in the instillation of contrast agents. They are beveled just like phlebotomy needles and have to be rather acutely angled so that they can reach the target easily and in a straight line. In addition, cutting-core biopsy needles have a cutting edge to excise and core the solid tissue needed for histological examination.

In simple cases with a short track, standard phlebotomy needles may be sufficient, e.g., for diagnostic thoracentesis of pleural effusions and paracentesis of ascites, or for cytological aspiration of the thyroid gland. For longer routes, an inner sheath plus outer-cannula combination must be used, such as the Chiba needle (Fig. 5.**4a**), developed for percutaneous transhepatic cholangiography (PTC) at Chiba University in Japan. The inner notched sheath prevents collection of undesired tissue along the access route, stabilizes the needle, and reduces the risk of injuries. For targets at intermediate distances, one inexpensive alternative is the spinal needle. A blind-ended needle with side-holes is used for therapeutic ethanol instillations into hepatic lesions (Fig. 5.**4b**).

Histological specimens are collected with cutting-core biopsy needles, which are based on two different principles:

- In the full-cut technique, also known as "Menghini" or aspiration/suction technique, the desired tissue cylinder is either cored out by the tip of the needle or cut out, depending on the sharpness of the tip edge (Fig. 5.**4c–f**). Here, the tissue cylinder will have the same diameter as the inside diameter of the needle. Large-caliber needles, such as the Menghini needle for liver biopsies, have a less acutely angled end in order to lower the risk of hemorrhage (Fig. 5.**4c**), while in contrast small-caliber needles have an acutely angled, beveled tip (Fig. 5.**4e–f**). Safe aspiration and biopsy requires several millimeters to 1 cm of negative suction in the needle, which is accomplished by pulling back on the attached syringe or the tight fitting stylet. The principle of cutting biopsy by moving a needle with crownlike tip in the lesion in a rotatory motion, which was popular at one time, has largely been abandoned (Fig. 5.**4d**).
- In the "Tru-Cut," "Vim-Silvermann," or "cutting" technique the stylet with its sampling notch is advanced into the target tissue. The outer cannula advancing over the trocar then cuts the tissue sample, resulting in a small piece of tissue being trapped within the notched area of the stylet (Fig. 5.**4g**). Here, the diameter of the tissue cylinder will be smaller than the inside diameter of the needle. In order to obtain tissue cylinders of the same diameter, the size of the Tru-Cut needle must therefore be bigger than that of a full-cut needle.

While both systems combine cutting and coring, the cutting action is more pronounced in the Tru-Cut technique. This makes specimen collection more reliable, but it also somewhat increases the risk of hemorrhage. The clinical relevance of the benefits and drawbacks of both biopsy techniques has been studied for large-bore needles in liver biopsies (Judmaier et al., 1989; Piccinino et al., 1986), but not for small-caliber needles.

Tru-Cut type needles entail the additional disadvantage that the tip of the needle reaches beyond the zone of sampling, which may cause problems with small lesions adjacent to structures prone to hemorrhage.

With either system, better results are obtained the faster the coring or cutting action takes place. Special spring-loaded high-speed automated biopsy needles (so-called biopsy guns) and handles have been developed for both techniques. The latter can be mounted on syringes (Fig. 5.**5a, b**) or come as a unit complete with syringe and needle (Fig. 5.**5c, d**). When spring-loaded biopsy guns are fired, the biopsy is taken in fully automatic fashion. There are commercial biopsy guns wherein a needle has to be mounted (Fig. 5.**5e–f**) as well as disposable ready-to-use units (Fig. 5.**5g**). In our experience, in most cases the quality of the results obtained with the handle will match that of a biopsy gun.

Multiple specimens from one and the same mass are best taken with so-called coaxial systems. Here, the outer cannula remains within the lesion while an inner needle is withdrawn and advanced repeatedly (Jeffrey 1988; Skamel et al., 1998).

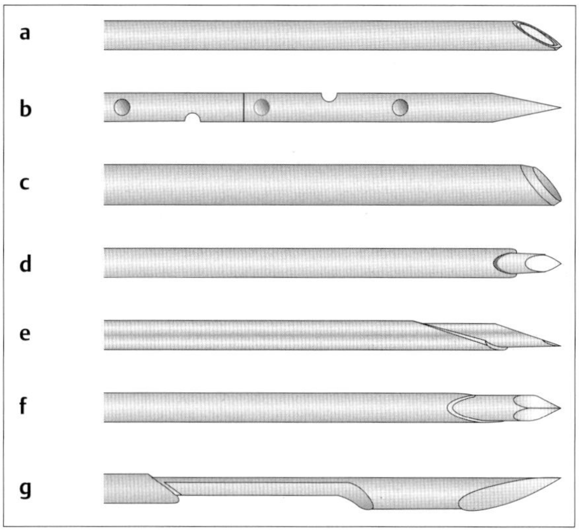

Fig. 5.**4** Needle types.
a Chiba needle with stylet
b Needle with lateral holes, for ethanol instillation
c Menghini biopsy needle
d–g Small-caliber cutting biopsy needles, each with stylet
d With crownlike tip
e, f With sharpened tip edge
g Tru-Cut biopsy principle

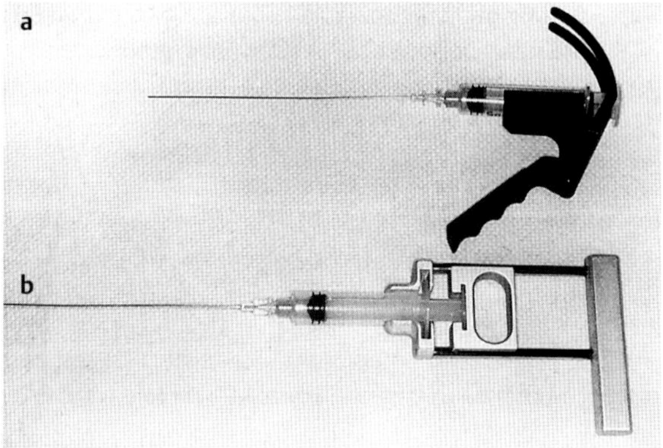

Fig. 5.**5** Handles and guns for small-caliber needles.
a, b Handles for mounting of full-cut (aspiration) needles

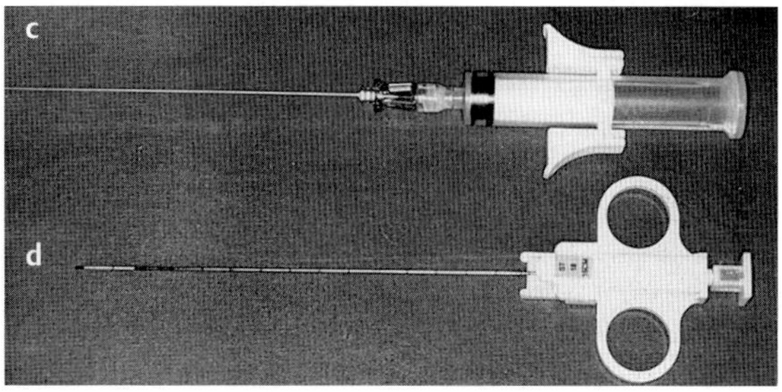

Fig. 5.**5 c** Integrated handle for full-cut needles.
Fig. 5.**5 d** Integrated handle for Tru-Cut type needles.

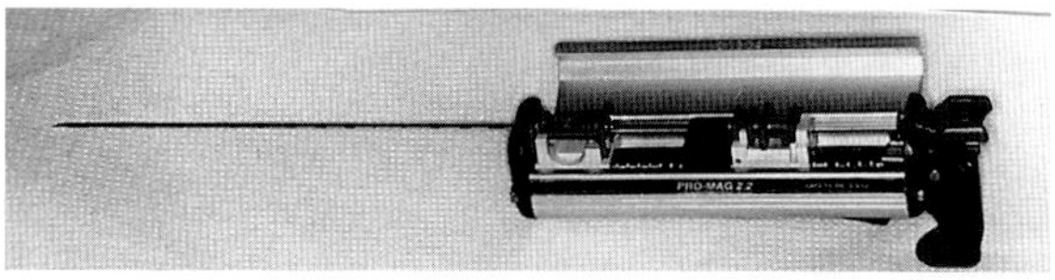

Fig. 5.**5 e** Opened biopsy gun for mounting of Tru-Cut type needles.

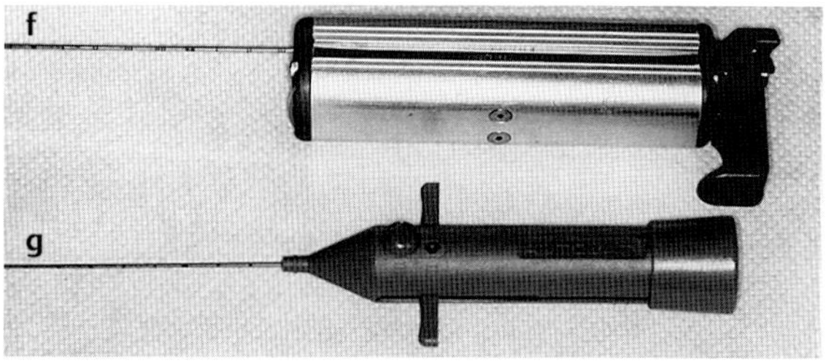

Fig. 5.**5 f** Biopsy gun for mounting of Tru-Cut type needles, ready for operation.

Aspiration of Pathological Fluid Collections

Fine-needle aspiration usually suffices for ascites; pleural, pericardial, and joint effusions; seroma, biloma, abscess; etc. Depending on the risk involved, purulent or mucous contents may call for a 17 or 18 gauge needle (diameter 1.4 or 1.2 mm). Usually, sonography cannot differentiate the kind of fluid based on the image alone. Depending on the issue in question, the specimen may undergo histopathological and laboratory study including: cell count, sediment smear, protein level, LDH, bacterial culture and microscopy, enzyme panel, tumor markers, etc.

Aspiration Biopsies in Diffuse Parenchymal Organ Disorders

Diffuse hepatic and renal disease is best biopsied for histopathological evaluation with large-caliber needles. The most common size chosen is 16 or 17 gauge (diameters 1.6 and 1.4 mm, respectively).

- For liver biopsies, the Menghini technique has stood the test of time (McGill et al., 1990; Menghini, 1970). Today, it is performed as a two-stage freehand procedure. The optimum site and direction of entry are determined sonographically, while the subsequent needle insertion and biopsy collection are carried out without real-time ultrasound control. This US-marking technique results in fewer complications than the previously common "blind liver biopsy" (Caturelli et al., 1996; Greiner and Franken, 1983; Lindor et al., 1996; Riley, 1999).
- Since biopsy of the kidney is more difficult and risk prone, real-time US-guidance of the entire procedure is usually aimed for. Over the years, biopsy guns employ-

ing Tru-Cut type needles have become standard (Chan et al., 2000; Nass and O'Neill, 1999; Nyman et al., 1997).

Histological specimens may also be obtained with fine-needles, and their use represents a suitable option for histopathological evaluation of diffuse parenchymal disease in critically ill patients with an increased risk of complications, e.g., in the presence of coagulation disorders. The complication rate of FNA is significantly lower than for a 17 gauge (diameter 1.4 mm) Menghini needle (Glaser et al., 1995). However, even the 16 gauge (diameter 1.6 mm) Menghini needle is considered safe in liver transplant patients (Lang et al., 1999).

Biopsy of Solid Lesions

In principle, any focus amenable for sonographic visualization is a potential target for biopsy, depending on the risk-benefit analysis. This analysis has to include the above conditions to be met by the patient as well as the risks and contraindications mentioned below. In most cases, a 19 gauge (diameter 1 mm) needle or smaller, i.e., fine needle, will suffice. Needles of 21 or 20 gauge (diameter 0.8 mm and 0.9 mm, respectively) are commonly used.

The procedure must be expected to have a significant impact on further management. Lesions to be resected by surgery no matter what the result of the biopsy should not be biopsied. FNA can, however, frequently accelerate diagnostic workup by obviating additional imaging procedures, if performed as the immediate next step after imaging has demonstrated a suspected lesion.

The Histopathological Result in Context

In general, evaluation of benignancy vs. malignancy is easier than histological typing and determination of the primary. While confirmation of malignancy has a specificity of almost 100%, malignancy cannot be definitively ruled out by FNA cytology. Reported sensitivities of FNA for diagnosing malignancy range from 60% to 100%. In centers with extensive experience, rates of 90% have become routine (Holtkamp et al., 1990; Weiss and Duntsch, 1996). The role of FNA cytology and histopathology cannot be assessed in general; it depends on the various organs and diseases (see corresponding chapters). For example, the diagnostic sensitivity for pancreatic cancer is usually lower, at 70–80%, than the rate of around 90% for other abdominal organs (Holtkamp et al., 1990). Possible technical errors resulting in a false-negative diagnosis include missing the target, insufficient specimen volume, or the collection of exclusively necrotic material, most common in tumors with central necrosis. Larger tumors should therefore be biopsied near their outer margins. Histopathological assessment of a malignant lesion may present a problem, for instance, when it comes to differentiating malignancy from chronic inflammation (e.g., chronic pancreatitis) or epithelial regeneration (e.g., in hepatic cirrhosis). Thus, the pathologist would prefer also to have samples of tissue remote from the lesion, e.g., when dealing with hepatic masses.

When pooling the experience gained for various organs, the success rate of correct typing averages about 70% (Wernecke et al., 1991). Cancer is easier to diagnose in FNA samples than lymphoma or mesenchymal tumors. Typing and grading of lymphoma based on FNA alone is not possible, but usually requires excisional lymph node biopsy. Ultimately, a comprehensive review of all clinical, laboratory, and imaging findings will determine whether the FNA result can be regarded as definitive diagnosis.

Risks

The most important and most frequent complications are pain, hemorrhage, infection, and, in case of malignancy, needle track seeding. This can be compounded by organ-specific complications, including pancreatitis, pneumothorax, and abortion. The risk of organ injury, especially hemorrhage, increases with the diameter of the needle (Glaser et al., 1995; McGill et al., 1990; Menghini, 1970; Weiss et al., 1988). The very low complication rates reported for diagnostic punctures have only been verified for fine needles (Table 5.**2**). Hemorrhage accounts for over three-quarters of severe complications after fine-needle aspiration and biopsy, excluding pneumothorax and abortion. More than 90% of all bleeding episodes are seen in liver procedures, but this also reflects the frequency per se of the liver as a target organ. Hemorrhage after hepatic procedures accounts for the majority of all lethal complications, followed by pancreatitis.

Needle track seeding has been reported for various organs and malignancies. The most recent poll by DEGUM (German Association of Ultrasound in Medicine) revealed an incidence of 0.0063% (6 cases in 95 070 procedures). According to this report, needle track seeding is significantly more common with large-caliber than with fine-needles.

Minimizing Risk by Proper Selection of Target Site and Needle Track

Needles may not safely transverse the following organs without subsequent damage, and thus adequate precautions must be taken to prevent entry of the needle.

- Heart: Injury of coronary vessels results in hemopericardium. Pericardiocentesis requires real-time monitoring of the entire procedure.
- Larger vessels, and aneurysms in particular: Fluid filled structures should be checked by color-flow Doppler imaging for possible perfusion or adjacent blood vessels. For example, splenic artery aneurysm should be ruled out prior to aspiration of a suspected pancreatic cyst. Although the epigastric artery cannot be demonstrated by

the probes commonly used in transabdominal sonography, the normal anatomical course should be taken into account when performing paracentesis or biopsy.
- Lungs: The needle track into organs such as the liver and spleen must be planned in such a way that it will not traverse any lung tissue even under maximum respiratory motion. Sonographically visualized pulmonary lesions with unequivocal adherence between parietal and visceral pleura may be punctured with impunity, as well as pleural processes themselves. If the risk of pneumothorax is low, pulmonary lesions are also amenable to CT-guided percutaneous biopsies.
- Central nervous system and larger nerves: Nerve injuries are rare.
- Hydatid cysts: Due of the risk of dissemination and anaphylactic shock, they may be aspirated–if at all–only after pretreatment with anthelmintics.
- Pheochromocytoma: As biopsy can induce hypertensive crisis, it should only be performed after adequate diagnostic workup and appropriate pretreatment (see Adrenal Glands, p. 214).
- Peripheral hepatic and splenic lesions: The needle track should traverse at least 1 cm of healthy tissue.
- Intra-abdominal organs in the presence of ascites: Coagulation is impaired by the plasminogen activators, among others, found in ascites. This contraindication is relative and should be weighed against the potential benefits of the procedure.
- Lesions at risk for infection through access via nonsterile tissue: This is particularly relevant when intestinal structures must be traversed before sterile fluid collections can be aspirated.

FNA of mural lesions in the GI tract is regarded as a safe procedure. It is indicated particularly in those situations where the pathological process cannot be accessed by endoscopy (e.g., in the small bowel or in severe stenosis of the upper colon (Carson et al., 1998). Omental invasion can be biopsied safely and easily (Sistrom et al., 1992).

Aspiration of the gallbladder for evaluation of cholecystic masses (Wu et al., 1996) or for treatment of cholecystitis involves the risk of bile leakage. However, this risk is rather low if transhepatic access into the body of the gallbladder is sought, as the gallbladder usually adheres to the liver in this area.

The right adrenal gland and pancreas must in some cases also be approached through the liver (Fröhlich et al., 1995; Teichgräber et al., 2000). In biopsies of the left adrenal gland, the spleen should be spared, if at all possible.

Although FNA biopsy of splenic masses carries a higher inherent risk of hemorrhage, a large study still found this procedure to be low in complications (Venkataramu et al., 1999).

In pancreatic biopsies one has to weigh the risk of induced acute pancreatitis. This risk is rather low, as long as pancreatic masses are sampled rather than normal parenchyma.

Cooperating with the Pathologist

The issue of FNA cytology versus biopsy is still not settled in the literature (Brown et al., 1993; Di Stasi et al., 1998). One option would be to combine both techniques, e.g., by employing a coaxial system. The pathologist should be involved in the decision-making process from the very outset. With the ongoing improvements in the design of needles for FNA biopsy, this technique will be increasingly favored.

The tissue cylinder is fixed in formalin immediately upon collection; if desired, it can be rolled on a slide beforehand for cytology.

Cytological samples are smeared on slides and air-dried or fixed while wet. In order to obtain material for cytology from fluids, the specimens are centrifuged. The type of fixation should also be specified by the pathologist. Ideally, cytological material would be collected in the presence of a partner experienced in cytology who can immediately assess the quantity and quality of the sample.

Table 5.**2** Complication rates in FNA procedures

Reference	Country and Year of Study	Complication Rate	Mortality		
		Percentage	Number of Cases	Percentage	Number of Cases
Smith (1984)	1983, USA			0.006	4/63108
Smith (1991)	1986/1987, USA			0.031	5/16381
Fornari et al. (1989)	1979–1987, Italy	0.18	20/10766	0.018	2/10766
Nolsoe et al. (1990)	1970,1990, Denmark	0.2	7/3500	0.028	1/3500
Weiss et al. (1988)	1988, Germany	0.55*	337/60949	0.0075	5/60949
Weiss and Duntsch (1996)	1996, Germany	0.81*	765/95070	0.0011	1/95070

* Major and minor complications pooled.

Principles of Drainage in Surgery

In the treatment of intra-abdominal abscess and fluid collection, interventional percutaneous drainage frequently offers an excellent alternative to the common surgical approach. Owing to the rapid development of sonography into an extremely sensitive instrument for diagnosis and guidance in interventions, percutaneous drainage has often become possible without radiation exposure, and even as a bedside procedure in the severely ill patient in the ICU. The successful realization of percutaneous drainage procedures requires comprehensive knowledge of the indications, contraindications, and limitations of this method, which is far less invasive than open surgery.

Basic Background

- Indications reported in the literature cover a rather broad spectrum and are centered on the abdomen, chest, and retroperitoneal space (Table 5.**3**).
- Principal indications in general surgery: postoperative intra-abdominal abscess formation, biloma, and pleural effusion.
- Intra-abdominal abscess: following various abdominal procedures, with a reported incidence of 11% after ileal pouch-anal anastomosis, 6.9% after liver resection, and 2.6% after open appendectomy for perforated appendicitis (Mathey et al., 1993; Paik et al., 1997; Xing et al., 1995).
- Typical abscess localizations in general surgery: Table 5.**4**
- If possible, written informed consent should be obtained from the patient. In elective drainage procedures, this should take place at least 24 hours prior to the intervention.
- General conditions:
  - Quick's PT assay > 50%
  - PTT not prolonged
  - Platelets > 100 000/μl
  - Low-dose heparin does not constitute a contraindication (drains may still be placed with poor coagulation parameters, but will then have a presumed higher risk of complication).
- Equipment:
  - Aspiration-dedicated probe or convex scanner (freehand technique), skin preparation, sterile draping.
  - Local anesthetic, scalpel (no. 11 blade), long aspiration needle, disposable syringe.
  - Sterile drainage kit (e.g., Medi-tech, Boston Scientific Corporation) either for guide wire exchange (Seldinger) or trocar technique, with different size drains (8–14 French).
  - Sutures, sterile needle holder, sterile scissors, dressings, sterile gloving.

Table 5.**3** Possible surgical indications for US-guided percutaneous therapeutic drainage

Postoperative intra-abdominal abscess
Liver abscess
Splenic abscess
Abscess in left-sided diverticular disease of the colon
Pleural and pulmonary abscess
Tubo-ovarian and other pelvic abscess
Appendicular abscess
Retroperitoneal abscess (psoas abscess, perirenal abscess)
Biloma
Pleural effusion
Postoperative intra-abdominal fluid collection
Pancreatic pseudocyst, symptomatic hepatic cyst
Percutaneous transhepatic cholangiography and drainage (PTCD)
Renal puncture (percutaneous nephrostomy; PCN)
Aspiration of ascites

Table 5.**4** Typical abscess localizations (modified from Jansen et al. 1999; $n = 62$)

Subdiaphragmatic on the left	29%
Subhepatic	29%
Intrahepatic	18%
Paracolic	10%
Pouch of Douglas/small pelvis	6%
Subdiaphragmatic on the right	5%
Retroperitoneal	3%

  - Sedatives (e.g., midazolam) and/or analgesics may be useful.
- Applicable techniques (Figs. 5.**6**, 5.**7**):
  - In the freehand technique, the needle can be placed perpendicular or almost perpendicular to the ultrasound beam, which improves needle visualization to the point where almost its entire length will become visible.
  - The trocar technique is faster, but should be reserved for superficial lesions adhering extensively to the abdominal wall.

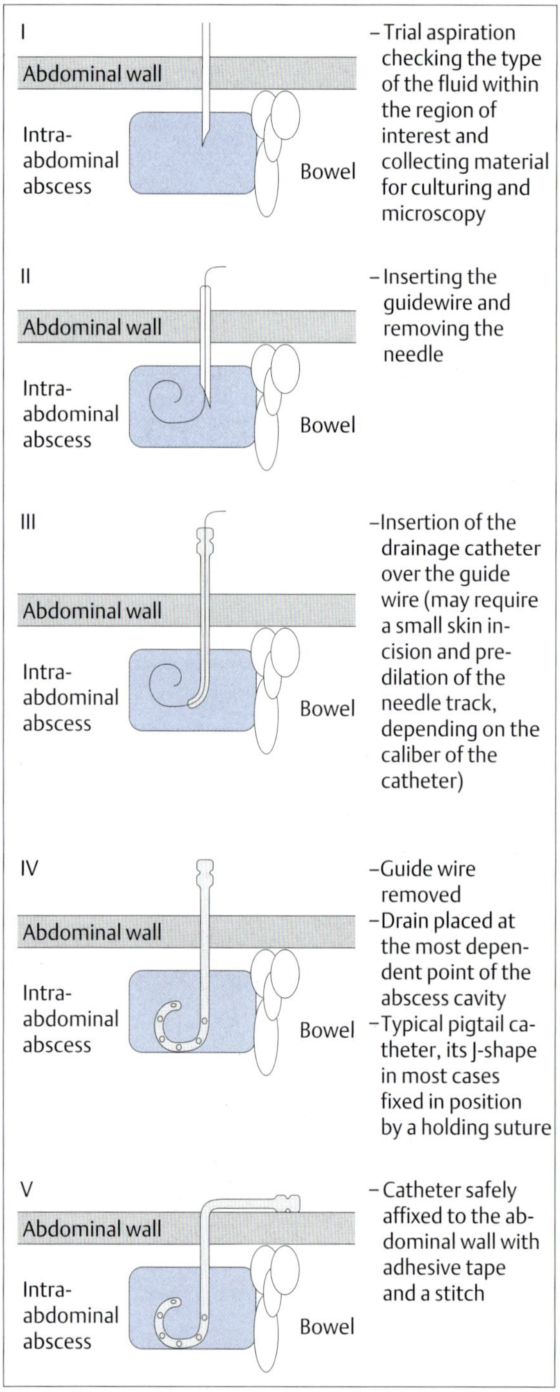

Fig. 5.**6** Drainage placement in the guide wire exchange (Seldinger) technique.

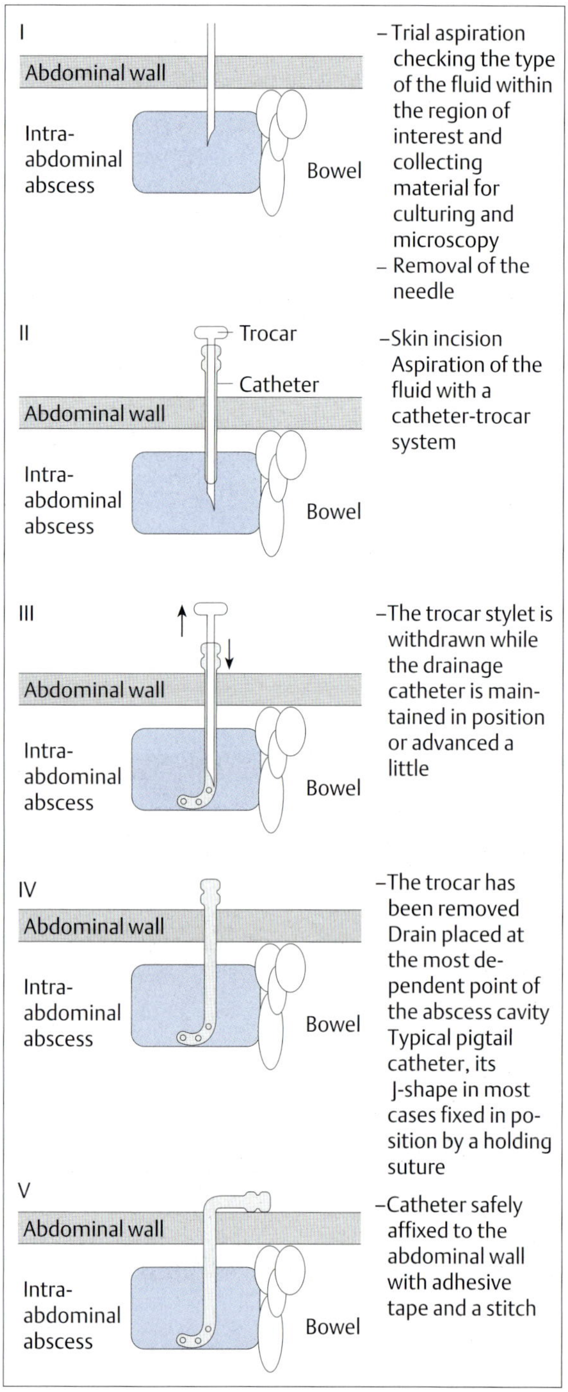

Fig. 5.**7** Drainage placement in the trocar technique.

– After insertion of the needle, the abscess cavity is irrigated with saline until clear fluid only is aspirated.
– Insert needle insertion during breath holding.
– Compared with diagnostic punctures, in drainage procedures no other organs should be traversed at all (possible risk of seeding contaminated material).

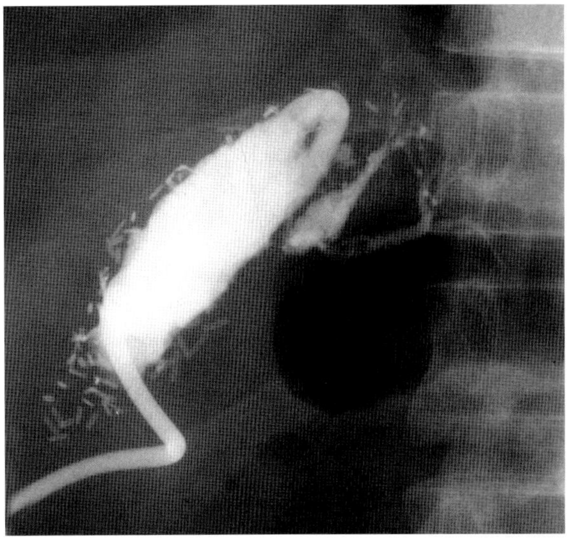

Fig. 5.**8a** Infected subhepatic biloma 2 weeks following left hemihepatectomy for Caroli disease. The abscess cavity is filled with contrast agent after US-guided pigtail catheter insertion; the fistula with the biliary tree causing the superinfected biloma is clearly delineated.

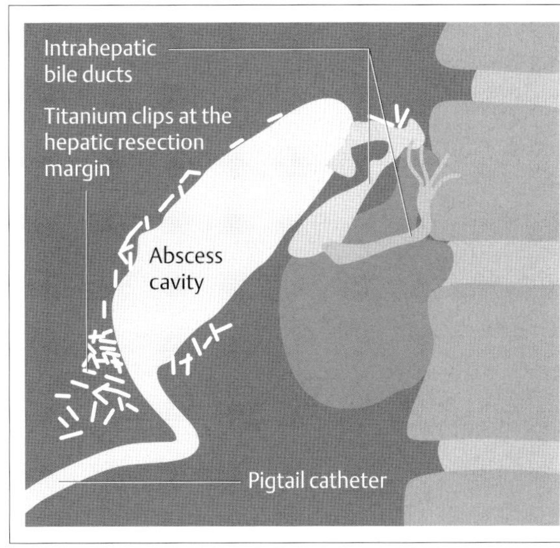

Fig. 5.**8b** Line drawing.

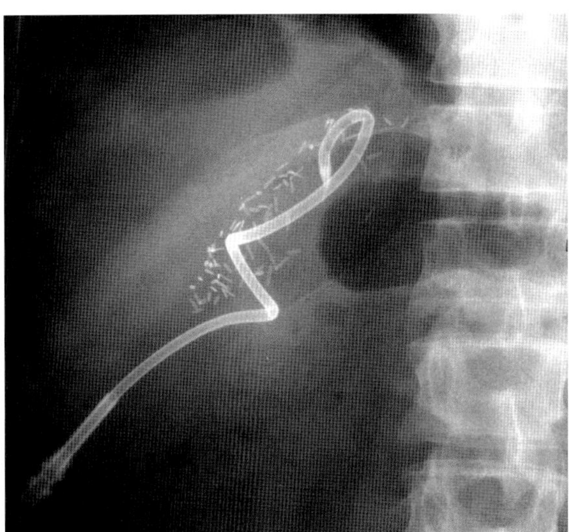

Fig. 5.**9a** Radiographic visualization of the pigtail catheter without contrast enhancement; on comparison with the subsequent contrast study, the tip should be placed in a more posteroinferior position, if possible.

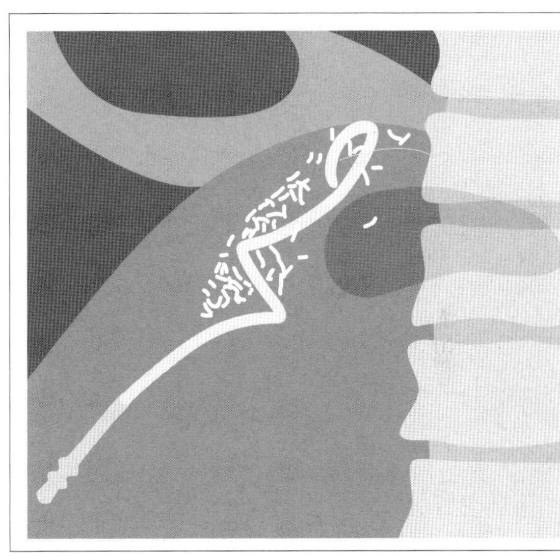

Fig. 5.**9b** Line drawing.

- The position of the drain and any possible fistula with the GI tract is confirmed by contrast-enhanced fluoroscopy with a water-soluble agent (Figs. 5.**8**, 5.**9**).
- Depending on the viscosity and type of secretion, the abscess cavity is irrigated once or twice daily with sterile saline; apart from the rinsing effect per se, this prevents occlusion of the drainage tubes.
- Abscess cavities should be irrigated 3 to 5 times per day (possibly even with an antiseptic solution).
- In case of systemic reaction to an abscess, treatment should be expanded by an antibiotic regimen; following successful drainage of the abscess the fever should abate, the WBC should start to fall, and the patient should exhibit signs of general recovery.

Table 5.**5** Potential complications in percutaneous drainage

Hemorrhage
Induction of sepsis
Perforation of the abscess membrane with diffuse intra-abdominal spread of pus
Pneumothorax
Skin infections
Dislocation or occlusion of the catheter
Organ perforation
Recurrent abscess formation after catheter removal

- The drainage kits vary in terms of the maximum permissible duration of catheter placement as well as the manufacturer's instructions to be followed in removal.
- Drainage related complications: Table 5.**5**.
- Sonography will detect abscess formations in the upper abdomen, pelvis, and retroperitoneal space with a sensitivity of about 90%, with significantly lower levels for bowel loop abscesses.
- Suspicion of an abscess/septic focus mandates examination of the entire abdomen including the pelvis. Anastomotic failure, central venous line sepsis, wound infection, pneumonia, and urinary tract infection must be considered as possible alternative causes of fever and elevated WBC.
- Computed tomography (with oral and possibly intravenous contrast enhancement) is superior to sonography in the diagnosis of intra-abdominal abscess formation, and should be undertaken if the sonographic findings are equivocal, or if inflammatory signs persist despite drainage. Under certain circumstances, CT guidance may be safer for placement of a pigtail catheter.
- The typical limitations of sonographic evaluation, including extreme obesity, intestinal gas, and bowel obstruction or ileus, may render ultrasound-guided drainage impossible.
- Treatment of nonseptated, well-delimited intra-abdominal abscess formations achieves overall success rates of 80–90% (Table 5.**6**).
- Consideration of the indication for interventional therapeutic drainage must include the localization, etiology, and morphology of the area to be drained as well as the clinical signs and physical condition of the patient (Table 5.**7**).
- Mortality rates by technique as reported in the literature: 0% (Jansen et al., 1999; Civardi et al., 1998; $n = 948$), <1% (Göhl et al., 1999).
- Mean duration of treatment was 9–30 days (Bouali et al., 1993; Göhl et al., 1999; Jansen et al., 1999); Bouali et al. found a mean interval of 17 days between surgery and interventional drainage in 121 patients. In 14% drainage did not suffice and reoperation became necessary; 33% of the patients required several drains inserted either simultaneously or in subsequent interventions. Perforations of small and large bowel were without consequence, as the needles were withdrawn as soon as this complication was recognized.
- Double-lumen drains may be inserted, permitting continuous irrigation and aspiration.
- The better results obtained with continuous drainage of abscess formations favor this technique over one-time aspiration.
- Assessing the type of fluid involved: Trial puncture before drain insertion is useful to elucidate the type of fluid in a symptomatic serous collection without signs of infection; here, one-time aspiration may be sufficient.
- The shrinking abscess cavity can be followed up by sonography and/or contrast-enhanced radiography.
- Abscess cavities should be irrigated until the returning solution is almost clear; before removal, the inserted tube is used only for spontaneous drainage (a small amount of saline should still be instilled daily to ascertain patency of the tubing).
- Therapeutic drains may be removed once the daily volume of secretion has dropped significantly (to < 10–20 ml/day) or has subsided completely, in parallel with a significant reduction in the size of the abscess cavity. Prior to removal of the drain, the exudate must be clear and there must be no clinical evidence of persisting infection.

Special Indications

- **Cyst:** Primarily symptomatic cysts (in liver, spleen, kidney, and pancreas) may also be treated by aspiration, even though by definition they are invested with epithelium possessing potential secretory ability. If they persist, particularly in the liver, injection of highly concentrated ethanol may be attempted (removing about ⅓ of the cyst contents and replacing it with the ethanol, followed 15–20 minutes later by complete evacuation of the contents).

Table 5.**6** Reported success and complication rates in percutaneous abdominal drainage

Author/Year	Patients (*n*)	Success Rate (%)	Complication Rate (%)
Van Sonnenberg et al. (1984)	250	836	104
Civardi et al. (1998)	886	904	66
Jansen et al. (1999)	62	85	64

Table 5.7 Indications for therapeutic drainage (adapted from Göhl et al. 1999)

	Favorable Conditions	Unfavorable Conditions
Localization	Subhepatic, subdiaphragmatic, intrahepatic, retroperitoneal, small pelvis, and paracolic retentions easily accessible	Completely surrounded by vessels or bowel; abscess without direct access from the abdominal wall
Etiology	Postoperative abscess and other symptomatic fluid collection, such as seroma, lymphocele, retained secretions at resection margins of the pancreas and liver as well as in the small pelvis	Primary hollow viscus perforation or extensive postoperative anastomotic breakdown without diversion ostomy
Morphology	Liquid formations on imaging, homogeneous, lacking septation, no communication with any other structure	Organized formations without significant liquid parts, encapsulated retentions with multiple septation, sequestration

- **Pleural effusion/empyema:** Pleural effusion in the posterior costodiaphragmatic recess can be sized quite well by sonography, which thus may contribute to the decision for or against thoracentesis. The sonograms can then be used to optimize the access route, minimizing possible complications of pleural punctures (see Chapters 4 and 8).
  - In US-guided thoracentesis as well, the needle must always be advanced over the upper margin of the rib in order to avoid possible injury to the intercostal neurovascular bundle.
  - The success rate of 70–80% in interventional treatment of pleural empyemas by drain insertion and irrigation resembles that in abscesses.
- **Biloma:** Bilomas may appear after hepatic and biliary surgery or trauma. They may become symptomatic by sheer mass, peritoneal irritation, or superinfection. Local limitation is similar to that of an abscess, but bilomas are always closely related to the surgical field as they form by bile leaking from the biliary tree.
  - The diagnostic and therapeutic protocol is identical to that for an intra-abdominal abscess.
  - In addition to radiography of its cavity with contrast enhancement via the inserted drainage catheter, localization of the leak should be attempted.
  - If the leak cannot be pin-pointed and there is persistent bile leakage: diagnostic/therapeutic endoscopic retrograde cholangiography (ERC) is advised.
- **Percutaneous transhepatic cholangiodrainage (PTCD):** If the bile cannot be diverted from the leak by ERC and stenting of the duct, employ transabdominal US-guided (TAUS) drainage of the bile duct system.
  - Following localization and aspiration, preferably of the left hepatic duct, and fluoroscopy with a water-soluble contrast agent, a guide wire is advanced into the extrahepatic bile duct system. After dilation, a drainage catheter is introduced for external bile drainage.
  - If the bile duct obstruction can be passed with the guide wire, a self-expanding metal stent can be deployed, reestablishing internal drainage along the physiological pathway (only in malignancy!).
- *Additional workup:* contrast-enhanced CT, MRI, contrast-enhanced radiography of the abscess cavity.

Sonographic Criteria

- An abscess has a markedly heterogeneous echotexture, is locally circumscribed and hypoechoic, and is sometimes surrounded with an abscess membrane. It may exhibit floating internal echoes and gas bubbles, which appear as small hyperechoic structures. In longer-standing abscesses, a larger fraction of particulate debris is encountered inside the abscess cavity (Figs. 4.**10**, 5.**10**, 5.**11**).
- Bilomas commonly present as ovoid anechoic fluid collections, similar to seromas; suspicion is based on history and localization, and confirmation is obtained by aspiration (Fig. 5.**12**).
- The route of access must be selected and measured prior to any aspiration.
- After insertion, needle placement must be checked sonographically (Fig. 5.**13**).
- Placement of the catheter is also checked sonographically (Fig. 5.**14**).
- A seroma is seen as a circumscribed anechoic mass. Definitive diagnosis requires aspiration.
- Hematomas exhibit different characteristics depending on their age. Fresh hematomas are hypoechoic to anechoic. They later become heterogeneous with both hypoechoic and hyperechoic parts (Fig. 5.**15**).

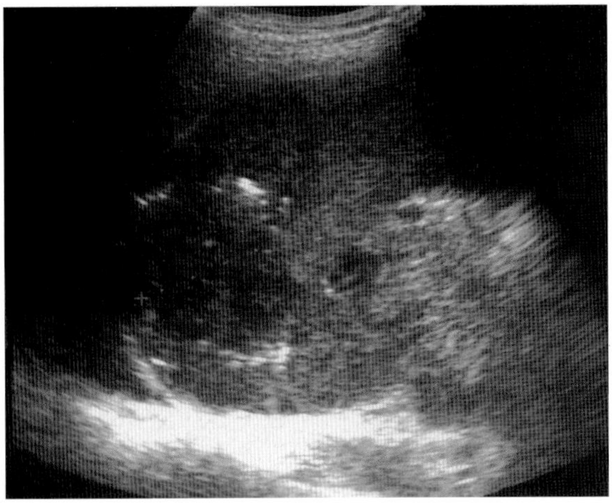

Fig. 5.**10 a** Round 46 mm heterogeneous splenic abscess in a sepsis patient. This usually requires splenectomy, although drainage alone may suffice in selected cases.

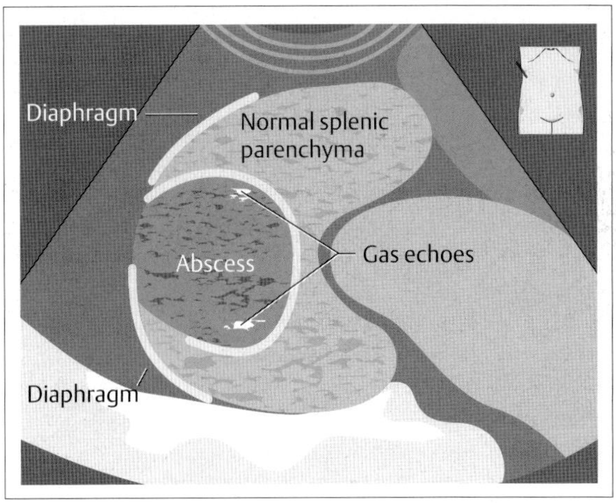

Fig. 5.**10 b** Line drawing.

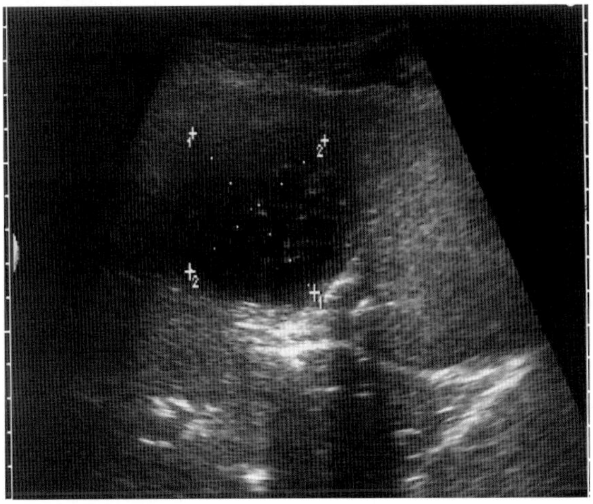

Fig. 5.**11 a** Heterogeneous 6 cm abscess in the left hepatic lobe with floating internal echoes and gas bubbles, prior to pigtail catheter drainage.

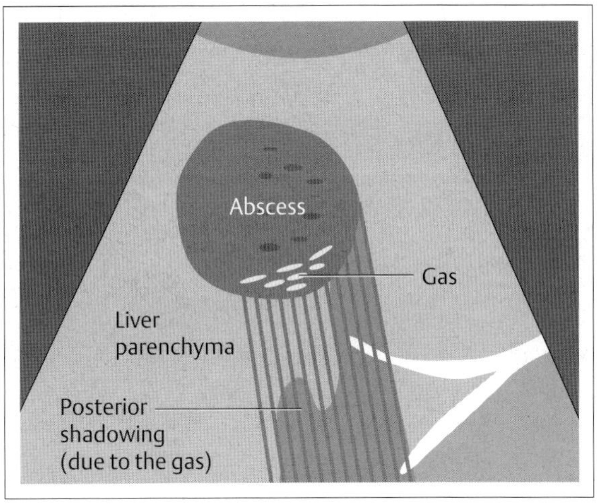

Fig. 5.**11 b** Line drawing.

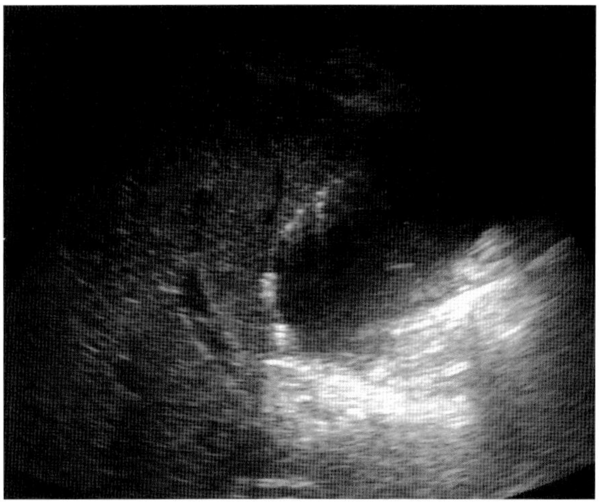

Fig. 5.12 a Large biloma of about 4 × 9 cm, two weeks after left hemihepatectomy–hypoechoic formation in relation to the margin of resection.

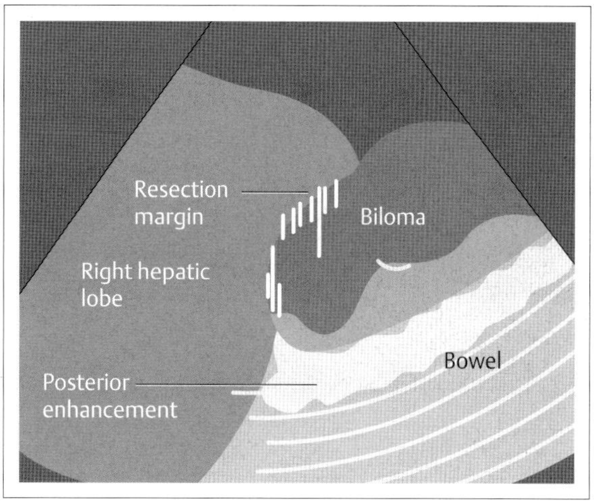

Fig. 5.12 b Line drawing.

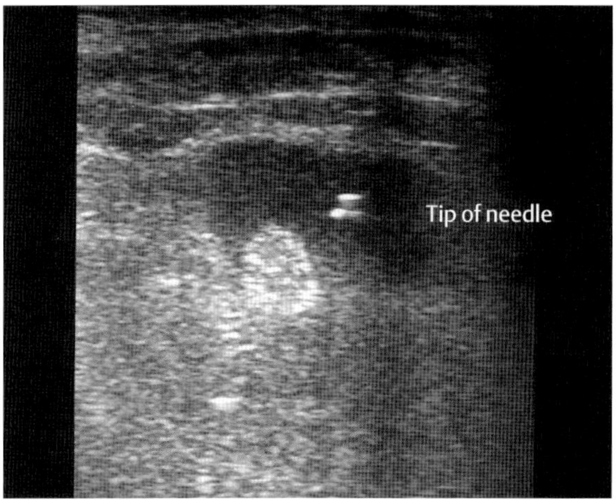

Fig. 5.13 a The biloma of Fig. 5.8, now with central needle through which a guide wire may be advanced for the Seldinger technique. The anechoic liquid formation adheres to the abdominal wall.

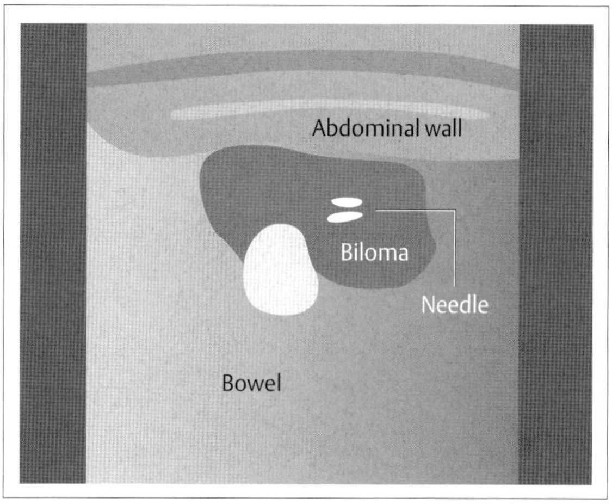

Fig. 5.13 b Line drawing.

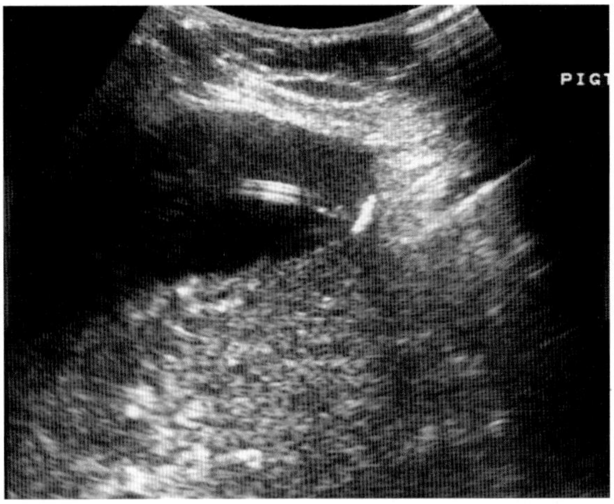

Fig. 5.**14 a** Placement control of the pigtail catheter after drainage of a biloma adhering to the abdominal wall.

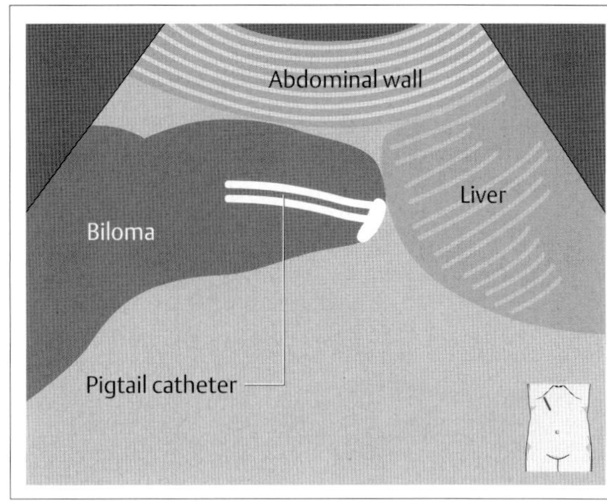

Fig. 5.**14 b** Line drawing.

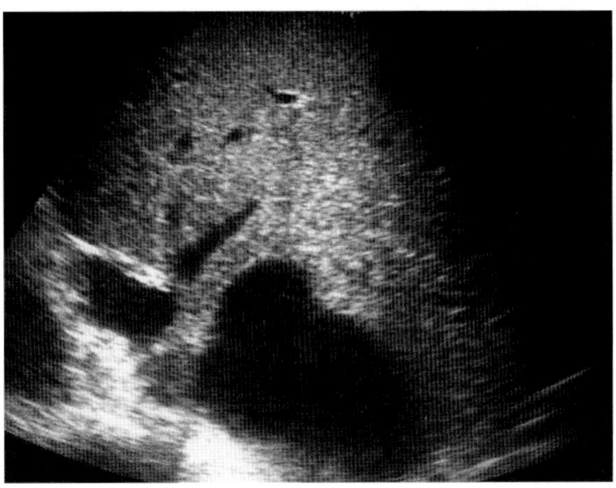

Fig. 5.**15 a** Anechoic homogeneous paracaval hematoma of 5 cm, 12 hours after liver transplantation.

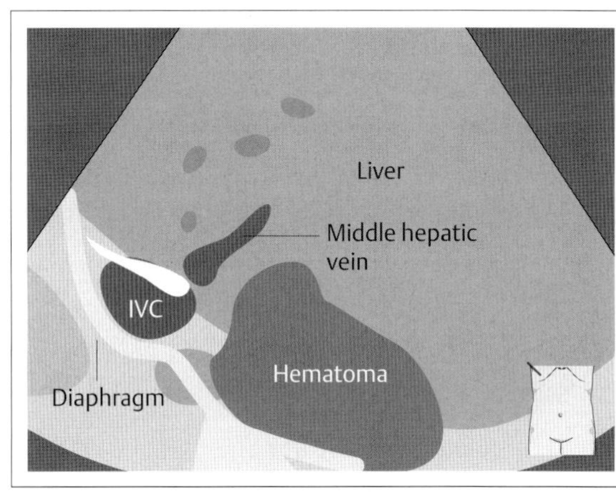

Fig. 5.**15 b** Line drawing.

Consequences for Surgical Treatment

Diagnosis	Characteristic Findings	Management
Cyst	Symptomatic in liver, pancreas, spleen, and kidney; unequivocal findings without evidence of a cystadenoma or malignancy	Therapeutic aspiration (elevated CA19-9 in the cyst fluid is suspicious of cystadenoma). In recurrences, in particular of hepatic cysts, ethanol (99.5%) injection, surgical ablation, or for pancreatic cysts internal drainage, are possible
Intra-abdominal abscess	Well defined, unilocular, or only partially septated, accessible without risk, possibly related to a small anastomotic leak	Percutaneous drainage with a pigtail catheter, in case of systemic reactions supplemented by antibiotics
Intra-abdominal abscess	Bowel loop abscess, infected necrotic tumor, multilocular abscess (hydatid disease, ameboma), large organized infected hematoma, infected pancreatic necrosis, abscess due to extensive anastomotic breakdown, previously unsuccessful attempts at intervention	Classical surgical evacuation with the advantages of safe access and possible causal therapy and/or necrectomy, in case of systemic reactions supplemented by antibiotics
Biloma	Symptomatic (local peritoneal irritation, infection clinically presenting like an abscess), due to lesion of small bile ducts, locally limited process without peritonitis	Percutaneous drainage, ERC with papillotomy, and possibly stenting to decrease outflow resistance, perhaps administration of octreotide
Biloma	Symptomatic (local peritoneal irritation, infection clinically presenting like an abscess), due to partial lesion of larger intra- and extrahepatic bile ducts, locally limited process without peritonitis	Percutaneous drainage, ERC with papillotomy, and possibly stenting to decrease outflow resistance or for bridging the leak, possibly attempt at surgical repair in case of persisting leakage In case of peritonitis, surgical revision becomes mandatory

Bibliography

Bouali K, Magotteaux P, Jadot A, Saive C, Fontaine F. Percutaneous catheter drainage of abdominal abscess after abdominal surgery. Results in 121 cases. J Belge Radiol. 1993; 76 (1): 11–4.

Brown KT, Fulbright RK, Avitabile AM, Bashist B. Cytological analysis in fine-needle aspiration biopsy: smears vs. cell blocks. Am J Roentgenol. 1993; 161: 629–31.

Carson BW, Brown JA, Cooperberg PL. Ultrasonographically guided percutaneous biopsy of gastric, small bowel, and colonic abnormalities: efficacy and safety. J Ultrasound Med. 1998; 17: 739–42.

Caturelli E, Giacobbe A, Facciorusso D, et al. Percutaneous biopsy in diffuse liver disease: increasing diagnostic yield and decreasing complication rate by routine ultrasound assessment of puncture site. Am J Gastroenterol. 1996; 91: 1318–21.

Chan R, Common AA, Marcuzzi D. Ultrasound-guided renal biopsy: experience using an automated core biopsy system. Can Assoc Radiol J. 2000; 51: 107–13.

Civardi G, Di Candio G, Giorgio A, et al. Ultrasound guided percutaneous drainage of abdominal abscesses in the hands of a clinician: a multicenter Italian study. Eur J Ultrasound. 1998; 8(2): 91–9.

Daltrey IR, Kissin MW. Randomized clinical trial of the effect of needle gauge and local anaesthetic on the pain of breast fine-needle aspiration cytology. Br J Surg. 2000; 87: 777–9.

Dameron RD, deLong DM, Fisher AJ, deLong DM, Dodd LG, Nelson RC. Indeterminate findings on imaging-guided biopsy: should additional intervention be pursued? Am J Roentgenol. 1999; 173: 461–4.

Di Stasi M, Lencioni R, Solmi L, et al. Ultrasound-guided fine needle biopsy of pancreatic masses: results of a multicenter study. Am J Gastroenterol. 1998; 93: 1329–33.

Fornari F, Civardi G, Cavanna L, et al. Complications of ultrasonically guided fine-needle abdominal biopsy. Results of a multicenter Italian study and review of the literature. The Cooperative Italian Study Group. Scand J Gastroenterol. 1989; 24: 949–55.

Fröhlich E, Rufle W, Strunk H, Stuckmann G, Seeliger H. Stellenwert der Feinnadelpunktion bei Nebennierentumoren. Ultraschall Med. 1995; 16: 90–3.

Glaser J, Mann O, von Eiff M, Pfahlberg A, Pausch J. Inzidenz sonographisch nachweisbarer Leberhämatome nach ultraschallgezielter Feinnadelpunktion mit der 0, 95-mm-Schneidbiopsiekanüle im Vergleich zur perkutanen Leberbiopsie mit der 1, 4-mm-Menghini-Nadel. Med Klin. 1995; 90: 131–3.

Glaser J, Pausch J. Zur Frage des Risikos von Leberbiopsien. Z Gastroenterol. 1995; 33: 673–6.

Göhl J, Gmeinwieser J, Gusinde J. Intra-abdominelle Abszesse. Zentralbl Chir. 1999, 124: 187–94.

Greiner L, Franken FH. Die sonographisch assistierte Leberbiopsie. Dtsch Med Wochenschr. 1983; 108: 368–72.

Herget EJ, Saliken JC, Donnelly BJ, Gray RR, Wiseman D, Brunet G. Transrectal ultrasound-guided biopsy of the prostate: relation between ASA use and bleeding complications. Can Assoc Radiol J. 1999; 50: 173–6.

Holtkamp W, Theilmeier A, Droese M, Ebert R, Reis HE. Ultraschallgesteuerte Feinnadelpunktion. Grenzen der Methode im Abdomen und Retroperitonealraum. Dtsch Med Wochenschr. 1990; 115: 809–12.

Jansen M, Truong S, Riesener KP, Sparenberg P, Schumpelick V. Ergebnisse der sonographisch-gesteuerten percutanen Drainage intra-abdomineller Abszesse im chirurgischen Alltag. Chirurg. 1999, 70: 1168–71.

Jeffrey RB Jr. Coaxial technique for CT-guided biopsy of deep retroperitoneal lymph nodes. Gastrointest Radiol. 1988; 13: 271–2.

Judmaier G, Prior C, Klimpfinger M, et al. Ist die perkutane Leberbiopsie mit der Trucut(Travenol)-Nadel der Menghini-Punktion überlegen? Z Gastroenterol. 1989; 27: 657–61.

Lang M, Neumann UP, Muller AR, Bechstein WO, Neuhaus R, Neuhaus P. Komplikationen der perkutanen Leberbiopsie bei Patienten nach Lebertransplantation. Z Gastroenterol. 1999; 37: 205–8.

Lindor KD, Bru C, Jorgensen RA, et al. The role of ultrasonography and automatic-needle biopsy in outpatient percutaneous liver biopsy. Hepatology. 1996; 23: 1079–83.

Mathey P, Ambrosetti P, Morel P, et al. The Swiss experience of ileo-anal anastomosis with reservoir. Complications and functional results. Ann Chir 1993; 47(10): 1020–5.

McGill DB, Rakela J, Zinsmeister AR, Ott BJ. A 21-year-experience with major hemorrhage after percutaneous liver biopsy. Gastroenterology. 1990; 99: 1396–400.

Melotti MK, Berg WA. Core needle breast biopsy in patients undergoing anticoagulation therapy: preliminary results. Am J Roentgenol. 2000; 174: 245–9.

Menghini G. One-second biopsy of the liver–problems of its clinical application. N Engl J Med. 1970; 283: 582–5.

Nass K, O'Neill WC. Bedside renal biopsy: ultrasound guidance by the nephrologist. Am J Kidney Dis. 1999; 34: 955–9.

Nolsoe C, Nielsen L, Torp-Pedersen S, Holm HH. Major complications and deaths due to interventional ultrasonography: a review of 8000 cases. J Clin Ultrasound. 1990; 18: 179–84.

Nyman RS, Cappelen-Smith J, Suhaibani H, et al. Yield and complications in percutaneous renal biopsy. A comparison between ultrasound-guided gun-biopsy and manual techniques in native and transplant kidneys. Acta Radiol. 1997; 38: 431–6.

Paik PS, Towson JA, Anthone GJ, Ortega AE, Simons AJ, Beart RW Jr. Intra-abdominal abscesses following laparoscopic and open appendectomies. J Gastrointest Surg. 1997; 1(2): 188–93.

Peterson P, Hayes TE, Arkin CF, et al. The preoperative bleeding time test lacks clinical benefit: College of American Pathologists' and American Society of Clinical Pathologists' position article. Arch Surg. 1998; 133: 134–9.

Piccinino F, Sagnelli E, Pasquale G, Giusti G. Complications following percutaneous liver biopsy. A multicentre retrospective study on 68, 276 biopsies. J Hepatol. 1986; 2: 165–73.

Reddy KR, Jeffers LJ. Evaluation of the liver. B: Liver biopsy and laparoscopy. In: Schiff ER, ed. Schiff's diseases of the liver. Philadelphia: Lippincott-Raven; 1999: 245–65.

Riley TR III. How often does ultrasound marking change the liver biopsy site? Am J Gastroenterol. 1999; 94: 3320–2.

Schafer AI. Effects of nonsteroidal anti-inflammatory therapy on platelets. Am J Med. 1999; 106: 25S–36S.

Sheafor DH, Paulson EK, Simmons CM, deLong DM, Nelson RC. Abdominal percutaneous interventional procedures: comparison of CT and US guidance. Radiology. 1998; 207: 705–10.

Shiffman ML, Farrel MT, Yee YS. Risk of bleeding after endoscopic biopsy or polypectomy in patients taking aspirin or other NSAIDS. Gastrointest Endosc. 1994; 40: 458–62.

Sistrom CL, Abbitt PL, Feldman PS. Ultrasound guidance for biopsy of omental abnormalities. J Clin Ultrasound. 1992; 20: 27–36.

Skamel HJ, Hanusch A, Mathias K. CT-gesteuerte Punktionen: Feinnadel-Aspirations-Biopsie versus automatisierte koaxiale Schneid-Biopsie. Aktuelle Radiol. 1998; 8: 273–7.

Smith EH. The hazards of fine-needle aspiration biopsy. Ultrasound Med Biol. 1984; 10: 629–34.

Smith EH. Complications of percutaneous abdominal fine-needle biopsy. Review. Radiology. 1991; 178: 253–8.

Teichgräber UK, Benter T, Schultz HJ, Kluhs L, Gutberlet M, Felix R. Ultraschallgesteuerte Punktionstechnik von zentral-venösen Gefäßen in Ein-Personen-Technik. Ultraschall Med. 2000; 21: 132–6.

Tikkakoski T, Ta-avitsainen M, Paivansalo M, Lahde S, Apaja-Sarkkinen M. Accuracy of adrenal biopsy guided by ultrasound and CT. Acta Radiol. 1991; 32: 371–4.

Venkataramu NK, Gupta S, Sood BP, K et al. Ultrasound guided fine needle aspiration biopsy of splenic lesions. Br J Radiol. 1999; 72: 953–6.

Wagner T. ASS und das operative Risiko. Internist. 1998; 39: 220.

Weiss H, Duntsch U. Komplikationen der Feinnadel-Punktion–DEGUM-Umfrage II. Ultraschall Med. 1996; 17: 118–30.

Weiss H, Duntsch U, Weiss A. Risiken der Feinnadelpunktion–Ergebnisse einer Umfrage in der BRD (DEGUM-Umfrage). Ultraschall Med. 1988; 9: 121–7.

Wernecke K, Mertens G, von Bassewitz DB, Peters PE. Möglichkeiten und Grenzen der perkutanen Nadelbiopsie in der histologischen Klassifikation von malignen Tumoren. Röfo Fortschr Geb Röntgenstr Neuen Bildgeb Verfahr. 1991; 155: 538–44.

Wu SS, Lin KC, Soon MS, Yeh KT. Ultrasound-guided percutaneous transhepatic fine needle aspiration cytology study of gallbladder polypoid lesions. Am J Gastroenterol. 1996; 91: 1591–4.

Xing X, Wu ZD. The retrospective study on high risk factors of subphrenic infection after hepatectomy. J Tongii Med Univ. 1995; 15(3): 158–61.

6 Technical Principles

U. Peitz

Introduction

When sound is below 20 Hz, it is inaudible to the human ear and is therefore called infrasound; sound above the threshold of human hearing (i.e., above 20 000 Hz) is classified as ultrasound.

Medical sonography makes use of reflection and diffraction of ultrasound waves on body structures in order to gain information about these very same structures. A so-called transducer, converting electronic signals into acoustic vibrations as well as turning acoustic waves back into electrical signals, transmits a brief ultrasound pulse lasting just one millionth of a second and subsequently records the reflected echoes ("pulse-echo mode"). This cycle of transmitting pulses and receiving echoes can be repeated many thousand times per second. By sweeping the ultrasound beam across the viewing plane, a two-dimensional image can be created on the monitor depicting the structures within the scanned body section true to scale. In Doppler imaging, the acoustic ultrasound measurements obtained from moving structures are displayed not only visually but also acoustically; in other words, they are transformed into audible sound waves.

Since the first half of the last century, the principle of imaging three-dimensional structures and their movements by recording the reflection of sound waves impinging on them has been used in navigation for measuring sea depth and locating submarines as well as fish shoals, and in industry for materials testing. It was introduced into medical diagnostics in 1940 by Gohr and Wedekind, and in 1942 by Dussik.

Physical Principles

Sound is defined as the propagation of pressure waves through matter. Since sound requires a substance through which to propagate, it cannot move through a vacuum–something which electromagnetic waves such as light can do. The propagation of the sound waves in gas and fluids and the motion of the particles affected both take place in the same direction, which characterizes sound waves as *longitudinal* mechanical waves. In the soft tissues of the human body, the behavior of sound waves resembles that in viscous fluids. Sound essentially moves in a straight line, and can therefore be sent out in a set direction as a sound beam. Sound waves are reflected, scattered, refracted, diffracted, and absorbed, just like light.

Sound waves are reflected at the interface between two media differing in their sound transmission resistance, also termed impedance. Acoustic impedance (Z) is defined as the product of the speed of sound in the tissue (v) and the density of the tissue (ρ). Both parameters, speed of sound (v) and density (ρ), are specific for each material (Table 6.**1**). The greater the difference in impedance between two media, the more energy is reflected at their interface. The ratio of the reflected sound energy (E_r) and the transmitted energy (E_e, or emission energy) is defined as:

$$E_r/E_e \sim [(Z_2 - Z_1)/(Z_2 + Z_1)]^2$$

where $Z = v \times \rho$ and the subscripts refer to the different media.

This relationship applies to ideal smooth interfaces perpendicular to the direction of sound wave propagation. In the reality of the human body with its irregularly shaped boundaries, apart from reflection, scattering contributes significantly to the acoustic energy returning to the transducer. Artifacts trace their origin to diffraction and refraction.

While the differences in impedance of various soft tissues are large enough to define the external contours and internal structures of organs, they are still small enough to permit a significant proportion of the energy to pass into deeper layers, where further interfaces result in additional echoes returning to the transducer. However, once the sound encounters a medium in the human body with a very low or very high impedance, such as gas and bone respectively, the very large difference in impedance will result in almost total reflection of the sound energy in both cases, as can be seen from the above equation for the energy of the reflected sound and the impedances listed in Table 6.**1**.

Table 6.**1** Typical values for the speed of sound v, density ρ, and impedance $Z = v \times \rho$ (Doessel, 2000)

Material	**v** (m/s)	ρ (g/cm^3)	Z (g/[cm^2 s])	**Absorption** (dB/MHz cm)
Air	331	0.0013	43	
Fat	1470	0.97	1.42×10^5	0.5
Water	1492	0.9982	1.49×10^5	0.002
Liver	1540	1.055	1.66×10^5	0.7
Muscle	1568	1.04	1.63×10^5	1
Compact bone	3600	1.7	6.12×10^5	30–90

Pulse-Echo Mode

The small difference in acoustic velocity between various organs and organ structures allows for the use of a set velocity (1540 m/s) for calculating the distance between the reflecting interface and the probe. In echo ranging based on the pulse-echo mode, a brief pulse of about two wavelengths is transmitted. For a transmission frequency of about 3.5 MHz this would correspond to a pulse duration of one millionth of a second (10^{-6} s).

The returning echoes are recorded during the interval until the next transmission pulse is emitted. The distance to the reflecting interface equals one half the transit time multiplied by the set acoustic velocity of 1540 m/s.

The sound energy is expressed in terms of the amplitude of the sound wave pressure. The propagating sound energy undergoes exponential attenuation by transformation into heat–also referred to as absorption. The amount of absorption is characteristic for each material, and, for example, is very high in bone. It does not vary much in the different soft tissues (Table 6.**1**). In order for echoes from similar interfaces, but at different distances, to be displayed with the same intensity, the absorption must be numerically compensated by a transit time-dependent amplification of the sound pressure amplitude (TGC = "time gain compensation"). Absorption is also the reason why sound has a limited depth of penetration. Since there is a linear relationship between absorption and sound frequency, the depth of penetration is inversely proportional to the frequency of the transmitted sound wave.

Spatial Resolution

The advantage of gaining a large depth of penetration by choosing a low transmission frequency is paid for in a loss of spatial resolution with decreasing transmission frequency. Spatial resolution is defined as the smallest distance between two points at which both can still be discriminated. The resolution along the direction of the ultrasound beam, i.e., axial resolution, is on the order of one sound wavelength, λ. The wavelength of the sound wave is given by the acoustic velocity (v) and the frequency of the sound (f):

$$\lambda = v/f$$

Selection of the transmission frequency thus requires a compromise between optimal depth of penetration and resolution (Table 6.**2**). Lateral resolution, or the discrimination of two objects in all axes perpendicular to the direction of sound propagation, also improves with higher sound frequency. In addition, it also depends on the shape of and energy distribution within the ultrasound field. The ultrasound field connotes that volume in space in which the sound waves transmitted by the transducer will propagate. The narrower the ultrasound field, the better the lateral resolution. Whereas a spherical source of sound will emit waves in all directions, a planar emitter will generate a directional ultrasound field. Near the transducer, in the so-called near field, the waves will travel almost in parallel, albeit with an inhomogeneous energy distribution (Fig. 6.**1 a**). In the far field, the sound waves diverge. While increasing the diameter of the ultrasound source broadens the near field, the sound waves will become less divergent. The diameter of the ultrasound source therefore also reflects a compromise between the probe-near width of the sound field and the probe-distant divergence of the beam. In technical terms, the ultrasound field is additionally narrowed by so-called focusing. With focusing, the sound pulses in the focal zone between near and far field will converge, thus resulting in a narrower field (Fig. 6.**1 b**). The field of a planar source with focusing takes the shape of a lobe ("sound lobe") (Fig. 6.**1 b**).

Table 6.**2** Choice of transmission frequency as a compromise between optimal depth of penetration and resolution

Transmission Frequency (MHz)	Wavelength (mm)	Depth of Penetration, One Way (cm)	Lateral Resolution (mm)	Axial Resolution (mm)
2	0.78	12.5	3	0.8
3.5	0.44	7	1.7	0.5
5	0.31	5	1.2	0.35
7.5	0.21	3.3	0.8	0.25
10	0.16	2.5	0.6	0.2

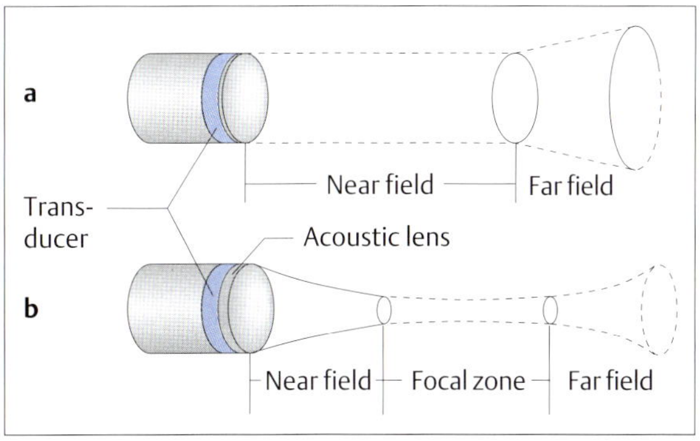

Fig. 6.**1** Schematic diagram of a transducer with circular transmission area and the contours of the sound field. Transducer without focusing (**a**): parallel propagation of the sound waves in the near field, divergence in the far field. Transducer with focusing (**b**): converging sound waves in the near field, small focal zone, and diverging sound waves in the far field.

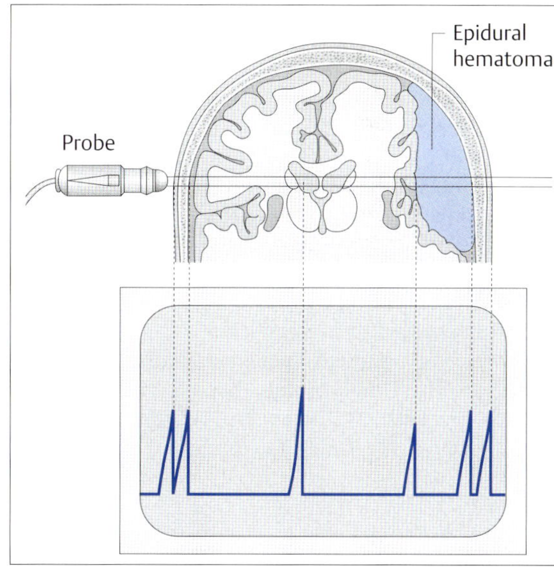

Fig. 6.**2** Typical application of A-mode sonography: echoencephalography. Detection of epidural hematoma characterized by displacement of the midline echo and an accessory echo from the brain–hematoma interface.

Piezoelectric Effect

Ultrasound waves may be generated by the reverse piezoelectric effect (from the Greek term *piezein* = to press). When a pressure wave, in this case an ultrasound wave, deforms a certain type of crystal, a voltage is generated; this phenomenon is referred to as the piezoelectric effect. In the reverse process, when such a crystal has a voltage applied to it, the crystal becomes deformed. By modulating the voltage applied, ultrasound waves can be generated. In diagnostic ultrasound, the piezoelectric transducers are made of ceramic and act as transmitters as well as receivers.

Imaging Modalities

A-Mode

The oldest and simplest imaging method is the A-mode, where 'A' stands for amplitude. In A-Mode imaging, pulses are transmitted in one direction only, and therefore spatial information is only one-dimensional. The sound pressure amplitudes of the echoes received are plotted on the vertical (*Y*-) axis of the screen ("oscilloscope") as a function of the transit time represented on the horizontal (*X*-) axis. The differences in amplitude represent true-to-scale differences in distance to the interfaces and may be used, for instance, in echoencephalography for visualization of hematomas (Fig. 6.**2**).

B-Mode

Two-dimensional spatial information is supplied by B-mode imaging (where 'B' stands for brightness), the modality underpinning all of the images in this book. In B-mode imaging, the sound pressure amplitudes are plotted not as deflections along the vertical axis of the screen but rather as pixels, the intensity (brightness) of which represents the level of the amplitude. The brightness is graded by means of a so-called "gray-scale." Thus, the echoes of a sound pulse will yield a line of pixels the distances of which will be a true-to-scale representation of the distances to the various interfaces. The direction of the pulse-echo train is changed mechanically or electronically such that it can be steered within a cross-sectional plane of the body. On the screen, the resulting lines of pixels are arranged in such a fashion that they reproduce a true-to-scale two-dimensional image of the viewing plane. In the language of the sonographer the pixels on the screen are referred to as "echoes" or "reflections."

In the now more or less historical "compound scan mode" the transducer, mounted on a mechanical swivel arm, was moved by hand across the surface of the body along the scan plane chosen. Based on the position of the swivel arm and the echo data, the computer generated a frozen picture resembling that of a CT scan. Nowadays, ultrasound scanning is usually performed in "real-time" mode. Here, the change in direction of the pulse-echo train is triggered within the transducer itself. Since the pulse-echo train may be generated many thousand times per second, its sweep across the viewing plane can be repeated at such a rate that this will result in jitter-free "real-time" image sequences.

M-Mode

The M-mode or TM- ("time motion") mode resembles the A-mode in that it is a one-dimensional spatial modality. Here, the direction of the pulse-echo train is kept constant. As in B-mode scanning, the sound pressure amplitude is encoded in terms of pixel brightness. The distance of the echoes from the transducer is plotted along the vertical axis of the screen. The horizontal axis represents the transit time. M-mode imaging is particularly useful when examining rapid interface motion, such as that encountered in cardiac valves.

Doppler Imaging

The audible and visual representation of blood flow is based on the so-called Doppler shift. This refers to the shift in frequency resulting from a change in distance between the source and the receiver of sound waves. If both move toward each other, the receiver will record a higher frequency than that of the source, while the frequency will be lower when both move apart; one well known example in everyday life is the sound of a passing train. In Doppler sonography the frequency shift is caused by the motion of the reflecting blood cells relative to the transducer. Thus, only this Doppler shift in frequency is amplified and translated into audible and visible signals. The relationship of the returning ultrasound frequency to the velocity of the reflector is governed by the Doppler equation:

$$f_d = f_1 - f_0 = 2 \cdot f_0 \frac{V_B \cdot \cos\Theta}{V_u}$$

where:

f_d Doppler shift frequency
f_0 frequency of the sound transmitted by the source
f_1 frequency of the ultrasound recorded by the receiver
v_B velocity of the reflecting blood cells
$\cos\Theta$ cosine of the angle between the direction of blood flow and the direction of propagation of the ultrasound beam
v_U speed of propagation of the ultrasound

According to this equation, the Doppler shift frequency will increase with the frequency of the transmitted ultrasound. This implies that for slow flow rates the sound source should transmit at the highest frequency possible. Unfortunately, just as in the pulse-echo mode, a high frequency of transmission will limit the depth of penetration. If the transmission frequencies are chosen such that the Doppler shift will result in a frequency within the range of human hearing, this frequency can be rendered audible by appropriate amplification.

It is possible to determine the velocity of the blood flow based on the Doppler equation and the Doppler shift frequency measured. However, the angle Θ between the sound field and the direction of blood flow has to be considered as well; this angle may be approximated by determining the axis of the blood vessel on a B-mode image scanned in the same plane. For an angle $\Theta = 0°$, i.e., ultrasound beam and blood flow directions are parallel, the Doppler shift will reach its maximum, while for $\Theta = 60°$ it is half the maximum, and for $\Theta = 90°$ it is nil. If the ultrasound beam is perpendicular to the blood flow, Doppler imaging will not yield any flow velocity at all.

Any velocity measurement of the blood flow is complicated by the fact that the flow is pulsatile in nature and that it is the resultant of a gamut of different velocities within the flow profile of the vessel. The pulsatility behavior and the velocity spectrum provide essential information on the behavior of the blood flow, permitting the differentiation of physiological flow within the various branches of the vascular tree, e.g., internal versus external carotid artery, as well as the diagnosis of pathological blood flow. Doppler imaging maps the spectrum and temporal pattern of the velocities in terms of the spectrum and pattern of the Doppler shift frequencies. The sound pressure amplitude of each Doppler shift frequency is a measure of the number of blood cells moving at the corresponding velocity. Over the time of the pulse train, the spectrum of frequencies can easily be assessed as an acoustic process. Here, the pitch of the tone represents the velocity of the blood cells. In the additional visual recording ("frequency analysis"), the horizontal axis represents the time elapsed. The vertical deflection of the pixels represents the level of frequency as well as the sign of the Doppler shift (positive or negative, depending on whether the flow is toward or away from the transducer). As the sound pressure amplitude correlates with the number of blood cells, it is encoded as pixel brightness.

Continuous Wave (CW) Doppler Mode

There are two types of Doppler excitation: continuous wave (CW) and pulsed wave (PW) Doppler. CW Doppler offers the advantage of being able to measure slow as well as fast blood flow velocities. For the continuous transmission and reception of sound waves, two separate but closely spaced piezoelectric crystals are needed. The major drawback is that all flow velocities will be recorded along the ultrasound beam, irrespective of their actual distance from the transducer.

Pulsed Wave (PW) Doppler Mode, Duplex Sonography

With pulsed wave Doppler ultrasound, the distance between the blood cell reflectors and the transducer can be determined by measuring the transit times for pulsed ultrasound waves based on the pulse-echo mode. In pulsed-wave imaging, each individual piezoelectric element functions both as transmitter and receiver. When this is combined with the B-mode image ("duplex sonography"), the vessel of interest is first depicted conventionally as a two-dimensional image. A marker–the so-called "gate" or "sample volume"–is then positioned on the screen inside this vessel. This gate defines the localization, length, and angle of the sample volume. Only those Doppler frequencies within this sample volume are measured and transformed into visual and audible signals.

The transit time of the ultrasound defines the length of the sample volume and its distance from the transducer, while the lateral scope of the gate is given by the width of the sound field. The angle of the beam used to measure the Doppler signal is steered by the combined phase-shifted activation of several piezoelectric crystals ("phased array").

Pulsed wave Doppler imaging has one drawback in that measurement of high flow velocities is limited by the so-called pulse repetition frequency, that is, by how often the pulses are repeated. Only those Doppler frequencies not exceeding one-half the pulse repetition frequency ("Nyquist frequency") can be measured accurately. Exceeding the Nyquist frequency results in "aliasing," whereby the measured Doppler frequencies are too low and point in the opposite direction. The pulse repetition frequency needs to be adjusted depending on the flow velocity expected.

Color Flow Doppler

In pulsed wave Doppler imaging the sample volume may be steered along the scan plane at a high speed. To the human eye it appears as if the data from a large number of small sample volumes arrive simultaneously. Instead of being displayed as a function of time, the Doppler frequency may be depicted as a brightness-coded colored pixel in a B-mode image obtained simultaneously (in "real-time"). Here, the color represents the direction of flow. By convention, flow toward the probe is displayed in red, while flow away from it appears blue. Higher velocity is displayed by increased brightness. There is the additional benefit of being able to measure turbulence, which is most often encoded as a yellow admixture. Aliasing can also be seen in color flow Doppler imaging and may result in the wrong flow direction and velocity. One further disadvantage of this method is that, owing to the enormous number of pulses needed to construct the B-mode and color flow Doppler images, the frame rate may fall below the temporal resolution of the human eye, i.e., below approximately 15 images per second. The frame rate can be increased by reducing the size of the viewing sector.

Power Doppler

Power Doppler is one variant of color flow Doppler imaging. Here, too, moving blood cells are displayed as colored pixels in a B-mode image, based on the Doppler shift frequencies measured. However, compared to color flow Doppler sonography, in this case pixel display does not depend on the velocity or direction. Only one color is used to encode direction, and by convention this is usually yellow. While in color flow Doppler sonography the brightness of the color encodes the Doppler shift frequency, in power Doppler mode it encodes the sound pressure amplitude. Power mode Doppler imaging therefore quantifies the blood flowing within the scan plane. The image resembles a standard or MRI angiogram.

■ Probe Types

While a pen-shaped transducer is sufficient for one-dimensional A-mode and CW Doppler imaging, there are numerous variations on the B-mode probe types, described below, the selection of which depends on the application in question. Almost all of the present B-mode probe types can be combined with duplex and color flow Doppler mode.

As described for B-mode scanning, the pulse-echo train is steered mechanically or electronically from within the transducer. In a mechanical probe the rotating transducer transmits the pulses in a radial direction. The resulting image has the shape either of a sector (mechanical sector scanner, Fig. 6.**3a**) or a circle, for instance, as in endosonography (Fig. 6.**3b**). In array scanners, the ultrasound probe is composed of a large number (usually around 200) of adjacent, closely spaced small piezoelectric elements (width about 1–4 wavelengths). These are activated in sequence. A straight line of piezoelectric crystals results in a rectangular image (linear array probe, Fig. 6.**3c**), while a curved line produces a fan shaped image (curved array probe, Fig. 6.**3d**). Furthermore, with array scanners, pulse train steering is also possible by activating adjacent piezoelectric crystals in coordinated fashion, i.e., by phasing ("phased array"). This generates a sound field that does not leave the transducer at a right angle but rather at an oblique angle. Changes in angle of up to 45° can be realized electronically. The electronic phased array principle thus permits sector (Fig. 6.**3e**) and trapezoidal (Fig. 6.**3f**) images as well as beam steering in pulsed wave Doppler imaging (see above).

The shape of the probe not only defines the shape of the B-mode image but also possible coupling at the anatomical region of interest. A small contact area is required for narrow ultrasound windows, for example, the intercostal space in echocardiography or for special intracavitary probes (endosonography). For these purposes, the sector scanners

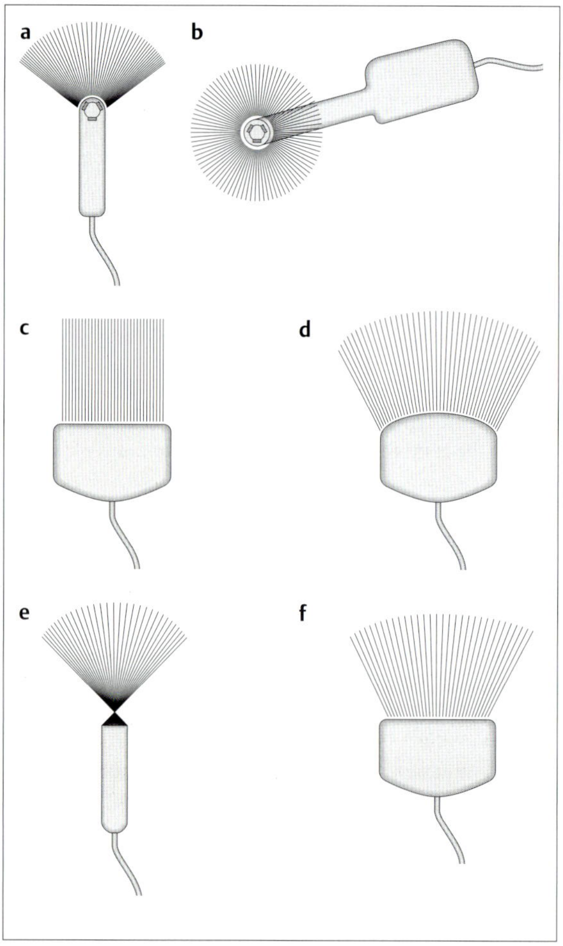

Fig. 6.3 Probe types with different types of image generation
a Mechanical sector scanner
b Endosonography probe
c Linear array probe
d Curved array probe
e Electronic sector scanner (phased array)
f Linear array probe with phased array activation

covering a small image section close to the transducer which widens into a fan shape with increasing distance from the probe are most suitable. A wider image section close to the transducer calls for a wider probe, i.e., a linear array scanner, as is used for the more superficial structures such as the thyroid, breast, scrotum, or musculoskeletal system. For the abdomen, the curved array probe represents a compromise between the size of the contact area and the image width close to the transducer.

Focusing

Lateral resolution is improved by focusing of the sound field. Focusing at constant depth is realized by a concave contact area of the probe or built-in acoustic lenses. Modern ultrasound probes utilize electronic focusing. Here, adjacent piezoelectric crystals are phase-activated in such a fashion that the individual pulses merge at the focal zone. This permits the depth of the focal zone to be varied according to the needs of the operator, as well as the combination of several focal zones.

Image Optimization

Basic settings of the ultrasound unit are best adjusted by referring to the organ of a healthy volunteer–in abdominal sonography most commonly the liver. The brightness of the monitor should be set such that the black background is almost as dark as the black margin of the screen. Contrast is adjusted so that the displayed gray scale covers a wide range of discernible shades of gray. In B-mode imaging, the highest possible ultrasound frequency is selected for which the depth of penetration still allows evaluation of the region of interest (reference values for the depth of penetration are listed in Table 6.**2**). One prerequisite is that the focal zones of the probe will cover the region of interest. In order to utilize the optimum depth of penetration, the depth gain control is adjusted to the scanned structures and total gain is increased. Should this be insufficient to depict sufficiently bright and sharp echoes, the radiated power is increased, which should otherwise be left at the low presettings in order to keep the applied ultrasound energy at lower levels for safety reasons.

Even though no clinically noticeable damage induced by ultrasound has been demonstrated, mechanical stress such as cavitation or noticeable warming in pulsed Doppler sonography may be produced.

Depending on the model of ultrasound unit, the contrast of the resulting image may be controlled by various parameters. The parameters take effect before or after image information is collected ("preprocessing" and "postprocessing," respectively).

The image section should be restricted to the region of interest. Smaller image sections will result in higher frame rates. This is particularly true for the window size in color flow Doppler imaging.

New Developments

Current technical refinements include three-dimensional ultrasound, panoramic view modes, harmonic imaging, and parametric sonography (Gebel, 2000). In the first two techniques the transducer is moved manually, and the information from multiple slices is stored and reconstructed in three dimensions or side by side, respectively. Harmonic imaging makes use of data from harmonics to improve resolution and contrast. When combined with ultrasound contrast agents, the resonance of the bubbles in the contrast medium permits a more sensitive delineation of foci with aberrant vascularization. Parametric sonography complements the operator-dependent image assessment by objectively quantifying image information. The clinical usefulness of these methods still needs further appraisal.

Documentation

One of the consequences of contract between patient and physician is the need to document findings as text and images. In Germany, formal requirements regarding documentation in sonography are defined only by the regional medical associations for outpatient treatment (Kassenärztlichen Vereinigung) and by the licensing bodies for private practice. Any written or image documentation must clearly identify the patient information and indicate the date of the examination as well as the institution at which it was performed.

In addition, the written documentation must specify the type of investigation, the operator performing the examination, the clinical issue to be addressed, the findings, and the assessment. The documentation must also indicate all organs examined, mention any reservations regarding assessment, and detail any pathological findings. The latter may–depending on the organ–refer to site, size, shape, contour, texture and vascular supply, and perhaps also to motility, tenderness, deformability, and positional variations. The terms *hyperechoic* and *hypoechoic* describe a region in a sonographic image where the echoes are respectively brighter or less bright than normal. A hyperechoic echo pattern can be generated by strong (i.e., bright) echoes with large amplitudes as well as by a high echo density, or both. When describing parenchymatous organs or masses, these two phenomena do not have to be differentiated, and quite often this is impossible, so that the term hyperechoic or hypoechoic is based on the overall impression. Objective measurement of echo density and intensity has proved of little use so far because of the multitude of interfering factors inherent in the individual patient. However, echo strength (i.e., brightness) may be used to characterize individual echoes, for instance, in bile ducts containing gas ("pneumobilia"). The term anechoic can largely be regarded as being objective; however, when assessing anechogenicity the ultrasound unit has to be at its optimum setting and the artifacts described below must be minimized. The national institutes of ultrasound in medicine strive for a uniform nomenclature (Heyder, 1994).

Images can be documented by means of photographs, particularly Polaroid prints or multi-format cameras, video prints, as well as videotapes. Lately, digital storage media have become an option as well. Aspects of safety and data privacy also have to be adhered to. Documented images must be accessible at all times and be comprehensible to others. Postprocessing of the documented images should not be possible. Apart from the sonographic image proper and the information mentioned above, the image should include a scale, usually with centimeter gradation, the time and place of the examination, and the basic parameter settings of the ultrasound unit. The position of the viewing plane may be indicated by appropriate pictograms and/or labeling of the organs depicted. Any pathological findings should, if at all possible, be documented, marked, and measured in at least two orthogonal planes.

Practical Example–Abdominal Sonography

Prerequisites

In general, the patient does not have to be prepared. However, when assessing the organs of the upper abdomen, in particular gallbladder and pancreas, the patient should be fasting. Administration of anti-foaming medication prior to the examination has not proved of any benefit. Filling of hollow viscera such as the stomach, colon, and especially the bladder, with fluid may sometimes be beneficial for assessment of mural details of these organs or for evaluation of more deeply sited structures, when the fluid will serve as an echo window.

Examination Sequence in Abdominal Sonography

The clinical questions to be answered predetermine the sequence of the examination. Nevertheless, since the benefit of sonography as a screening modality is so high, complete assessment of all abdominal organs should always be attempted. The sonographer can also check for any pleural and pericardiac effusions without too much additional work.

For a complete abdominal examination a standardized course is recommended, which may be tailored to the sonographer, or better the department, and should then be followed routinely. In our department, rather than stipulating a sequence of viewing planes to run through, it has proved more effective to assess the organs in standardized scan planes, and we therefore simply work through the list of organs to be evaluated. The viewing planes to be acquired for each organ are outlined in the chapters on the individual organ systems. Each organ should be scanned completely in at least two orthogonal (mutually perpendicular) planes. Limitations apply to those organs that are partially or completely covered by bone (ribs, pelvis). These call for additional special planes adapted to the limited access, e.g., intercostal views where the probe is placed into the intercostal space, or subcostal planes immediately inferior to the costal arch. From such positions the probe is tilted through as many planes as possible until the organ disappears from the viewing plane or the interference from the ribs starts to mask the image.

One of the advantages of sonography over CT scanning is the free choice of scan planes. However, at the same time this freedom increases the requirements for precise documentation. The possibility of moving the probe through an almost infinite number of angles makes it clear that simply stating the probe position (e.g., "right subcostal view") does not define the viewing plane exactly. The statement "right subcostal view" only describes the line of contact of the probe, as specified by the pictogram and detailed further with the use of terms such as "transverse upper abdominal view," "flank view," "longitudinal suprapubic view," etc. As the additional variations by tilting of the probe are almost impossible to put into writing, the topographic relationship to organs and anatomical landmarks should be used to further document the findings.

The most important landmarks for finding organs as well as for documentation are the major vessels, usually visualized as tubelike anechoic structures, which can be traced with little difficulty. Tubular structures such as the common bile duct or an enlarged ureter are easily differentiated from blood vessels by their anatomical relationships.

The freedom of choice of viewing planes may also hamper the repeatability of pathological findings. This becomes particularly evident in follow-up of measurements of distance, e.g., when determining the diameter of masses. Any follow-up measurement must be performed along the identical axis and within the same plane as in the initial workup. In turn, this requires a combination of image documentation and a detailed description of the findings. The descriptive part of the measurement is guided by the topographic relationship to the anatomical landmarks. If at all possible, the measurements should also be related to the anatomical axes (longitudinal, sagittal, transverse axes), and in two-dimensional measurements to the three planes of the human body (sagittal, frontal, and transverse plane). In such cases the measurements can be repeated more accurately than by simple designation of the line of contact for the probe.

Artifacts

Artifacts are those elements of the image which lack any anatomical or pathoanatomical correlation. They may limit the assessment or even obstruct it completely but on the other hand may also be used as part of image interpretation, especially in sonography (Steiner, 1993).

Posterior Shadowing

Behind strongly attenuating or reflecting structures such as bones, calculi (e.g., gallstones; Fig. 6.**4**), and sometimes also behind gas (Figs. 6.**4**, 6.**10**), the echo amplitudes may be reduced or even missing altogether. In this context "behind" means posterior to the structure in question, the transducer being anterior. The correct term is posterior (acoustic) shadowing. Large differences in impedance between these structures and the surroundings result in such reflection of the ultrasound waves, in addition to strong absorption in bone, that the sound energy transmitted beyond the structure is too low to generate any useful echoes. The degree of shadowing depends not only on the density, and thus on the impedance, of the structures, but also on the position of these structures within the ultrasound field. For instance, gallstones quite often exhibit more severe posterior shadowing than intestinal gas. Any calculus not located completely within the ultrasound field will result in incomplete posterior shadowing (Fig. 6.**4**).

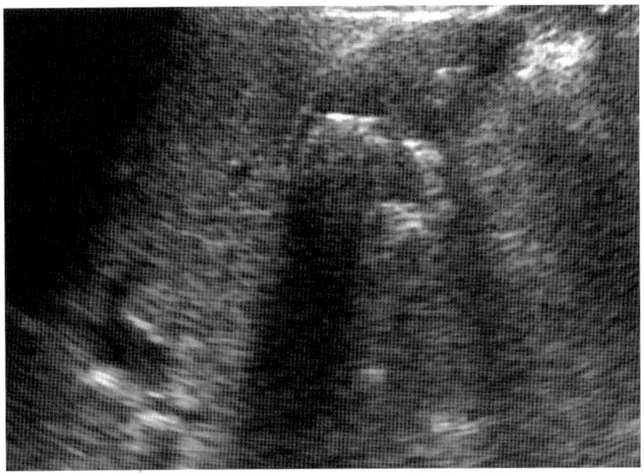

Fig. 6.4a Gallbladder with two calculi. The larger gallstone results in complete and the smaller one in incomplete posterior shadowing. Incomplete posterior shadowing is also evident posterior to the intestinal gas within the adjacent colon. The image of those parts of the gallbladder facing the transducer are marred by artifacts due to electronic noise.

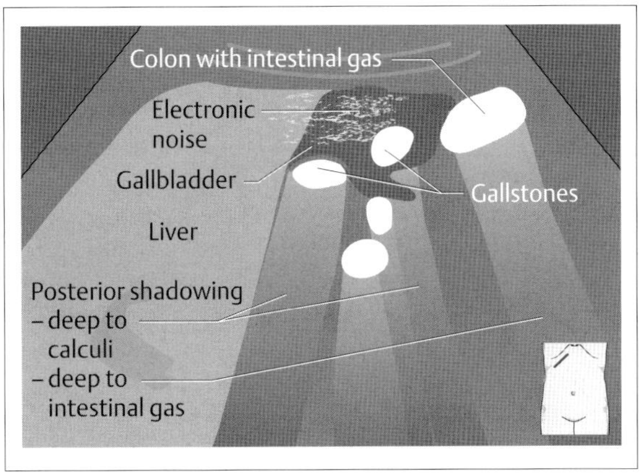

Fig. 6.4b Line drawing.

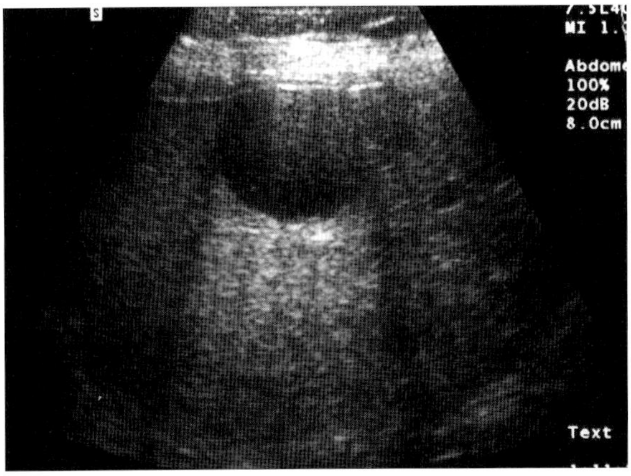

Fig. 6.5a Hepatic cyst with lateral shadowing, posterior acoustic enhancement, and electronic noise in those parts of the cyst close to the transducer.

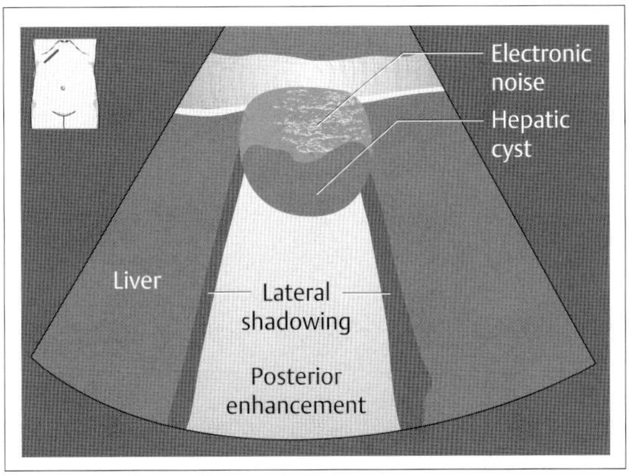

Fig. 6.5b Line drawing.

Lateral Shadowing

Several types of artifacts, some of which hamper while others facilitate interpretation, are demonstrated quite nicely by this hepatic cyst (Fig. 6.5). Acoustic shadowing quite often originates at the lateral edge of a cyst by refraction and diffraction of ultrasound waves. Such lateral shadowing can help identify cystic and fluid-filled structures, but should not be mistaken for posterior shadowing encountered, for instance, behind gallstones.

Posterior Enhancement

The echoes generated deep to a cyst will be brighter than those from the surrounding tissue, e.g., in the liver (Fig. 6.5). While traveling through the cyst, the sound waves generating these brighter echoes will undergo less attenuation by absorption and reflection than in the adjacent liver tissue. Apart from their anechogenicity, this posterior enhancement is a typical characteristic of fluid-filled cysts.

Electronic Noise

In the near-field of the lobe-shaped sound field, i.e., proximal to the focal region, the ultrasound energy exhibits a nonhomogeneous distribution, resulting in numerous small echoes. This signal noise should not be mistaken for sedimentation in the gallbladder or a cyst (Figs. 6.**4**, 6.**5**).

Beam Width (Synonyms: Image Averaging or Slice Thickness) Artifact

As detailed above, lateral resolution is lower than axial spatial resolution. Due to the thickness of the sound field, the viewing plane is not a true plane but rather a slice with a certain thickness. All anatomical structures located within this slice will add to image formation. If, for example, the gallbladder wall crosses this slice volume obliquely, the wall as well as the lumen will contribute to the final image, resulting in an ill-defined wall with finely dispersed intraluminal echoes close to it. This can easily be misinterpreted as sedimentation (Fig. 6.**6**).

Reverberation

Strongly reflecting interfaces, especially the tissue–gas interface, deep to the transducer may induce not only echo attenuation but also repeated images of such a strongly reflecting interface. This type of artifact arises when the ultrasound beam is reflected so strongly that the waves run back and forth several times between the interface and the probe or other interfaces. The ultrasound unit therefore records a multiple of the transit time, thereby computing a corresponding multiple of the distance, and thus projects evenly spaced repeated echoes beyond the interface.

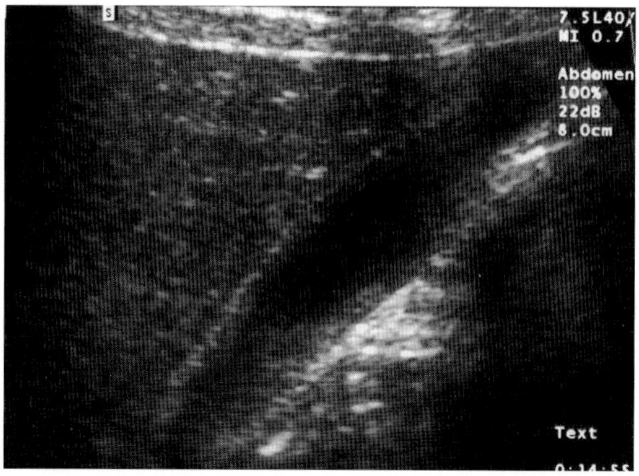

Fig. 6.**6 a** Gallbladder with beam width artifact, an ill-defined wall, and the illusion of sedimentation.

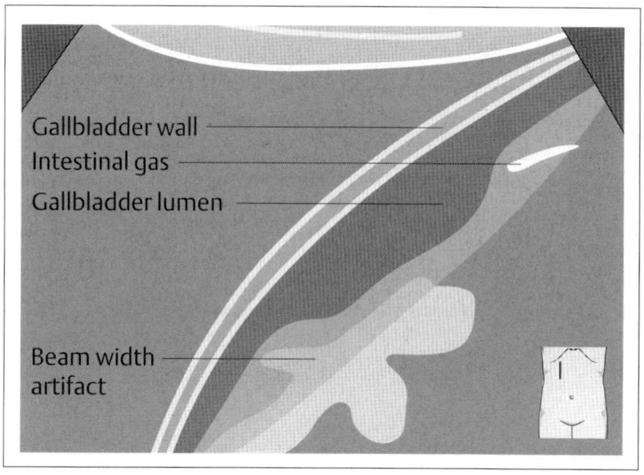

Fig. 6.**6 b** Line drawing.

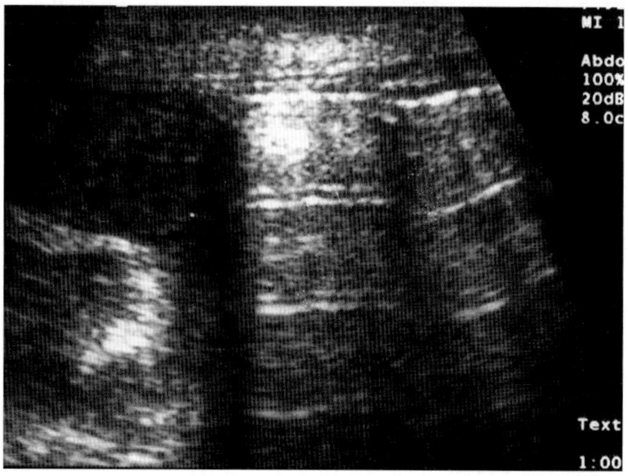

Fig. 6.**7 a** Intestinal gas with reverberation. On the left there are bowel loops without gas.

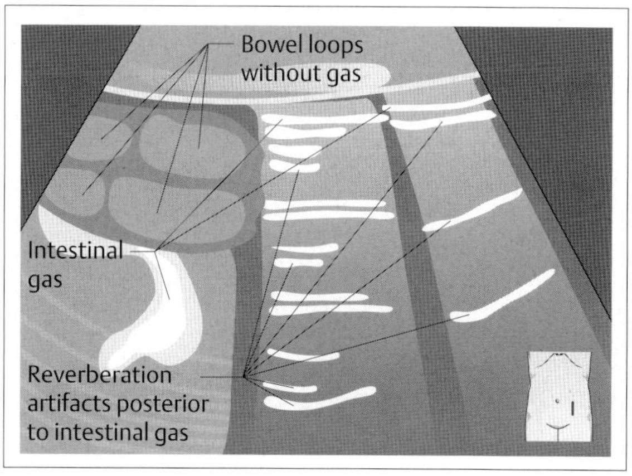

Fig. 6.**7 b** Line drawing.

Comet-Tail (Synonyms: Resonance or Ring-Down) Artifact

The images of so-called comet-tail artifacts strongly resemble those due to reverberation. Here, a tail of contiguous bright, dense echoes appears, once again posterior to a strongly reflecting interface. The explanation for this phenomenon is seen in the ultrasound induced resonance of the reflector. Comet-tail artifacts are frequently observed deep to gas (Fig. 6.**8**), cholesterol deposits, and metallic foreign bodies but are rarely triggered by calcified structures.

Mirror Image Artifact

Strongly reflecting interfaces may give rise to mirror images of entire organs. The most important example is mirroring of the hepatic structures at the diaphragm–lung interface, where the hepatic structures appear to be within the chest cavity (Fig. 6.**9**). This is due to sound being reflected at the diaphragm–air interface. Since the sound waves are reflected on their way to the interface as well as on their return, based on the transit time of the echoes the computer calculates the hepatic structures to be localized beyond the diaphragm, i.e., within the thorax. When costal cartilage is mirrored into the liver, arising from reflections at the interface between cartilage and liver capsule, this may mimic an intrahepatic mass (Fig. 6.**10**).

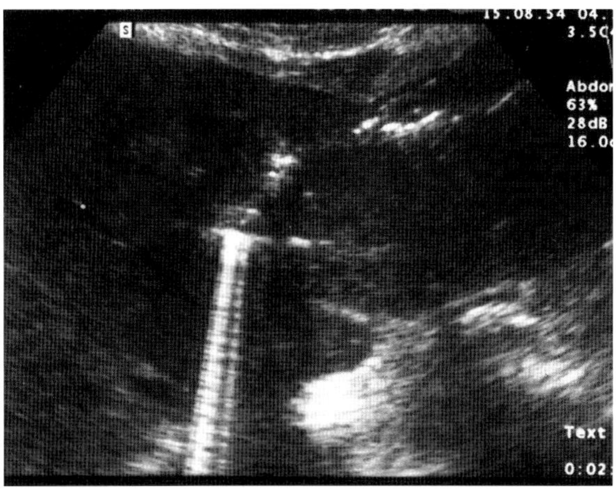

Fig. 6.**8 a** Comet-tail artifact deep to gas within the biliary tree ("pneumobilia"), to be differentiated from intraductal cholesterol deposits.

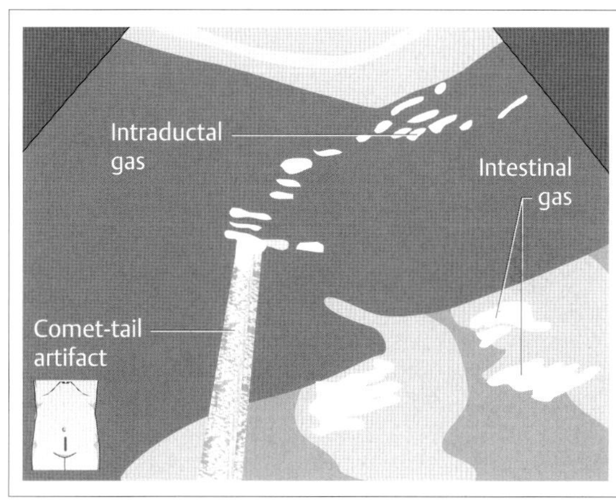

Fig. 6.**8 b** Line drawing.

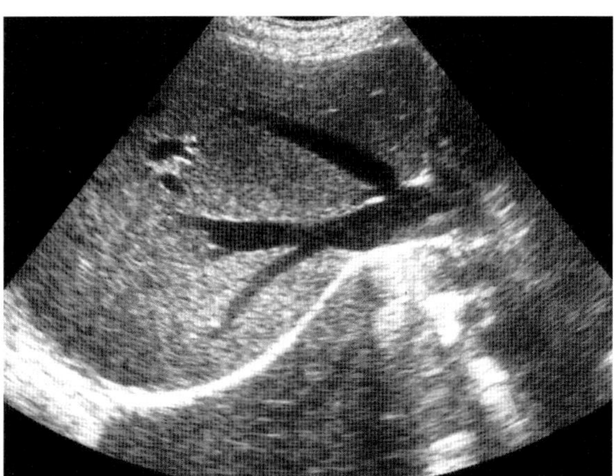

Fig. 6.**9 a** Mirror image artifact, originating at the interface between the diaphragm and the lungs. Flow artifacts in the hepatic veins.

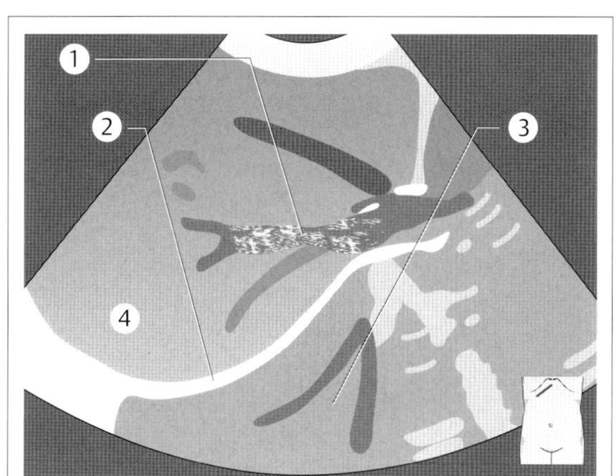

Fig. 6.**9 b** Line drawing. 1 Flow artifact; 2 Gas echo of lung; 3 Mirror image artifact; 4 Liver with hepatic vein.

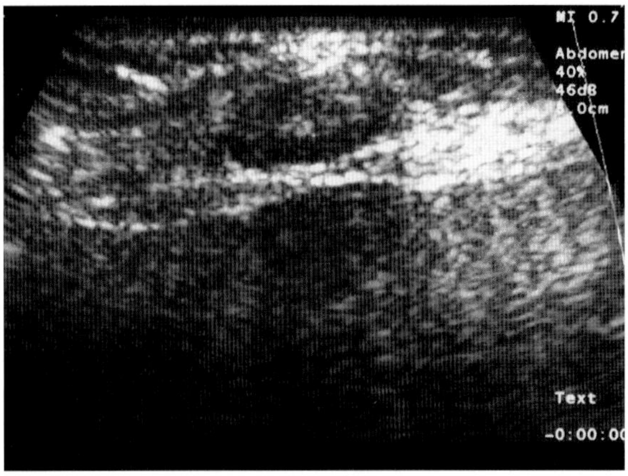

Fig. 6.10 a Transit time artifact inferior to the costal cartilage. The bulging contour of the liver is not real but feigned by the artifact. In addition, at the cartilage interface the costal cartilage is mirrored into the liver, thereby mimicking a mass.

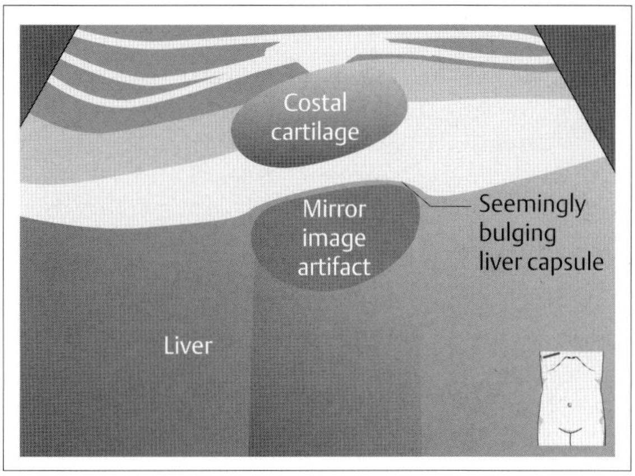

Fig. 6.10 b Line drawing.

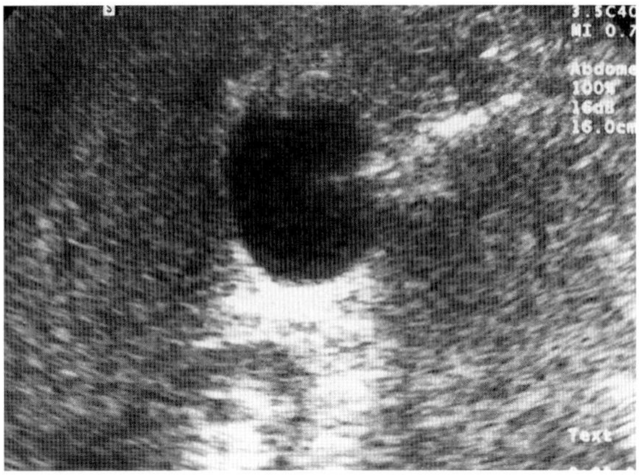

Fig. 6.11 a Side-lobe artifact in the gallbladder, originating from neighboring intestinal gas.

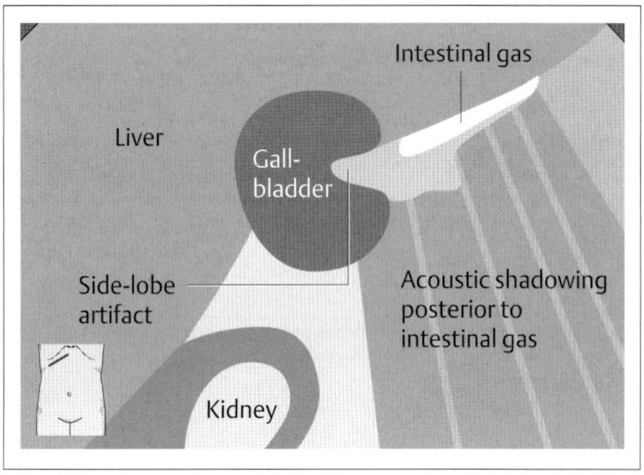

Fig. 6.11 b Line drawing.

Side-Lobe Artifact

Strongly reflecting interfaces, such as those with gas or bone, will sometimes appear again next to the genuine structures. Since this lateral copy is attenuated, it will be displayed primarily in anechoic structures, e.g., the gallbladder or urinary bladder (Fig. 6.**11**). It may be caused by refracted sound waves or by echoes originating from the so-called side-lobes that regularly arise next to the main sound field.

Transit Time Artifact

When structures conduct sound with a speed faster or slower than 1540 m/s, any structures deep to the transducer will appear correspondingly closer or farther away. Thus, a rather fatty structure will sometimes result in apparent posterior displacement, while cartilage will seemingly produce anterior displacement (Fig. 6.**10**).

Flow Artifacts

Slow blood flow, particularly when encountered in the hepatic veins (Fig. 6.**9**) will result in streaky moving echoes not to be confused with thrombi. When seen within the right atrium in the presence of atrial fibrillation, this so-called spontaneous contrast indicates an increased risk of thrombus formation.

Lessons to be Learned for the Examination

Most of the artifacts described above will be displayed posterior to the structures from which they originate. This implies the necessity to vary the scanning direction of the ultrasound probe: quite a number of these artifacts will be eliminated simply by moving the probe somewhat. Furthermore, the real structures deep to the transducer can be visualized only by this very movement of the probe. Imaging in at least two different planes is also mandatory in order to benefit from optimal axial resolution. Beam attenuation and enhancement can be partially compensated for by resetting the depth gain compensation (DGC; see above).

Electronic noise and beam width artifacts can be curtailed, but not always eliminated, by selecting the highest ultrasound frequency possible, by positioning the focal zone into the region of interest, and by reducing the overall gain.

■ Bibliography

Doessel O. Bildgebende Verfahren in der Medizin: von der Technik zur medizinischen Anwendung. Berlin: Springer; 2000; 191–225, 622–79.

Gebel MJ. Neue Modifikationen und Verfahren der Sonographie und ihre praktische Bedeutung. Internist. 2000; 41: 3–8.

Heyder N. Befundung und Nomenklatur bei Ultraschalluntersuchungen innerer Organe. Berlin: Springer; 1994.

Steiner E. Ultraschallbildartefakte. Physikalische Grundlagen. Radiologe. 1993; 33: 1–10.

7 Abdominal Sonography

U. Peitz, R. Mantke, H. U. Schulz, H. Lippert

Gastrointestinal Tract

Fundamentals and Indications for Sonography

Although in the past the gastrointestinal (GI) tract was considered more of a nuisance in abdominal sonography because of its highly reflective gas contents, nowadays complete sonographic assessment from the lower esophagus to the rectum is possible and strived for. However, visualization in continuity is still impossible. Intraluminal gas has remained the essential impediment to delineation of the GI tract; only those wall segments can be assessed that are between the ultrasound probe and the gas masking the echoes. Under favorable conditions, one may succeed in sufficiently compressing or displacing gas-filled bowel loops with small transducers to allow visualization of parts of the GI tract farther from the probe as well. One more factor, appraisal of the fatty tissue surrounding the bowel, is becoming increasingly important in the pathology of IBD.

Intraintestinal fluid, be it physiological or pathological, improves the conditions for assessment of the GI tract wall considerably. Oral or peranal fluid loading for diagnostic purposes ("hydrosonography"), while in experienced hands permitting sensitive and detailed evaluation of the gastric mucosa (Worlicek et al., 1989) or colon (Limberg, 1998), has not gained acceptance because it is time-consuming and has to compete with endoscopy and EUS. In the small bowel, fluid loading may offer possibilities that so far have been underestimated (Bin et al., 1992).

In the majority of patients with problems related to the GI tract, sonography is the initial imaging modality of choice. Accordingly, it often points the diagnostic workup in a particular direction and complements any further diagnostic imaging. In some diseases, such as appendicitis or diverticulitis, sonography furnishes enough information on its own to confirm the suspected clinical diagnosis.

Specific Technique and Diagnostic Evaluation

- The patient is routinely examined supine; special investigative questions may require a change in position (lateral decubitus, prone, erect), in particular for assessment of intraluminal or intraperitoneal fluid shift.
- Standard 3.5 MHz and 5 MHz probe; in slim subjects and children a 7.5 MHz transducer may provide more detail.
- Selection of the viewing plane is adapted to the organ; the intestinal wall should be visualized at least in two planes, on cross-section with the typical target sign (Figs. 7.**2**, 7.**7**) or in the presence of gas as an incomplete ring, and in the longitudinal view as a ribbonlike structure (Fig. 7.**1**, 7.**3**). The descriptive term "cockade" for a ring-type structure stems from the days when any visualization of the bowel wall as a hypoechoic ring was regarded as manifest wall thickening. Since nowadays the normal gastrointestinal wall will always be displayed as a target sign, the term "cockade" should be abandoned or at least amended by a statement defining it as physiological or pathological.
- Intercostal views demonstrate the gastric fundus and body as well as the left and right colonic flexures.
- Organ identification relies on the anatomy of the intraluminal folds (circular folds of the small intestine and the circular folds of the colon, Fig. 7.**3**, 7.**4**) and the presence of sphincters (lower esophageal sphincter, pylorus (Fig. 7.**1**), ileocecal valve (Figs. 7.**17**, 1.**8**).
- In addition, the rectum may be visualized from the perineum and by EUS.
- The liver, spleen, urinary bladder, and intraluminal fluid can be used as acoustic windows.
- When scanning with a high-resolution or endoluminal probe it may be possible to differentiate five layers within the bowel wall (Kimmey et al., 1989) (Figs. 7.**1**–7.**3**):
  1. Hyperechoic: interface between adventitia and muscularis propria, "entrance echo."
  2. Hypoechoic: muscularis propria (note: high-resolution probes can differentiate the outer longitudinal from the inner circular muscle layer, both being separated by a hyperechoic band (Fig. 7.**14**; chapter 1, Figs. 1.**30**, 1.**31**); this is the wall layer best recognized as it is the thicker of the two hypoechoic structures and, because of its low echogenicity, contrasts well with the adjacent connective tissue.
  3. Hyperechoic: submucosa, outer parts of the mucosa.
  4. Hypoechoic: inner parts of the mucosa.
  5. Hyperechoic: interface between mucosa and intestinal contents, "exit echo", often impossible to differentiate from the bowel contents.
- By convention, wall thickness is measured from entrance to exit echo. Differentiation between inflammatory and simple edematous swelling is frequently impossible and is therefore derived from the clinical context, e.g., diffuse bowel wall swelling encountered in hydropic states (portal hypertension, cardiac or renal failure). Considering these qualifications, the normal thickness of the (noncontracted) gastrointestinal wall is:
  - Stomach 6 mm maximum
  - Small and large bowel 3 mm maximum
- **Caveat:** Wall thickness depends greatly on its tension and hydration, i.e., despite inflammatory mural invasion

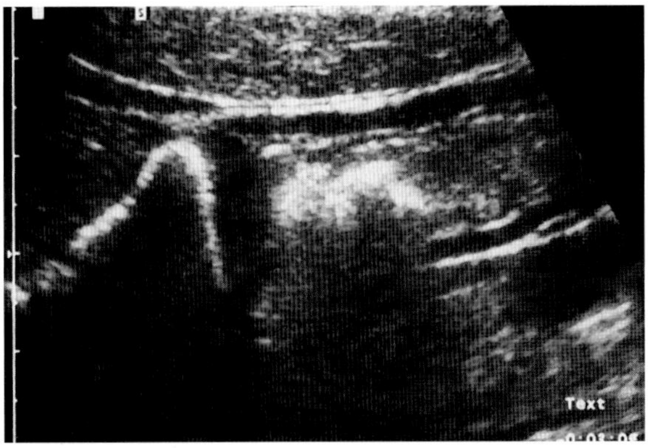

Fig. 7.1 **a** Longitudinal view of the gastric antrum, pylorus, and duodenal bulb. In the stomach, typical five-fold GI wall layering with the strong muscularis.

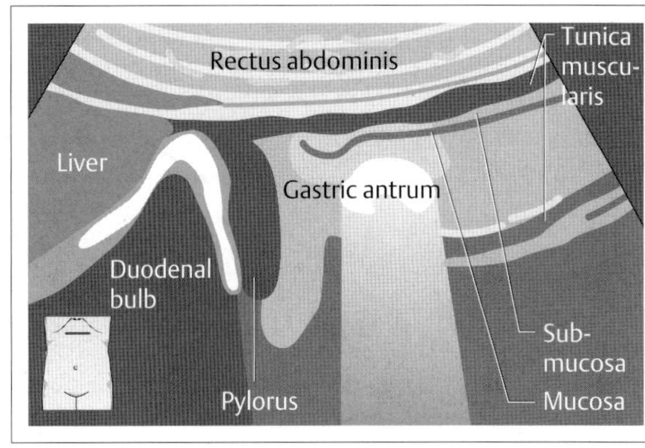

Fig. 7.1 **b** Line drawing.

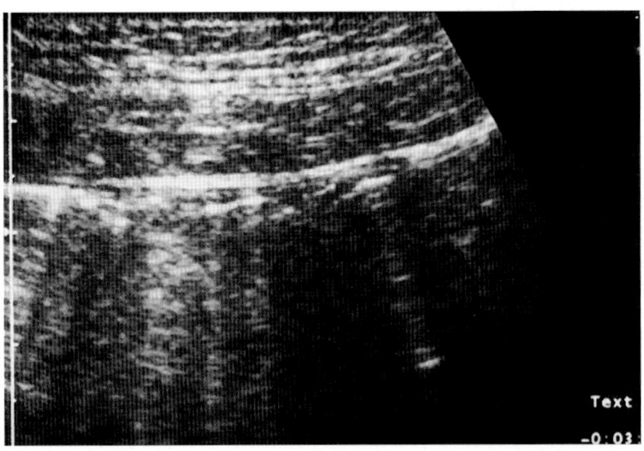

Fig. 7.2 **a** Small bowel loops, some filled with gas and others with chyme. The five layers of this thin-walled intestinal segment may be demonstrated in some areas with a 7.5 MHz probe.

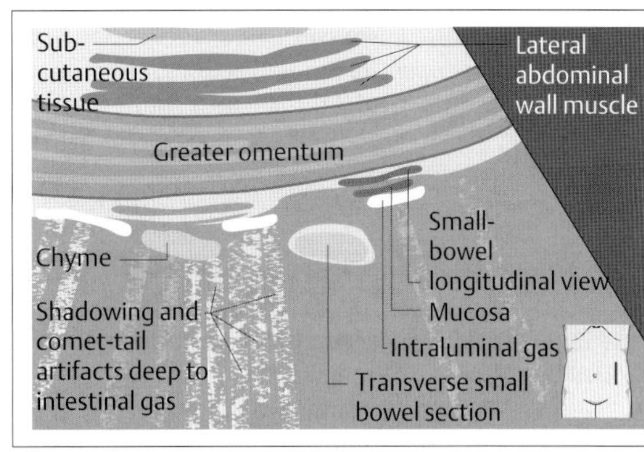

Fig. 7.2 **b** Line drawing.

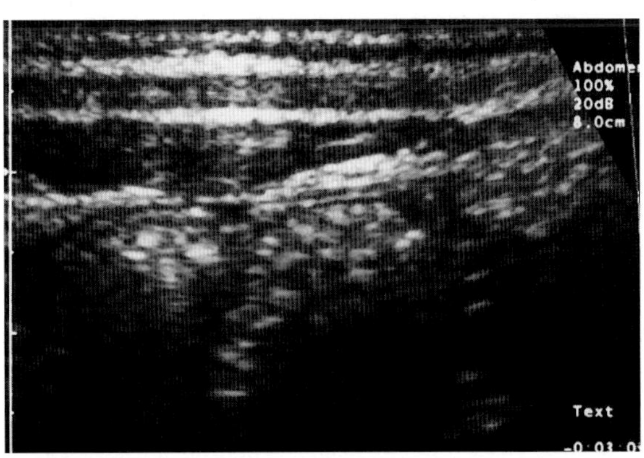

Fig. 7.3 **a** Descending colon, discernible by its semilunar folds and the five wall layers of the GI tract.

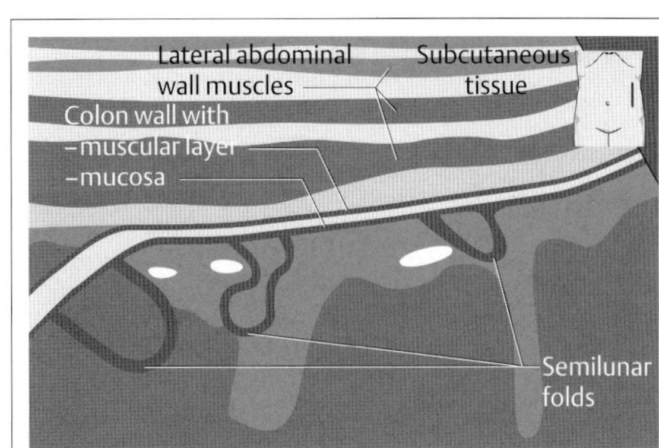

Fig. 7.3 **b** Line drawing.

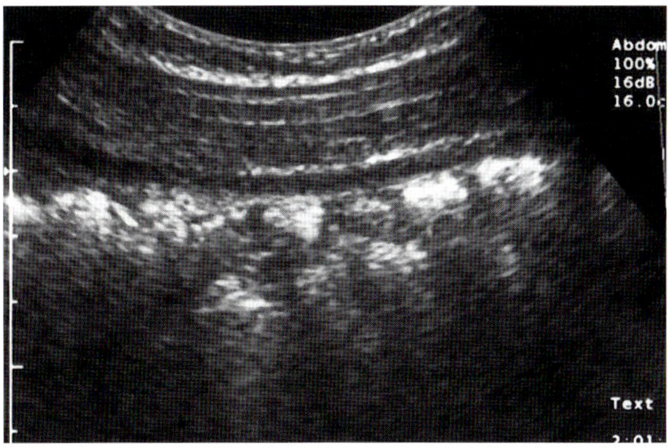

Fig. 7.4 a Ascending colon, discernible by the two parallel rows of gas-filled haustra. At this lower resolution the typical wall-layering can no longer be demonstrated.

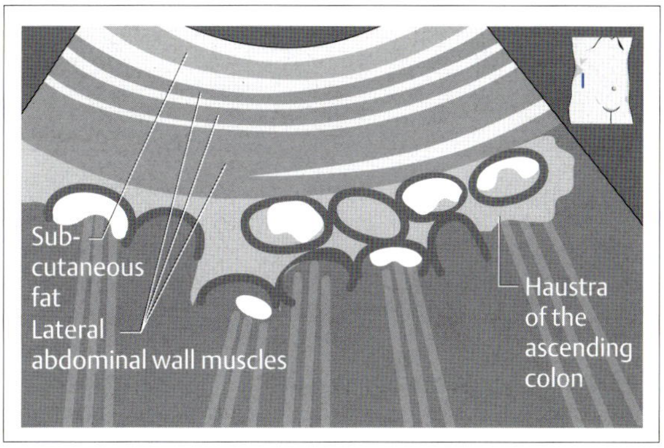

Fig. 7.4 b Line drawing.

there may be little thickening of the wall, or none whatsoever, if the GI segment concerned is distended at the same time. The opposite is also true: diffuse wall thickening may be mimicked if the lumen is totally empty, in other words, when the bowel is collapsed or undergoing peristalsis.

- The diameter of the lumen and the gas as well as fluid contents are assessed.
- Assessment of motility: Normoperistalsis, hypoperistalsis, and hyperperistalsis, as well as paradoxical pendulating peristalsis and localized wall rigidity.
- Assessment of the surrounding fatty tissue of the mesentery and omentum regarding its volume, shape, density, and mobility in relation to the peritoneum. Localized inflammation, such as appendicitis or diverticulitis, results in compaction of adjacent fatty tissue and capping of the site of inflammation.
- Demonstration of free intraperitoneal gas or fluid.

Gastroduodenal Peptic Ulceration

Basic Facts

- Nonspecific clinical signs: Diagnostic workup of upper GI complaints has to include sonography. While definitive ulcer diagnosis relies on endoscopy, sonography may, in some patients, raise the suspicion of peptic ulcer (Danneels et al., 1990; Garcia, 1999).
- Incidence:
  - Prevalence: Peptic gastric ulcer 0.3%, duodenal ulcer 1.4%.
  - Lifetime incidence: 10%, peaking between age 35 and 55; in men, the incidence of peptic duodenal ulcer is 2–3 times that in women.
- Endoscopic findings may be complemented by additional sonographic information, e.g., possible invasion of neighboring structures, or in the case of malignant ulcers depth of invasion and lymph node status. For this, EUS has proved much more sensitive than TAUS.
- For perforated ulcer, see Chapter 1, p. 18, Perforation of the Gastrointestinal Tract.
- *Additional workup:* Esophagogastroduodenoscopy, in case of suspected penetration CT, possibly exploratory endoscopy with contrast-enhanced fluoroscopy.

Sonographic Criteria

- **Inflammatory thickening of the gastric or duodenal wall around the ulcer**, sonographically visualized as circumscribed eccentric hypoechoic thickening of the wall (Fig. 7.5).
- **The ulcer itself** may appear as a sessile bright gas echo in the wall, corresponding to the suppurating base of the ulcer (Fig. 7.5).
- **Invasion of neighboring organs** is characterized by a fistula with intraluminal gas, possibly with abscess formation in the invaded organ (Fig. 7.6).
- **Perforation:** See Chapter 1, p. 18, Perforation of the Gastrointestinal Tract.

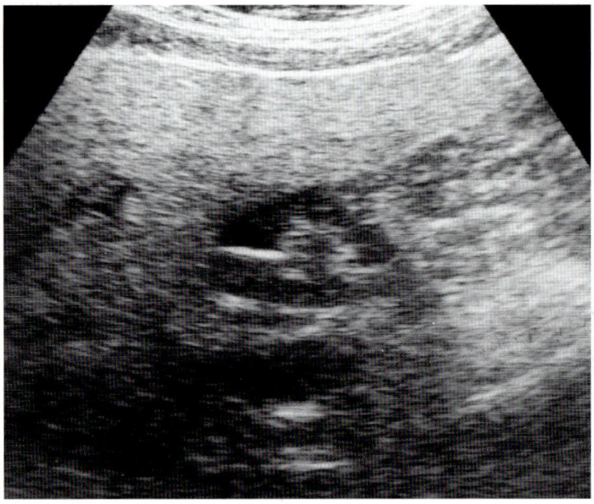

Fig. 7.**5 a** Peptic duodenal ulcer with eccentric hypoechoic wall thickening and sessile intramural gas echo. Incidental finding: fatty liver.

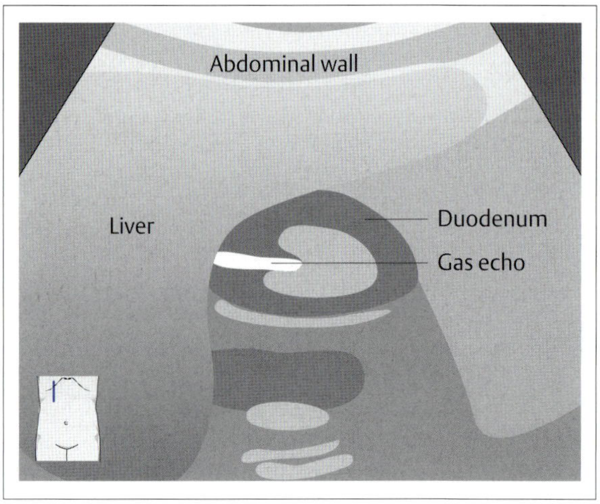

Fig. 7.**5 b** Line drawing.

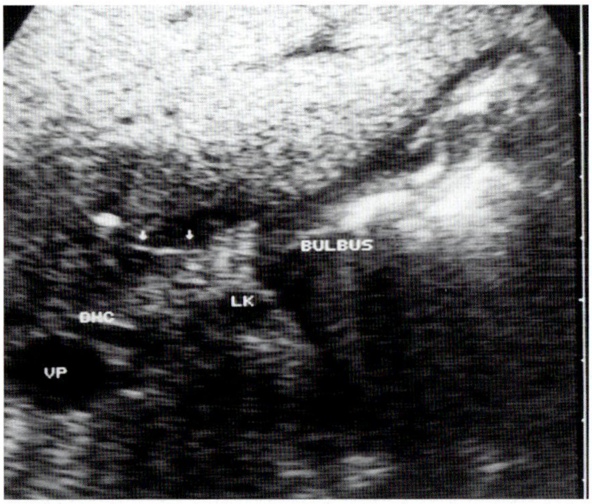

Fig. 7.**6 a** Peptic duodenal ulcer invading the liver: thickened hypoechoic wall of the duodenal bulb with a hypoechoic fistula displaying gas in its center, feeding a hepatic abscess. Compact fatty tissue between duodenal bulb and liver with lymphadenopathy. Course: After gastroscopic irrigation the abscess resolved under antibiotics.

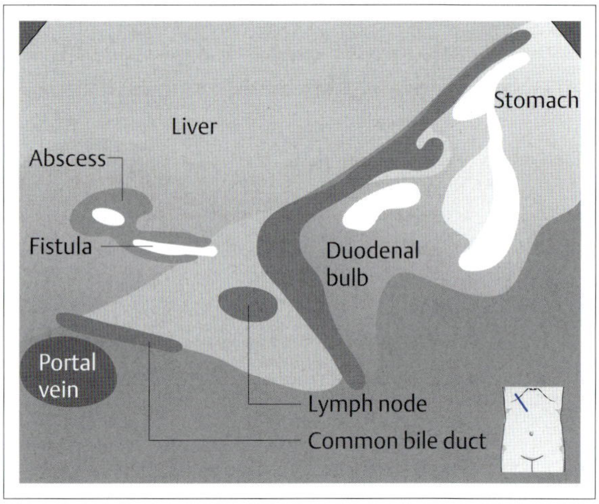

Fig. 7.**6 b** Line drawing.

Consequences for Surgical Treatment

Diagnosis	Characteristic Findings	Management
Suspected gastric or duodenal ulcer	Duodenal wall > 3 mm Gastric wall > 6 mm With or without the normal 5 wall layers	Additional diagnostic workup: esophagogastroduodenoscopy
Suspected ulcerous invasion of neighboring organs	Hypoechoic fistula with intraluminal gas	Esophagogastroduodenoscopy Diagnosis confirmed by CT or fistulography, endoscopic drainage or surgical resection
Suspected perforation: see Chapter 1, p. 18, Perforation of the Gastrointestinal Tract.		

Tumors

Basic Facts

- In the GI tract, sonography is not sensitive enough to be the sole modality for tumor screening.
- Any focal wall thickening not otherwise explained must arouse suspicion of malignancy (Dietrich et al., 1998a; Limberg, 1998; Tous and Busto, 1997). Sonographic evidence of tumor mandates further workup.
- Although sonography cannot differentiate between a malignant and benign process or type a tumor, it can provide some clues:
  - Usually, malignant bowel wall thickening is hypoechoic.
  - Extensive, relatively homogeneous bowel wall thickening (Fig. 7.**9**) suggests a malignant lymphoma of the GI tract (MALT lymphoma).
- If endoscopic biopsies are impossible or not desired, one option would be ultrasound-guided FNA of the GI tract wall (Bin et al., 1992; Carson et al., 1998).
- In case of known histology and favorable sonographic conditions, staging information may be gathered regarding depth of invasion, lymph node involvement, and intra-abdominal metastasis.
- Transabdominal sonography is of particular value when intestinal segments are not accessible by EUS, e.g., in the small bowel or proximal to colonic stenoses blocking passage of a colonoscope.
- *Additional workup:* Endoscopy; CT; diagnostic laparoscopy; in case of small bowel involvement, small bowel enteroclysis.

Sonographic Criteria

- **Localized wall thickening**, which in most cases is less echogenic than normal submucosa or the surrounding connective tissue (Figs. 7.**7**–7.**11**), and eccentric or asymmetric on transverse views (Fig. 7.**7**–7.**11**).
- **Loss of the typical wall layering** (Fig. 7.**7**–7.**11**); for sonographic staging of mural invasion, see Chapter 10, Endosonography.
- **Rigid wall**
- Possible **stenosis** is characterized by a narrow intraluminal gas echo, with distension and paradoxical pendulating peristalsis upstream.
- Cap-shaped compact mass of fatty tissue as possible **concomitant inflammatory reaction** (Fig. 7.**11**).
- **Malignant lymphomas** originating in the GI tract (**MALT lymphomas**) usually spread along the submucosa and appear as extensive, rather homogeneous hypoechoic wall thickening, often displaying a circular shape in the small bowel (Fig. 7.**9**).
- **Lymphadenopathy** in known GI cancer has to be regarded as lymph node metastasis. While a lymph node diameter ≥ 1 cm is regarded as evidence of metastasis, differentiation between benign and malignant change is hardly ever possible in lymph nodes ≤ 1 cm. Malignancy is suggested (borrowing from EUS experience with high-frequency probes, i.e., at least 5 MHz) by the presence of homogeneous hypoechoic structure and round contour (Fig. 7.**8**) rather than the physiological kidney shape with its definite hilum. The incidental finding of some abdominal lymphadenopathy of up to 2 cm in a number of asymptomatic volunteers emphasizes the need to take into account the clinical context when enlarged lymph nodes are found (Dietrich et al., 1998 b).
- **When spread is beyond the organ itself**, the hypoechoic mass extends into adjacent fatty tissue or neighboring organs (Fig. 7.**11**), and mobility in relation to omentum, peritoneum, and adjacent organs is lost.
- **Peritoneal carcinomatosis** is suggested, though not proved, by ascites, diffuse hypoechoic bowel wall thickening, possible wall rigidity, compact fatty tissue, irregular peritoneal surface, and/or evidence of intestinal obstruction (Fig. 7.**12**).

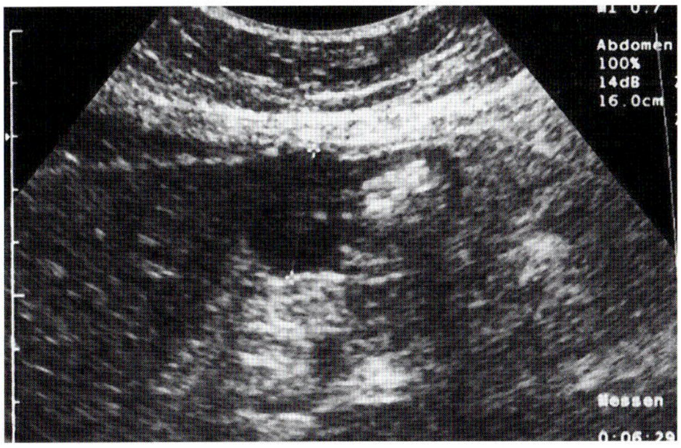

Fig. 7.**7 a** Neuroendocrine tumor of the gastric submucosa: Hypoechoic round thickening of the gastric wall on a transverse view of the antrum with visceral slide in relation to the liver and abdominal wall; definite submucosal localization on EUS.

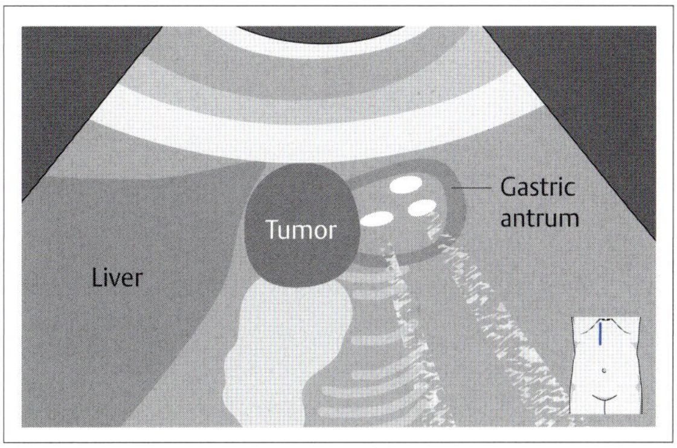

Fig. 7.**7 b** Line drawing.

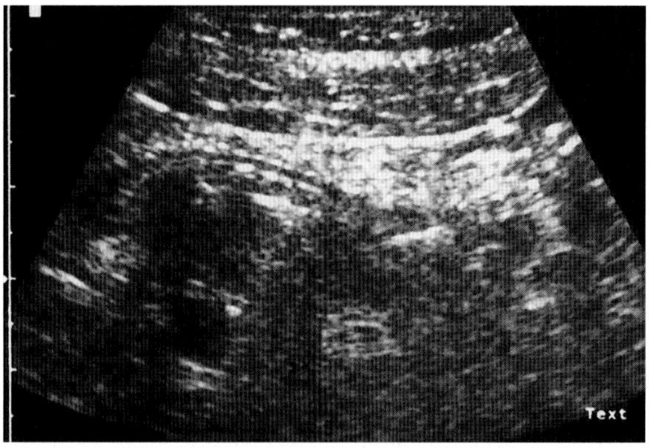

Fig. 7.**8 a** Carcinoid tumor of the ileum with lymph node metastasis: Hypoechoic ileal mass with irregular lobulated contour, partial destruction of the wall, and a hypoechoic enlarged lymph node (15 mm) in the mesentery.

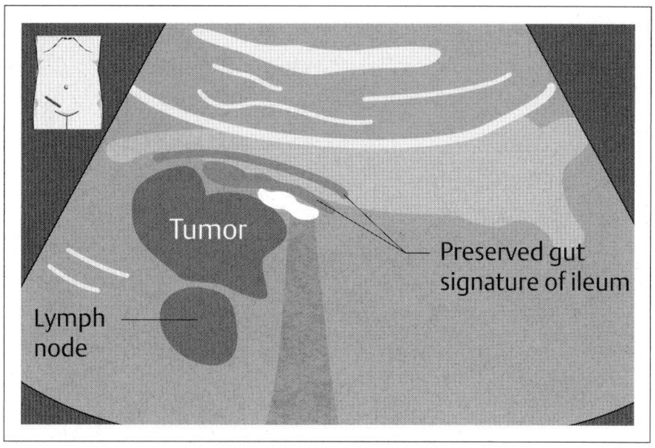

Fig. 7.**8 b** Line drawing.

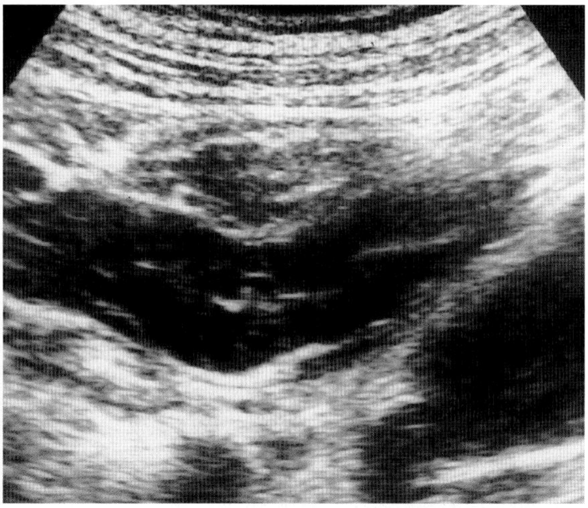

Fig. 7.**9 a** Malignant non-Hodgkin lymphoma of the ileum: Longitudinal view of the ileum with extensive, rather hypoechoic thickening of submucosa and mucosa; the severely compressed lumen is identified by the gas echoes. The muscle layer is still intact.

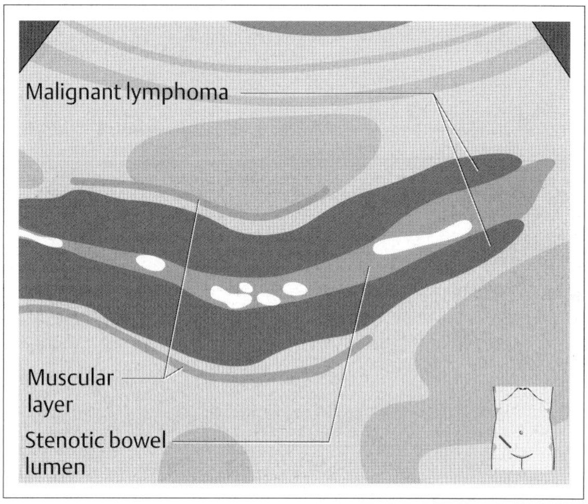

Fig. 7.**9 b** Line drawing.

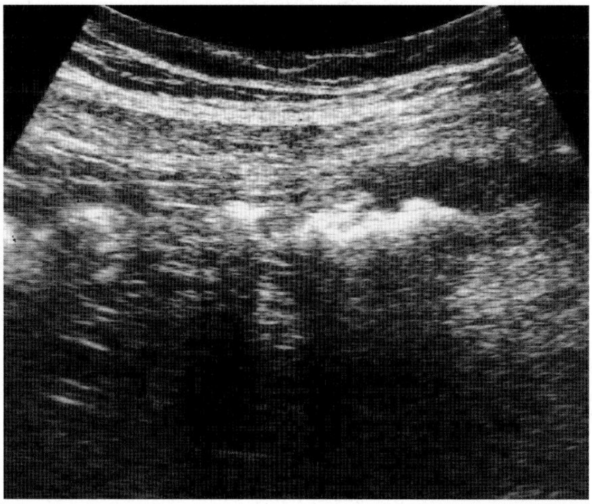

Fig. 7.**10 a** Cancer of the descending colon, stage T3. Longitudinal view of the colon with haustra, localized hypoechoic thickening of the wall with destruction of all layers, and irregular contour.

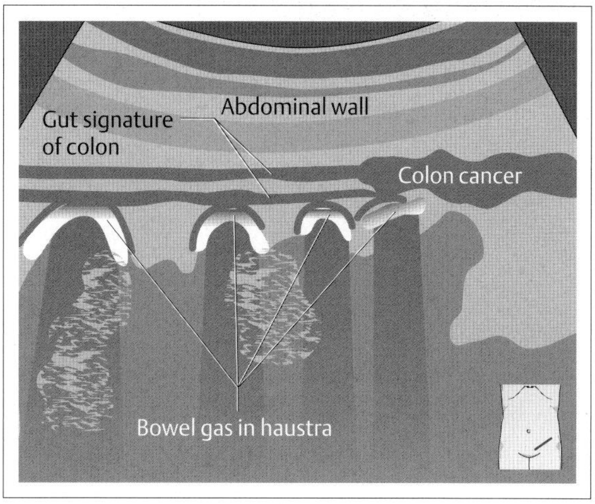

Fig. 7.**10 b** Line drawing.

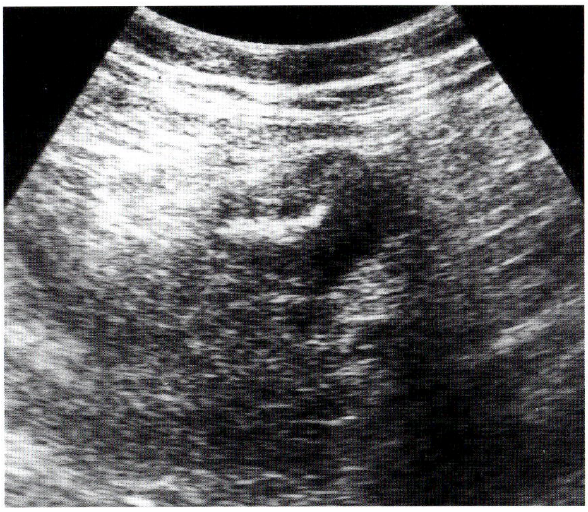

Fig. 7.**11 a** Same patient as in Fig. 7.**10**; transverse view of the descending colon with eccentric hypoechoic wall thickening, breaching the contour in some places. Compact fatty tissue capping the process, indicating concomitant inflammation of the omentum or mesocolon.

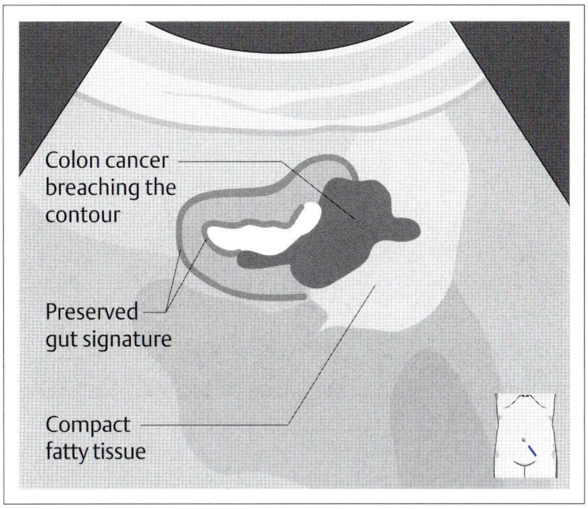

Fig. 7.**11 b** Line drawing.

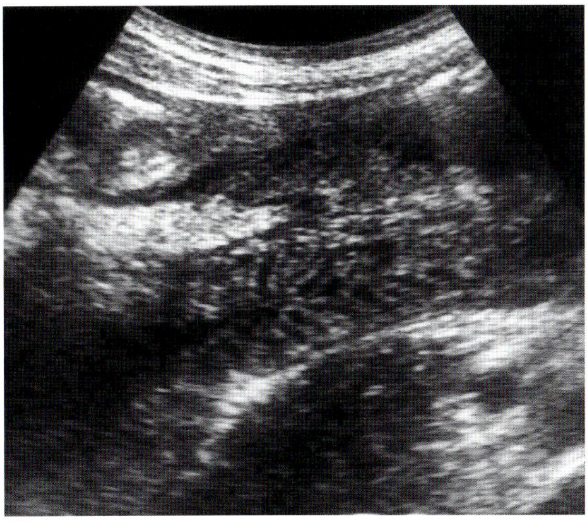

Fig. 7.**12 a** Peritoneal carcinomatosis. Diffuse hypoechoic thickening of the jejunal wall, contrasting with the compact fatty tissue. Diffuse swelling of the circular folds; bowel motility and visceral slide are reduced.

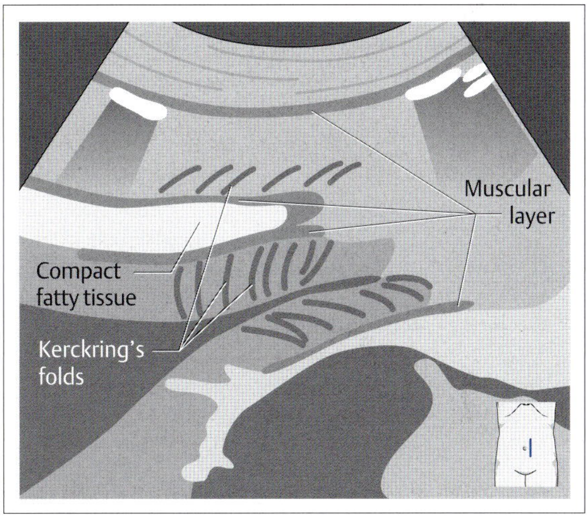

Fig. 7.**12 b** Line drawing.

Consequences for Surgical Treatment

Diagnosis	Characteristic Findings	Management
Suspected malignancy of GI wall	Localized thickening of the GI wall, e.g., during diagnostic workup of unspecific abdominal complaints or other general symptoms of malignancy.	Additional workup: endoscopy, contrast-enhanced fluoroscopy, CT
Lymphadenopathy	During general search for a tumor, without sonographic evidence of malignancy	Additional diagnostic workup: Endoscopy, contrast-enhanced fluoroscopy, CT

Mechanical Bowel Obstruction and Paralytic Ileus

See Chapter 1, Acute Abdomen.

Chronic Inflammatory Bowel Disease

Basic Facts

- *Leading symptoms:* abdominal pain and diarrhea; hematochezia common in ulcerative colitis.
- *Differential diagnosis* of Crohn disease and ulcerative colitis is based on the clinical course, laboratory tests, endoscopic and histological picture; in about 10% of cases differentiation between these two entities is impossible. Distinction between mild or early forms of chronic inflammatory versus infectious bowel disease (e.g., Crohn disease vs. yersiniosis, ulcerative colitis vs. salmonellosis) sometimes becomes possible only over the course of the disease.
- Both diseases have almost identical sex and age distributions, with preponderance of primary manifestation in the age group 15–40 years.
  - *Ulcerative colitis:* Contiguous diffuse inflammation of the mucosa, beginning at the rectum and involving the upstream colon to a varying degree, in rare cases extending into the terminal ileum as so-called backwash ileitis; with multiple ulceration in flare-ups. Since the sonographic presentation is the same as that in infectious colitis, the value of sonography rests more with the follow-up.
  - *Crohn disease:* Segmental inflammation of the small and/or large bowel, interspersed with segments of normal mucosa, results in the picture of "skip lesions" transmural spread of the inflammation is possible often with easily visualized fistulas, abscesses, and stenoses. Valuable additional information complementing the endoscopic and radiological findings, particularly regarding possible involvement of the small bowel. As in ulcerative colitis, the main role of sonography lies in long-term follow-up.

Sonographic Criteria

- **Ulcerative colitis** (Bozkurt and Lux, 1998; Meckler and Herzog, 1989; Truong et al., 1998):
  - Extensive circular wall thickening, typically involving the mucosa and submucosa (Fig. 7.**13**).
  - The rectum is always involved, the disease extending upstream contiguously over varying distances.
  - Long-term chronic disease may result in complete loss of haustration (Fig. 7.**14**).
- **Crohn disease** (Bozkurt and Lux, 1998; Gasche et al., 1999; Limberg, 1998; Meckler and Herzog, 1989)
  - Segmental wall thickening of the small or large bowel (Fig. 7.**15**), on transverse sections frequently eccentric rather than circular (Fig. 7.**16**).
  - Sometimes involving the mucosa and submucosa with wall layering preserved, while in others the layered gut signature is destroyed by transmural hypoechoic infiltration (Figs. 7.**15**, 7.**16**).
  - In case of transmural spread, the compact fatty tissue of the surroundings mirrors the inflammatory involvement (Figs. 7.**16**, 7.**17**); hypoechoic "inflammation lanes" in the omentum or mesentery signify increasingly severe inflammation.
  - Lymphadenitis (Fig. 7.**16**).
  - Fistulas may be visualized as hypoechoic strands with bright central intraluminal gas echoes (Fig. 7.**18**).
  - An abscess appears as a paraintestinal fluid collection, sometimes containing gas echoes, in most cases walled off by compact fatty tissue (Fig. 7.**19**).
  - Stenoses are characterized by the narrowed intestinal lumen with passage of intraluminal gas echoes; paradoxical pendulating peristalsis upstream. Causes may be (reversible) inflammatory wall thickening (Figs. 7.**15**, 7.**18**) or (fixed) scarring without wall thickening (Fig. 7.**20**).
- Quite often, differentiation between **infectious** and **chronic inflammatory bowel disease** is not possible on the basis of sonomorphology alone (Figs. 7.**13**, 7.**17**).

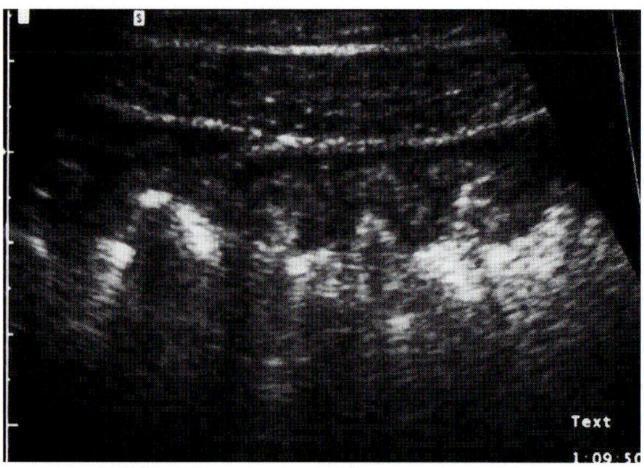

Fig. 7.**13a** Acute ulcerative colitis. Long-axis view of the descending colon with wall thickening, primarily of the mucosa and submucosa. Colitis: further specification is not possible with sonography but relies on clinical and endoscopic features.

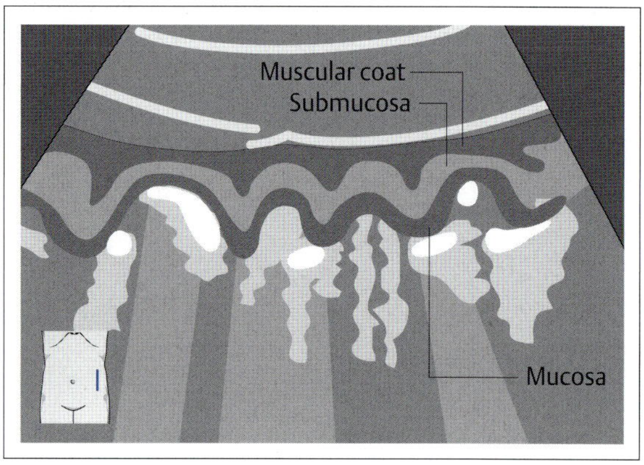

Fig. 7.**13b** Line drawing.

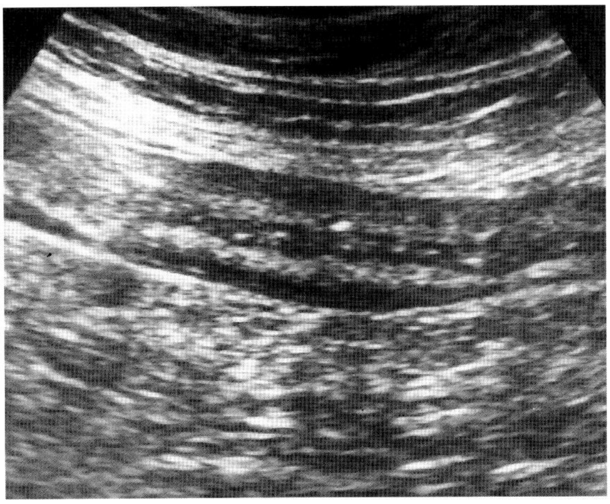

Fig. 7.**14a** Acute-on-chronic ulcerative colitis of many years' standing. Long-axis view of the sigmoid colon with wall thickening, primarily of the mucosa and submucosa. The lumen is empty, haustra are missing. The accompanying edema of the muscularis propria has separated the inner circular from the outer longitudinal muscle layer by a narrow hyperechoic band.

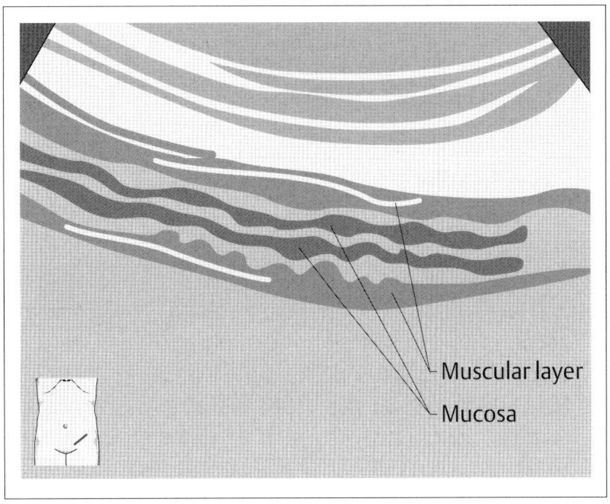

Fig. 7.**14b** Line drawing.

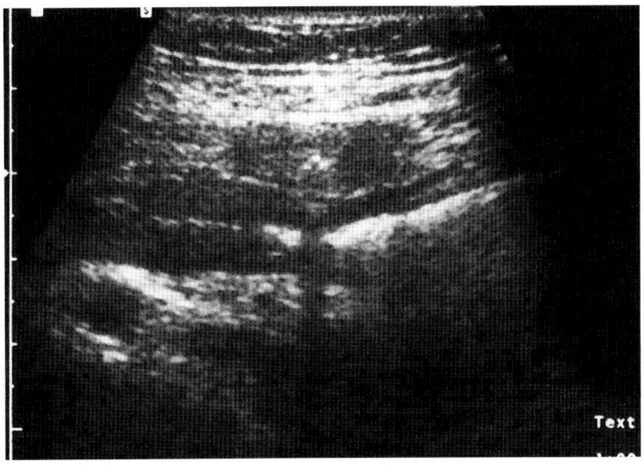

Fig. 7.**15a** Acute episode of Crohn disease of the small bowel with inflammatory stenosis. Small bowel with two criss-crossing loops; the transverse view of the loop closer to the transducer exhibits slight thickening of the wall and gut signature with preserved layering. The longitudinal view of the loop away from the probe is characterized by significant segmental wall thickening of up to 12 mm with loss of layering and hypoechoic transformation of the wall. This wall thickening results in luminal stenosis and distension of the upstream segment (right half of the image). Preserved layering in the distended bowel segment with only moderate thickening (≤ 5 mm) of the wall.

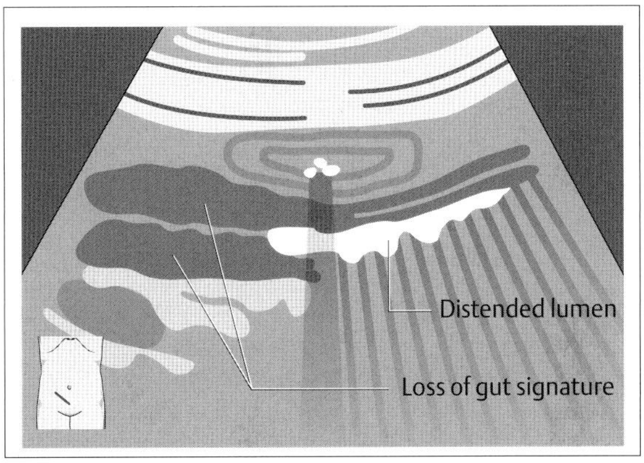

Fig. 7.**15b** Line drawing.

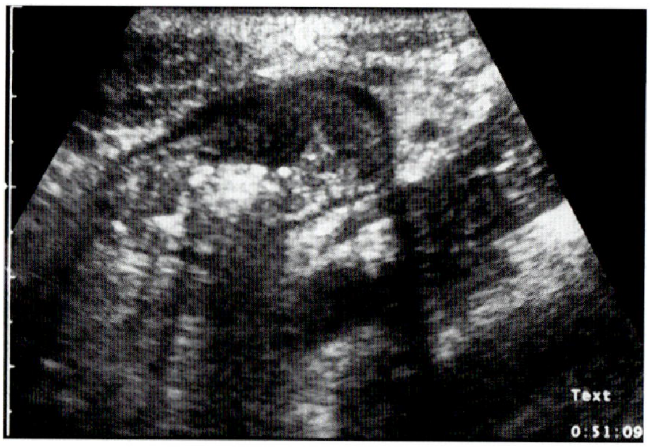

Fig. 7.**16a** Acute episode of Crohn disease of the large bowel with transmural inflammation. Transverse view of the ascending colon with eccentric wall thickening (≤ 15 mm) and loss of layering. Inflamed enlarged mesenteric lymph node (7 mm) in the fatty tissue of the mesocolon.

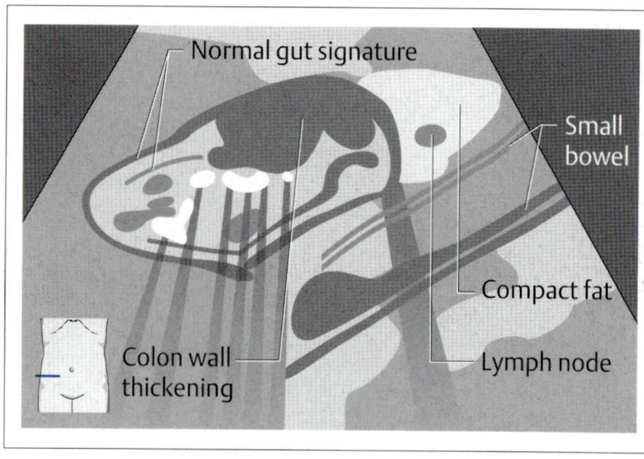

Fig. 7.**16b** Line drawing.

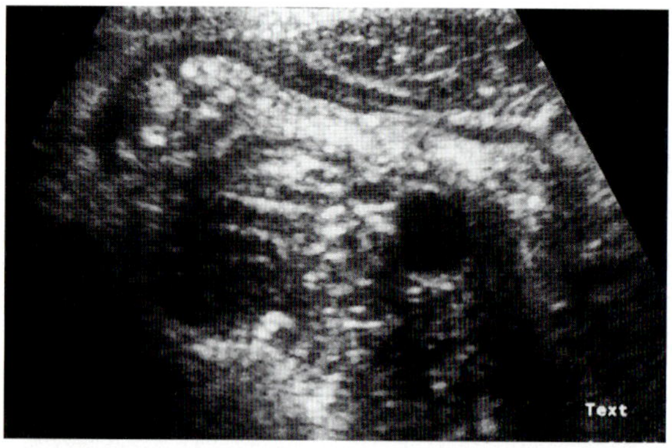

Fig. 7.**17a** Same patient as in Fig. 7.**16**. Ileocecum with thickened wall of the terminal ileum and cecum. Swollen ileocecal valve with preserved wall layering. Differentiation from infectious ileocecitis is not possible by sonography alone.

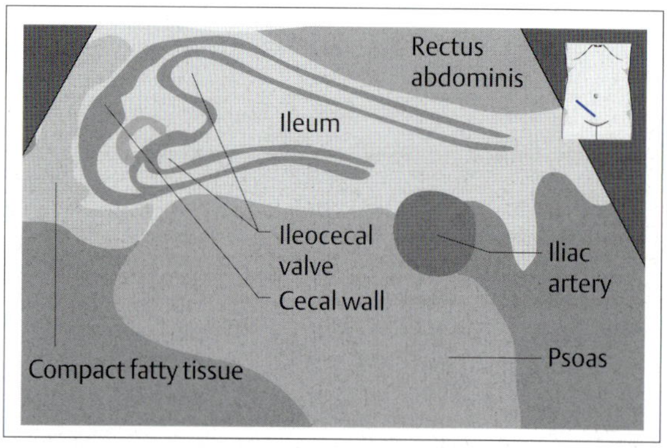

Fig. 7.**17b** Line drawing.

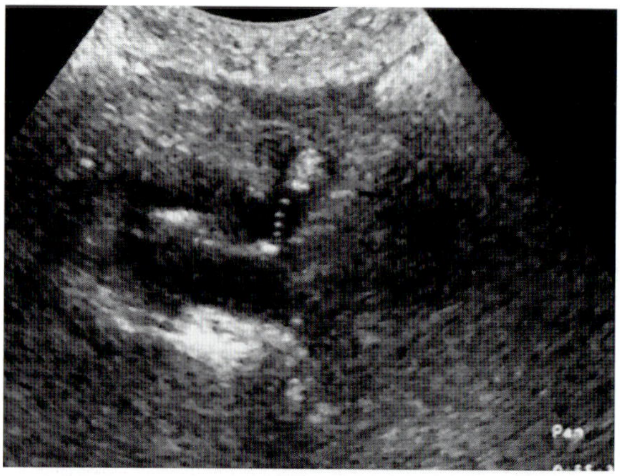

Fig. 7.**18a** Enteroenteric fistula with a small bowel conglomerate in Crohn disease: The hypoechoic mass can be palpated in the right lower quadrant. Loss of layering, the intestinal walls of adjacent loops can no longer be separated. The narrowed lumen is identified by the central intraluminal gas echoes. The thin trail of gas bubbles between the lumina signifies a fistula.

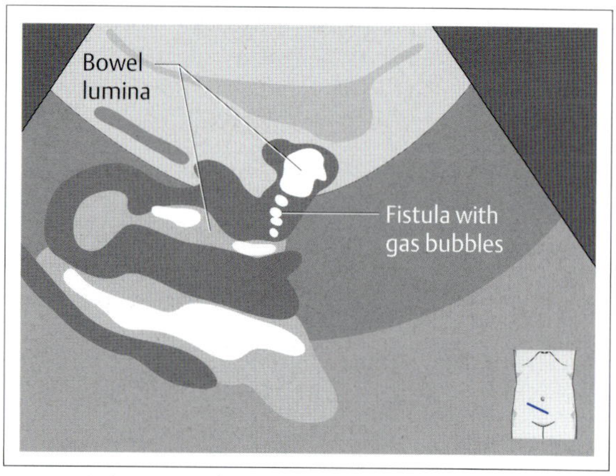

Fig. 7.**18b** Line drawing.

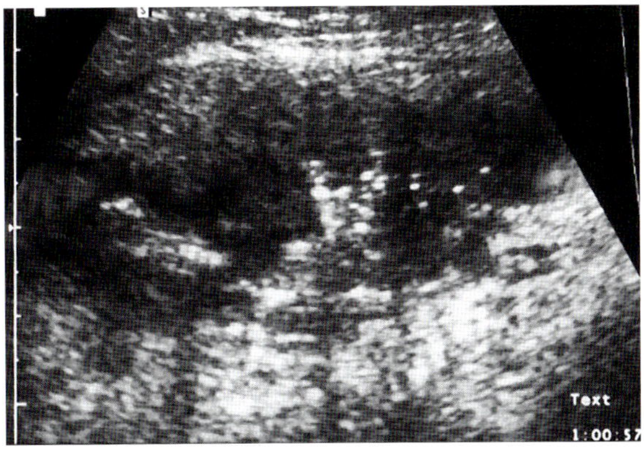

Fig. 7.**19 a** Crohn disease with fistula from the small bowel to an abscess in the abdominal wall. Hypoechoic mass with an almost anechoic center in the abdominal wall of the right lower quadrant. Within the mass there is a web of gas echo trails. Individual bowel loops can no longer be separated from the hypoechoic mass. Fine-needle aspiration of the hypoechoic mass yielded pus.

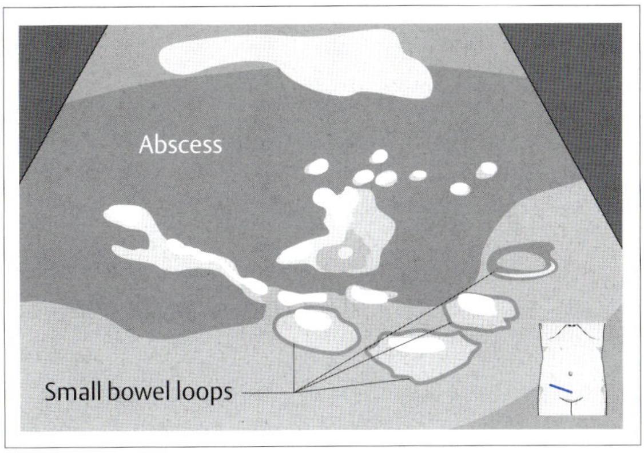

Fig. 7.**19 b** Line drawing.

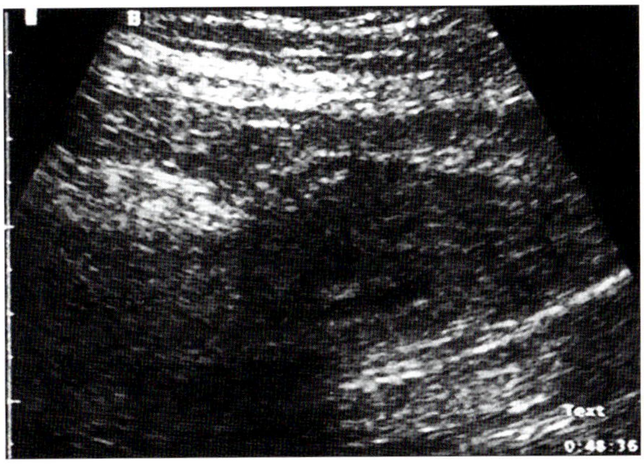

Fig. 7.**20 a** Stenosis of the terminal ileum due to scarring in chronic, but currently inactive, Crohn disease: On the right, short-segment wall thickening of the terminal ileum with preserved wall layering. On the left, severe stenosis of the terminal ileum without wall thickening, surrounded by fatty tissue.

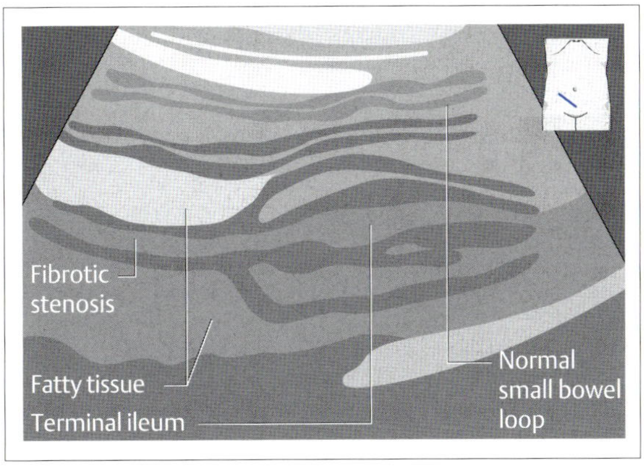

Fig. 7.**20 b** Line drawing.

Consequences for Surgical Treatment

Diagnosis	Characteristic Findings	Management
Abscess	Extraintestinal hypoechoic/anechoic mass, possibly with gas inclusion, often surrounded by compact fatty tissue	Interventional drainage; if drainage is impossible or does not suffice, surgical evacuation
Fistula	Enteroenteric or enterocutaneous hypoechoic straplike structure with central gas echoes	MRI or contrast-enhanced radiological fistula delineation; attempt at nonsurgical management with drug treatment of the underlying disease; surgery in case of persistence or complications
Inflammatory stenoses without ileus	Stenosis of the intestinal lumen with hypoechoic bowel wall, no signs of obstruction (see Chapter 1, Acute Abdomen)	Attempt at conservative management
Symptomatic fibrotic stenosis	Narrowed intestinal lumen without wall thickening	Limited surgical resection

Appendicitis

See Chapter 1, Acute Abdomen.

Diverticulitis

Basic Facts

- **Diverticula** may arise anywhere along the GI tract.
  - Congenital diverticula (rare): herniation of all wall layers.
  - Acquired diverticula: herniation of just the mucosa ("pseudodiverticula") through a gap in the muscle coat, especially around the papilla of Vater as well as in the sigmoid and descending colon.
- The incidence of acquired diverticula in the population aged 50 years and older is 20–50%, most often associated with thickening of the muscle layer ("myochosis"), contraction of haustra, and luminal narrowing.
- Diverticulitis (inflammation mainly of just one diverticulum) is seen almost exclusively in the colon, and there mostly in the sigmoid, except for: Meckel's diverticulum (ileum).
- Diverticulitis is **diagnosed** on clinical grounds in patients presenting with localized pain and guarding, usually in the left lower quadrant, occasionally associated with a palpable inflamed bowel segment.
- Sonography confirms the suspected diagnosis and aids in the detection of complications (abscess, fistula, perforation, stenosis) (Schwerk et al., 1993; Truong et al., 1998), but is of no help in diverticular hemorrhage.
- *Additional workup:* Colonoscopy or barium enema after the acute episode has subsided, in order to rule out malignoma.
  - Suspected abscess: CT, possibly paracentesis.
  - Suspected fistula: contrast-enhanced fluoroscopy or MRI.
  - Suspected perforation: abdominal films, possibly laparoscopy.

Sonographic Criteria

- **Diverticula** and **muscular hypertrophy** can frequently be visualized sonographically even in the absence of diverticulitis.
  - Diverticula: round structures containing gas, either intramural or budding the colonic wall, frequently multiple and arranged along the tenias (Fig. 7.**21**).
  - Myochosis (muscular hypertrophy): thickening of the hypoechoic muscularis propria, haustra shortened, possible luminal narrowing (Fig. 7.**21**).
- **Diverticulitis** (Figs. 7.**22**, 7.**23**):
  - Compact fatty tissue (mesentery, omentum, epiploic appendices) capping a diverticulum.
  - In contrast, the lumen of the diverticulum is hypoechoic; due to the inflamed diverticular wall there is intraluminal exudate.
  - Within the diverticular lumen there are frequently also bright echoes with posterior shadowing, corresponding to enteroliths or gas.
  - Local thickening of all gut wall layers; on transverse views this swelling appears eccentric, and there may be mild luminal narrowing (Fig. 7.**24**).
- Complications of diverticulitis that may be demonstrated sonographically:
  - *Abscess:* By erosion of the wall and inflammation of the cellular debris in its lumen, diverticulitis always results in diverticular empyema; only if the suppuration extends beyond the original diverticulum will abscess formation take place. The sonographic criteria are identical to those of the inflamed diverticulum, only bigger and possibly farther away from the intestinal lumen; when in doubt–FNA of the hypoechoic mass.
  - *Fistula:* Frequently only minor signs of inflammation because the diverticular contents will drain via the fistula. The fistula may sometimes be demonstrated as a hypoechoic strap with central gas echoes surrounded by compact fatty tissue; for example, gas within the urinary bladder would indicate an enterovesical fistula (Fig. 7.**25**).
  - *Perforation:* Evidence of free intraperitoneal gas, quite often hampering assessment of the bowel.
  - *Stenosis:* The size of the lumen can be determined sonographically, although its capacity to distend cannot be gauged. Since quite often the lumen is only narrowed by inflammation, this process can be reversed. Fibrotic stenosis, on the other hand, is permanent and can be demonstrated indirectly through prestenotic distension of the colon after the diverticulitis has subsided.

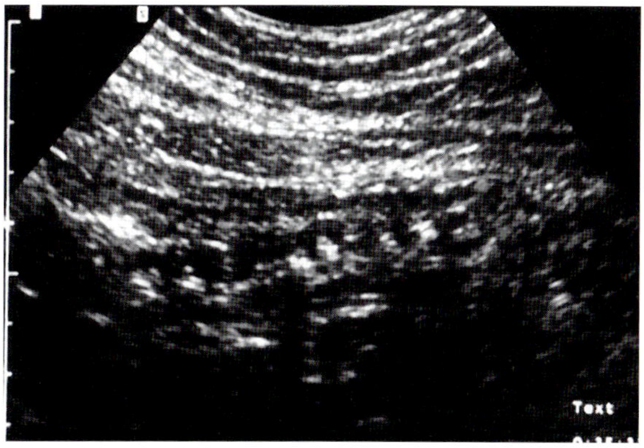

Fig. 7.21 a Longitudinal view of diverticula of the sigmoid colon. Multiple round structures containing gas and abutting the colon. Myochosis: hypoechoic thickening of the muscularis propria with shortened haustration and slightly narrowed colonic lumen.

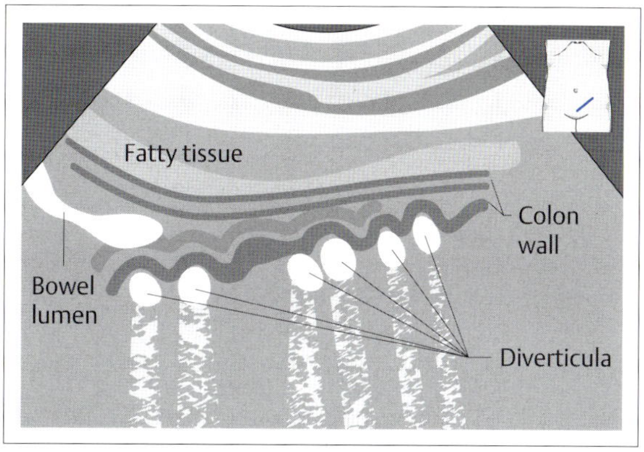

Fig. 7.21 b Line drawing.

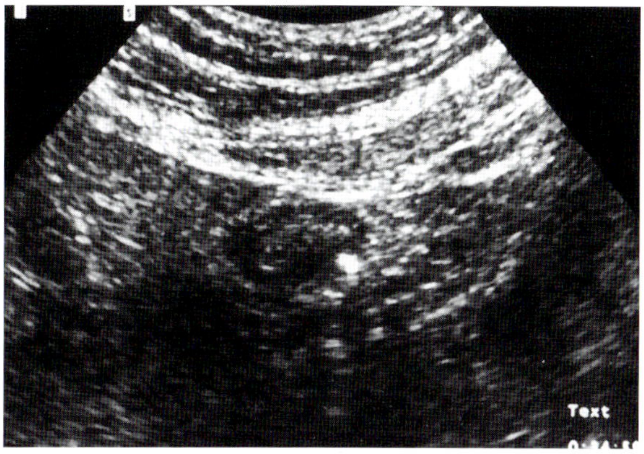

Fig. 7.22 a Same patient as in Fig. 7.21. Transverse view of the sigmoid colon with one of the gas-containing diverticula budding from the colonic wall.

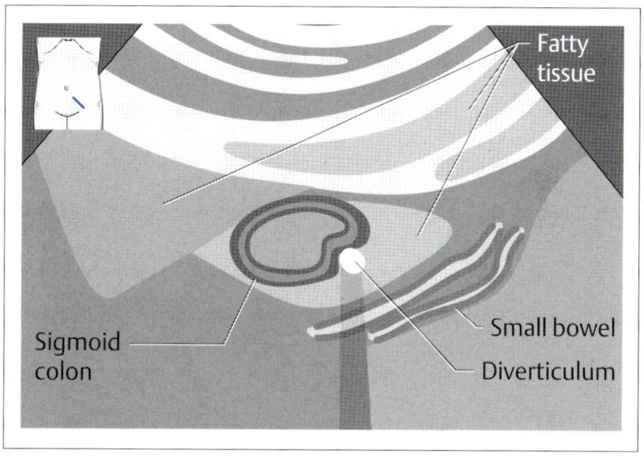

Fig. 7.22 b Line drawing.

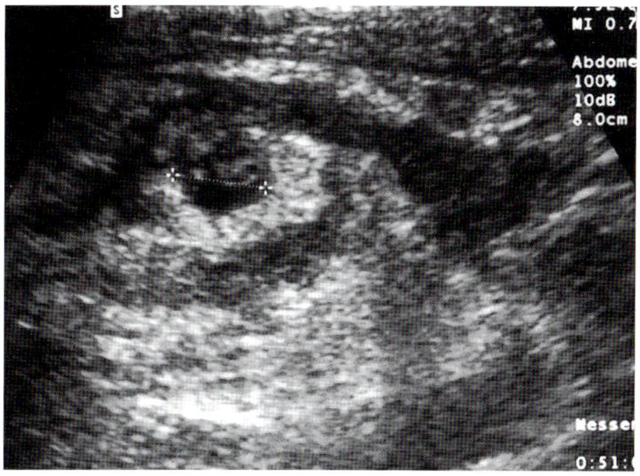

Fig. 7.23 a Acute diverticulitis. Longitudinal view of the sigmoid colon with mostly hypoechoic diverticular contents and compact adjacent fatty tissue capping the diverticulum. Curving compression of the colon by this compact fatty tissue and asymmetric segmental thickening of the colonic wall.

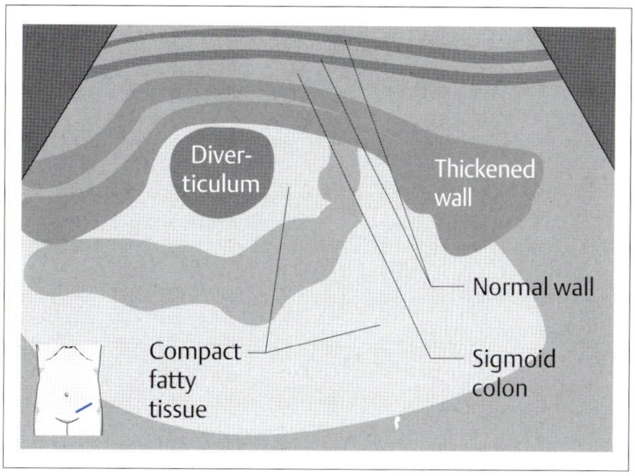

Fig. 7.23 b Line drawing.

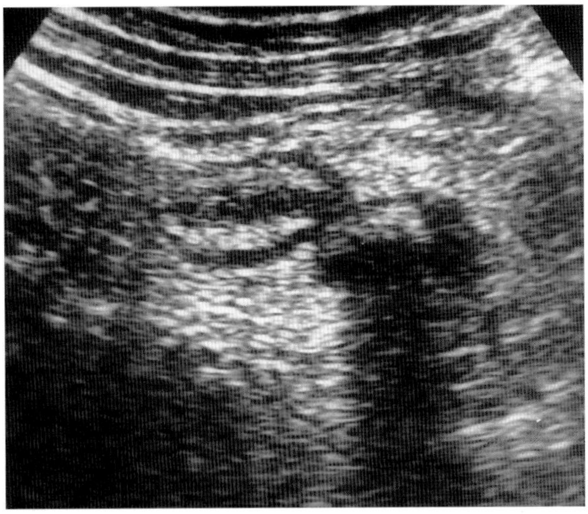

Fig. 7.**24 a** Acute diverticulitis. Transverse view of the sigmoid colon with hyperechoic diverticular contents (i.e., gas or enterolith), but also with hypoechoic parts of the diverticulum (beginning abscess formation possible) and compact fatty tissue in the surroundings.

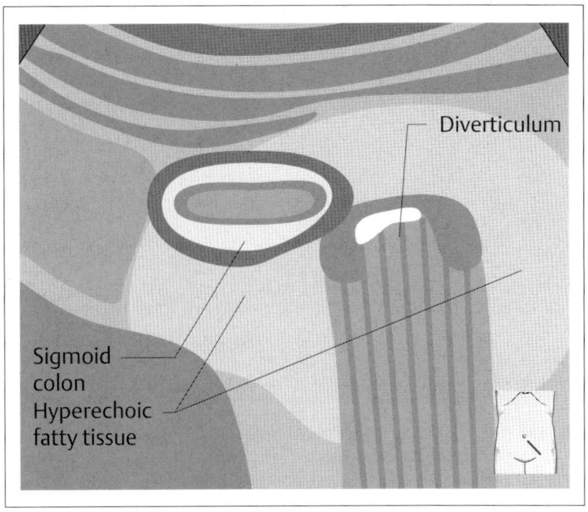

Fig. 7.**24 b** Line drawing.

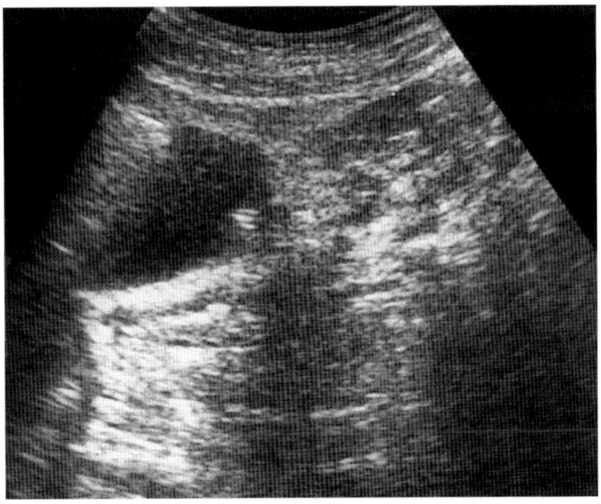

Fig. 7.**25 a** Fistula from the sigmoid colon to the urinary bladder in diverticular disease. Gas within the bladder, compact fatty tissue between bladder and sigmoid colon, multiple diverticula of the sigmoid. Hypoechoic strap with central gas echoes in the compact fatty tissue, running from the sigmoid colon to a polypoid structure at the left posterior wall of the urinary bladder, corresponding to the opening of the fistula.

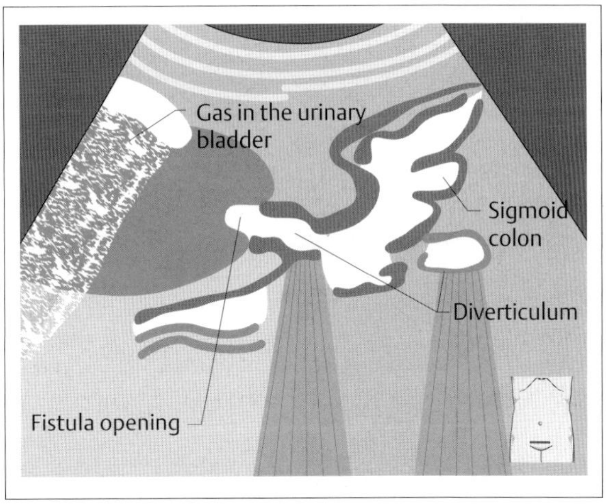

Fig. 7.**25 b** Line drawing.

Consequences for Surgical Treatment

Diagnosis	Characteristic Findings	Management
Uncomplicated diverticulitis	Local tenderness, sonography reveals an inflamed gas- or fluid-filled diverticulum with compact adjacent fatty tissue	No oral intake, antibiotics; colonoscopy once inflammation has subsided; when abscess is suspected, CT and possibly paracentesis or drainage
Diverticular abscess	Signs of diverticulitis with liquid mass, usually within the surrounding fatty tissue	Drainage
Diverticular fistula	Signs of diverticulitis, hypoechoic fistula tract with central gas echoes	Resection of fistula plus segmentectomy of the bowel
Perforated diverticulitis	Signs of diverticulitis, also free gas	Bowel resection with anastomosis or end colostomy in severe peritonitis (Hartmann's procedure)
Diverticular stenosis	Demonstration of diverticula, possibly with diverticulitis, distended bowel upstream	Segmentectomy, if diverticulitis persists after antibiotic regimen

■ Liver

Indications for Sonography

- Sonography is the imaging modality of choice whenever liver disease is suspected.
- The liver offers excellent conditions for sonography owing to its parenchyma, compact shape, and large area of contact with the thoracic and abdominal wall.
- Since the findings are often incidental, especially in masses, the liver should always be scanned during abdominal sonography. Sonography provides the definitive diagnosis in some cases and directs the choice of further workup in others.
- **Main indications:**
  - Upper quadrant pain, jaundice.
  - Clinical signs of hepatomegaly, cirrhosis, or hepatic failure.
  - Equivocal abnormal blood chemistry tests of the liver.
  - Tumor screening in patients at risk, e.g., looking for hepatocellular carcinoma in known chronic viral hepatitis or cirrhosis.
  - Search for metastases in patients with a known primary.
  - Fever of unknown origin, other signs of inflammation.
  - Suspected involvement of the liver in systemic or metabolic disease.
  - Thoracic or abdominal trauma.
  - Monitoring of liver biopsies for histology or cytology.
  - Follow-up for known liver pathology, e.g., monitoring the size of metastases during and after chemotherapy.

Specific Technique and Diagnostic Evaluation

- Relationships of the liver in the right upper quadrant:
  - Convex surface (diaphragmatic aspect; Fig. 7.**26a**) facing the diaphragm.
  - Flat surface, in parts concave (visceral aspect; Fig. 7.**26b**), in contact with the adjacent intra-abdominal organs.
  - Attached to the diaphragm, inferior vena cava, stomach, and duodenum by ligaments that normally sonography cannot differentiate from the surrounding fasciae and fatty structures of the lesser sac; they do, however, become delineated in the presence of ascites.
- 3.5 MHz probes are preferred, with higher-frequency transducers (5 or 7.5 MHz) for those parts of the liver close to the thoracic or abdominal wall. Due to the large size of the liver, the focal zones need to be depth-adapted to the regions of interest.
- In the epigastrium and right upper quadrant, the probe scans in the longitudinal plane (Fig. 7.**27a, b**) and along both costal arches, i.e., right subcostal (Fig. 7.**27c**), subxiphoidal (Fig. 7.**27d**), and left subcostal view (Fig. 7.**27e**), and on the right also in the intercostal plane (Fig. 7.**27f**). Additional views are adapted to the structures of interest, e.g. for visualizing the tubular structures in the hepatoduodenal ligament; see below (Fig. 7.**27g**).
- Epigastrium and right upper quadrant are examined with the patient supine and in left semi-lateral decubitus position. Subcostal views are best performed with the liver as far caudad as possible, i.e., with contraction

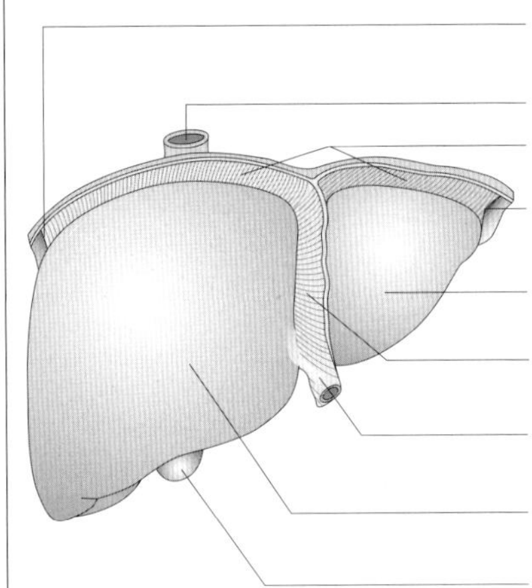

Fig. 7.**26 a** Shape and surface of the liver with fissures and ligaments: Diaphragmatic surface.

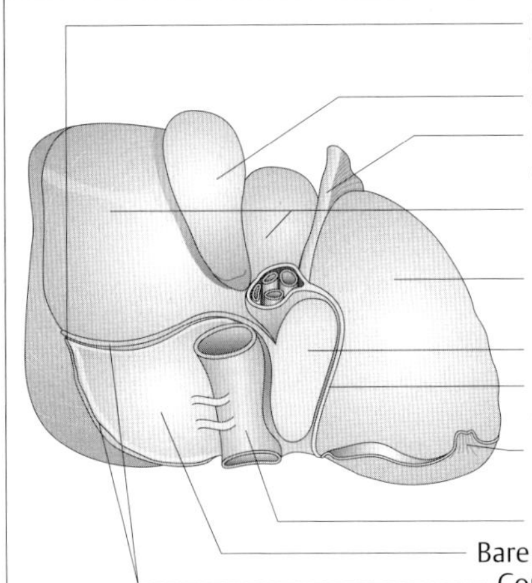

Fig. 7.**26 b** Shape and surface of the liver with fissures and ligaments: Visceral surface.

of the diaphragm–in other words, with the patient exhaling (sometimes the patient should be asked to push out the abdomen).

- Intercostal imaging is performed with the patient supine, using all intercostal spaces in contact with the liver, in the middle of respiration or while breath-holding. Stretching the right side of the body by placing the right hand behind the neck also helps.
- Always scan the entire organ at each point of probe contact by moving and tilting the transducer. The superior aspects of the liver immediately inferior to the diaphragm may only be visualized by tilting the probe as far cephalad as possible.
- The capsule of the liver is rather thin and cannot be separated from the reflections of the hepatic surface. The normal liver surface appears as a thin, bright, straight echo line, to be differentiated from the neighboring structures only with respiratory motion or in the presence of ascites.
- The inferior border of the liver, i.e., the caudal transition from the diaphragmatic to the visceral aspect, forms an acute angle of 30–45° in the left lobe, increasing to up to 75° in the right lobe.
- The size of the liver represents an important parameter in numerous hepatic diseases, especially diffuse ones; however, this measurement suffers from potential errors inherent in the procedure.
  - Shape and especially length along the three axes of the body demonstrate significant variation between people; the best reference parameter is the liver volume, which is determined precisely by the summation of parallel slices (same concept as in CT).
  - Longitudinal and sagittal dimensions are strongly influenced by the depth of the chest and by body constitution: In a light, thin body with a shallow chest, the liver will be short in the sagittal plane but rather long in the longitudinal dimension (Fig. 7.**28 b**). In barrel-chested patients, e.g., in pulmonary emphysema or in those with a pyknic build, the liver will be short along the longitudinal axis and long in the sagittal dimension (Fig. 7.**28 a**).
  - Upper normal limits discounting variations in shape. Height at the medioclavicular line: 11 cm from the liver–lung interface (line x in Fig. 7.**28**) and 13 cm from the bare area to the inferior margin of the liver (line y in Fig. 7.**28**) (Niederau and Sonnenberg, 1984).
- It is rather rare for the left lobe of the liver to extend so far to the left that on left intercostal views it will appear superior to the spleen. It may then be confused with a crescent-like splenic mass, e.g., subcapsular hematoma.
- Variations in shape may be due to additional lobes, protruding from the normal hepatic contour from a broad base or pedicle, e.g., Riedel's lobe projecting caudad from the inferior border of the right lobe. Diaphragmatic hiatus may result in liver parenchyma protruding into the thoracic cavity. Ostensible further subdivisions of the hepatic lobes by additional fissures not corresponding to intersegmental boundaries are common in the left lobe (Martinoli et al., 1992). Impressions on the diaphragmatic aspect due to individual diaphragmatic cords must not be confused with hepatic lesions!
- Normal hepatic echotexture is homogeneous, of identical echodensity irrespective of the distance from the transducer, hyperechoic compared with the normal kidney, and usually less echogenic than spleen and pancreas.
- Portal vein: The trunk of the portal vein stretches from the confluence of the splenic and superior mesenteric veins to the porta hepatis, representing the largest and most posterior tubular structure in the hepatoduodenal ligament. A right upper quadrant view along an oblique line joining right shoulder and navel best delineates the

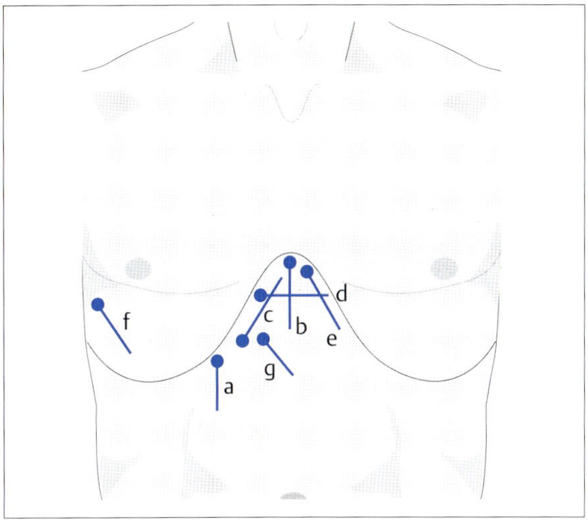

Fig. 7.**27** Lines for probe positioning in sonography of the liver.
a Longitudinal epigastric
b Longitudinal right upper quadrant
c Subcostal right
d Subxiphoidal
e Subcostal left
f Intercostal
g Organ-specific for visualizing the portal vein, CHD, and CBD

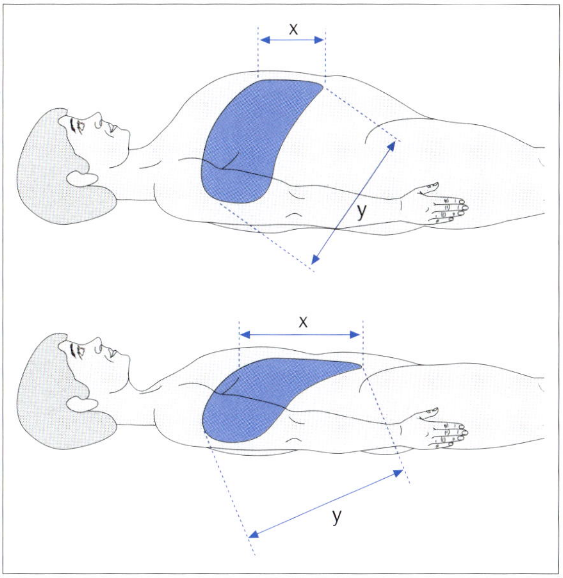

Fig. 7.**28** Position and shape of the liver depending on body build and shape of the chest. In barrel-chested patients, e.g., in pulmonary emphysema or in those with a pyknic build, the liver will be shorter in the longitudinal axis.
a Pyknic build.
b Thin, long build.

course of the vein (Fig. 7.**27 g**), supplemented by additional right intercostal views through the hepatic parenchyma (Fig. 7.**27 f**). The inferior vena cava (IVC) is seen running posterior to the portal vein. Normal diameter of the portal vein is 11 ± 2 mm.

- The common duct (CHD + CBD) is the most anterior structure in the hepatoduodenal ligament (see Biliary System, Biliary Tree, p. 159).
- Subject to numerous variations, the hepatic artery may be traced from its origin at the celiac trunk. Usually, the right branch of the hepatic artery proper runs between the common duct and portal vein (see Biliary System, Bile Ducts, p. 158; Fig. 7.**71**).
- Intrahepatic portal vein branches and hepatic veins can be reliably differentiated by their course and wall structure:
  - At the porta hepatis the trunk of the portal vein divides into the left and right branches, with more dichotomous branching further on, the intrahepatic vascular bed taking on a staghorn-like appearance. Integral part of the hepatic triads, i.e., accompanied by arteries and bile ducts, although unless dilated these can only be visualized as additional tubular structures when close to the porta hepatis.
  - Hepatic veins take a straight or mildly curved course and join the inferior vena cava at the star-shaped confluence (Fig. 7.**29 b**). There are three trunks: Left, right, and middle hepatic vein, usually demonstrated in one plane (Fig. 7.**30 a**) by subcostal scanning (Fig. 7.**27 d**) with the probe directed cephalad to the confluence with the IVC.
  - Further differentiation between portal vein branches, arteries, and bile ducts can be made by color-flow Doppler imaging.
  - The hyperechoic wall of the portal vein branches is thicker than that of the hepatic veins. Bile ducts and the branches of the portal vein as well as hepatic arteries are encased by common connective tissue, which appears hyperechoic on sonography.
- Hepatic lobes and segments:
  - The anatomical description of the liver and localization of hepatic lesions is rendered difficult by complex anatomy, variability of shape, and the rich variety of the vascular supply, and is further hampered by nonstandard use of the nomenclature between medical specialties.
  - Couinaud's functional anatomy, so important in hepatectomy, subdivides the liver into eight segments (Lafortune et al., 1991; Rieker et al., 2000); prior to surgery every attempt should be made to assign any focal mass as precisely as possible to one of these segments.
  - Segmental boundaries can be demonstrated sonographically based on the blood supply, since each segment is supplied via the vessels of the hepatic triad (no collaterals). The branches of the portal vein run in the center of the segments (Figs. 7.**29 a**, 7.**30 a**), while

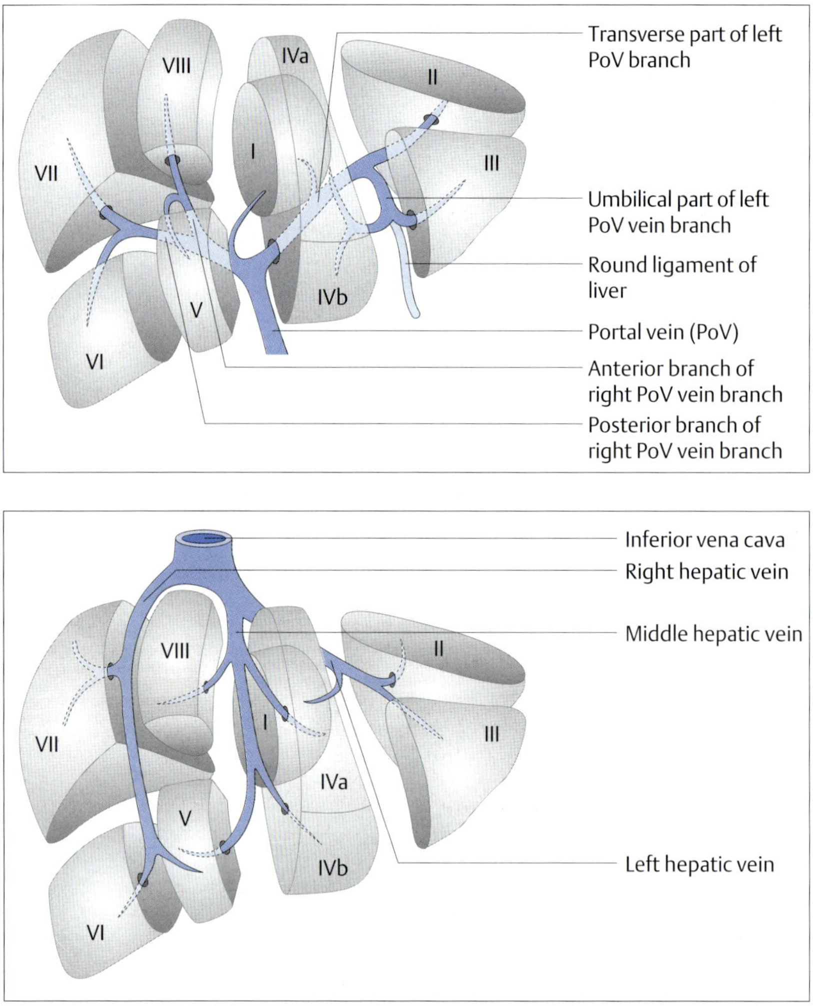

a

b

Fig. 7.**29** Segmentation of the liver. Vascular variants with additional branches are common, particularly in the hepatic veins. Numbering and nomenclature of the segments:

I Caudate lobe
II Laterosuperior
III Lateroinferior
IVa mediosuperior (subsegment)
IVb medioinferior (subsegment)
V Inferoanterior
VI Posteroanterior
VII Posterosuperior
VIII Anterosuperior

a With the course of the portal vein (PoV) branches.
b With the course of the hepatic veins.

the hepatic veins (left, right, and middle) course between the segments (Figs. 7.**29 b**, 7.**30 a**), thus marking the segmental boundaries in the longitudinal direction. This results in two lateral, medial, anterior, and posterior segments each (Figs. 7.**29 b**, 7.**30 a**), with additional subdivisions into individual superior and inferior segments by a transverse plane at the level of both main branches (Fig. 7.**29 a**).

- Due to the numerous anatomical variants of the hepatic veins, especially in terms of additional branching, the consistent course of the portal vein branches assumes greater importance for segmental mapping (Figs. 7.**29 a**, 7.**30 b, c**).
- The caudate lobe (segment I) takes a unique position in that it is usually supplied from both branches of the portal vein (primarily via the transverse part of the left portal branch; Figs. 7.**26 b**, 7.**29 a**) and drains via veins joining the IVC separately (Fanney et al., 1990).

– Fissures and ligaments divide the liver macroanatomically into three lobes: the small left (segments II and III) and large right lobe (segments IV–VIII), and the caudate lobe (segment I) (Fig. 7.**26**).
  - The term "lobe" connotes different meanings: a macroanatomical lobe based on contour or a functional lobe based on the dichotomous blood supply via the left and right portal vein branches. When discussing function, the less ambiguous term "left/right liver" rather than "lobe" will be used below with the meanings left liver = segments I–IV and right liver = segments V–VIII. The anatomical fissures between the lobes also mark segmental boundaries, but most of these cannot be discerned on the surface of the liver.
  - Ligaments run in these fissures. The falciform ligament runs in the umbilical fissure of the diaphragmatic aspect; the round ligament of the liver courses along the inferior border of the visceral surface, and the ligamentum venosum along the superior border. The round ligament of the liver corresponds to the ob-

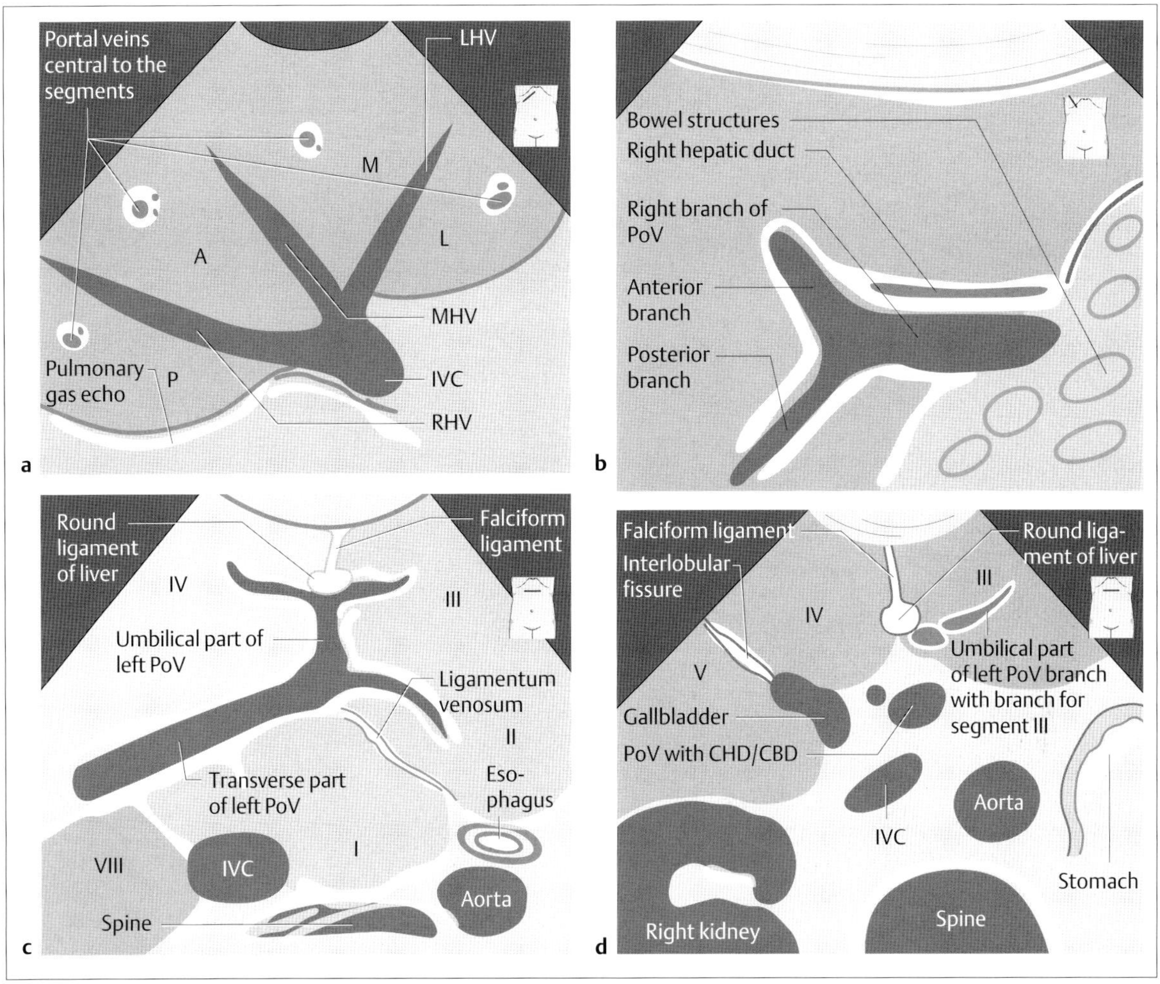

Fig. 7.**30** Schematic typical sonographic views of the liver, essential for identification of the liver segments. (PoV, portal vein.)
a Right subcostal view: hepatic veins segmenting the liver in longitudinal direction. P = posterior, A = anterior, M = medial, L = lateral segments.
b Right intercostal view. Right main portal branch with branching into a posterior as well as anterior second-order vein.
c Subxiphoidal view: Left main portal branch marking the anterior border of the caudate lobe (segment I). Boundary between right (segment IV) and left (segments II and III) hepatic lobes marked by the falciform ligament and the umbilical part of the left portal branch; the boundary between the caudate lobe and segment II runs along the ligamentum venosum.
d Subxiphoidal view further caudad than in **c**: The gallbladder and main portal fissure mark the boundary between segments IV and V, and the falciform ligament that between segments III and IV.

literated umbilical vein at the posteroinferior border of the falciform ligament, and the ligamentum venosum to the obliterated duct of Arantius.

- Both the round ligament and ligamentum venosum join the umbilical part of the left portal vein branch (Figs. 7.**29 a**, 7.**30 c**); since the round ligament is encased in connective and fatty tissue, it is hyperechoic on sonography, partly resulting in posterior acoustic shadowing. Its diameter varies between patients, and it may be mistaken for a hepatic mass (Fig. 7.**30 b, c**). The ligamentum venosum separates the caudate lobe (segment I) from segment II of the left lobe (Fig. 7.**30 c**).

- The boundary between right and left liver, corresponding to the boundary between segment IV of the left liver and segments V and VIII of the right liver, cannot be discerned on the diaphragmatic surface; on the visceral surface it correlates with the course of the IVC and the gallbladder ("gallbladder–IVC line"). In the parenchyma close to the gallbladder, a small hyperechoic septum is frequently seen, the interlobular ligament (Fig. 7.**30 d**) corresponding to the boundary between segments IV and V.
- The following classification into diffuse, focal, and vascular hepatic pathology applies more to sonographic

Table 7.1 Differential diagnosis of diffuse liver disease, based on size and echotexture

Enlarged liver (hepatomegaly)	Fatty liver, acute hepatitis (usually just mild hepatomegaly; typical in EBV hepatitis), congestive liver disease, fibrosis and cirrhosis (usually in the early stages), diffuse malignant invasion (diffuse metastasis, primary HCC, malignant lymphoma, invasion in leukemia), storage disease, e.g., glycogenosis
Small liver	Cirrhosis (usually in the late stages), severe hepatitis, extensive hepatocellular necrosis, atrophy in portal vein thrombosis
Diffuse hyperechoic hepatic texture ("bright liver"), frequently combined with distal attenuation	Fatty liver, cirrhosis, storage disease, e.g., glycogenosis
Diffuse hypoechoic hepatic texture, less echogenic than the kidney	Congestive liver disease, acute hepatitis (usually just slightly hypoechoic), hepatic edema of other causes, amyloidosis
Differential diagnosis in mottled heterogeneous echotexture of the liver	Fibrosis, cirrhosis, heterogeneous fatty infiltration, diffuse malignant invasion (diffuse metastasis, primary HCC, malignant lymphoma, invasion in leukemia)

phenomena than to disease entities; in a clinical setting combinations and overlap are common. Pathologies difficult to differentiate sonographically include macronodular cirrhosis versus multilocular intrahepatic metastases, both of which demonstrate a diffuse patchy echotexture (Table 7.1).

Diffuse Liver Disease–Basic Facts

- Sonography may detect alterations in size, shape, surface, angle of the inferior border of the liver, consistency, and internal texture, as well as vascular and perivascular structures. Consistency is assessed by gently compressing the liver surface with the probe or finger.
- Most diffuse hepatic conditions, however, at least in their early stages, do not result in changes detectable by sonography, e.g., acute hepatitis, hemochromatosis. Objective measurement of the hepatic echotexture has so far not become routine in clinical practice (Oosterveld et al., 1993).
- Sonography is extremely sensitive for detecting fatty infiltration of the liver (see below).
- If sonographic signs of diffuse liver pathology are present, they are frequently nonspecific and do not offer inferences as to the cause (Sanford et al., 1985), resulting in a purely descriptive sonographic finding that is of little avail: the general diagnosis of "diffuse parenchymal liver damage."
- Etiological clues are usually derived from clinical and laboratory information (see below).
- While definitive diagnosis frequently requires biopsy, stage and potential complications can often be well defined by sonography, e.g., cirrhosis, portal hypertension, ascites, thrombosis, and focal liver lesions.
- Hepatic fibrosis without cirrhosis cannot be diagnosed reliably by sonography, as differentiation either from normal echotexture or from fatty infiltration (and other diffuse pathology) is fraught with problems. Only broadening of the periportal structures has certain, though low, specificity (Joseph et al., 1991).

Fatty Liver

Basic Facts

- **Causes:**
  - Common: diabetes, alcohol consumption, disorders of lipid metabolism.
  - Uncommon: Wilson disease, pregnancy, medication, etc.
- Histologically, in most cases fatty infiltration is of the large-drop and rarely of the fine-drop variety, e.g., in acute fatty liver of pregnancy.
- Depending on the patient population, incidence may reach 30% and is frequently associated with not yet diagnosed abnormal glucose tolerance or lipid metabolism disorder (Schlottmann et al., 2000).
- *Additional workup:* Laboratory testing, consultation with internist, liver biopsy.

Sonographic Criteria

- Quite often enlarged liver with a rounded inferior border.
- Increased consistency, but much less marked than in cirrhosis of the liver.
- Hyperechoic homogeneous echotexture, i.e., increased echogenicity. "Bright" liver (for the physical basis of this hyperechogenicity, see Chapter 6, Technical Principles).
- Distal echo attenuation, i.e., constant reduction in the echodensity of the parenchyma so that assessment of parts more distant to the probe may prove impossible.
- Rarefied intrahepatic vascular bed, secondary to the increase in organ volume and also to reduced visualization of the vessels due to scattering from the many reflecting interfaces.
- The no longer quite homogeneous appearance of the echotexture is caused by less compaction, i.e., focal fat sparing (Caturelli et al., 1992), of:
  - Subcapsular parts of the parenchyma. In rather heterogeneous fatty infiltration the hepatic veins are encased in flamelike or tonguelike, more compact tissue (Fig. 7.**31**), easily mistaken for focal masses, but this heterogeneous fatty infiltration never displaces the vessels.
  - Ribbon-shaped or angular parenchymal areas around the gallbladder (see Fig. 7.**68 a**) and along (in most cases anterior to) the main portal vein branches (Aubin et al., 1995).
- Much less common is the opposite kind of change in echodensity, i.e., more compact parenchyma, corresponding to focal fatty infiltration around portal vein branches, gallbladder, and falciform ligament. Important in differential diagnosis of hyperechoic hepatic masses.
- Sometimes focal fatty infiltration does not involve the lobes or segments to the same degree; usually, it is more severe in the right liver and the hepatic veins delineate the boundaries.
- The degree of fatty infiltration correlates with the increase in echogenicity.

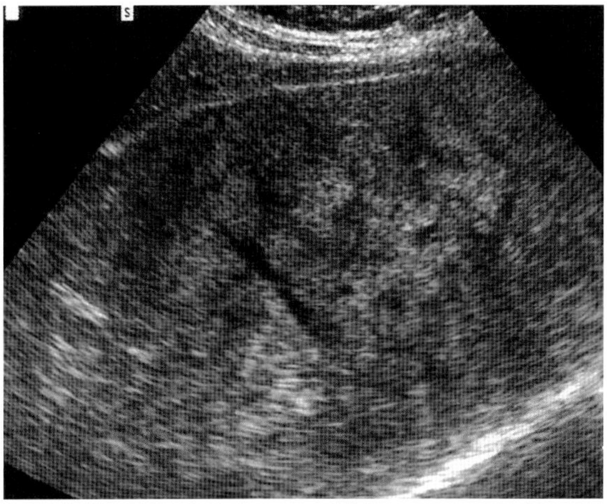

Fig. 7.**31 a** Heterogeneous fatty infiltration of the liver. Right hepatic lobe with flamelike zones of compact echotexture. The subcapsular areas of the liver are typically spared. Echogenicity decreases with the distance from the transducer ("distal echo attenuation").

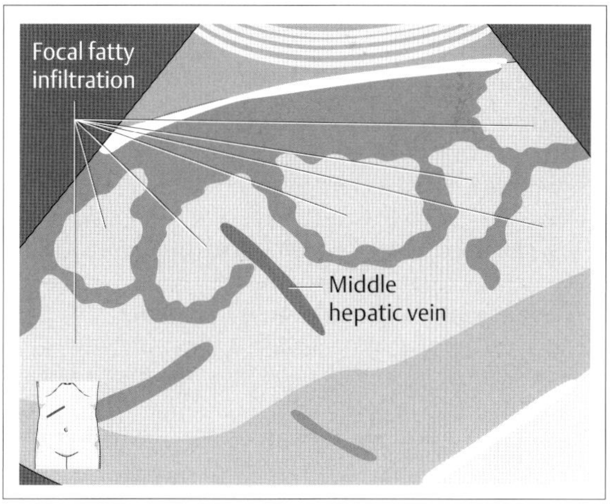

Fig. 7.**31 b** Line drawing.

Cirrhosis

Basic Facts

- Terminal stage of a diverse group of chronic hepatic disorders.
- **Definition:** Diffuse increase in the connective tissue with portoportal and portocentral fibrous bridging and nodules of regenerating hepatocytes.
- The size of the nodules depends on the etiology:
  - Micronodular < 3 mm.
  - Macronodular > 3 mm to several centimeters.
- Portosystemic venous shunting along the fibrous bridges.
- Hemodynamics: increased cardiac output and splanchnic blood flow, increased overall resistance in the portal system.
- Pathophysiological consequences: portal hypertension, liver failure.
- Prevalence: 4–10% in autopsy series, depending on the prevalence of the underlying disease.
- Male preponderance of 2 : 1.
- **Causes:**
  - In Germany, alcohol consumption accounts for 40–60%.
  - Chronic viral hepatitis accounts for 25–30%.
  - Uncommon: inborn errors of metabolism (e.g., hemochromatosis, Wilson disease, alpha$_1$-antitrypsin deficiency, hepatic porphyrias, glycogen storage disease), autoimmune mechanisms (autoimmune hepatitis, primary biliary cirrhosis, etc.), diseases of the biliary system (primary and secondary sclerosing cholangitis, cystic fibrosis, etc.), cardiovascular pathology (right ventricular failure, Budd–Chiari syndrome, veno-occlusive disease, etc.); cryptogenic about 10% (Bahr and Manns, 1999).
- **Complications:**
  - Liver failure.
  - Variceal hemorrhage, ectatic veins, or gastrointestinal ulcers.
  - Hepatocellular carcinoma.
- **Symptoms:** Cutaneous liver signs, edema, ascites, splenomegaly, gastrointestinal hemorrhage, generalized bleeding diathesis, hepatic encephalopathy.
- Staging according to Child based on these five clinical/biochemical parameters: encephalopathy, ascites, INR, bilirubin, and albumin levels.
- **Aims of sonography:**
  - To assist in the establishment of a diagnosis
  - To provide information on staging and hemodynamics, permitting conclusions to be drawn regarding prognosis, indications, and follow-up of treatment: medication (e.g., diuretics), shunting (TIPSS), transplantation.
  - Screening for hepatocellular carcinoma.

Sonographic Criteria

- Depending on stage and etiology, **enlargement or reduction in size of the entire liver**.
  - Enlargement is common in cirrhosis secondary to fatty liver and primary biliary cirrhosis.
  - A small liver is frequently found in cirrhosis secondary to hepatitis.
- The left and caudate lobes become **disproportionately large** and plump, while the right lobe of the liver becomes disproportionately small (Goyal et al., 1990).
- **Rounding of the inferior border** of the left lobe to an angle > 45°; the visceral surface is no longer concave but becomes biconvex. The inferior border of the liver is drawn posteriorly or anteriorly; on longitudinal views the liver resembles an animal head (Fig. 7.**32**).
- **Nodular surface**, ranging in size from micro- to macronodular. Especially in micronodular cirrhosis of the liver, resolution should be as high as possible, necessitating a high-frequency probe (5 MHz, or better still 7.5 MHz). Assessment of the diaphragmatic surface, best done from the epigastrium, proves more reliable in evaluation of the visceral surface, as the former is closer to the transducer. In the healthy patient the surface is smooth and flat, orthogonal to the ultrasound beam, and is not marred by echoes from intestinal gas. In cirrhosis, the bright, even echo line of the hepatic surface is broken; when the probe is shifted, the nodular structure generates an undulating surface echo. (Di Lelio et al., 1989; Simonovsky, 1999) (Fig. 7.**32**).
- The individual images exhibit a patchy echotexture of the organ, with a nodular element on dynamic scanning; the connective-tissue structures between the nodules are usually hyperechoic. Differentiation from malignant liver lesions is difficult.
- Rarefaction, displacement, and irregular delineation of the hepatic veins; on Doppler sonography the triphasic waveform of the hepatic veins is lost (Teichgräber et al., 1996).
- The peripheral branches of the **intrahepatic portal vein branches** appear rarefied but dilated **at the center** (resembling a "gnarled tree").
- **Broad** hyperechoic **periportal structures**, ill-defined against the parenchyma. Diameter of the vessels at the porta hepatica > 2 cm, including the hyperechoic periportal structures. Broadening of the hyperechoic periportal connective tissue is a sign of hepatic fibrosis (also present in noncirrhotic fibrosis). In conjunction with a compatible history, massive broadening is pathognomonic of the late stages of schistosomiasis.
- **Dilatation of the hepatic arteries**, the intrahepatic segments of which may become the widest vessels of the portal triads.
- Signs of portal hypertension (see below).

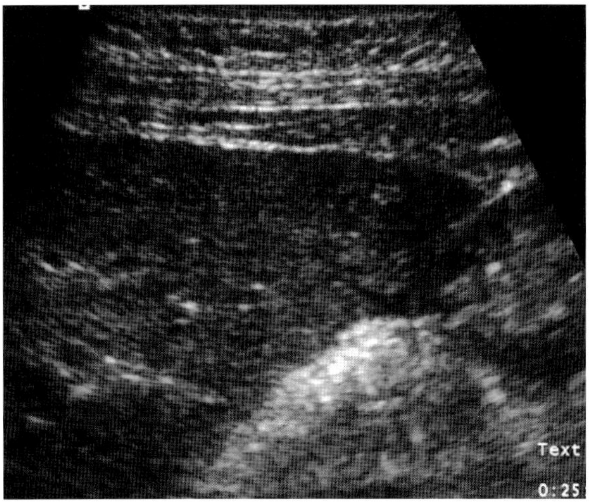

Fig. 7.**32a** Cirrhosis of the liver. Longitudinal view of the left hepatic lobe along the medial plane. Rounded inferior border of the lobe, pulled posteriorly. The two-dimensional view demonstrates a wavy surface that resolves into a nodular surface when the probe is tilted through the planes. Patchy echotexture of the organ, the connective tissue between the regenerating nodules being somewhat hyperechoic.

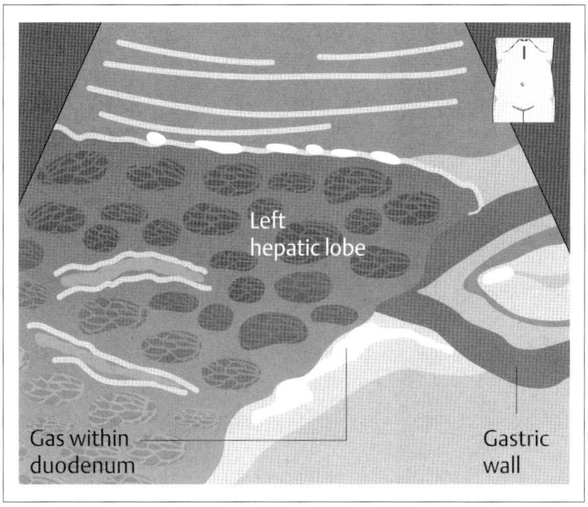

Fig. 7.**32b** Line drawing.

- *Additional workup:* Laboratory tests to assess liver function and establish potential causes; GI endoscopy for varices; hepatic histopathology of percutaneous or laparoscopic biopsies; laparoscopy; additional cross-sectional imaging modalities if cancer is suspected.

■ Portal Hypertension

Basic Facts

- Normal portal vein pressure is 3–10 mmHg; portal vein pressure > 12 mmHg indicates portal hypertension.
- **Pathophysiological consequences:** Portosystemic collaterals (clinically apparent as Medusa's head), ascites, splenomegaly.
- Complications: Bleeding from portosystemic shunts, most commonly from esophageal and gastric varices, rarely from varices in other parts of the GI tract, e.g., from rectal or duodenal varices or from ectatic veins in the gastric mucosa, i.e., in portal-hypertensive gastropathy or "watermelon stomach" (gastric vascular ectasia [GAVE]).
- **Pathogenesis:**
  - Increased resistance in the portal vein system or downstream of it.
  - Increased inflow secondary to vascular dilatation or splanchnic arteriovenous shunts.
  - Combined mechanisms: Common, especially in cirrhosis. The increased resistance usually has a higher impact on the pathogenesis.

Table 7.**2** Cause and site of increased resistance in portal circulation

Prehepatic	Splenic vein thrombosis Portal vein thrombosis (see below) Arteriovenous fistula
Intrahepatic presinusoidal	Congenital hepatic fibrosis Schistosomiasis Myelo- and lymphoproliferative disorders Metastases Primary biliary cirrhosis etc.
Intrahepatic sinusoidal	Cirrhosis (see above) Fatty liver (see above) Hepatitis Storage disorders, etc.
Intrahepatic postsinusoidal	Veno-occlusive disease
Posthepatic	Budd–Chiari syndrome (see below) Right ventricular failure

- Depending on where the increase in vascular resistance occurs, B-mode imaging and Doppler sonography can differentiate between a prehepatic, intrahepatic, and posthepatic type (Table 7.**2**).
- The site in relation to the sinusoids is of low clinical importance and can only be defined invasively.

Sonographic Criteria

- **Portal vein pressure increased** to > 13 mmHg; the diameter of the portal vein correlates poorly with portal vein pressure. Specificity > 90%, sensitivity only about 50% (Cottone et al., 1986; Seitz and Wermke, 1995).
- **Dilatation of the superior mesenteric vein** and the **splenic vein** to > 10 mm is seen in about half the patients with portal hypertension.
- These venous diameters are determined during inspiration: The physiological dilatation of the splanchnic veins during inspiration becomes lost in portal hypertension (Abu-Yousef, 1992).
- **Reduction of flow velocity and flow volume** in the portal vein is seen on Doppler sonography.
  - The normal range of peak flow velocity is 12–20 cm/s (Mohr et al., 1998); measurement depends on the operator and the equipment employed, and requires standardization and validation in one's own laboratory (Sabba et al., 1995).
  - Flow is also altered by respiration (being maximal on inspiration), oral intake, cardiac output, and body position. In reopened periumbilical veins (see below) this flow must be subtracted from the flow in the portal vein (Domland et al., 2000; Sacerdoti et al., 1995).
  - The drop in flow velocity in the portal vein correlates with portal vein pressure, measured as critical closing pressure of the hepatic veins (Schepke et al., 2000; Taourel et al., 1998).
- **Retrograde flow or paradoxical pendulating flow** in the portal vein or the splenic/mesenteric veins is pathognomonic for portal hypertension, but becomes evident only in severe hypertension; this sign is observed in about 8% of all cirrhotic patients (Gaiani et al., 1991).
- **Venous collaterals** also confirm the diagnosis:
  - Tortuous veins at the splenic hilum and perirenally, especially on the left.
  - Dilatation of the gastroesophageal and left gastric veins.
  - Recanalization of the paraumbilical veins in the round ligament of the liver, known as Cruveilhier–Baumgarten syndrome, enables blood flow from the left portal vein branch via the ligamentum teres to the umbilicus. In the true sense the term "reperfused umbilical vein" is a misnomer, because the true umbilical vein usually remains obliterated.
  - Often, the veins mentioned above can only be visualized by color-flow Doppler imaging.
- Nonspecific signs:
  - Splenomegaly; see Spleen, later in this chapter).
  - Ascites, in supine position primarily between right hepatic lobe and right kidney, i.e., in Morison's pouch, around the spleen, and in the lower abdomen.
  - Diffuse hypoechoic thickening of the gastric and intestinal wall due to engorgement with blood.

Portal Vein Thrombosis

Basic Facts

- **Potential sites:** Portal vein and its intrahepatic branches or the splanchnic veins. Combined forms are common.
- **Causes:** Liver disorders (particularly those associated with portal hypertension and/or malignancy), umbilical vein catheters, phlebitis of the umbilical vein, venous compression or invasion (e.g., in pancreatic cancer), pylephlebitis (e.g., in appendicitis, pancreatitis), thrombophilic conditions (e.g., polycytemia), etc.
- Malignant infiltration can rarely be differentiated sonographically from thrombosis. The combination of thrombosis and adjacent malignancy, e.g., hepatocellular carcinoma (see Malignant Hepatic Mass: Hepatocellular Carcinoma, below) or pancreatic cancer is highly indicative of malignant invasion of the vessels.

Sonographic Criteria

- **Non-anechoic vein.** Thrombotic material is most often mildly echogenic.
- **Noncompressible vein.**
- More accurate assessment with color-flow Doppler imaging: **Color-flow Doppler signal missing** despite an angle of incidence < 60°; when in doubt, the color-flow Doppler signal may be enhanced with a sonographic contrast agent.
- Compared to thrombosis, **malignant invasion of the vein** is confirmed if duplex ultrasound demonstrates pulsatile arterial signals within the echogenic lumen of the vein (Fig. 7.**33**).
- **Venous collaterals** are seen in long-standing thrombosis, their distribution depends on the site of the thrombosis.
- **Cavernous transformation** of the portal vein: Post-thrombotic partial recanalization of the portal vein, together with collaterals around it, forms a coil of veins that may be difficult to delineate from the actual vena portae (Fig. 7.**34**).

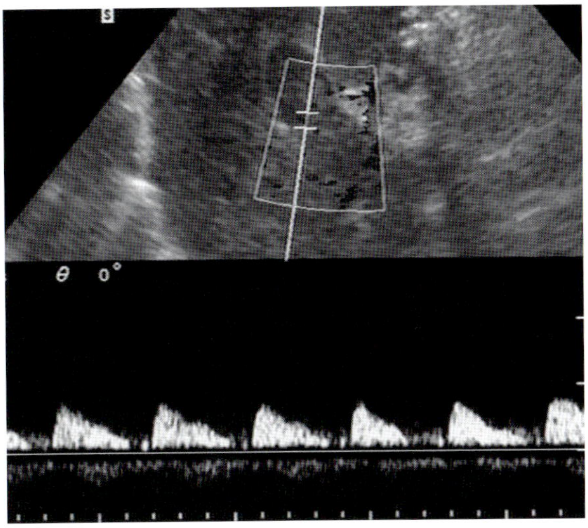

Fig. 7.**33 a** Malignant invasion of the right branch of the portal vein. Echogenic structure in the right portal branch, impossible to differentiate from thrombosis without Doppler sonography. On duplex ultrasound the arterial flow signals within the echogenic structure confirm the malignant nature.

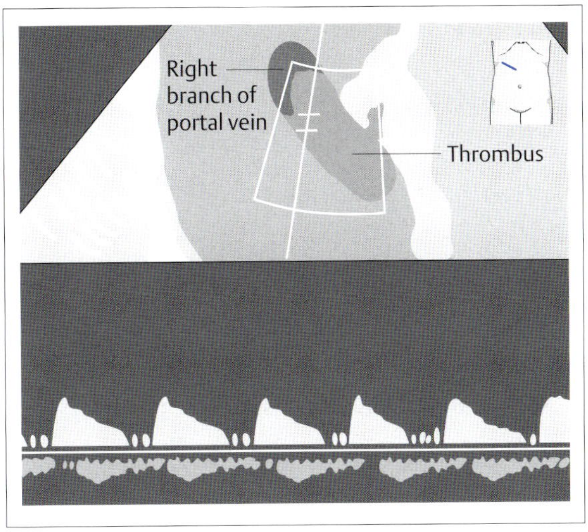

Fig. 7.**33 b** Line drawing.

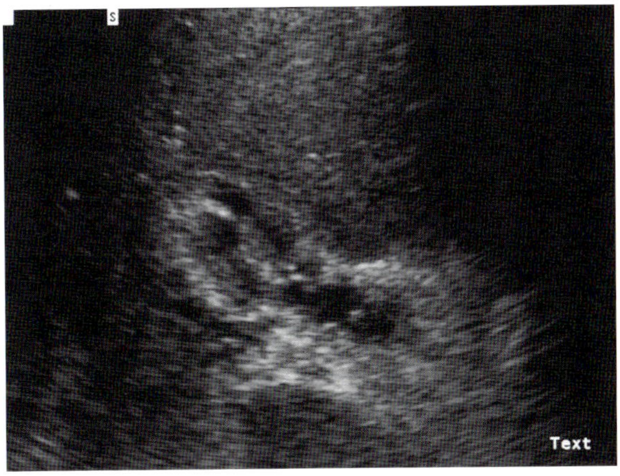

Fig. 7.**34 a** Postthrombotic cavernous transformation of the portal vein. The portal vein itself can no longer be identified; a broad coil of veins is encountered instead, with multidirectional flow on color-flow Doppler imaging.

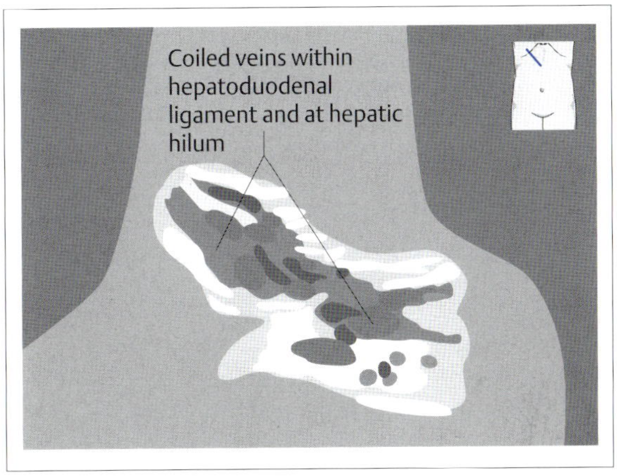

Fig. 7.**34 b** Line drawing.

Budd–Chiari Syndrome

Basic Facts

- Occlusion of the hepatic veins or the intrahepatic segment of the inferior vena cava.
- **Causes:**
  - Thrombosis related to thrombophilia (e.g., polycythemia, hypercoagulability, estrogen medication), malignant liver disease, trauma, or fibrous venous membranes.
  - Malignant invasion of the hepatic veins or the IVC (e.g., in renal cancer).
- Consecutive portal vein thrombosis is common.
- Acute onset triggers pain by hepatic capsule distension and may induce acute liver failure due to ischemic hepatocellular necrosis; chronic Budd–Chiari syndrome may progress to cirrhosis of the liver.
- Usually, the caudate lobe is spared because of its direct drainage into the inferior vena cava.
- **Management:** Treatment of the underlying cause; medical management of portal hypertension; surgical options: venous decompression, portosystemic shunt, liver transplantation (Ringe et al., 1995), and in selected cases, TIPSS (Blum et al., 1995).

Sonographic Criteria

- **Acute:**
  - Painful hepatomegaly.
  - Thrombi or tumors in IVC or hepatic veins; the latter might not be visualized at all and there is no color-flow Doppler signal.
  - Patchy heterogeneous echotexture (Kane and Eustace, 1995: Vilgrain et al., 1999) (Fig. 7.**35**).
- **Chronic–as above plus:**
  - Signs of cirrhosis (see above).
  - Hypertrophy of the caudate lobe.
  - Intrahepatic venous collaterals along the hepatic veins; possible retrograde flow in the hepatic veins.

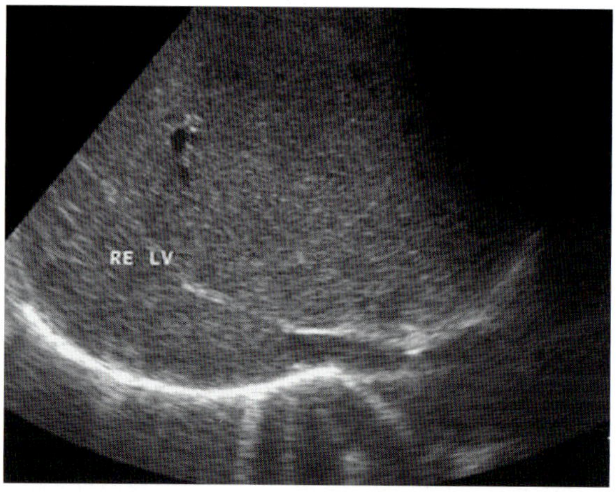

Fig. 7.**35 a** Budd–Chiari syndrome. Subcostal view of the right hepatic lobe. Except for a wall echo of the right hepatic vein, the hepatic veins cannot be differentiated from the parenchyma. The right hepatic vein (RE LV) is thrombosed up to the IVC; the liver is greatly enlarged and displays a patchy heterogeneous echotexture.

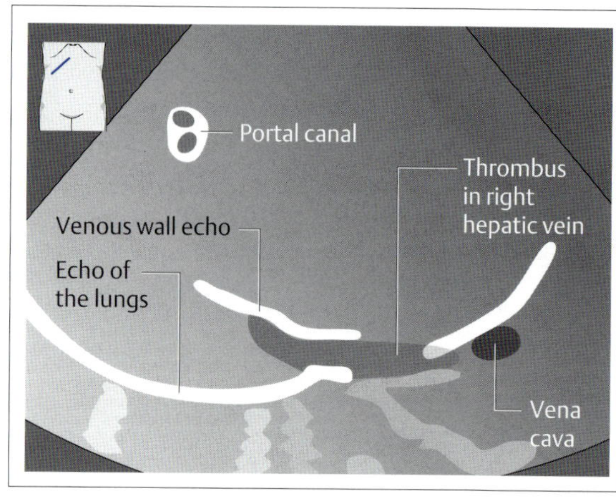

Fig. 7.**35 b** Line drawing.

Passive Hepatic Congestion

Basic Facts

- Increased venous pressure due to right ventricular failure.
- **Causes:** Acute cor pulmonale (most often due to pulmonary embolism); chronic cor pulmonale as sequela to lung disease; valvular defects; heart failure; constrictive pericarditis.
- **Histopathology:** Acute passive congestion results in centroacinar fatty infiltration and possible centroacinar hepatocellular necrosis. In chronic passive congestion there may also be fibrosis, and possibly cirrhosis of the liver (cardiac cirrhosis).

Sonographic Criteria

- Hepatomegaly, painful in acute congestion, with rounding of the hepatic border.
- Hypoechoic parenchyma in the acute stage.
- Distended hepatic veins, > 10 mm close to their junction with the IVC, easy to trace far into the hepatic periphery.
- Distension of the IVC with loss of respiration dependent caliber variation.
- Hypoechoic echotexture of the liver; in case of concomitant fibrosis, there may be a diffuse increase in echogenicity and possible signs of cirrhosis.

Focal Liver Disease–Basic Facts

Focal hepatic lesions are frequently asymptomatic and discovered incidentally, or they are revealed by systematic search. For the appraisal of a hepatic mass, the clinical context is as important as the sonographic criteria presented below (Lock and Schölmerich, 1997). The importance of history, physical examination, age, and sex need not be emphasized. The most important clinical conditions predisposing to focal hepatic masses are listed in Table 7.**3**. It is beyond the scope of this book to discuss the rich variety of rare congenital syndromes and the large number of exogenous factors that can give rise to focal hepatic masses. Especially when dealing with conditions associated with an in-

Table 7.**3** Clinical conditions associated with increased risk for liver masses.

Diagnosis	Interpretation of the Hepatic Mass
Known extrahepatic epithelial or mesenchymal malignancy	Metastases
Known extrahepatic malignant lymphoma	Focal or diffuse invasion by the lymphoma
Cirrhosis, chronic viral hepatitis, excessive alcohol consumption, hemochromatosis, aflatoxin exposure	Hepatocellular carcinoma
Primary sclerosing cholangitis, Caroli disease	Cholangiocellular carcinoma
Long-term estrogen or androgen medication	FNH Hepatocellular adenoma Peliosis hepatis
Glycogen storage disease type I	Multiple hepatocellular adenomas ("adenomatosis")
Septicemia, septic focus (especially within the splanchnic organs), cholangitis, immunodeficiency	Liver abscess
History of thorium dioxide (Thorotrast) administration, exposure to vinyl chloride	Hepatic carcinoma Angiosarcoma Hemangioendothelioma
Polycystic kidney disease	Hepatic cysts
Trauma, hepatic FNA, HELLP syndrome	Hepatic hematoma
Status post liver FNA	Arteriovenous fistula
Recent stay in the tropics	Amebic abscess Schistosomiasis Fasciola hepatica

creased risk of hepatic malignancy or in the presence of known malignant underlying disease, any newly detected mass in the liver must be considered malignant until proven otherwise.

Sonography plays a central role in the differentiation of benign and malignant hepatic masses. Irrespective of their benign or malignant nature, focal masses are characterized by their displacement of normal anatomical structures, in particular by their

- Displacement of hepatic vessels
- Buckling of the hepatic surface
- Indentation of adjacent organs, such as the gallbladder.

These signs may be the only obvious pathology of a mass that is isoechogenic with the unaffected hepatic parenchyma (e.g., focal nodular hyperplasia). The following characteristics indicate malignancy:

- Hypoechoic rim around the mass
- Destruction and invasion of adjacent organs, e.g. sudden termination of vessels.

Such a hypoechoic halo has positive and negative predictive values of 90% (Wernecke et al., 1992 b). The halo may comprise live tumor cells or edematous/compressed liver tissue (Wernecke et al., 1992a). For comparison on follow-up, the documentation must state whether the halo is included in the measurement. The majority of malignant masses are characterized by increased arterial vascularity (Gaiani et al., 2000). Doppler sonography, especially when enhanced by an intravenous contrast medium, can contribute to the differentiation between benignancy and malignancy, but it is a matter of debate whether vascular patterns are of sufficient specificity (Gaiani et al., 2000; Strunk et al., 1998; Rickes et al., 2002).

Based on their sonographic appearance, hepatic masses may also be classified as anechoic or echogenic lesions. Anechoic masses almost always are liquid. However, if they contain cells or detritus quite a number of fluid collections are not anechoic. Sedimentation phenomena are observed in liquids containing particulate matter, e.g., blood or debris. By itself sonography cannot type the fluid in a liquid mass, e.g., blood, pus, bile ("biloma"), or serous fluid (Gebel et al., 1997).

Echogenic masses are compared to the healthy liver tissue in terms of their echodensity and echointensity and are described accordingly as hypoechoic, isoechoic, hyperechoic, or of mixed/complex echogenicity. Most often they are solid. Diffuse changes in the texture of the liver obviously will alter the sonographic contrast to the echotexture of a mass. Thus, hypoechogenic lesions are more easily detected in fatty liver, while the more hyperechoic masses are harder to delineate.

When combined with new techniques of ultrasound transmission, such as stimulated acoustic emission (Albrecht et al., 2000; Harvey et al., 2000), and echo detection, e.g., harmonic imaging (Becker et al., 2000; Beissert et al., 2000), sonographic contrast-enhancement will result in higher detection rates for focal hepatic masses in the future.

In certain pathologies, the typical sonographic findings by themselves will suffice for the definitive diagnosis of the disorder, e.g. in dysontogenetic cysts or hemangioma. In all other cases, the suspected sonographic diagnosis must be confirmed by additional imaging modalities. Frequently, though, it is neither necessary nor desirable to employ the whole gamut of diagnostic imaging modalities but is better to strive for early histopathological assessment by FNA biopsy (Stölzel et al., 2000).

Benign Fluid Collections: Dysontogenetic Cysts

Basic Facts

- Dysontogenetic cysts are epithelium-lined fluid collections, supposedly originating from the biliary tree but without persisting connection with the biliary system.
- Clear colorless or yellow liquid.
- **Differentiation into two entities:**
  - Simple hepatic cysts: Solitary in up to 75% of cases, multiple in 25%. Presumably congenital, but number and size increase with age; they are rarely detected before midlife. Overall prevalence is 4%, rising to 7% by the age of 80 years. They are seldom symptomatic: pain from bleeding or sheer volume, if the cyst is large (tense liver capsule, compression of neighboring organs), possible obstruction of the IVC. Rarely infection; hemorrhage is usually self-limiting.
  - Polycystic liver disease: Liver riddled with cysts, dominant autosomal inheritance (manifesting in adulthood) or recessive autosomal inheritance (presenting in childhood); around 60% of patients suffer from polycystic kidney disease as well. In polycystic kidney disease 50–75% of patients harbor hepatic cysts, and in 25–50% of cases polycystic liver disease is found as well. Complications are the same as for simple hepatic cysts: Sometimes portal hypertension, while congenital hepatic fibrosis or Caroli disease ("fibropolycystic disease") is uncommon (Nicolau et al., 2000).
- Ultrasound alone usually suffices for unequivocal diagnosis.
- Important differential diagnoses: Hydatid cyst (see below), arteriovenous fistula.
- *Additional workup:* CT, MRI, serological tests for hydatid disease.

Sonographic Criteria

- Round to ellipsoid masses, sometimes with clustering of neighboring cysts and sometimes confluent with adjacent lesions.
- Anechoic contents, posterior enhancement, edge shadowing.
- Sharp demarcation in the shape of a bright, rather narrow interface echo, particularly if the cyst wall is orthogonal to the ultrasound beam ("cyst entrance and exit echoes"). Intracystic hemorrhage causes bizarre polypoid texture or sedimentation.
- Color-flow Doppler imaging reliably distinguishes arteriovenous fistulas from cysts.

Consequences for Surgical Treatment

Diagnosis	Characteristic Findings	Management
Asymptomatic dysontogenetic cyst or polycystic liver disease	Round anechoic mass with typical artifacts and simple thin wall	None Follow-up while asymptomatic
Chronic symptomatic dysontogenetic cysts or polycystic liver disease	Chronic upper abdominal pain, symptoms due to compression of adjacent organs, e.g., IVC syndrome, sonographically numerous and/or large cysts	Paracentesis and sclerotherapy (recurrence common), laparoscopic fenestration (always send cyst wall for histology), consider indication for LTx (especially in polycystic liver disease and hepatic failure)
Atypical hepatic cysts	Cysts with irregular wall or septation, cysts with mucinous contents	Resect atypical cysts since cystadenoma or cystadenocarcinoma can only be ruled out by histology.

Benign Fluid Collections: Hydatid Disease

Basic Facts

- Infection with larvae of the dog tapeworm *Echinococcus granulosus*.
- Geographic distribution: Mediterranean countries, Middle East, Africa, South America, Australia, also sporadic occurrence in the more northern regions.
- Annual **incidence**: Switzerland 0.38, Greece 13, Kenya 220 per 100 000 inhabitants. Anonymized case reporting to the public health authorities has been mandatory in Germany since 1 January 2001.
- The liver is infested in more than 60% of patients, the lungs in 20%; rarely other organ systems including bones and the CNS.
- Doubled cystic wall: host cyst with fibrous wall, larval endocyst. Within the endocyst there is endoluminal budding of brood capsules containing protoscolices that release several generations of cysts, the endocyst collapsing later. Calcified cysts usually do not contain any viable parasites.
- **Symptoms:** upper abdominal pain, fever, intrahepatic mass, rarely portal hypertension, jaundice
- Slow growth rate of 1–5 cm per year; 90% of cysts measure < 7.5 cm in diameter.
- **Complications:**
  - Perforation into bile ducts, peritoneal cavity, GI tract, pleural space, and lungs
  - Risk of anaphylactic shock
- **Diagnosis:**
  - Based on sonography, CT, and serological tests, the latter having a sensitivity of 60–80%. The six stages of the WHO classification are based on sonographic findings (see www.medicalweb.it/aumi/echinonet).

Sonographic Criteria

- **Stage 1:** Unilocular anechoic cystic mass in the liver with posterior acoustic shadowing. Sonography cannot differentiate between dysontogenetic and recent cysts.
- **Stage 2:** Unilocular cystic mass with hyperechoic wall, partly with layering ("double line" sign; Fig. 7.**36**), sometimes "hydatid sand" (a mixture of viable and nonviable parasitic material) resembling sludge in the gallbladder.
- **Stage 3:** Multivesicular or septated cysts with characteristic "wheel-like" or "honeycomb" appearance, comprising fertile daughter cysts with viable protoscolices (Fig. 7.**36**).
- **Stage 4:** Cysts with floating hyperechoic membrane that has sloughed off the pericyst ("water lily" sign), sometimes also a few hypoechoic daughter cysts.
- **Stage 5:** Rather heterogeneous cyst texture with hyperechoic, hypoechoic, or mixed hyper-/hypoechoic contents ("ball of wool" sign). Usually without any viable protoscolices.
- **Stage 6:** Partially or completely calcified mass without any viable protoscolices.

- *Additional workup:* CT, MRI, serological testing for hydatid disease.

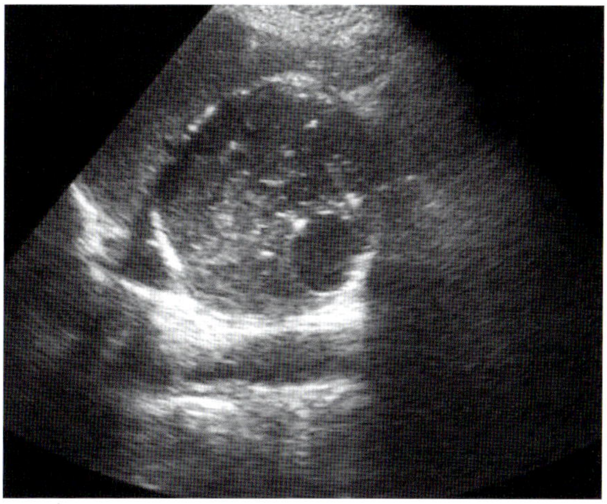

Fig. 7.**36 a** Hydatid cyst, WHO stage 3. Longitudinal view of the left hepatic lobe. Double-layered hyperechoic cyst wall; multiple large and small daughter cysts within the lumen. Typical artifact: edge shadowing.

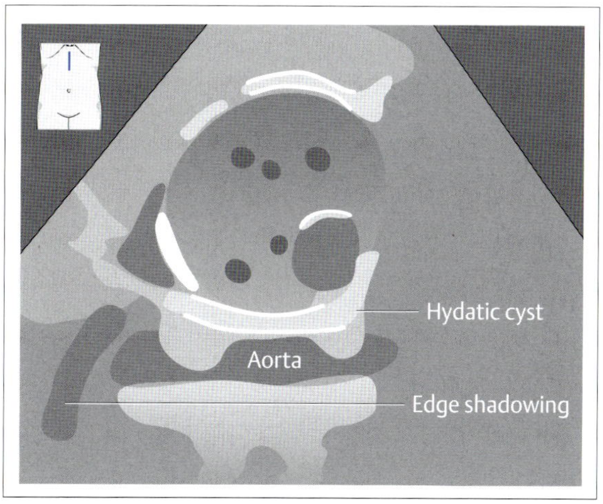

Fig. 7.**36 b** Line drawing.

Benign Fluid Collections: Alveolar Hydatid Disease

Basic Facts

- Infection with larvae of the less common fox tapeworm *Echinococcus multilocularis*.
- Characterized by invasive growth with destruction of the liver and correspondingly poor prognosis.
- Cystic or solid hyperechoic echotexture, which does not always permit differentiation from malignancy. Calcification is seen in 50% of cases.
- The diagnosis is confirmed serologically (Kern et al., 2000).

Consequences for Surgical Treatment

Diagnosis	Characteristic Findings	Management
Hydatid cyst	Cyst with double-layered wall, possibly with sedimentation, calcification, membranes or daughter cysts, serological testing positive for hydatid disease	Pericystectomy, liver resection, closed toal cystectomy

Benign Fluid Collections: Liver Abscess

Basic Facts

- **Important differential diagnosis:** pyogenic versus amebic abscess.
- Amebic abscess is rare in industrialized countries and is usually acquired in the tropics. Worldwide it is the more common form.
- In 50% of cases pyogenic abscess is secondary to cholangitis and the other 50% are arterial or portal borne.
  - Portal venous spread is often triggered by a focal splanchnic infection (e.g., appendicitis, pancreatic abscess).
  - Invasion of the liver in continuity (e.g., in cholecystitis or penetrating peptic ulcer) is rare.
  - Superinfection of an existing hepatic mass, e.g., metastasis, cyst, or hematoma, is possible and also most often secondary to cholangitis.
- **Clinical presentation:** septicemia, upper abdominal pain, possibly palpable hepatomegaly.
- *Additional workup:* blood culture, FNA, CT, serological testing if amebic abscess is suspected.

Sonographic Criteria

- **Pyogenic abscess:**
  - The initial stage with phlegmon presents with an ill-defined hypoechoic mass that may progress to a true abscess, visualized as a rather hypoechoic (possibly anechoic) mass, also poorly delineated. Surrounding hepatic tissue is hypoechoic due to edema; usually, sonography cannot delineate the abscess membrane from the hypoechoic hepatic texture (Fig. 7.**37**).
  - Smaller abscesses are most often round, while larger ones are lobulated or ramified like a cloverleaf (Fig. 7.**37**).
  - Hematogenous abscesses often come in multiples.
  - Within the abscess there may be sedimentation phenomena and/or gas echoes, the latter characterized by bright signals with posterior shadowing and comet-tail artifacts.
- **Amebic abscess:**
  - Similar to pyogenic abscess.
  - Size: 3–40 cm.
  - Shape: round or oval.
  - Typically a finely mottled hypoechoic hepatic texture, but more echogenic than a pyogenic abscess.
  - A hypoechoic wall is uncommon.
  - Brown creamy contents on aspiration. As response to medical therapy tends to be good, paracentesis is only indicated in case of threatening complications, e.g., rupture or therapeutic failure, or for a very large abscess.

Consequences for Surgical Treatment

See Chapter 5, p. 85, Principles of Drainage in Surgery.

Benign Fluid Collections: Hematoma

See Chapter 2, Thoracic and Abdominal Trauma.

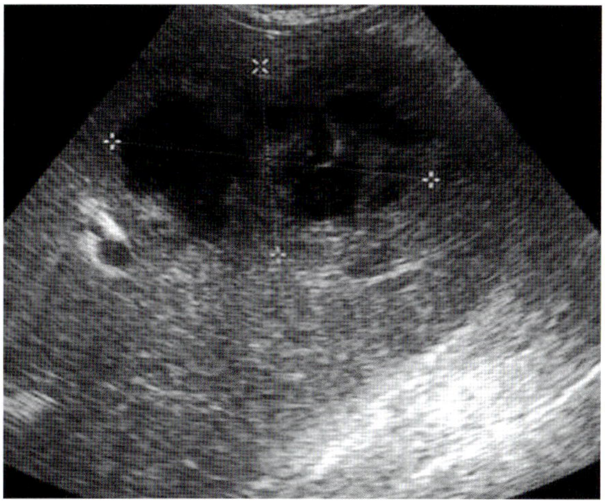

Fig. 7.**37 a** Pyogenic hepatic abscess. Almost anechoic lobulated mass, poorly delineated from the hypoechoic liver tissue. Diameter 10 cm.

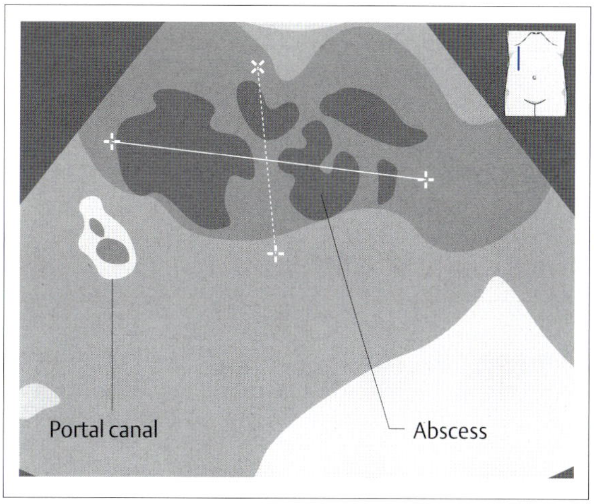

Fig. 7.**37 b** Line drawing.

Benign Solid Masses: Hemangioma

Basic Facts

- Benign arteriovenous malformation.
- **Prevalence**: about 8 %; female preponderance by a factor of 5 : 1
- Although there is no or little increase in size with age, estrogen medication or pregnancy may trigger growth.
- 90 % are solitary.
- Most measure < 3 cm in diameter but may reach sizes > 20 cm.
- Often **localized** in the right hepatic lobe with a predilection for the subcapsular region.
- **Most hemangiomas are asymptomatic**; upper abdominal pain, thrombocytopenia, or in infants intravascular coagulation (Kasabach–Merritt syndrome), are rare; arteriovenous fistula, jaundice, abscess, or rupture with intraperitoneal hemorrhage are rather uncommon.
- **Sonography alone is frequently diagnostic**. Because of the rim of > 1 cm of healthy liver tissue, FNA carries a low risk but is of little benefit cytologically and histologically.
- *Additional workup:* MRI (most precise), CT, erythrocyte scintigraphy.

Sonographic Criteria

- Round or polygonal mass without destruction of surrounding tissue or vessel displacement (Fig. 7.**38**).
- Sharp demarcation, small efferent vessels may be visualized along the rim (Fig. 7.**38**).
- Hyperechoic texture otherwise resembling that of the liver (Fig. 7.**38**); sometimes small tubular structures are seen corresponding to vessels, but owing to the slight flow there is almost no signal on Doppler sonography.
- Posterior enhancement in some cases, since hyperechoic structures such as fatty liver or lipomas usually result in echo attenuation.
- Atypical hemangiomas: hypoechoic echotexture. Central hypoechogenicity is usually due to thrombosis or cavernous regions, while a totally hypoechoic texture is seen if the entire lesion is cavernous.
- In typical hemangiomas without risk for liver lesions of other etiology, sonography is diagnostic and further investigations are unnecessary (Gandolfi et al., 1991; Leifer et al., 2000; Shamsi et al., 1993).

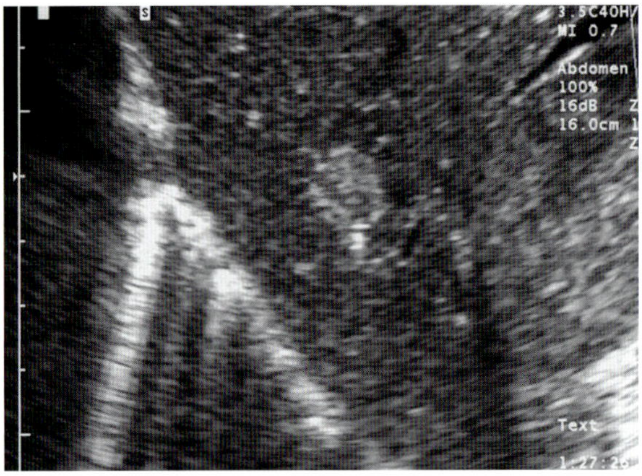

Fig. 7.**38 a** Typical hemangioma: sharply delineated polygonal mass. Hyperechoic texture, typically somewhat less echogenic at the center. Small efferent vessels along the rim. Intercostal view of the right hepatic lobe.

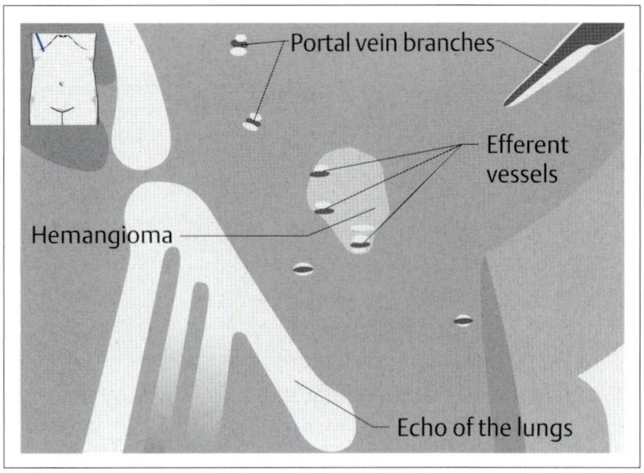

Fig. 7.**38 b** Line drawing.

Benign Solid Masses: Focal Nodular Hyperplasia (FNH)

Basic Facts

- Usually solitary nodular mass.
- Histology is similar to inactive cirrhosis with hepatocytes, bile ducts, Kupffer cells, and fibrous septa.
- 90% of patients are women, mostly in their second or third decade of life, often associated with long-term use of contraceptive medication.
- In 20% of cases there is multiple FNH.
- Occurrence in childhood is rare, there may also be vascular malformation.
- Epidemiologically, FNH is three times as common as hepatic adenoma, its incidence increasing faster than in adenomas (Cherqui et al., 1995).
- Partial spontaneous regression is possible after hormonal contraceptives have been discontinued (Di Stasi et al., 1996).
- No malignant transformation.
- *Additional workup:* hepatobiliary scintigraphy, CT, MRI, FNA (histologically, differential diagnosis from cirrhosis of the liver is difficult). In case of persisting doubt, laparoscopy and possibly resection.

Sonographic Criteria

- Round or ellipsoid mass, frequently close to the capsule, sometimes having a pediculated surface.
- Displacement of neighboring structures, no infiltration.
- Almost isoechoic with healthy liver tissue, sometimes hypoechoic.
- Border sharply delineated, sometimes with hypoechoic halo where, in contrast to metastases, Doppler sonography will reveal vessels (von Herbay et al., 1997); however, on color-flow Doppler imaging it may be mistaken for HCC (see below).
- In structural detail, FNH is less homogeneous than normal liver; in 20–50% of patients, a confluent star-shaped hyperechoic structure ("wheel-like" structure, Fig. 7.**39**) is seen corresponding with fibrous strands (Di Stasi et al., 1996).
- Arteries follow this radial structure, with centrifugal arterial flow on color-flow Doppler imaging (Bartolozzi et al., 1997). Acoustic contrast agents may enhance visualization of the vessels. Masses < 3 cm lack this wheel-like vascular structure (Uggowitzer et al., 1999).

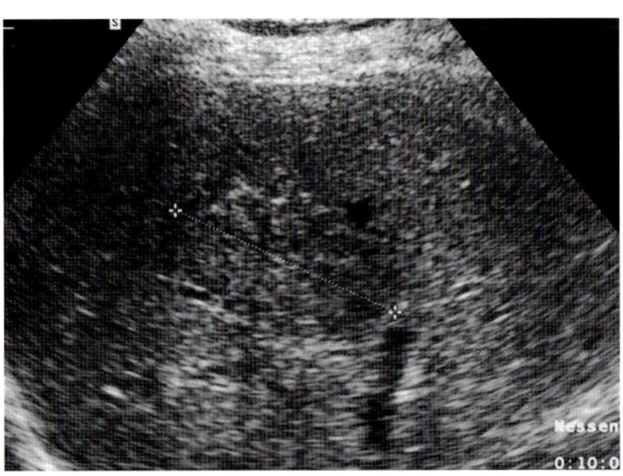

Fig. 7.**39 a** Focal nodular hyperplasia. Sharply delimited mass, almost isoechoic with the liver; typical wheel-like structure.

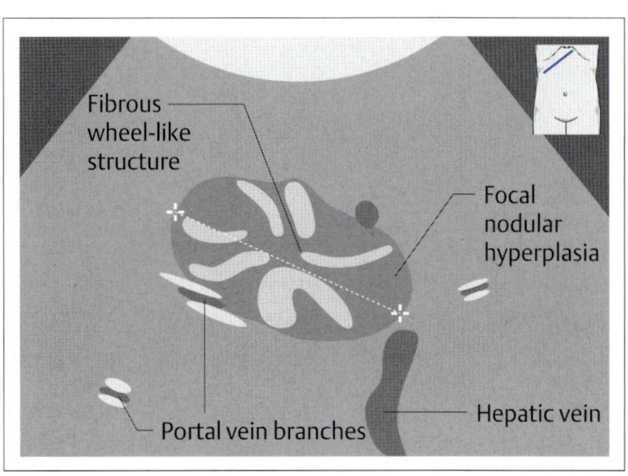

Fig. 7.**39 b** Line drawing.

Benign Solid Masses: Hepatocellular Adenoma

Basic Facts

- Bands of hepatocytes lacking portal triads; Kupffer cells are absent or few. Some central necrosis or hemorrhage.
- Rare before the advent of oral contraceptives. In addition to long-term (> 5 years) use of oral hormonal contraceptives, hepatocellular adenomas are also seen in androgen therapy and pregnancy, and may run in families.
- Multiple adenomas are rare, only occasionally related to hormones, but with a positive family history or seen in glycogen storage disease type I (van Gierke) (Chiche et al., 2000; Grazioli et al., 2000).
- Mostly subcapsular and **localized** in the right hepatic lobe, sometimes pediculated.
- **Presentation:** pain due to capsular tension, hemorrhage, possible bleeding into the peritoneal cavity.

Sonographic Criteria

- Round or ellipsoid mass.
- Sharply delimited, usually without capsule.
- Nodular echotetxure, poorly contrasted to the normal liver; hypoechoic in about 40% of cases (Fig. 7.**40**), hyperechoic in approximately 30%, the remainder being isoechoic or of mixed echogenicity (Al Otaibi et al., 1995). Lipid induced massive hyperechogenicity is rare.

- **Long-term malignant transformation** is seen in about 10% of the patients (Al Otaibi et al., 1995; Foster and Berman, 1994); regression upon termination of hormonal contraception is rare (Daldrup et al., 1995).
- *Additional workup:* CT, MRI, FNA (for diagnostic confirmation).

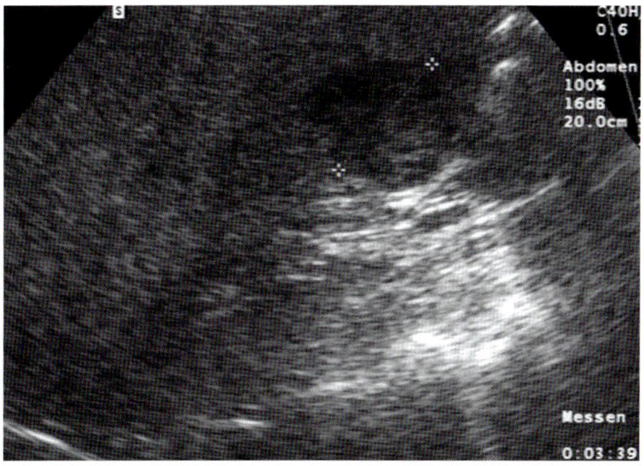

Fig. 7.**40 a** Hepatocellular adenoma: sharply delimited hypoechoic mass with nodular echotexture, diameter 3.7 cm.

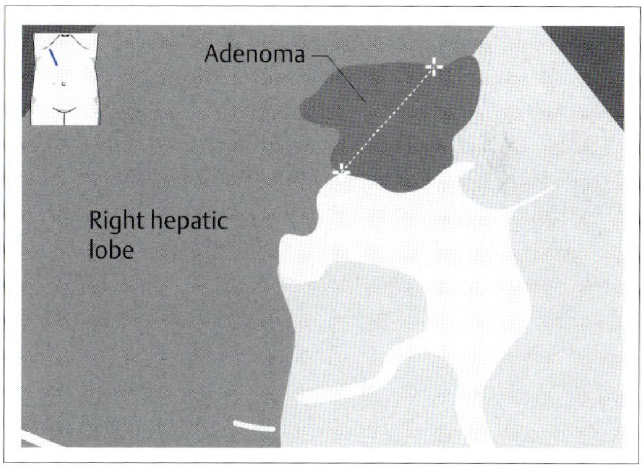

Fig. 7.**40 b** Line drawing.

Consequences for Surgical Treatment

Diagnosis	Characteristic Findings	Management
FNH	Asymptomatic, small	No excision indicated if diagnosed by imaging, follow-up; if possible confirm diagnosis by histology; if diagnosed during surgery decision is left to the surgeon
FNH	Symptomatic, size > 10 cm, with hemorrhage	Relative indication for resection
Hepatocellular adenoma	Inherent risk of rupture/malignant transformation regardless of size and symptoms	Resection
Hemangioma	< 5 cm, asymptomatic	Follow-up
Hemangioma	Very large symptomatic hemangiomas (risk of bleeding) increasing in size (DD: hemangioendotheliosarcoma)	Hepatic resection; possibly embolization if surgery is contraindicated

Uncommon Benign Liver Tumors

Lipoma, Angiomyolipoma

- Far less common than hemangioma.
- Histology is related to hemangioma; mixed forms vary in the amount of endothelium, smooth muscle, and fat.
- Less common than, but sometimes associated with, renal angiomyolipoma, possibly as part of tuberous sclerosis.
- The mass itself cannot be differentiated from a hemangioma sonographically, but in contrast to hemangioma there is posterior echo attenuation rather than enhancement.
- No further diagnostic workup is needed if findings are typical; possibly conformation by CT, MRI, FNA.

Biliary Cystadenoma

- Intrahepatic localization or along the extrahepatic biliary tree.
- Affects mainly middle-aged women.
- Tends to undergo malignant transformation.
- Mucinous contents; expresses CA 19–9.
- On sonography, a thick-walled multiseptated cystic mass, partly with nodular or papillomatous mural structures.

Mesenchymal Hamartomas

- Fibrous mass with cystic parts lined with bile duct epithelium.
- Affects mainly children below the age of 2 years.
- On sonography, a somewhat hyperechoic, partly multiseptated cystic mass about 5–20 cm across.

Meyenburg's Complexes

- Bile duct hamartoma, comprising dilated bile ducts within fibrous stroma.
- Usually seen in multiples, each < 1 cm.
- Very rarely malignant (Blanc et al., 2000; Jain et al., 2000).
- Quite diverse sonographic image: hyperechoic, hypoechoic, or cystic (Wohlgemuth et al., 1998).

Infantile Hemangioendothelioma

- Presentation in the first year of life.
- Rapid growth, with eventual spontaneous regression in most cases.
- Complications: cardiac failure due to arteriovenous shunting, anemia, thrombocytopenia, hemorrhage.
- Sonography: hyperechoic like hemangiomas or hypoechoic/cystic; usually multiple lesions.

Other benign mesenchymal or embryonic tumors are rare.

Malignant Hepatic Mass: Metastases of Solid Tumors

Basic Facts

- The liver frequently harbors metastases, especially those of gastrointestinal tumors.
- Hematogenous rather than lymphatic or contiguous spread (e.g., peritoneal expansion in ovarian cancer) is the most common form of dissemination.
- Correlation of the sonographic image with a specific primary tumor is hardly ever possible, although a certain pattern of metastasis may be more common in certain tumor entities (see below)
- Metastases are rare in cirrhotic livers.
- The size of the lesions is an important indicator in the follow-up of chemotherapy.
- *Additional workup:* CT, MRI, octreotide scintigraphy for neuroendocrine tumors.

Sonographic Criteria

- Hepatomegaly.
- **Multiple lesions** are more common than **solitary metastasis**.
- Most often round masses, polycyclic in case of confluent lesions.
- Hypoechoic halo ("target" sign) (Wernecke et al., 1992 a and b). Rather diverse texture, depending on the size and histology of the mass. Hyperechoic masses are common in **adenocarcinomas** of the GI tract, in particular colon cancer (Fig. 7.**41**), while hypoechoic metastases are characteristic of fast-growing tumors, e.g., **pancreatic cancer**.
- Large metastases tend to have a hyperechoic and heterogeneous structure due to, for example, necrosis, hemorrhage, or calcifications. In the latter there may be comet-tail artifacts, e.g., cancer of the colon.
- Liquefaction of necrosis results in a hypoechoic to anechoic center ("bull's eye" sign), e.g., in fast-growing tumors or in hyperechoic metastases of neuroendocrine tumors.
- Truly cystic metastases are rare; they are seen in **cystadenocarcinomas**.
- Multiple small metastases may be difficult to differentiate from diffuse liver disease, particularly cirrhosis.
- Multiple small hypoechoic metastases are more common in rapidly progressive tumors, e.g., small-cell **lung cancer, breast cancer**, and malignant **melanoma**.
- Displacement and interruption of vascular structures in the residual hepatic parenchyma.
- Destruction of the liver capsule echo.

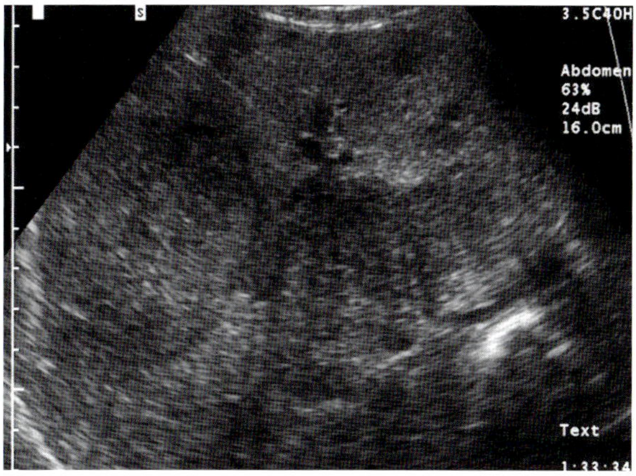

Fig. 7.**41 a** Metastases in cancer of the colon. Multiple round, sometimes confluent masses, hypoechoic rim. The hyperechogenicity of the mass texture increases with size.

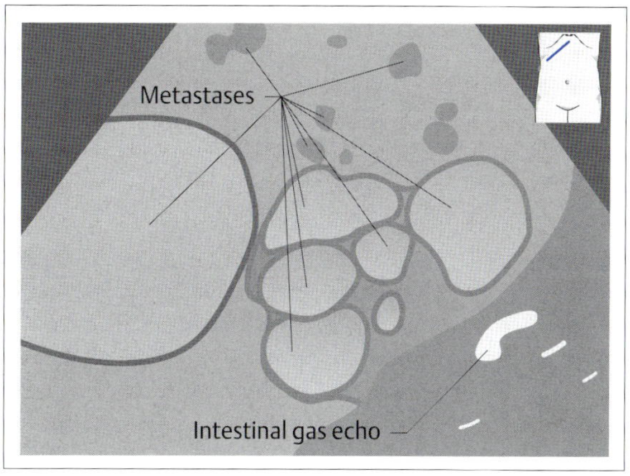

Fig. 7.**41 b** Line drawing.

Malignant Hepatic Mass: Liver Involvement in Malignant Hematological Disease

- **Acute leukemia:** frequently mild liver enlargement without other changes detectable by sonography.
- **Chronic leukemia**, myeloproliferative disorders: in most cases major hepatomegaly due to diffuse infiltration or extramedullary hematopoiesis.
  - Diffuse parenchymal infiltration cannot be identified sonomorphologically.
  - Extramedullary hematopoiesis may result in hypoechoic zones within the hepatic parenchyma.
- **Malignant lymphoma:**
  - Liver involvement in 50% of cases.
  - Infiltration is always hypoechoic.
  - Frequently micro- or macronodular infiltration, less commonly diffuse or localized invasion of the tumor (Görg et al., 1994).

Malignant Hepatic Mass: Hepatocellular Carcinoma (HCC)

Basic Facts

- Adenocarcinoma of the hepatocytes.
- Percentage of all carcinomas in Germany: men 2.7%, women 1.6% (Caselmann et al., 1999). Mortality 1995: men 4.7/100 000, women 2.1/100 000
- Much higher incidence in Asia and the sub-Saharan parts of Africa, reaching 150 per 100 000, where HCC is sometimes is the most common malignancy.
- Main risk factors: chronic hepatitis B and C (incidence in hepatitis B is about 0.5%/year); aflatoxin exposure; and, historically, application of thorium dioxide (Thorotrast).
- Cirrhosis of the liver is a risk factor by itself with an HCC incidence of 1–6% per year.
- The risk in cirrhosis depends on the etiology:
  - High: chronic viral hepatitis, hemochromatosis, tyrosinemia.
  - Medium: chronic alcohol abuse, autoimmune hepatitis, and alpha$_1$-antitrypsin deficiency.
  - Low: primary biliary cirrhosis, primary sclerosing cholangitis, and Wilson disease (Kubicka et al., 1997; 2000).
- 70% of the tumors express alpha-fetoprotein (AFP), which also rises nonspecifically in cirrhosis.
- The AFP level and sonography are the two most important components in the screening of patients with chronic hepatitis and/or cirrhosis (Chalasani et al., 1999).
- Sonography is also the imaging modality of choice for percutaneous regional treatment, such as ethanol injection (Giorgio et al., 2000; Hargreaves et al., 2000; Livraghi et al., 1998; Orlando et al., 2000) or thermocoagulation (Curley et al., 2000; Holtkamp and Müller, 2000; Livraghi et al., 2000).
- *Additional workup:* serum AFP level, CT, MRI, FNA.

Sonographic Criteria

- **Unilocular, multilocular**, or **diffuse** growth.
- Commonly arises in one site, and then develops lymphogenic metastases as satellite lesions.
- The echotexture varies, more often hypoechoic than hyperechoic; in most cases heterogeneous complex echotexture, characteristic pattern of "tumors in the tumor" (Fig. 7.**42**).
- Typical sign of malignancy: hypoechoic rim (Fig. 7.**42**).
- Portal vein thrombosis close to the tumor is common.
- Malignant invasion of the portal vein occurs early, less commonly into the hepatic veins, and rarely into the right atrium.

- B-mode sonography cannot reliably differentiate malignant vascular infiltration from thrombosis, the latter often preceding the former. Echogenic mural structures within the vein are visualized in both thrombosis and invasion, and in this area normal flow signals are lacking on color-flow Doppler imaging. Arterial Doppler signals in such a suspected thrombus signify malignant invasion (see Portal Vein Thrombosis, above; Fig. 7.**33**).
- Color-flow and power Doppler sonography usually reveal a highly vascularized tumor with arterial waveforms, especially in its rim; however, these modalities do not permit sufficiently reliable discrimination either from benign lesions or from other malignancies (Gaiani et al., 2000; Strunk et al., 1998).

- Percutaneous ethanol injection: Fluid injected into HCC distributes almost selectively in the malignant mass, as becomes evident sonographically by bright gas echoes in the fluid (Fig. 7.**43**). Alcohol 95% is injected via fine needles with lateral openings (Livraghi et al., 1998). An injection volume of around 50–90% of the tumor volume is required, with a maximum volume of 10 ml per tumor per session. Complete tumor necrosis is usually attained only after repeated injections; power Doppler sonography and contrast-enhanced CT scans check for vital tumor residues. Some authors aim for complete eradication in a single session using injection volumes of up to 60 ml under general anesthesia (Giorgio et al., 2000).

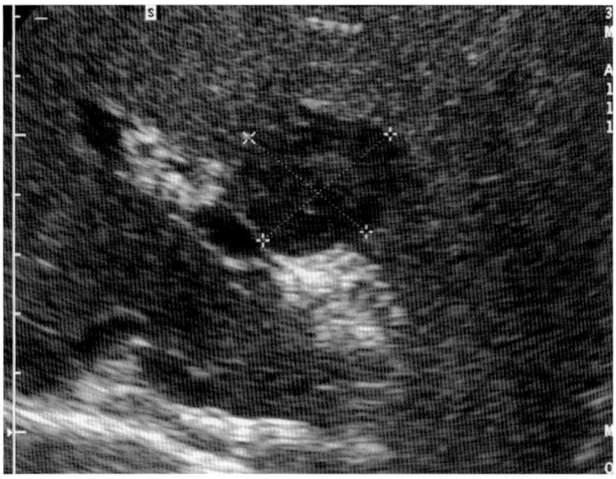

Fig. 7.**42 a** Hepatocellular carcinoma. Poorly delimited polycyclic lesion, measuring 29 mm across. Hypoechoic heterogeneous echotexture resembling a "tumor within a tumor." Compression of a portal vein branch.

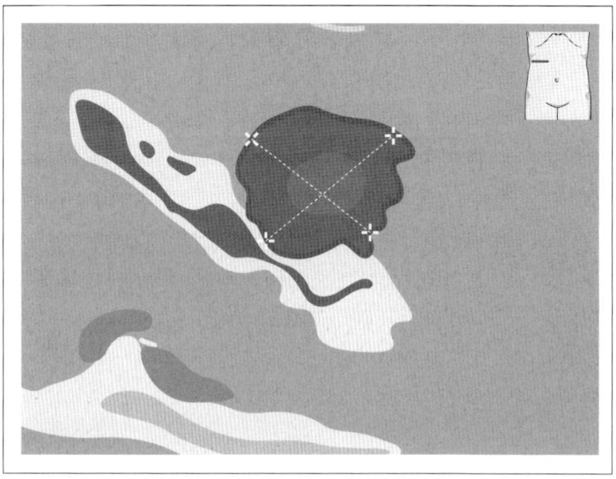

Fig. 7.**42 b** Line drawing.

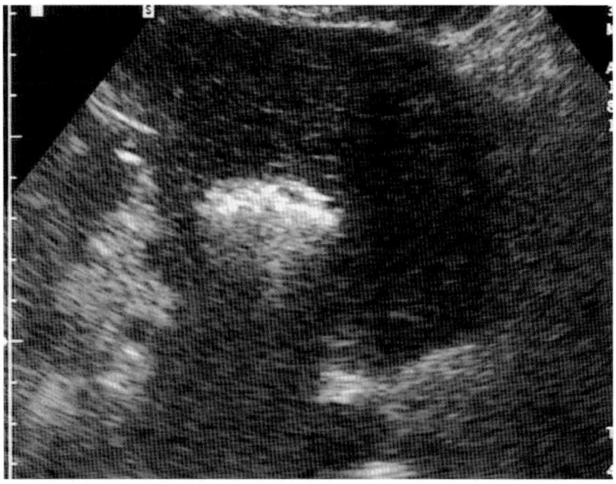

Fig. 7.**43 a** Hepatocellular carcinoma: percutaneous ethanol injection. The alcohol 95% has dispersed throughout the entire carcinoma, as demonstrated by the hyperechoic gas bubbles in the fluid.

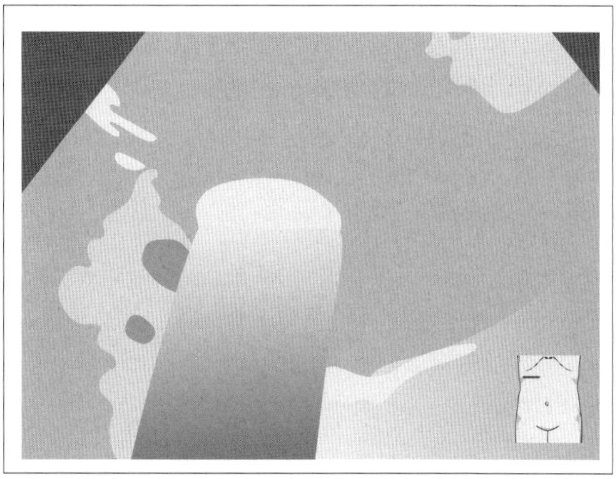

Fig. 7.**43 b** Line drawing.

Consequences for Surgical Treatment

Diagnosis	Characteristic Findings	Management
Hepatic metastasis of colorectal cancer	Solitary or multiple spread, primarily unilateral, no extrahepatic involvement	Resection with curative intent; determining factor in liver resection is the amount of healthy liver remaining, and not the hepatic involvement per se
Hepatic metastasis of colorectal cancer	Diffuse spread in all segments	Confirmation by histology, palliative systemic chemotherapy
HCC	< 5 cm, solitary, unilateral, enough remaining parenchyma (often cirrhotic)?	Resection will depend on the extent of the cirrhosis, residual liver function, and portal hypertension; patient-specific evaluation for LTX
HCC	> 5 cm, metastatic, in severe cirrhosis	Palliative local or systemic therapy (chemotherapy, arterial chemo-embolization, thermal ablation, alcohol injection)

Pancreas

Indications, Specific Technique, and Diagnostic Evaluation

- The pancreas makes a mild S-shape in the retroperitoneal space, rising slightly from the curve of the duodenum to the splenic hilum (Fig. 7.**44**).
- A slim patient after an overnight fast offers the best examination conditions.
- Standard views are the transverse and longitudinal planes in the upper abdomen.
- The splenic vein is the landmark for this organ, which is assessed from the head to body and tail.
  - The *head* comprises all pancreatic tissue to the right of the left wall of the superior mesenteric vein.
  - The *body* extends from the left wall of the superior mesenteric vein to the left wall of the aorta.
  - The pancreatic *tail* extends from the left wall of the aorta to the splenic hilum.
- Localization of the gastroduodenal artery at the anterior right pancreatic border helps with differentiation from the duodenum; the CBD can be delineated in the posterior part of the pancreatic head as a further tubular structure aiding orientation (Fig. 7.**45**).
- Transsplenic views help in scrutinizing the tail region.
- If access is impaired by superimposed stomach or intestines, graded compression with the probe or deep inspiration may displace the viscera; gastric filling with 100–300 ml of water may facilitate pancreatic assessment (the water should be administered with a straw to avoid swallowing air), as may scanning with the patient erect.
- Pancreatic pathology is subdivided into diffuse and localized changes (Table 7.**4**).

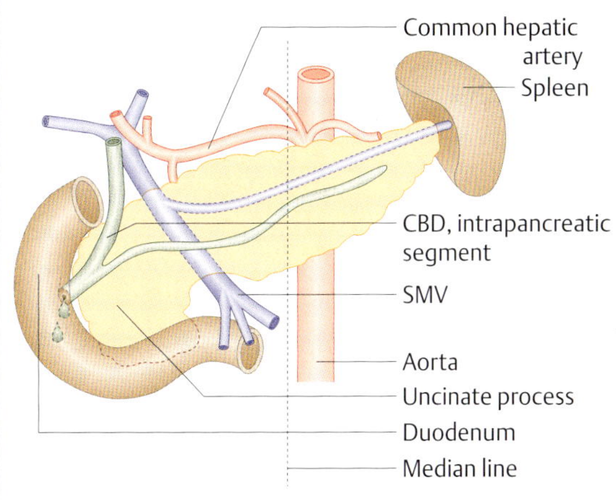

Fig. 7.**44** Anatomical relationships of the pancreas.

Table 7.**4** Common pancreatic pathology important in sonography

Primarily Diffuse	Primarily Localized
Chronic pancreatitis	Pancreatic cancer
Acute pancreatitis	Pseudocyst
Fibrolipomatosis	Necrosis related to pancreatitis
Aging pancreas	Pancreatic duct calculi/calcification
	Cystadenoma

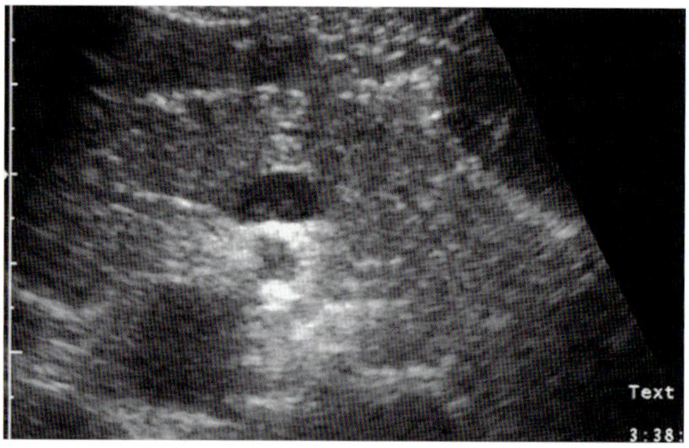

Fig. 7.**45 a** Transverse epigastric view of the normal pancreas.

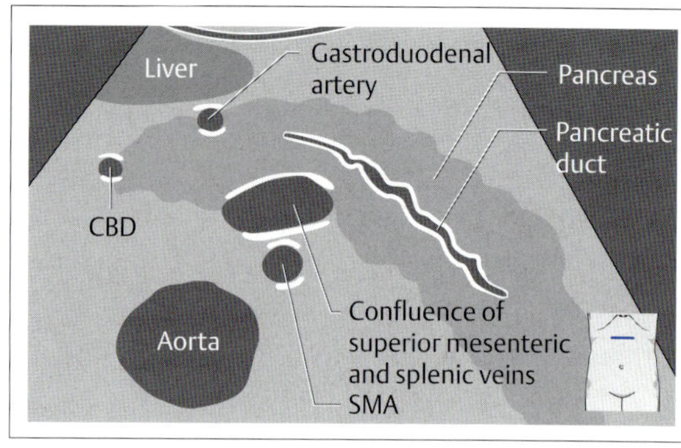

Fig. 7.**45 b** Line drawing.

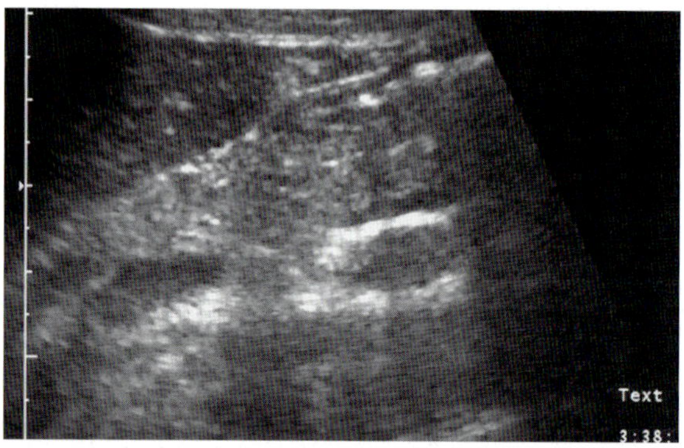

Fig. 7.**46 a** Longitudinal epigastric view of the normal pancreas including the superior mesenteric artery.

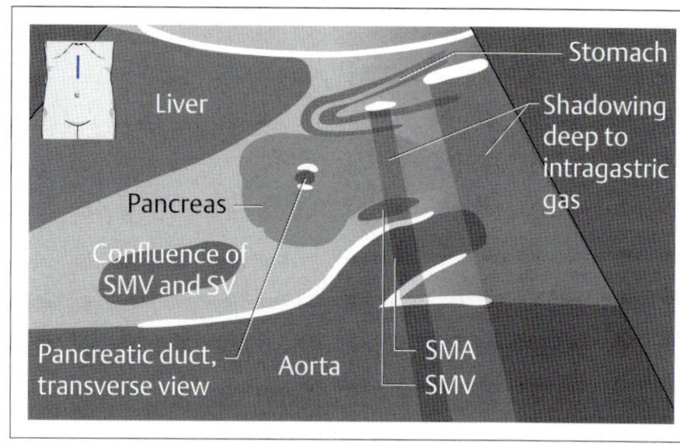

Fig. 7.**46 b** Line drawing.

General Criteria for Sonographic Assessment

- The normal pancreas has a homogeneous finely grained echotexture, usually somewhat hyperechoic to the hepatic parenchyma (Figs. 7.**45**, 7.**46**).
- Normal dimensions:
  - Head: < 30 mm, body < 18 mm, tail < 30 mm, duct < 2–3 mm.
  - Since the pancreas is not situated exactly within the transverse plane, the diameter should always be determined in the plane of the organ (Fig. 7.**47**).
- The healthy pancreas is elastic and deformable.
- The juvenile pancreas is hypoechoic, while the aging pancreas is clearly more echogenic.
- The pancreatic duct does not always course along the center of the organ.

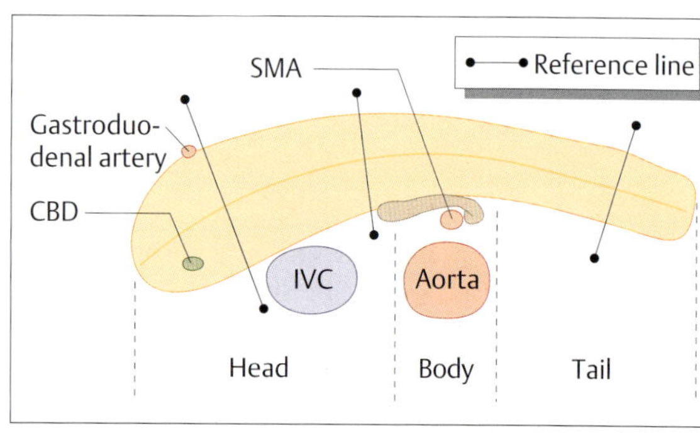

Fig. 7.**47** Determining the diameter of the pancreas in a plane orthogonal to the pancreatic axis. Transverse upper abdominal view, line drawing.

Acute Pancreatitis

See Chapter 1, Acute Abdomen.

Chronic Pancreatitis

Basic Facts

- Sometimes intermittent progressive inflammation of the pancreas with destruction of the parenchyma, which is replaced by fibrotic tissue.
- Chronic alcohol abuse is the most common etiological factor in Germany (80–90%).
- Highly variable course; most often intermittent pain attacks, less commonly chronic persistent pain or asymptomatic course.
- May involve the entire organ, or just individual segments, with different intensity (= segmental chronic pancreatitis).
- During active inflammation the pancreas is frequently swollen.
- In the late stages the organ becomes smaller because of the fibrotic transformation.
- Fibrosis results in stenosis and distension in the ductal system; after inflammatory episodes, pseudocysts may arise with formation of ductal calculi, first within the branches and later in the main pancreatic duct.
- The excruciating upper abdominal pain of some patients is attributed to the increased pressure in the pancreatic duct as well as to the inflammation itself.
- Exocrine and endocrine pancreatic failure is also characteristic of advanced chronic pancreatitis (with diarrhea, steatorrhea, and weight loss).
- About 10% of cases experience an asymptomatic course or present with only minor upper abdominal pain.
- The incidence in Central Europe averages 0.04–5 per 100 000 per year with a male preponderance; the peak lies between the age of 35 and 45 years.
- Common local complications: bile duct stenosis; duodenal narrowing secondary to fibrosis, inflammatory mass, or pseudocysts.
- Pancreatic pseudocysts are cavities filled with fluid or debris and surrounded by a fibrous capsule (lacking an epithelial lining compared with true cysts).
- Pseudocysts develop in around 20% of patients with chronic pancreatitis, may remain asymptomatic, and can regress spontaneously; treatment is needed only in case of complications.
- After acute pancreatitis, pseudocysts are mostly filled with hemorrhagic or greenish secretion, and in chronic pancreatitis with clear fluid rich in enzymes.
- Pancreatic necrosis and pseudocysts can extend into all areas of the abdomen and even into the pleural cavity.
- Vascular erosion may lead to hemorrhage into the pancreatic duct or pseudocysts.
- In the late stages of chronic pancreatitis there may be exocrine and endocrine pancreatic failure.
- *Additional workup:* plain abdominal films, spot film of the pancreas, ERCP, CT, EUS, MRI, MRCP, fecal fat quantitation, glucose tolerance testing, fecal elastase, pancreolauryl test, and direct tests of pancreatic function.

Sonographic Criteria

- The diameter of the pancreatic duct frequently exceeds 2–3 mm (Fig. 7.**48**).
- **Irregular pancreatic outline** and enhanced textural echoes due to scarring; mixed forms are possible, in particular during acute exacerbation (Fig. 7.**48**).
- **Fibrosis** renders the pancreas more echogenic than in a normal setting.
- **Pancreatic duct stones** are characterized by bright echoes and posterior shadowing; they may be solitary or lined up like a string of beads (Figs. 7.**48**, 7.**49**).
- Calculi within the side branches mimic "**parenchymal calcification**" (Fig. 7.**48**).
- **Bile duct dilatation** secondary to stenosis of the distal intrapancreatic segment of the CBD.
- **Pseudocyst** visualized as an anechoic, almost round, structure with posterior shadowing and lined with a hypoechoic membrane; floating echoes correspond to debris, while gas echoes may indicate infection (Fig. 7.**50**).
- In case of **hemorrhage** into the pseudocyst, the contents become more echogenic; color-flow Doppler imaging may pinpoint the bleeding directly (Fig. 7.**51**).

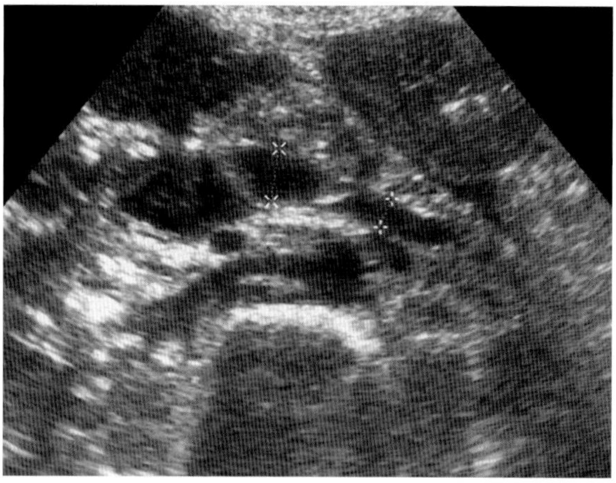

Fig. 7.**48 a** Transverse epigastric view in chronic pancreatitis. Pancreatic duct distended to 12 mm; intraductal stone, inflammatory hypoechoic swelling next to hyperechoic areas and calcification, sometimes with posterior shadowing.

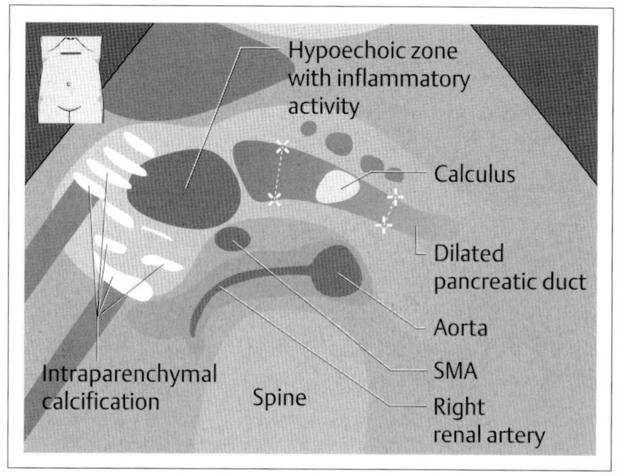

Fig. 7.**48 b** Line drawing.

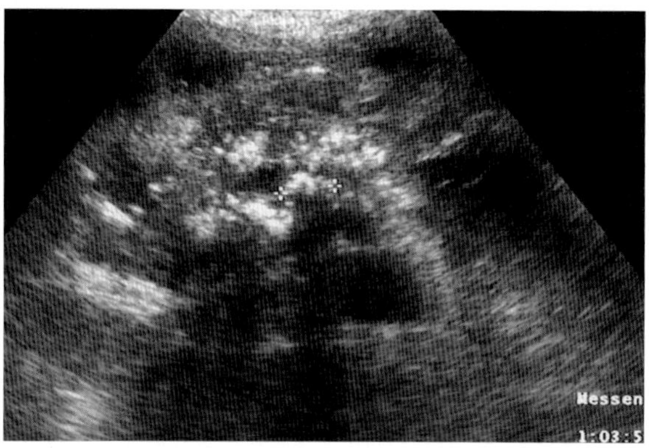

Fig. 7.**49 a** Transverse epigastric view in chronic pancreatitis. Pancreatic duct distended; intraductal calculus with posterior shadowing; mixed pattern with hypoechoic and hyperechoic areas and parenchymal calcification.

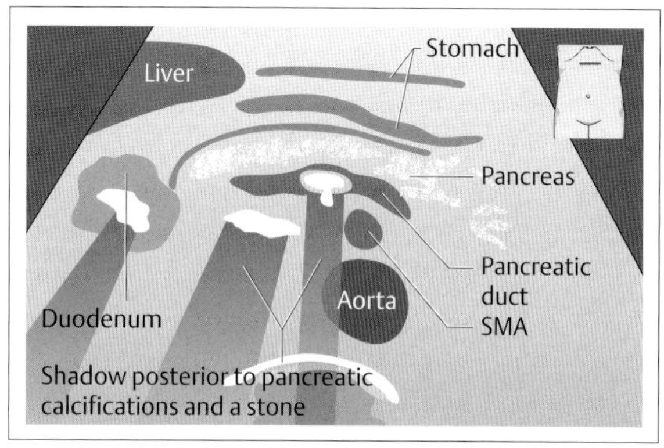

Fig. 7.**49 b** Line drawing.

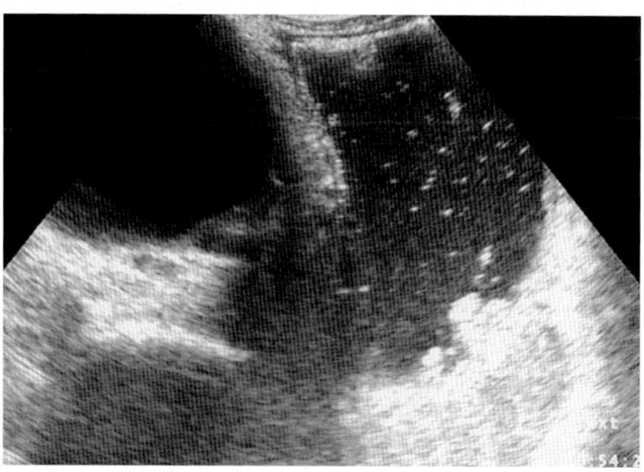

Fig. 7.**50 a** Large anechoic pseudocyst in chronic pancreatitis compressing the stomach and leading to gastric outlet obstruction.

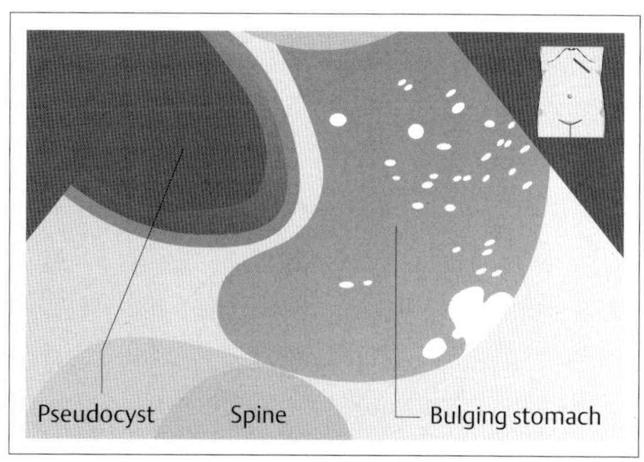

Fig. 7.**50 b** Line drawing.

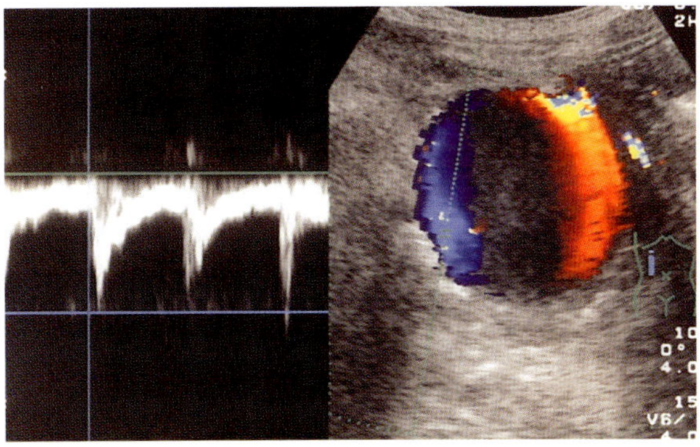

Fig. 7.51 a Color-flow Doppler imaging of acute hemorrhage into a pancreatic pseudocyst in chronic pancreatitis; arterial flow signal due to bleeding from the pancreaticoduodenal artery into the pseudocyst.

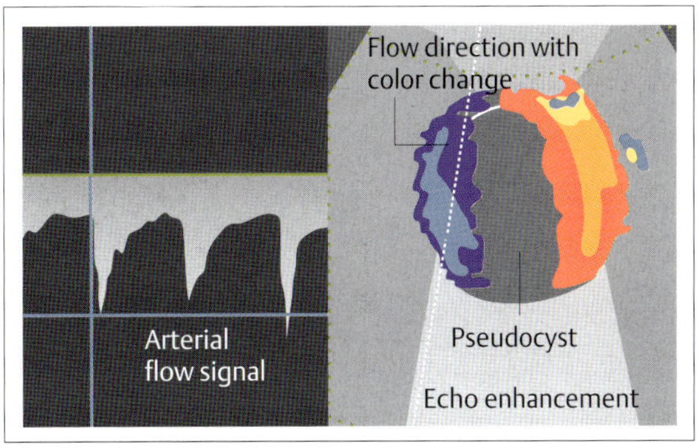

Fig. 7.51 b Line drawing.

Consequences for Surgical Treatment

Diagnosis	Characteristic Findings	Management
Chronic pancreatitis with inflammatory mass at the pancreatic head	Stenosis of the CBD or duodenum No pseudocysts or ductal stenosis in body and tail of pancreas	Duodenum-preserving resection of the head of the pancreas (Beger procedure) or pylorus-preserving Whipple procedure
Chronic pancreatitis with inflammatory mass at the pancreatic head	Stenosis of the CBD or duodenum with stenosis of the pancreatic duct and stasis at the body or tail	Duodenum-preserving resection of the pancreatic head and side-to-side pancreatico-jejunostomy (Frey procedure)
Pancreatic pseudocyst	Symptomatic (e.g., pain, CBD stenosis, impaired intestinal passage, abscess) and persistent over the long run	Surgical drainage (e.g., pseudocysto-jejunostomy) or endoscopic drainage

Pancreatic Cancer

Basic Facts

- Pancreatic cancer may alter the size, shape, and texture of the pancreas.
- Adenocarcinomas originating from the ductal epithelium are by far the most common tumors of the pancreas, with about 75% arising in the head of the pancreas.
- Men in the seventh decade of life are most commonly affected (men : women = 5 : 1), with a rising incidence (about 10/100 000 per year).
- Quite often, tumor invasion into the distal CBD, resulting in painless jaundice, will be the initial symptom leading to the diagnosis.
- Other symptoms: weight loss, asthenia, indigestion, abdominal and back pain, Courvoisier's law.
- Around 33% of pancreatic head cancers and 75% of tumors of the body/tail already have detectable metastases at the time of diagnosis.
- As they remain clinically silent for a very long time, carcinomas in the tail and body of the pancreas are usually much larger at the time of diagnosis than those within the head.
- CA 19–9 is elevated in over 70% of all pancreatic cancers (however, elevated levels are also possible in benign conditions).
- New-onset diabetes in patients with known chronic pancreatitis is suspicious for evolving pancreatic cancer.
- Main role of sonography in suspected pancreatic cancer (Table 7.**5**):
  - Detection of pancreatic masses, differentiation between chronic pancreatitis and malignant mass.
  - In case of strong suspicion of pancreatic malignancy, assessment of the anatomical relationships and possible inoperability.

- Criteria of inoperability include:
  - Peritoneal carcinomatosis
  - Distant spread (most commonly to the liver)
  - Extraregional lymphatic spread
  - Tumor growth beyond the pancreatic head with invasion of neighboring organs (except for the duodenum)
  - Extensive invasion of the portal vein/superior mesenteric vein or superior mesenteric artery (relative indication because of possible graft interposition)
- Only 40% of patients undergoing surgery will be resected with curative intent (5-year survival rate about 5–10%).
- Apart from direct tumor demonstration with its sensitivity of 67–85% (Brambs et al., 1993; Niederau and Grendell, 1992; Rösch et al., 1992), indirect signs of pancreatic head cancer also aid in the diagnosis:
  - Dilatation of bile and pancreatic ducts
  - Liver metastases
  - Ascites
  - Delayed gastric emptying
  - Lymphadenopathy
- Series including only those patients in whom the entire pancreas could be fully viewed have reported detection sensitivities of 95–98% (Brambs and Claussen, 1993; Gandolfi and Fukuda, 1997).
- Differentiation between vascular compression and invasion is difficult in TAUS; because tumor staging by EUS with its accuracy of 92% is more sensitive, it has become standard in present-day clinical practice (Sugiyama et al., 1999 Table 7.**6**).
- Equivocal sonographic findings of the pancreas must always be elucidated by additional diagnostic measures.
- *Additional workup:* ERCP, EUS, contrast-enhanced CT scan, MRI, angiography, diagnostic FNA, exploratory laparoscopy/laparotomy.

Table 7.**5** Sonographic characteristics of pancreatic malignancies in a series of 62 patients (modified from Yassa et al., 1997)

Parameter	Frequency
Average size	4.5–3.5 cm
Largest tumor	14 × 19 cm
Smallest tumor	1.8 × 1.1 cm
Pancreatic head cancer	69%
Pancreatic body/tail cancer	26%
Diffuse growth	3%
Oval or round shape	60%
Irregular shape	40%
Breaching of pancreatic contour	65%
Homogeneous hypoechoic	55%
Homogenous hyperechoic	3%
Homogenous isoechoic	2%
Heterogeneous echotexture	40%
Calcified tumor	6%
Intratumoral cystic structures	15%
Portal vein thrombosis	5%
Vascular encasement	13%

Sonographic Criteria

- Often hypoechoic or isoechoic **tumor mass**; in early stages homogeneous, later breaching the normal contour of the pancreas, possibly with fine offshoots of the tumor (Fig. 7.**52**).
- Anechoic areas corresponding to **necrotic tumor** may occur in large tumors, with the latter possibly displaying a hyperechoic echotexture (Fig. 7.**53**).
- Possible **compression, displacement**, and **invasion** of neighboring structures (duodenum, portal vein, superior mesenteric artery/vein, celiac trunk) (Fig. 7.**54**).
- Possible **dilatation of the pancreatic duct** (> 2–3 mm) or the bile ducts (CBD, CHD > 9 mm) upstream of the tumor-induced obstruction (Fig. 7.**53**).

Table 7.**6** Comparison of different diagnostic modalities in suspected pancreatic carcinoma (modified from Sugiyama et al., 1999; 91 patients)

	IOS	TAUS	Contrast-Enhanced CT	EUS	Angiography	Parameter
Sensitivity (%)	100	79	81	95	54	Detection of pancreatic or biliary ductal tumors <2 cm
Sensitivity (%)	92	56	64	91	76	Detection of portal vein invasion
Specificity (%)	92	73	74	92	83	Detection of portal vein invasion

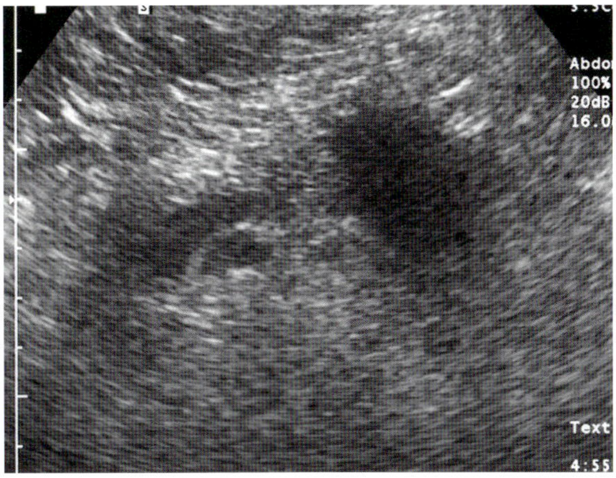

Fig. 7.52 a Transverse epigastric view: hypoechoic cancer of the pancreatic tail with irregular border breaching the normal pancreatic contour.

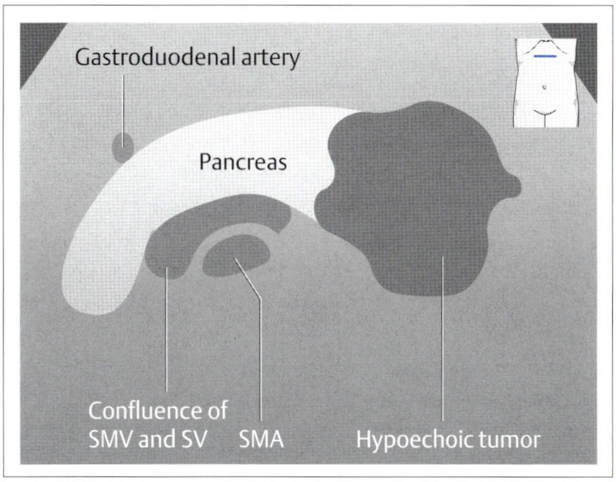

Fig. 7.52 b Line drawing. SMS = superior mesenteric artery; SV = splenic vein.

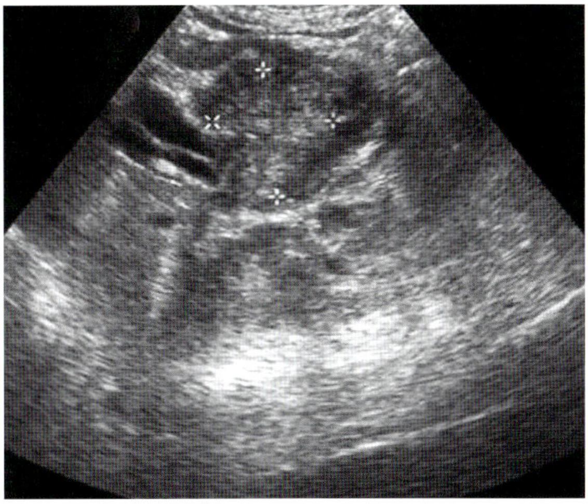

Fig. 7.53 a Oblique epigastric view: large hyperechoic carcinoma of the pancreatic head (5.5 × 4.5 cm) obstructing the CBD.

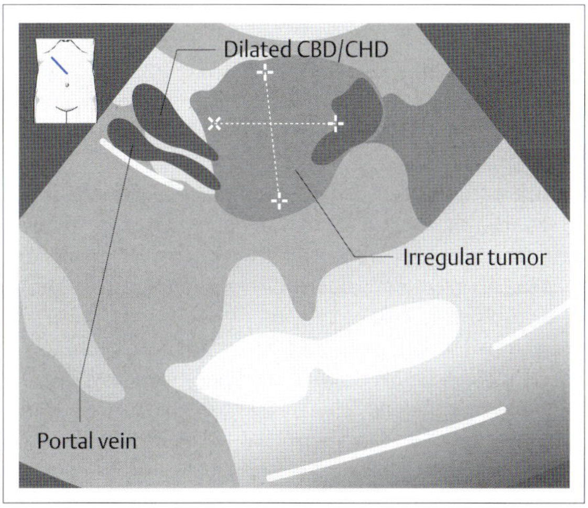

Fig. 7.53 b Line drawing. DHC = common bile duct (CBD).

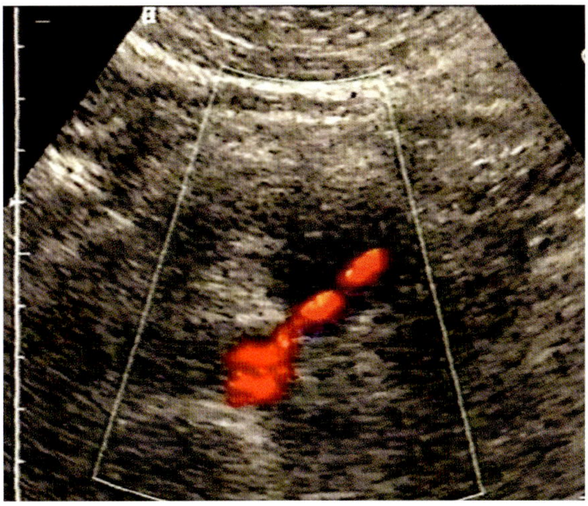

Fig. 7.54 a Oblique epigastric view, color-flow Doppler sonography: pancreatic carcinoma encasing the superior mesenteric artery.

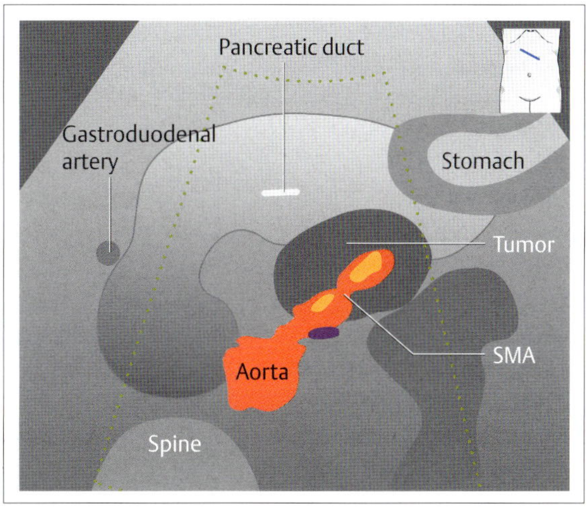

Fig. 7.54 b Line drawing. AMS = superior mesenteric artery.

Consequences for Surgical Treatment

Diagnosis	Characteristic Findings	Management
Cancer of the pancreatic head	No invasion of portal vein or superior mesenteric artery No distant lymphatic spread No organ metastasis	Partial pancreaticoduodenectomy with (Traverso–Longmire) or without (Whipple) preservation of the pylorus
Cancer of the pancreatic head	With limited invasion of portal vein or superior mesenteric artery	In some cases (only if R0!) extended partial pancreaticoduodenectomy with vascular grafting may be indicated
Pancreatic cancer (irrespective of site)	Extraregional lymphatic spread or distant metastasis	In general, resection of tumor not indicated In symptomatic cases, gastric bypass and/or choledochojejunostomy, palliative management
Pancreatic body/tail cancer	No distant lymphatic spread No organ metastasis	Left pancreas resection including spleen and local lymph nodes

Rare Tumors of the Pancreas

Basic Facts

- Serous and mucinous cystadenomas and cystadenocarcinomas comprise no more than 1% of all malignant pancreatic tumors and thus are rare findings in diagnostic sonography of the pancreas.
- Mucinous cystadenomas always carry a malignant potential or have already become malignant by the time of their discovery.
- As classification is impossible without complete histological work-up of the tumor, total en-bloc resection should always be attempted.
- Recurrent upper abdominal pain, sometimes radiating to the back, may be the initial symptom; other symptoms depend on the site of the tumor.
- Sonographic differentiation from pancreatic pseudocyst is difficult, but usually the typical history of pancreatitis is absent (Meyer et al., 1999).
- At the time of diagnosis the tumor diameter varies from 2 to 12 cm (mean 6.1 cm).
- In (*preselected*) patient series, cystic tumors have been reported to comprise up to 10% of all cystic lesions of the pancreas (Meyer et al., 1999).
- Cystadenocarcinomas seem to be localized predominantly in the pancreatic head, while cystadenomas exhibit no such preferential site.
- Cystadenocarcinomas grow more slowly and metastasize later than the far more common adenocarcinomas of the pancreas, so complete resection is frequently possible.
- Malignancy was regularly seen in cystic pancreatic tumors > 6 cm (Kimura and Makuuchi, 1999).
- The 5-year survival rate after cystadenocarcinoma is 52–63% (Hashimoto et al., 1998; Le Borgne et al., 1999)
- Approximately 20% of cystic pancreatic tumors are cystadenocarcinomas, about 80% of which are amenable to resection.
- Apart from complete resection, preservation of organ function is of primary interest in benign tumors; malignant tumors require resection according to oncosurgical protocols, and here intraoperative frozen sections are of particular importance.
- The indications for resection of a pancreatic cyst are given in Table 7.7.
- *Additional workup:* CT, MRI, ERCP, EUS, FNA cytology and biopsy:
  - Viscosity of secretion?
  - Tumor marker levels in the cyst contents (CA 19–9).
  - Cytology

Table 7.**7** Indications for resection of a pancreatic cyst (modified from Meyer et al., 1999)

Patient without a history of trauma or pancreatitis
Typical characteristics of cystic pancreatic tumors on sonography, CT, MRI–see text
Unsuccessful intervention
Elevated tumor marker levels in cyst contents
Positive cytology in cyst contents

Sonographic Criteria

- Round, usually cystic mass, frequently > 2 cm in diameter.
- Hyperechoic septations or posterior shadowing in the wall, induced by calcifications, differentiate them from pseudocysts.
- Small papillary offshoots of the tumor may protrude from the cyst wall into the lumen.
- Serous cystadenomas are frequently multilocular (> 6 cysts) and measure < 2 cm in diameter (sonographic sensitivity 80–93%).
- Mucinous tumors are usually composed of < 6 cysts and measure > 2 cm in diameter (sonographic sensitivity 93–95%) (Fugazzola et al., 1990; Gandolfi 1997).
- Apart from these cystadenomas there are other rare pancreatic tumors that lack characteristic sonographic features.

Consequences for Surgical Treatment

Diagnosis	Characteristic Findings	Management
Cystic pancreatic head tumor	Typical criteria of cystic tumors on sonography and additional diagnostic workup, possibly positive tumor markers or positive cytology of cyst contents	**Complete** resection of cystic tumor by duodenum-preserving resection of the pancreatic head; pancreaticoduodenectomy in case of malignancy (possibly preserving the pylorus)
Cystic pancreatic body tumor	Often involving the tail as well; typical criteria of cystic tumors on sonography and additional diagnostic workup; possibly positive tumor markers or positive cytology of cyst contents	In case of malignancy, **complete** resection of the cystic tumor (e.g., resection of body and tail with splenectomy and lymphadenectomy in case of malignancy)
Cystic pancreatic tail tumor	Typical criteria of cystic tumors on sonography and additional diagnostic workup; possibly positive tumor markers or positive cytology in cyst contents	In case of malignancy **complete** resection of the cystic tumor (e.g., resection of pancreatic tail with splenectomy and lymphadenectomy in case of malignancy)

Endocrine Tumors of the Pancreas

Basic Facts

- Only around 4% of all pancreatic tumors exhibit endocrine activity.
- The most common benign tumors of the pancreas are endocrine in nature, followed by cystic tumors.
- Mostly insulinomas (60%) or gastrinomas (18%); less common are glucagonomas, VIPomas, somastatinomas, or nonsecreting islet cell tumors.
- Size often 0.2–4 cm (mean 0.8 cm).
- Accordingly, unequivocal identification by TAUS is often impossible; intraoperative palpation and IOS are in fact more sensitive.
- 99% of all insulinomas are intrapancreatic, about 90% are solitary; there is no predisposition of any segment, and the rate of malignancy is < 10%.
- Sonography has a reported sensitivity of 25–63% for detection of insulinomas.
- Only about 30% of gastrinomas are intrapancreatic, primarily in the head of the pancreas, and their rate of malignancy is > 50%.
- About 70% of all gastrinomas are found in the duodenal wall–here, palpation is superior to IOS.
- 80% are solitary.
- Gastrinomas induce Zollinger–Ellison syndrome; multiple occurrence is common; one-third of patients suffer from multiple endocrine neoplasia (MEN I).
- Most gastrinomas are found in a triangle bordered by the following structures:
  - Junction of the cystic duct and the CBD
  - Inferior section of the third duodenal segment
  - Border between head and body of the pancreas
- *Additional workup:* CT, MRI, EUS, selective portal venous blood sampling, IOS and palpation, possibly octreotide scintigraphy.

Sonographic Criteria

- Most endocrine tumors are hypoechoic, round, and sharply delimited (Fig. 7.**55**).
- They usually do not breach the organ borders.
- Calcification or cystic/necrotic parts are rare occurrences.

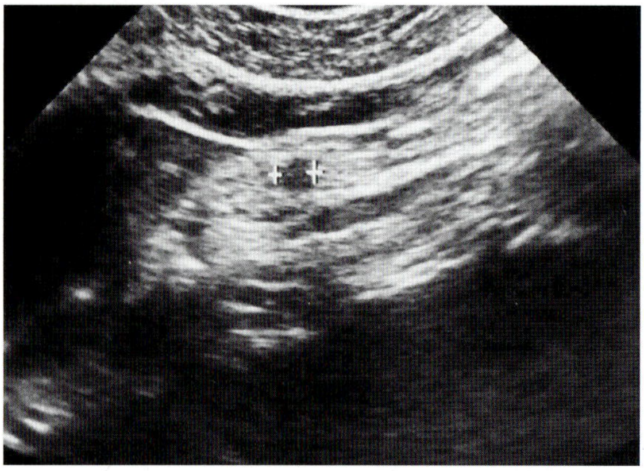

Fig. 7.**55 a** Hypoechoic endocrine tumor (10 mm) in the pancreatic body (insulinoma). Longitudinal epigastric view of the pancreas including the superior mesenteric artery. (Department of Endocrinology, University of Magdeburg Medical Center.)

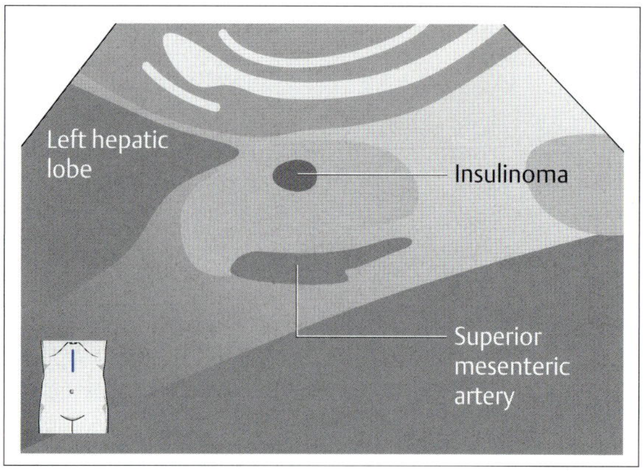

Fig. 7.**55 b** Line drawing.

Consequences for Surgical Treatment

Diagnosis	Characteristic Findings	Management
Endocrine tumor in pancreatic head or body	No malignancy on frozen section (sonography helps in the localization)	Excision or "coring out" (in case of tight relation to the pancreatic duct system, internal drainage via Roux-en-Y may be indicated) Segmental pancreatectomy (head or body), if complete excision is impossible.
Endocrine tumor in pancreatic head or body	Malignancy on frozen section	Adequate pancreatectomy according to surgical oncology protocols as for ductal adenocarcinoma
Endocrine tumor in the pancreatic tail	No malignancy on frozen section	Spleen-preserving resection of the pancreatic tail
Endocrine tumor in the pancreatic tail	Malignancy on frozen section	Adequate pancreatectomy according to surgical oncology protocols as for ductal adenocarcinoma (resection of pancreatic tail and/or body, usually with splenectomy)

Spleen

Basic Facts

- Sonography is the standard imaging modality when assessing the spleen.
- Causes of changes in splenic structure and size include:
  - Lymphatic and myeloproliferative disorders
  - Hemolytic anemias
  - Infections
  - Cirrhosis of the liver and venous congestion
  - Abscesses, infarctions, metastases, cysts
  - Hematomas, rupture
- The spleen is examined in oblique subcostal/intercostal views, and via flank access.
- Right lateral decubitus position with left arm elevated over the head opens up the intercostal spaces, thus improving visualization.
- On inspiration the spleen is pushed caudad, which facilitates visualization of the entire organ.
- Relationships: Left upper quadrant of peritoneal cavity, below the diaphragm (Fig. 7.**56**).
- Long axis paralleling the 9th–11th rib.
- Splenic abscess is rare, mostly occurring in the context of acute pancreatitis, endocarditis, or septicemia.
- Splenic calcifications develop mainly as late sequelae of hematoma, infarction, abscess, or infectious disease (more common in Mediterranean countries).

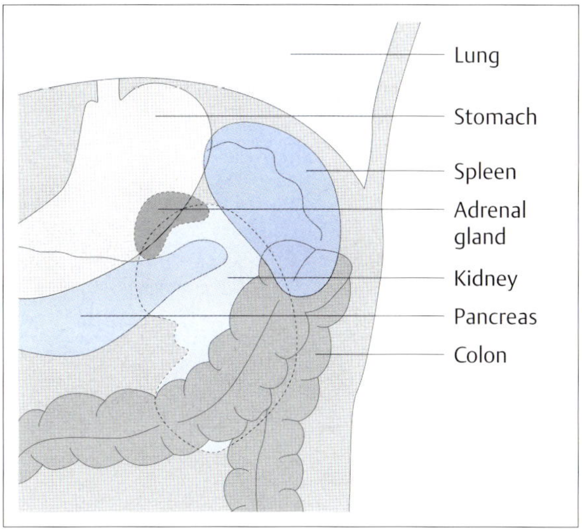

Fig. 7.**56** Schematic topography of the spleen and its relationships to the diaphragm, splenic flexure of the colon, stomach, kidney, and pancreatic tail.

- Intrasplenic arterial occlusion regularly results in regional infarction as the branches of the splenic artery are end arteries.
- Splenic infarctions may have a variety of causes, e.g., splenic artery aneurysm, leukemia, pancreatitis, or pancreatic carcinoma with splenic artery invasion.
- Hemangiomas are the most common benign tumors of the spleen.
- Hypersplenism is characterized by degradation of one or more blood cell lines within the spleen and often by splenomegaly; splenectomy usually results in recovery of the previously reduced blood cell line(s).
- Splenic metastases occur in only around 7% of all diffusely metastasized malignancies; about 50% of these are metastases of malignant melanoma.
- *Additional workup:* FNA, contrast-enhanced CT, MRI, scintigraphy, hematological workup.

Sonographic Criteria

- The normal spleen is hypoechoic and homogeneous, and vessels may be visualized at the splenic hilum (Fig. 7.**57**).
- Normal splenic dimensions: Depth < 4 cm (splenic hilum–lateral surface); length < 11 cm (longest cephalocaudal diameter); width < 7 cm (not measured routinely) (Fig. 7.**58**).
- **Splenomegaly** may be homogeneous (portal hypertension, portal vein thrombosis) or display an uncharacteristic echotexture (infectious and systemic diseases) (Fig. 7.**59**).
- **Splenic cysts** are round and anechoic with posterior enhancement.
- **Splenic rupture** may be characterized by a visible parenchymal defect, but a common isolated earlier sign is intraperitoneal fluid stemming from this defect; subcapsular hematoma encasing the spleen, initially hypoechoic and later on hypoechoic (Fig. 7.**60**); regression of the hematoma with hyperechoic capsule.
- **Splenic abscesses** may vary considerably–frequently heterogeneous with hypoechoic parts, at times including internal echoes (gas) (Fig. 7.**61**).
- **Lymphomas of the spleen** are often hypoechoic lesions of variable shape and size, frequently resulting in splenomegaly (Fig. 7.**62**).
- **Splenic infarction** may typically, though not always, be wedge-shaped with irregular borders, lacking vascularity on color-flow Doppler imaging.
- Most **metastases within the spleen** are hypoechoic; a hypoechoic rim and central necrosis are possible (Fig. 7.**63**).
- **Splenic calcifications** appear as bright echoes with posterior acoustic shadowing.

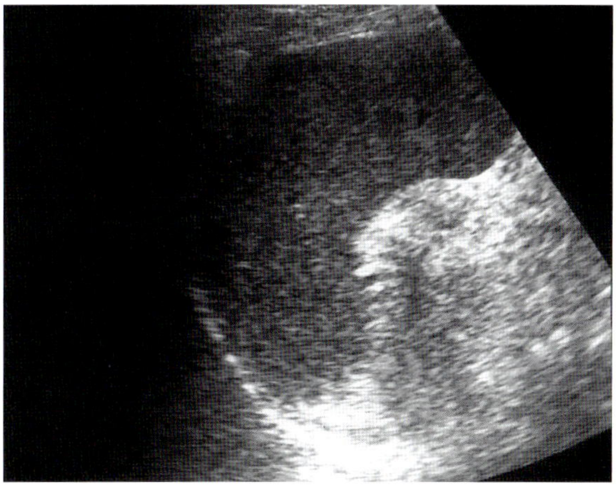

Fig. 7.**57 a** Intercostal view of the normal spleen, homogeneous parenchyma.

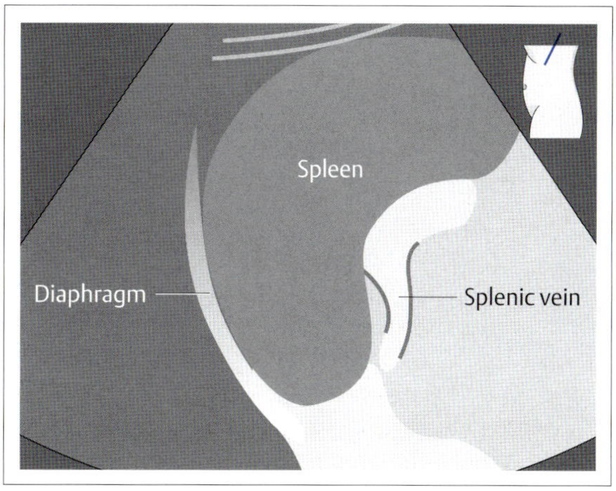

Fig. 7.**57 b** Line drawing.

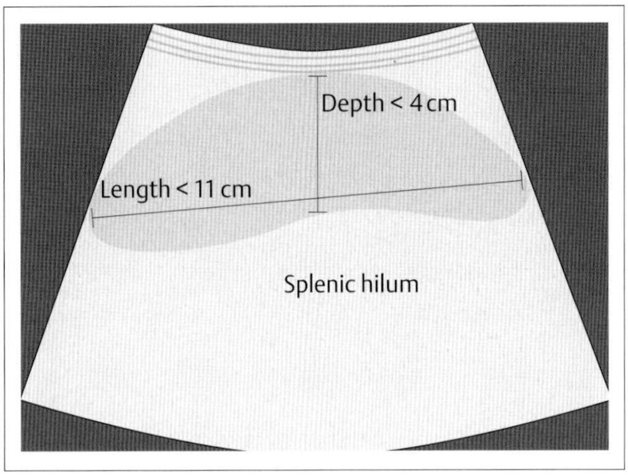

Fig. 7.**58 a** Schematic drawing of the reference lines for determining splenic size in intercostal views (depth and length).
Length = largest cephalocaudal diameter
Depth = splenic hilum–lateral surface.

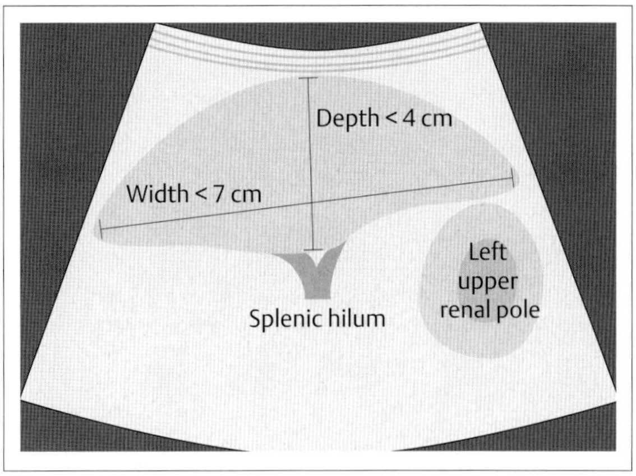

Fig. 7.**58 b** Schematic drawing of the splenic width, not mandatory in clinical routine, transverse view of the spleen.

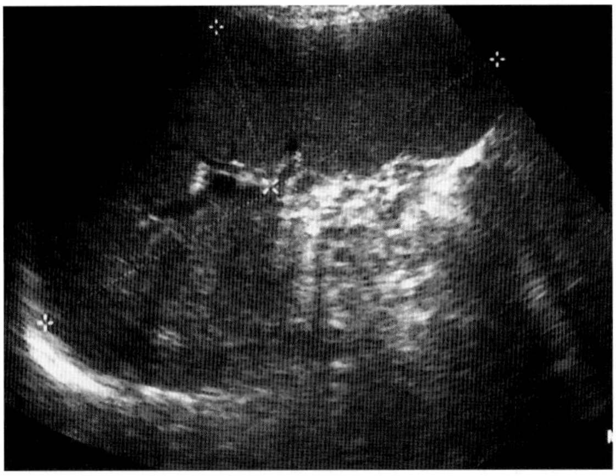

Fig. 7.**59 a** Splenomegaly secondary to portal hypertension (liver cirrhosis), homogeneous spleen, length 16.8 cm and depth 5.2 cm; intrasplenic vessels are well visualized due to venous congestion.

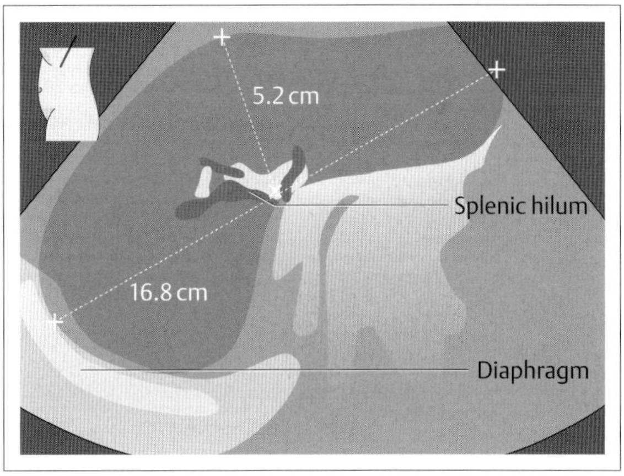

Fig. 7.**59 b** Line drawing.

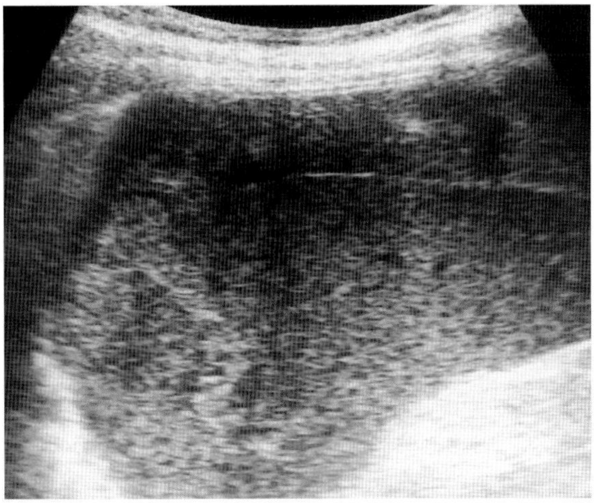

Fig. 7.**60 a** Posttraumatic intraparenchymal lesion of the spleen, hyperechoic to the other parenchyma and heterogeneous at the superior pole.

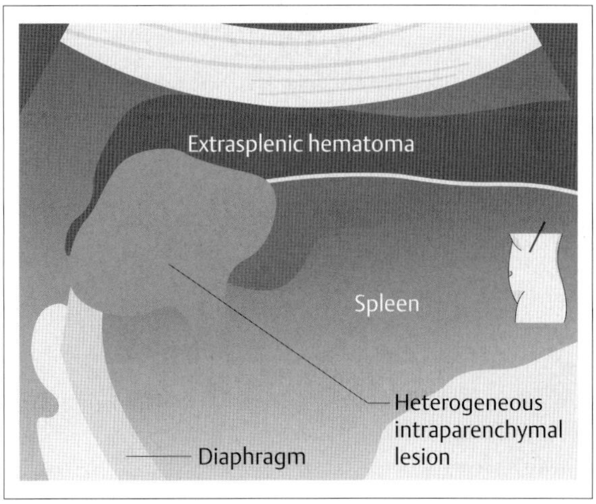

Fig. 7.**60 b** Line drawing.

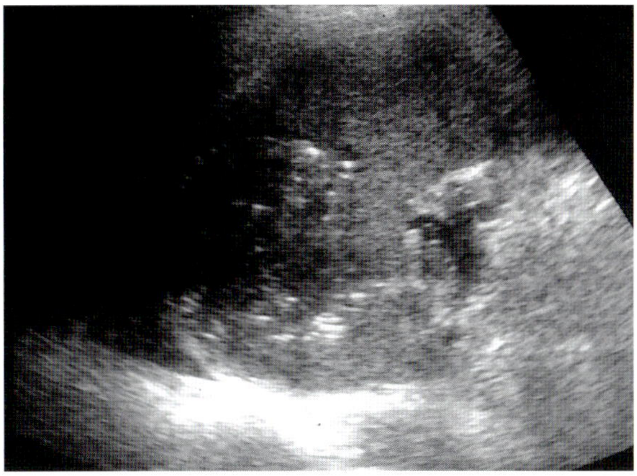

Fig. 7.**61 a** Splenic abscess after liver transplantation and immunosuppression. Heterogeneous focus with gas inclusions and rim.

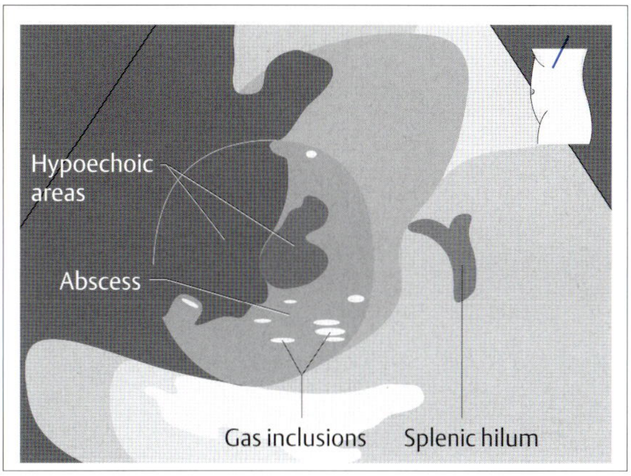

Fig. 7.**61 b** Line drawing.

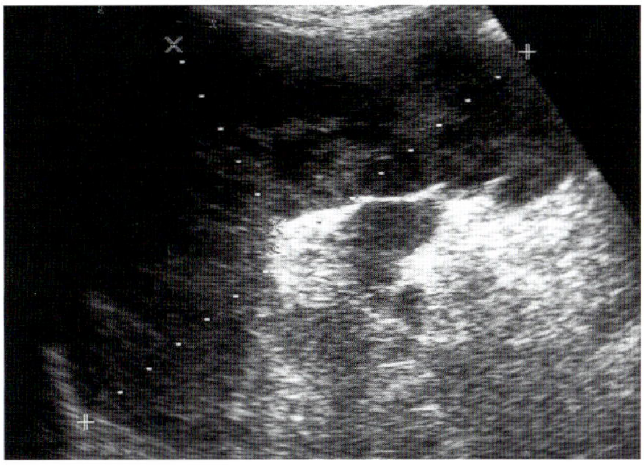

Fig. 7.**62 a** Splenic involvement in high-grade non-Hodgkin lymphoma with splenomegaly and hypoechoic masses within the parenchyma.

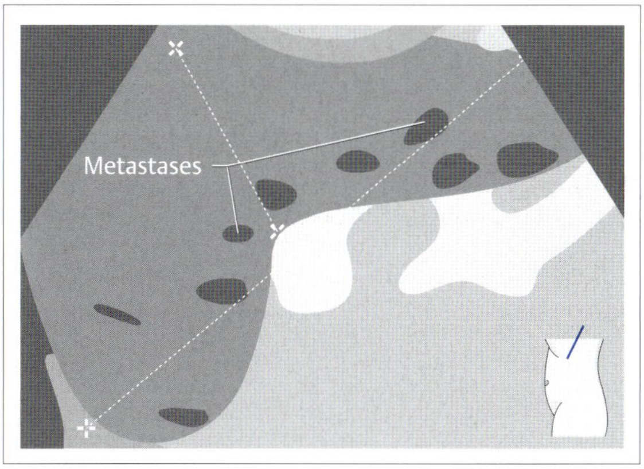

Fig. 7.**62 b** Line drawing.

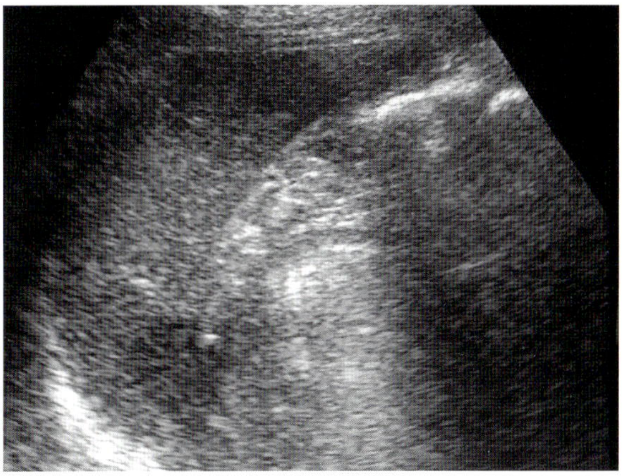

Fig. 7.**63 a** Hypoechoic splenic metastasis of anal carcinoma; diameter 1.5 cm.

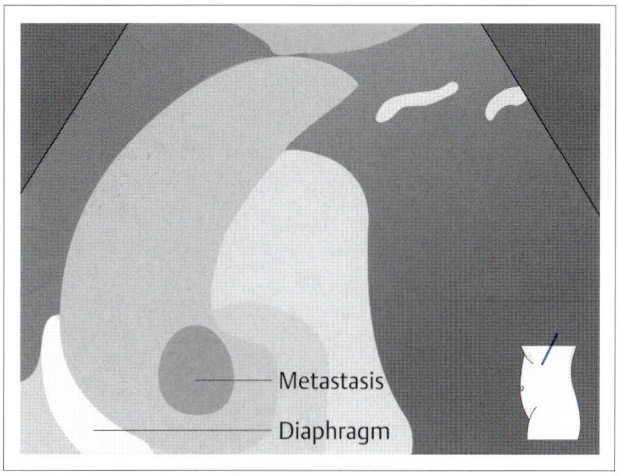

Fig. 7.**63 b** Line drawing.

Consequences for Surgical Treatment

Diagnosis	Characteristic Findings	Management
Splenomegaly	No hypersplenism (e.g., cirrhosis of the liver, right ventricular failure, infections)	Treatment of underlying disease
Splenomegaly	With hypersplenism (e.g., primary hypersplenism, hereditary spherocytosis, thalassemia major, warm autoantibodies, idiopathic/autoimmune thrombocytopenic), status after unsuccessful nonsurgical management	Laparoscopic (normal size or slightly enlarged) or open splenectomy
Splenic cyst	Parasitic (hydatid disease)	Splenectomy
Splenic cyst	No suspected tumor, no symptoms; not parasitic	Follow-up
Splenic tumor	Primary tumor or metastasis suspected, equivocal tumor without systemic disease	Histological confirmation via splenectomy; in selected cases FNA
Splenic tumor	As part of systemic lypmphatic disease	Specific lymphoma treatment, possibly splenectomy as part of staging laparotomy (controversial)
Splenic abscess	Manifestation with signs and symptoms characteristic of abscess	Splenectomy or possibly drainage

Biliary System

Indications for Sonography

- Sonography is the imaging modality of choice when there is clinical suspicion of biliary disease, particularly in cases with right upper quadrant pain and in jaundice.
- Sensitivity and specificity for gallstones are very high (Neubrand et al., 2000), so that nowadays in symptomatic gallstone disease sonography suffices as imaging modality prior to cholecystectomy.
- In obstructive jaundice, sonography is one diagnostic element complementing the various modes of cholangiography.
- Sonography also plays a role in screening of patients with an increased risk for malignancy, e.g., gallbladder cancer in long-standing cholecystolithiasis, or cholangiocarcinoma in primary sclerosing cholangitis or Caroli disease.

Specific Technique and Diagnostic Evaluation

- **Gallbladder**
  - 3.5 MHz probes are preferred, with higher-frequency transducers (5 or 7.5 MHz) for those parts of the gallbladder close to the abdominal wall.
  - As in the liver, the gallbladder is accessed by intercostal and subcostal scanning.
  - The gallbladder is contained in a fossa on the inferior surface of the liver as an extension of the interlobular fissure; the latter can be visualized as a narrow hyperechoic band between the liver segments IV and V (see Fig. 7.**30 d**).
  - Shape: piriform sac with fundus, body, and neck (synonym: infundibulum).
  - The normal gallbladder does not exceed 10 cm in length and 4 cm in width; larger sizes (particularly in the longitudinal axis) are without pathological significance in the aging gallbladder and after prolonged fasting.
  - Anechoic lumen except for artifacts characteristic of fluid collections (Fig. 7.**64**; Chapter 6, Technical Principles)
  - In the fasting patient, maximum wall thickness of the gallbladder is 3 mm; at high resolution, triple layering is clearly recognizable: hyperechoic – hypoechoic – hyperechoic. The inner and outer hyperechoic layers primarily correspond to entrance and exit echoes, i.e., they do not correlate with a defined anatomical layer (Weiss et al., 1993; see Gastrointestinal Tract, this chapter). After oral uptake of food, the gallbladder contracts, thus reducing the lumen and increasing the wall thickness in favor of the hypoechoic middle layer (primarily corresponding to smooth muscle).

- The gallbladder is often "folded over": at the fundus this is known as a Phrygian cap, or this kinking may be at the infundibulum (Fig. 7.**68**). Sonographically, this mimics an intraluminal septum but disappears with change of position. True septa or diverticula are rare.
- Anomalous position or orientation of the gallbladder can usually be detected by sonography:
  - Congenital: ectopy, e.g., intrahepatic site or in/at the left hepatic lobe.
  - Acquired: atypical position is possible due to fibrous adhesions after cholecystitis, e.g., at the anterior surface of the liver (Naganuma et al., 1998).
- Congenital anomalies: agenesis, duplication, septation.
- The gallbladder may be confused with walled-off intraperitoneal fluid collections, bowel loops, hepatic cysts, or other hepatic masses.

- **Biliary tree**
  - 3.5 MHz probes are preferred, with higher-frequency transducers (5 MHz) for slim patients.
  - Access to the intrahepatic and proximal extrahepatic biliary tree is via intercostal and subcostal views, as for the liver; for the distal extrahepatic biliary tree the probe is positioned in the epigastrium.
  - With a 3.5 MHz transducer the main trunks of the right and left hepatic ducts of the intrahepatic biliary tree can be visualized; further peripheral tributaries can only be delineated with higher-frequency transducers or when dilated. The intrahepatic bile ducts parallel the branches of the portal vein. Maximum normal diameter of the intrahepatic biliary tree is no more than 50% of the diameter of the portal vein. Dilatation of intrahepatic bile ducts results in the "double-barrel shotgun" sign, where a second tubular structure parallels the intrahepatic portal vein branches (Fig. 7.**70**). This double-barrel shotgun sign may also be seen in the peripheral portal vein branches due to dilated hepatic arteries, e.g., in arteriosclerosis and/or arterial hypertension. Bile ducts and arteries can be differentiated by following the tubular structures into the hepatic hilum and, more reliably, by duplex Doppler sonography.
  - The parts of the extrahepatic biliary tree that can be delineated by sonography are the CHD and CBD. Usually, the junction of the cystic duct cannot be identified because of its small caliber and tortuous and variable course. Since there is no clear-cut sonographic distinction between the CHD and the CBD, the working term "common duct" is increasingly being used in sonographers' circles. Initially, it runs with the portal vein (see Liver in this chapter) and often is the most anterior tubular structure in the hepatoduodenal ligament, where it may be mistaken for the hepatic artery, although origin at the celiac trunk and pulsations betray the nature of the artery. The arteries take quite a variable course. Frequently demonstrated is the left branch of the hepatic artery at the hepatic hilum where the common duct and portal vein cross (Fig. 7.**71**).
  - Posterior to the descending part of the duodenum, the CBD is frequently masked by bowel gas. The distal third of the CBD traverses the head of the pancreas posteriorly at the right lateral margin of this organ to end at the duodenal papilla (Fig. 7.**66**). Here, the course of the CBD parallels the longitudinal axis. The interfering bowel gas may be shifted by graded compression with the probe or by change in patient position. The pancreas itself serves as the echo window for the intrapancreatic part of the CBD.
  - Maximum diameter of the normal common duct is 6 mm (Niederau et al., 1984; Parulekar 1979). However, as this is age dependent (Wu et al., 1984); above 60 years the maximum diameter in millimeters corresponds to the number of decades of life (up to 70 years 7 mm, up to 80 years 8 mm, and so on); the maximum normal diameter post cholecystectomy is 10 mm. Sonographic normal values are lower than radiological ones, probably because of bile duct dilatation due to application of contrast medium and/or to magnification on radiographs. The common duct is widest in its middle third. Since this segment is frequently masked by bowel gas and studies determining the standard diameter have measured close to the hepatic hilum, values exceeding these normal values by just a few millimeters are likely to be of no pathological significance (Bowie, 2000). Especially when viewing this middle third, care also needs to be taken not to measure cystic and common duct conjointly, as the two frequently run in parallel for a stretch, the former usually posterior to the latter.

Gallstones

Basic Facts

- Gallbladder stones
  - Prevalence in the western world is 6–10%; female preponderance is 2 : 1. There is a positive correlation with age, body mass index, and family history (Kratzer et al., 1998).
  - Composition: 80% pure cholesterol or mixed stones with > 70% cholesterol content, 20% pigment stones > 80% of which consist of calcium bilirubinate.
- Gallbladder "sludge," frequently associated with gallbladder stones, may precede stone formation; sludge is mostly reversible, consists of mucinous matter and microcrystals, and is favored by hypomotility of the gallbladder and altered bile composition: during long fasting, e.g., after abdominal surgery, in pregnancy, liver cirrhosis, etc. (Boland et al., 2000; Chintapalli et al., 1999; Naganuma et al., 1998; Van Bodegraven et al., 1998; Wilkinson et al., 1996). Even in the absence of stones, sludge

is one potential cause of biliary pancreatitis (Lee et al., 1992).

- Lifetime incidence of symptomatic gallstone disease: around 30% of gallstone carriers, out of whom 10% present with complications, e.g., cholecystitis, cholangitis, or acute pancreatitis. The annual complication rate is 0.1–0.2% in asymptomatic gallstone carriers, rising to 1–2% after the first biliary colic (Neubrand et al., 2000).
- The slightly higher risk of gallbladder carcinoma in asymptomatic gallstone carriers does not justify preventive cholecystectomy. This is, however, indicated in the presence of gallstones > 3 cm, for gallbladder polyps > 1 cm, and for porcelain gallbladders, as these are associated with a significantly higher risk of cancer (Neubrand et al., 2000).
- Symptomatic cholelithiasis (based on a maximum normal diameter of 6 mm for the common duct) plus dilated bile ducts raises the probability of intraductal bile stones to 40% (Majeed et al., 1999). Therefore, whenever dilated bile ducts are encountered before planned cholecystectomy, additional cholangiographic imaging modalities should be performed: primarily ERCP, and if this is not possible, then MRCP, PTC, EUS and/or intraoperative cholangiography. EUS has a diagnostic quality index of > 90% for extrahepatic cholangiolithiasis (Aubertin et al., 1996). Bile duct imaging before cholecystectomy must also be considered if there is clinical evidence of cholangitis and if transaminase or bilirubin levels exceed 200% of the upper normal limit (Alponat et al., 1997).
- *Additional workup:* ERCP, spot film of gallbladder (looking for calcified stones or pneumobilia), MRCP, PTC, EUS, intraoperative cholangiography.

Sonographic Criteria

- **Gallbladder stone:** Bright, usually hemispherical echo with posterior shadowing and mobile intraluminal position.
- Acoustic shadowing depends on stone size, transmission frequency, and position of the calculus in relation to the focal zone (with 3.5 MHz, posterior shadowing is usually encountered in stones ≥ 2 mm; higher frequencies are desirable as long as the depth of penetration remains sufficient (see Chapter 6, Technical Principles). Possibility of error: Differentiate posterior shadowing from the edge shadowing artifact at the edge of the gallbladder (Fig. 7.**64**).
- Testing for change in position helps differentiate stones from **gallbladder polyps**. Calculi adhere to the wall only in case of encrustation or impaction in the neck. Otherwise they mainly sediment, though cholesterol stones may float (rarely).
- With the patient supine, gallstones are difficult to differentiate from Heister valves in the neck of the gallbladder (Fig. 7.**64**) or in the cystic duct; therefore, the patient should always be examined in left lateral decubitus position as well and while standing or sitting, if possible.
- Small stones impacted in the infundibulum or cystic duct are easily overlooked, but frequently result in **hydrops of the gallbladder** (see Chapter 1, p. 5, Acute Cholecystitis).
- Gallstones, which do not reflect the ultrasound waves completely but transmit part of them, demonstrate an internal echotexture (mainly cholesterol stones, Fig. 7.**65**). Differentiation of gallstone consistency based on sonographic reflection is not accurate enough, and in terms of treatment may just suffice for lithotripsy.
- If the gallbladder is filled completely with multiple stones or cast with one large stone, no gallbladder lumen can be outlined. Difficult differential diagnoses: stone-filled gallbladder versus **porcelain gallbladder** (see below) versus air in the gallbladder ("pneumobilia"). In all three conditions a sickle-shaped bright echo with posterior shadowing is seen, corresponding in shape and location to the gallbladder. Air in the gallbladder may be clinically associated with evidence of **gallstone penetration** into the GI tract with corresponding symptoms (see gallstone ileus, Chapter 1, p. 14, Mechanical Bowel Obstruction and Paralytic Ileus). Since porcelain gallbladder and stone-filled gallbladder often occur together, the former can be reliably ruled out only if the gallbladder wall can be well differentiated from the stones. In unclear cases, a spot film of the gallbladder will demonstrate mural calcification when porcelain gallbladder is present.
- **Gallbladder sludge:** Fine cloudy echoes in the bile without posterior shadowing (Fig. 7.**65**), usually shifting their position on compression or change in the patient's position; sometimes rather viscous consistency and adhering to the wall, in which case they can hardly be distinguished from polyps. Additional differential diagnoses: pus (Chapter 1, p. 5, Acute Cholecystitis), blood (hemobilia), milk calcium/limy bile or mucocele of the gallbladder in long-standing hydropic gallbladder, pneumobilia. In finely dispersed pneumobilia (e.g., after papillotomy) very bright reflections with comet-tail artifacts are seen, in marked pneumobilia posterior shadowing is seen as well.

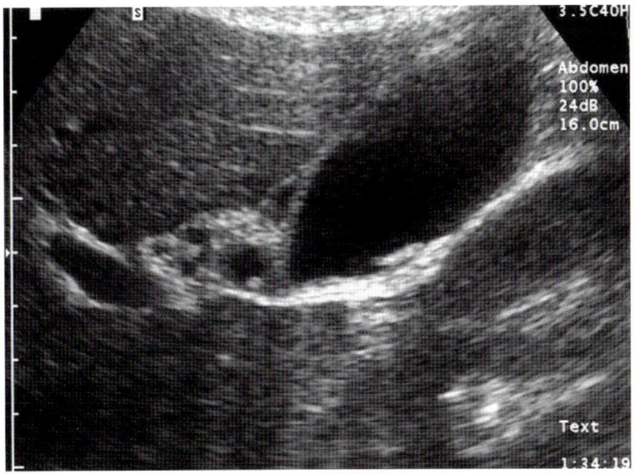

Fig. 7.**64a** Gallbladder stones in acute biliary colic. Bulging gallbladder with several small (diameter 2–3 mm) gallstones and one small calculus (3 mm) in the infundibulum. Gallbladder artifacts: electronic noise near the probe, acoustic shadowing posterior to the gallbladder, edge shadowing. Gallstone artifacts: posterior acoustic shadowing, faint because of the small size.

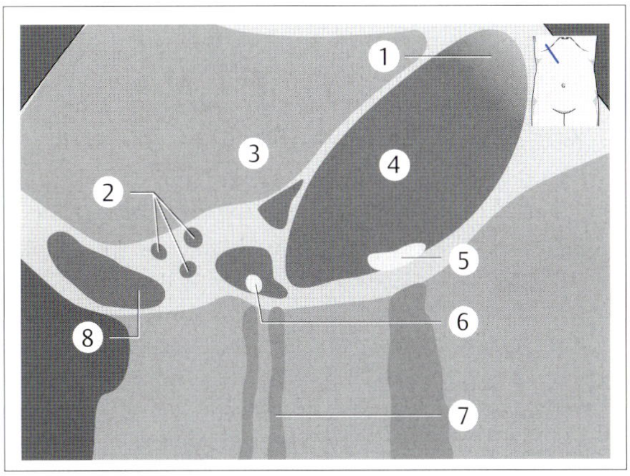

Fig. 7.**64b** Line drawing. 1 Electronic noise. 2 Cross-sectional view of vessels and cystic duct. 3 Liver. 4 Gallbladder lumen. 5 Stone with posterior shadowing. 6 Stone in neck with posterior shadowing. 7 Edge shadowing. 8 Portal vein.

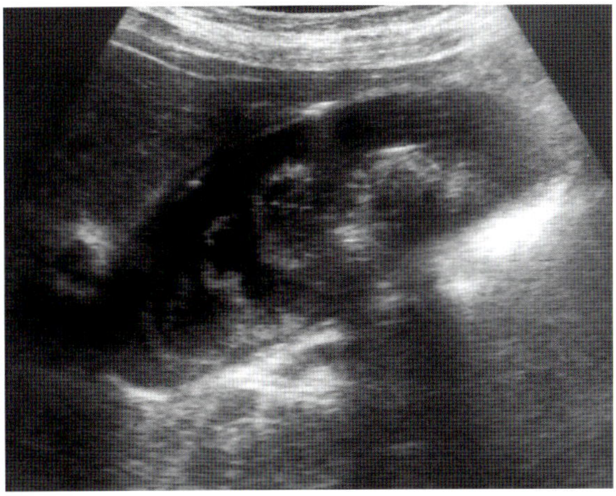

Fig. 7.**65a** Acute-on-chronic cholecystitis with cholesterol stones, incipient porcelain gallbladder. Bulging tender gallbladder. The gallstones are sonolucent but exhibit posterior shadowing; in addition there is sludge without shadowing. Slightly thickened triple layered wall, sporadic mural calcifications, some with comet-tail artifacts.

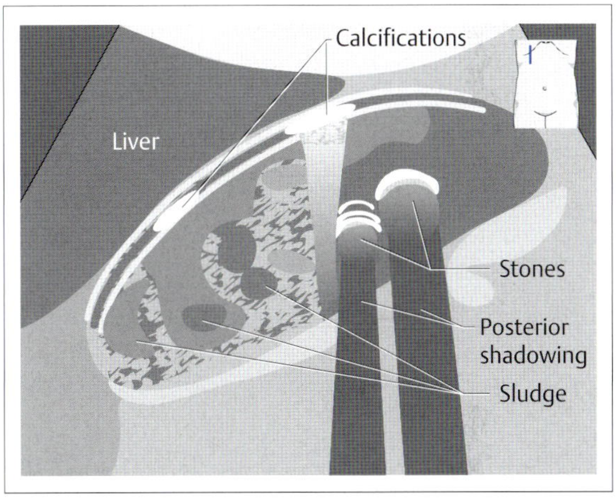

Fig. 7.**65b** Line drawing.

Consequences for Surgical Treatment

Diagnosis	Characteristic Findings	Management
Symptomatic gallbladder stones	Gallstone(s) or sludge with typical biliary colic or other complications (acute cholecystitis, biliary pancreatitis)	Laparoscopic cholecystectomy
Asymptomatic gallbladder stones with risk of carcinoma	Sonographic evidence of gallstones with porcelain gallbladder or gallstone carrier with stone > 3 cm, or polyp > 1 cm	Preventive cholecystectomy: when carcinoma is suspected, open surgery!

Bile Duct Stones

Basic Facts

- Pathogenesis of bile duct stones:
  - In most cases migration of small stones from the gallbladder (mainly cholesterol stones) into the bile ducts; 10% of cholecystolithiasis is associated with bile duct stones as well.
  - Intraductal stone formation is less common (primarily pigmented stones); often seen in bile duct obstruction, e.g., Caroli disease, bile duct cyst, ductal stenosis.
- Frequently encountered in the common duct, rarely within the liver (e.g., Caroli disease).
- More than half of the bile duct stones are symptomatic and often present with complications: obstructive jaundice, cholangitis, acute pancreatitis.
- Sonographic sensitivity is only 50%, while specificity is 90%.
- Gas in the bile ducts ("pneumobilia") strongly impairs visualization of bile duct stones. Causes of pneumobilia: common following bile duct intervention (papillotomy, choledochojejunostomy), rare in acute cholangitis with gas-forming bacteria.

Sonographic Criteria

- **Cholangiolithiasis**: intraductal echo characteristic of gallstones, frequently accompanied by dilated bile ducts. Calculi are commonly localized in the prepapillary area (Fig. 7.**66**); in supine position, ductal stones sometimes gravitate to the hepatic hilum. Sensitivity is limited mainly by gas in the duodenum. False-positive results are possible, in particular misinterpretation of the hepatic artery or duodenal gas as a prepapillary stone (Fig. 7.**71**).
- **Ductal pneumobilia:** Band-shaped, very intense echoes with comet-tail artifacts and posterior shadowing. Collection is contrary to gravity; for example, when the patient is supine, collection will be in the anterior segments of the intrahepatic bile ducts. In small bile ducts, the echoes are arranged like a string of beads, corresponding to a chain of gas bubbles (Chapter 6, p. 102, Artifacts).
- Both sensitivity and specificity of bile duct stone detection suffer greatly from pneumobilia, since the bright gas reflections mimic stone echoes or mask calculi by posterior shadowing.

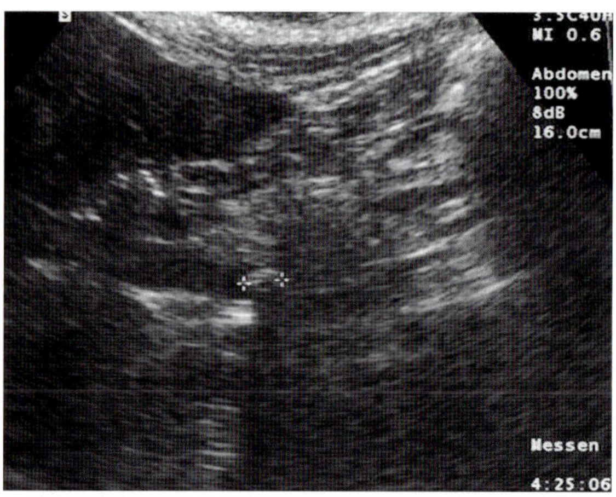

Fig. 7.**66 a** Cholangiolithiasis of the common duct with mechanical cholestasis. The common duct is distended to 10 mm, ductal stone (10 mm) posterior to the pancreatic head with distal acoustic shadowing.

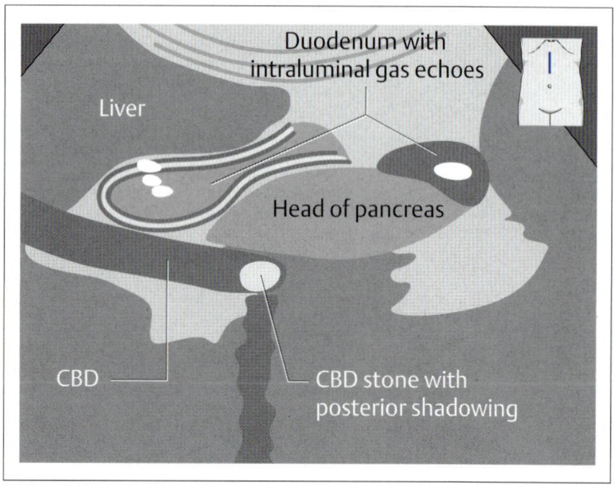

Fig. 7.**66 b** Line drawing. CBD = Common bile duct

Consequences for Surgical Treatment

Diagnosis	Characteristic Findings	Management
Ductal stones post cholecystectomy	On US, dilated bile ducts and/or evidence of bile duct stones (bright intraluminal echoes with posterior shadowing), confirmed by cholangiography (e.g., ERCP)	Endoscopic papillotomy with stone extraction Alternatives: temporary endoscopic drainage plus ESWL or percutaneous intervention If unsuccessful, surgical bile duct exploration
Ductal stones in cholecystolithiasis	Sonographic evidence of gallbladder and ductal stones, confirmed by cholangiography	Endoscopic papillotomy with stone extraction before surgery If unsuccessful, surgical bile duct exploration and cholecystectomy

Cholangitis

Basic Facts

- Acute purulent cholangitis:
  - Bacterial infection of the bile ducts with a high risk of septicemia and high mortality; it is usually a sequela of mechanical cholestasis and/or an abnormal bilioenteric communication via spontaneous fistula formation, or following previous bile duct intervention, e.g., papillotomy or choledochojejunostomy.
- Differential diagnosis of mechanical bile duct obstruction: See Bile Duct Tumors, below
- Secondary chronic cholangitis due to persistent bacterial infection and mechanical cholestasis leads to destruction and fibrotic ductal stenosis, ending in biliary cirrhosis of the liver.
- Primary sclerosing cholangitis: chronic autoimmune cholangitis with multiple stenoses, particularly of the intrahepatic but also extrahepatic biliary tree. Complications: cirrhosis of the liver, cholangiocellular carcinoma.

Sonographic Criteria

- **Acute cholangitis:** No specific sonographic signs, apart from rare pneumobilia by gas-forming bacteria. The combination of clinical signs (Charcot's triad) and sonographic demonstration of predisposing conditions (cholangiolithiasis, ductal dilatation, bile duct tumor, pneumobilia signifying a pathological bilioenteric communication) suggests the diagnosis.
- **In chronic cholangitis** there is an increase in hyperechoic structures around the intrahepatic bile ducts and, due to stenosis, various segments of the bile ducts may become dilated.

- *Additional workup:* ERCP or other cholangiographic modality, possibly CT and liver biopsy.

Consequences for Surgical Treatment

Diagnosis	Characteristic Findings	Management
Acute purulent cholangitis	Right upper quadrant pain, fever, jaundice: possibly dilated bile ducts and/or pneumobilia on US	Endoscopic papillotomy with elimination of the obstruction, endoscopic drainage, antibiotics. Surgical intervention, if possible, after inflammation has subsided

Chronic Cholecystitis

Basic Facts

- Recurrent cholecystitis, even if unnoticed, leads to mucosal atrophy and fibrosis of the gallbladder wall. However, fibrosis does not always result in thickening of the gallbladder wall and shrinkage.
- Complications of chronic cholecystitis:
  - Acute episodes
  - Mirizzi syndrome
  - Bilioenteric fistula, possibly gallstone ileus (see Chapter 1, p. 14, Mechanical Bowel Obstruction and Paralytic Ileus)
- Mural calcifications lead to "porcelain gallbladder," usually an asymptomatic variant of chronic cholecystitis. Porcelain gallbladder is a precancerous condition: 10–30% of patients develop gallbladder carcinoma (Ashur et al., 1978; Sheth et al., 2000; Shimizu et al., 1989).
- *Additional workup:* spot film of the gallbladder, ERCP, possibly MRCP, PTC, EUS, CT.

Sonographic Criteria

- **Chronic cholecystitis**
  - Hyperechoic wall with loss of triple layering; possibly gallbladder shrinkage, i.e., small gallbladder even when fasting. Possible gallbladder wall thickening with hyperechoic texture (Fig. 7.**67**).
  - Mirizzi syndrome: intrahepatic biliary tree and CHD dilated up to the level of the gallbladder. Obstruction of the CHD by scarring or compression due to a calculus in the gallbladder.
- **Porcelain gallbladder:** loss of the physiological triple layering of the gallbladder wall. Strong small echoes in the wall, some with posterior shadowing or comet-tail artifacts (Fig. 7.**65**) (Kane et al., 1984). (Differential diagnosis Table 7.**8**.)

Table 7.**8** Differential diagnosis of bright echoes in or along the gallbladder wall with posterior shadowing and comet-tail artifact

Causes	Sonographic Criteria
Pneumobilia of gallbladder	Intraluminal echoes, collecting contrary to gravity
Cholesterolosis	Polypoid echoes adhering to the wall and protruding into the lumen
Encrusted gallbladder stone	Usually in the neck of the gallbladder and with signs of chronic cholecystitis
Porcelain gallbladder	Together with gallbladder stones, echoes in a fibrosed wall
Emphysematous cholecystitis	Intraluminal echoes, collecting contrary to gravity; signs of acute cholecystitis
Adenomyomatosis	Numerous diverticulum-like eventrations in the thickened wall, some filled with cholesterol calculi

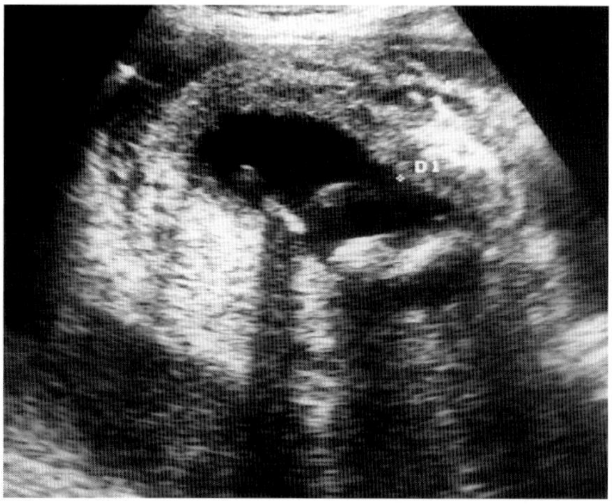

Fig. 7.**67a** Acute-on-chronic cholecystitis in cholecystolithiasis. Massive thickening (up to 20 mm) of the gallbladder wall, primarily hyperechoic; loss of wall layering. The hypoechoic regions in the wall are due to acute inflammatory edema. The gallbladder is partly encased by hyperechoic, i.e., inflamed, fatty tissue. Several calculi are visible within the reduced gallbladder lumen.

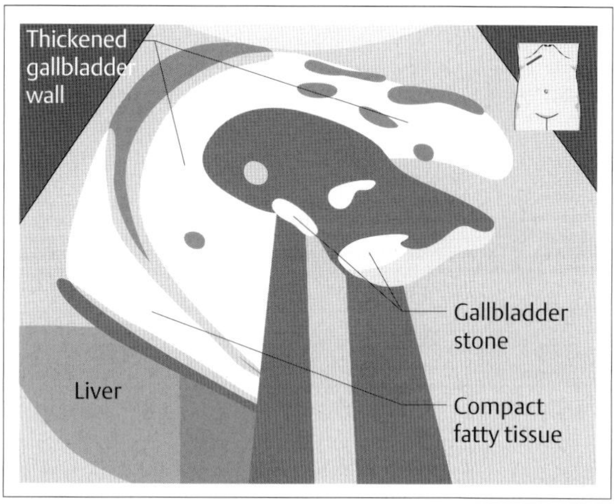

Fig. 7.**67b** Line drawing.

Consequences for Surgical Treatment

Diagnosis	Characteristic Findings	Management
Symptomatic chronic cholecystitis	Recurrent right upper quadrant pain; hyperechoic gallbladder wall with loss of triple layering	Laparoscopic cholecystectomy
Porcelain gallbladder	Calcification echoes in the gallbladder wall with posterior shadowing and comet-tail artifacts; calcifications on abdominal film	Open cholecystectomy (precancerous!)

Gallbladder Polyps, Cholesterolosis, Gallbladder Tumors

Basic Facts

- Of the gallbladder polyps visualized with ultrasound, 95% are cholesterol polyps (Heyder et al., 1990); they develop in the same way as diffuse cholesterolosis by cholesterol ester deposits in macrophages. Other polyps include adenomas, malignant tumors, adenomyomatosis, chronic cholecystitis; 90% of the malignant tumors are adenocarcinomas.
- Only one-quarter of these arise as polypoid lesions, the others exhibiting diffuse invasive growth from the onset. Risk constellation for cancer: broad-based polyp, size > 10 mm, patient older than 60 years, co-occurrence with cholelithiasis (Mainprize et al., 2000; Terzi et al., 2000).
- Malignant tumors of the gallbladder have few symptoms; thus, they tend to be detected only at the more advanced stages.
- TAUS staging of gallbladder carcinoma proves sufficiently accurate for size and hepatic invasion, but frequently "understages" peritoneal dissemination and lymph node metastases (Pandey et al., 2000). EUS seems promising for a more accurate diagnostic evaluation of polypoid gallbladder lesions, but has not been validated sufficiently (Fujita et al., 1999; Sugiyama et al., 2000).
- For differential diagnosis of focal gallbladder wall thickening, see Table 7.**9**, and for that of diffuse gallbladder wall thickening, see Acute Cholecystitis, Chapter 1, p. 5).
- Adenomyomatosis: diffuse hyperplasia of the smooth muscles and glands of the gallbladder wall. Dilated Rokitansky–Aschoff sinuses containing cholesterol deposits abound in the thickened wall. No malignant transformation, but frequent epigastric pain or discomfort.
- *Additional workup:* CT,, ERCP, EUS, laparoscopy, possibly MRCP, FNA.

Sonographic Criteria

- Typical **cholesterol polyps**: hyperechoic; pediculated (particularly, if size > 5 mm); multiple in 50% of cases; associated with fine granular contour of the gallbladder mucosa corresponding to cholesterolosis (Fig. 7.**68**); cholesterolosis sometimes with comet-tail artifact. Most cholesterol polyps remain constant in size over years, though disappearance or growth is also possible (Heyder et al., 1990).
- **Adenomas or adenocarcinomas** are broad-based in most cases, ill defined against the unaffected gallbladder wall, and usually solitary; they grow steadily in size (Fig. 7.**69**).
- In malignant invasion of the liver, the gallbladder wall is ill defined from the liver and there is usually hypoechoic invasion (Fig. 7.**69**). Lymphatic spread first arises in the hepatoduodenal ligament and celiac trunk.
- Differential diagnosis of **adenomyomatosis**: irregular wall thickening with small cystic structures resembling diverticula. Cholesterol deposits with echoes as in cholesterolosis or mural calcifications (Table 7.**9**). Diagnosis may be confirmed by contrast-enhanced radiography of the gallbladder (Hwang et al., 1998).

Table 7.**9** Differential diagnosis of focal gallbladder wall thickening

Gallbladder polyp, e.g., cholesterol polyp or adenoma
Gallbladder carcinoma, rarely metastases, lymphoma, or other neoplasm
Adenomyomatosis
Acute cholecystitis or chronic cholecystitis with intramural abscess formation
Gallbladder varices

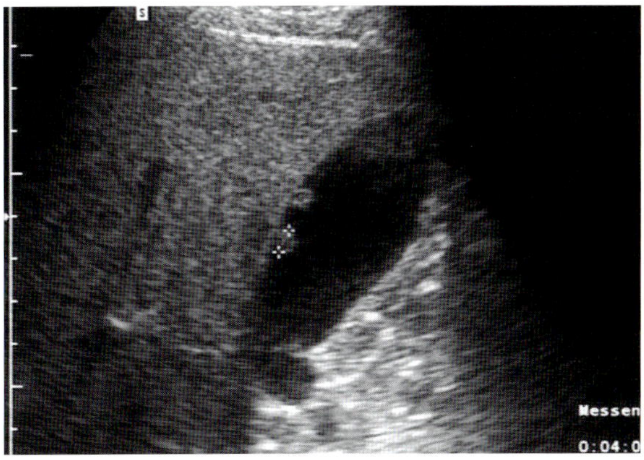

Fig. 7.**68 a** Two cholesterol polyps in the gallbladder: round structures with a maximum diameter of 6 mm, adhering to the wall but not deforming it. Kinking of the gallbladder infundibulum. Incidental finding: fatty liver with hyperechoic texture and characteristic focal sparing around the gallbladder.

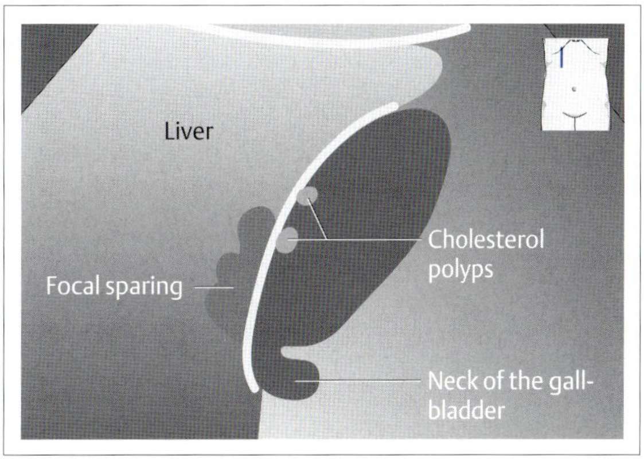

Fig. 7.**68 b** Line drawing.

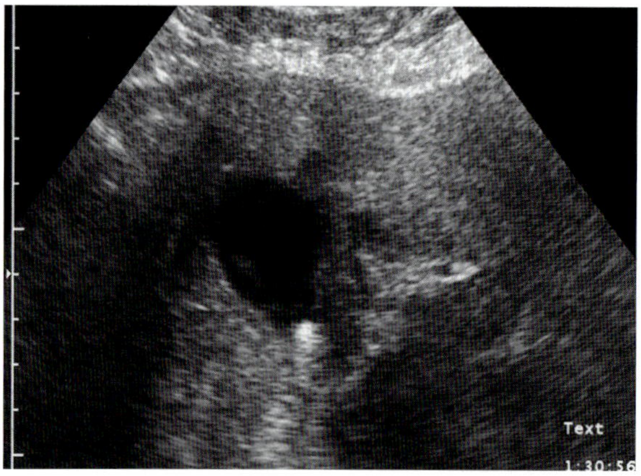

Fig. 7.**69 a** Carcinoma of the gallbladder invading the liver. Hypoechoic tumor of the gallbladder with mural destruction and invasion into the hepatic parenchyma. Gallstone impacted in the tumor.

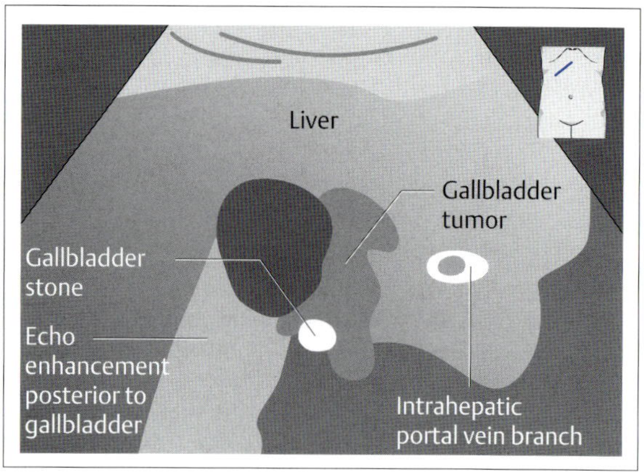

Fig. 7.**69 b** Line drawing.

Consequences for Surgical Treatment

Diagnosis	Characteristic Findings	Management
Cholesterol polyp	Hyperechoic texture, pediculated, < 5 mm; possibly multiple	Annual sonographic follow-up
Equivocal polyp, not classifiable	Broad-based, but clearly delineated to the gallbladder wall Size: 5–10 cm	Sonography every 3 months, cholecystectomy if growing
Polyp suspicious for adenoma or carcinoma	Size > 10 mm or ill-defined gallbladder wall	Open cholecystectomy
Gallbladder carcinoma amenable to resection	No sign of distant spread or invasion of hepatic artery and portal vein	En-bloc resection of gallbladder and liver segment V; lymphadenectomy
Gallbladder carcinoma not amenable to resection	Distant spread, invasion of the hepatoduodenal ligament	Possibly palliative irradiation or chemotherapy under study protocols. Endoscopic drainage

Bile Duct Tumors, Differential Diagnosis of Bile Duct Obstruction

Basic Facts

- Bile duct tumors are almost always carcinomas of poor prognosis, very rarely benign or mesenchymal tumors.
- Classification according to site:
  - Proximal bile duct tumors (hepatic duct bifurcation, Klatskin's tumor)
  - Tumors of the middle third (CBD)
  - Tumors of the distal third (retroduodenal and intrapancreatic CBD)
- Tumors of the papilla are frequently adenomas, but 60% are associated with adenocarcinomas. More favorable prognosis than in cholangiocellular carcinoma.
- Tumors at the hepatic hilum, of the extrahepatic bile ducts, and at the papilla almost always manifest with obstructive jaundice. This usually signifies advanced stages; incidental finding is very rare and mainly restricted to intrahepatic forms. Diagnosis is possible at an earlier stage by regular tumor screening in patients with risk factors for cholangiocellular carcinomas:
  - Primary sclerosing cholangitis
  - Caroli disease
  - Bile duct cysts
  - Familial polyposis
  - Infections with *Clonorchis sinensis* (a parasite prevalent in Asia)
- Comparably to CT, sonography can detect the level of obstruction in around 90% and its cause in about 70% of cases (Busse et al., 1993). ERCP or other cholangiographic

modalities are necessary for further clarification. For differential diagnosis of bile duct obstruction, see Table 7.**10**.

- Histopathological diagnosis is possible on biopsy or brush cytology samples collected via ERCP or FNA.
- TAUS does not suffice for staging; intraluminal (Wagner et al., 1995) and intraoperative (Bezzi et al., 1998) sonography have been added on a trial basis.
- *Additional workup:* ERCP or other cholangiographic modality, CT, biopsy or brush cytology on ERCP, FNA biopsies.

Table 7.**10** Causes of bile duct obstruction

Bile duct stones
Pancreatic neoplasm, frequently carcinoma, rarely adenoma
Bile duct tumor (most often cholangiocarcinoma)
Tumors of the duodenal papilla–adenoma and/or carcinoma
Lymph node compression or invasion, primarily malignant lymphadenopathy in the hepatoduodenal ligament or along the pancreas
Pancreatitis with CBD compression by edema or pseudocyst or by fibrotic tubular stenosis of the CBD
Fibrous stenosis after bile duct intervention
Parasites, e.g., ascaris or clonorchis, ascending from the GI tract
Congenital duct anomalies

Sonographic Criteria

- The level of **bile duct obstruction** corresponds to the transition between dilatation (Fig. 7.**70**) and normal bile duct caliber.
- Depending on the level of obstruction, the gallbladder is either collapsed or hydropic.
- Compared to the fatty and connective tissue at the hepatic hilum and hepatoduodenal ligament, the echotexture of **cholangiocarcinomas** usually is hypoechoic (Fig. 7.**71**), rarely isoechoic or hyperechoic. Echodensity frequently differs little from that of the hepatic parenchyma, but carcinomas are heterogeneous and some have a hypoechoic rim. Sonography cannot differentiate between intrahepatic bile duct carcinoma and hepatocellular carcinoma (see p. 143). It may destroy the shape and surface of the liver, and displace or invade vessels and adjacent structures.
- In extrahepatic tumors, cholangiocarcinoma may be difficult to differentiate from lymph node metastasis in the hepatoduodenal ligament as well as tumors of the papilla and pancreatic head.

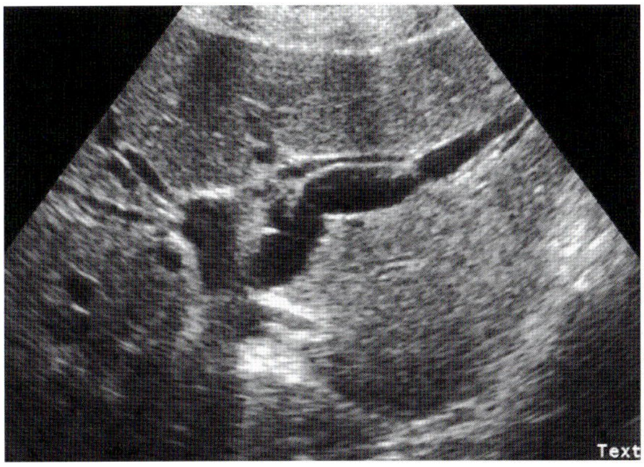

Fig. 7.**70 a** Intrahepatic bile ducts dilated due to ductal tumor at the hepatic hilum (Klatskin's tumor): "double-barrel shotgun" sign. The bile ducts are even wider than the portal vein branches they run with, and the hepatic artery can only be identified by Doppler sonography.

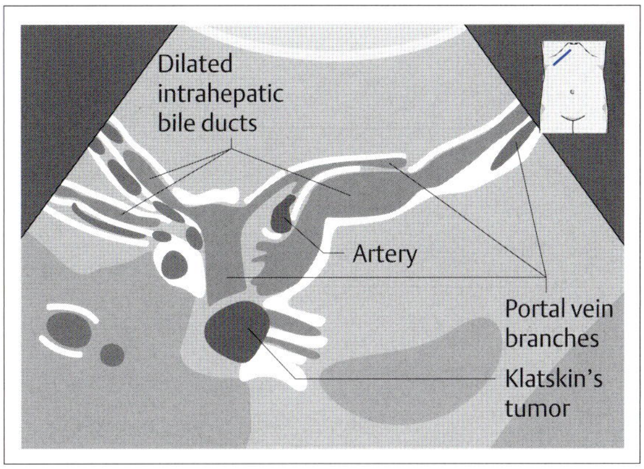

Fig. 7.**70 b** Line drawing.

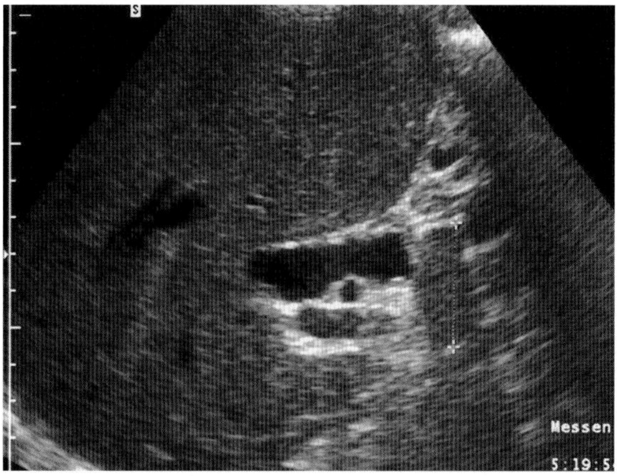

Fig. 7.**71 a** Dilated common duct cut off by obstructing tumor. Bile duct carcinoma (diameter 34 mm).

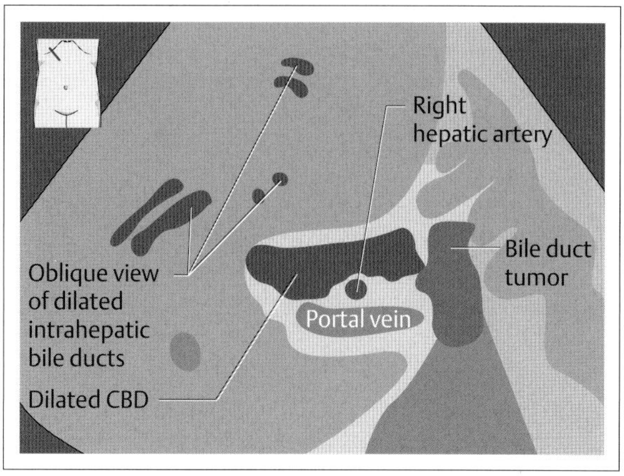

Fig. 7.**71 b** Line drawing.

Consequences for Surgical Treatment

Diagnosis	Characteristic Findings	Management
Tumors of the hepatic duct bifurcation (Klatskin's tumors), type Bismuth I	Tumor of the CHD sparing the bifurcation	Resection of the CHD + CBD, lymphadenectomy, (bi-)hepaticojejunostomy, lymphadenectomy
Tumors of the hepatic duct bifurcation (Klatskin's tumors), type Bismuth II	Tumor affecting the hepatic duct bifurcation but sparing the secondary left and right branches	Resection of CBD + bifurcation, lymphadenectomy, bihepaticojejunostomy, possibly combined with hepatectomy in order to achieve R_0
Tumors of the hepatic duct bifurcation (Klatskin's tumors), type Bismuth III	Tumor extending unilaterally to secondary branches	Hemihepatectomy + caudate lobe + bifurcation + hepatic + CBD, lymphadenectomy, hepaticojejunostomy
Tumors of the hepatic duct bifurcation (Klatskin's tumors), type Bismuth IV	Bilateral involvement of secondary branches, precludes R_0 resection; confirmation often requires exploration	Palliative interventional transtumoral bile drainage, LTX possible in selected cases, possibly palliative irradiation or chemotherapy under study protocols
Bile duct tumor	Middle third–corresponding to CBD	Whipple procedure, lymphadenectomy
Bile duct tumor	Distal third, retroduodenal and intrapancreatic CBD	Whipple procedure, lymphadenectomy

Congenital Anomalies of the Bile Ducts

Basic Facts

The following malformations may occur in isolation or in combination:

- Bile duct atresia or hypoplasia:
  - Usually involves the common duct.
  - Clinical presentation: progressive jaundice after the first weeks of life, pale stools.
  - Hepatic fibrosis/cirrhosis and recurrent cholangitis remain common complications after successful hepatoenteric anastomosis.
- CBD cysts, either as cystic dilatation or as mural diverticula at the intraduodenal segment; frequently associated with a "common channel" of CBD and pancreatic duct (Weishorn and Seitz, 1989; Weyant et al., 1998).
  - Complications: Reflux of pancreatic secretions into the CBD leads to inflammation and possibly fibrotic stenosis of the CBD with cholestasis and cholangitis; this reflux also increases the risk of ductal and gallbladder carcinomas (Misra and Dwivedi, 1990; Sheth et al., 2000). Therefore, even asymptomatic choledochal cysts necessitate regular screening for tumor.
  - Manifestation in different age groups.
- Cystic dilatation of the intrahepatic biliary tree (Caroli disease), frequently with calculi forming in these cystic dilatations. Sometimes combined with congenital hepatic fibrosis. Caroli disease may be limited to individual liver segments.
  - Usually manifests in midlife with cholangitis and/or liver abscess.
  - Long-term complications: secondary biliary cirrhosis, amyloidosis, bile duct carcinoma. Tumor screening is therefore indicated.
- *Additional workup:* ERCP, MRCP, MRI, CT.

Sonographic Criteria

- **Bile duct atresia** or **hypoplasia**: dilated bile duct up to the level of atresia.
- **Choledochal cysts:** Segmental dilatation or diverticular sacculation of the CBD.
- **Caroli disease:** segmental dilatation of the intrahepatic bile ducts: however, primary manifestation is frequently cholangitis. Intrahepatic ductal calculi, which may completely fill the cystic dilatation of the duct (Fig. 7.**72**). Ductal obstruction then adds to further dilatation of the intrahepatic biliary tree.

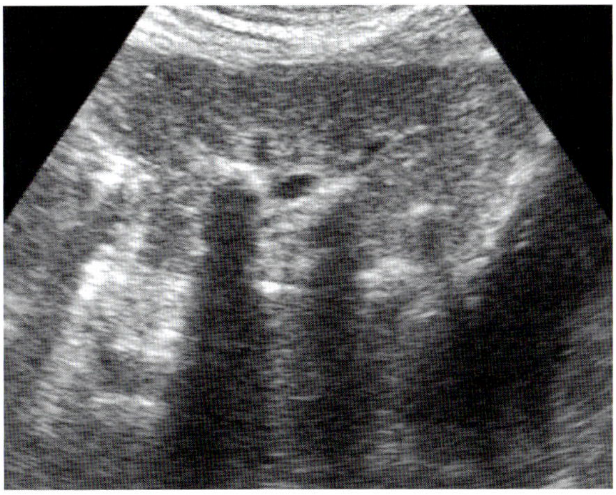

Fig. 7.**72 a** Caroli disease. Several intrahepatic ductal stones with posterior shadowing; cystic dilatation of the bile duct. Also post-papillotomy pneumobilia in some bile ducts and comet-tail artifacts.

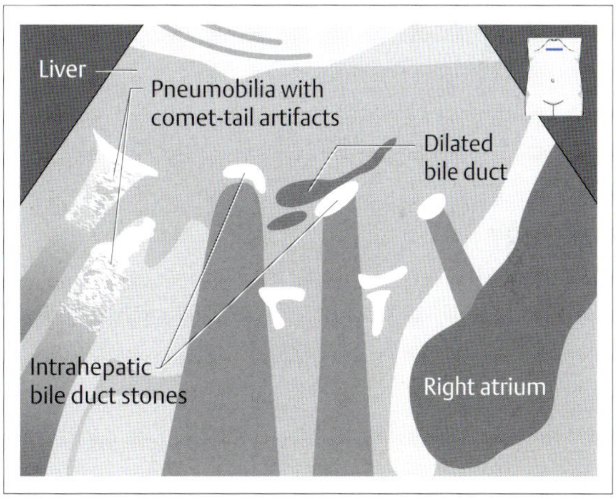

Fig. 7.**72 b** Line drawing.

Consequences for Surgical Treatment

Diagnosis	Characteristic Findings	Management
Bile duct atresia or hypoplasia	Dilated bile ducts in the newborn	Choledochojejunostomy or hepaticojejunostomy
Complicated choledochal cysts	Cystic or diverticular sacculation of the CHD with biliary colic or cholangitis	Resection of the cyst and hepaticojejunostomy
Symptomatic segmental Caroli disease	Cystic dilatation of the intrahepatic bile ducts, often with calculi	Hepatic segmentectomy

Bibliography

Abu-Yousef MM. Normal and respiratory variations of the hepatic and portal venous duplex Doppler waveforms with simultaneous electrocardiographic correlation. J Ultrasound Med. 1992; 11: 263–8.

Al Otaibi L, Whitman GJ, Chew FS. Hepatocellular adenoma. Am J Roentgenol. 1995; 165: 1426.

Albrecht T, Blomley MJ, Heckemann RA, et al. Stimulierte akustische Emission mit dem Ultraschall-Kontrastmittel Levovist: Ein klinisch nutzbarer Kontrasteffekt mit leberspezifischen Eigenschaften. Röfo Fortschr Geb Rontgenstr Neuen Bildgeb Verfahr. 2000; 172: 61–7.

Alponat A, Kum CK, Rajnakova A, Koh BC, Goh PM. Predictive factors for synchronous common bile duct stones in patients with cholelithiasis. Surg Endosc. 1997; 11: 928–32.

Ashur H, Siegal B, Oland Y, Adam YG. Calcified gallbladder (porcelain gallbladdecr). Arch Surg. 1978; 113: 594–6.

Aubertin JM, Levoir D, Bouillot JL, et al. Endoscopic ultrasonography immediately prior to laparoscopic cholecystectomy: a prospective evaluation. Endoscopy. 1996; 28: 667–73.

Aubin B, Denys A, Lafortune M, Dery R, Breton G. Focal sparing of liver parenchyma in steatosis: role of the gallbladder and its vessels. J Ultrasound Med. 1995; 14: 77–80.

Bahr MJ, Manns MP. Leberzirrhose. Internist. 1999; 40: 1308–22.

Bartolozzi C, Lencioni R Paolicchi A, Moretti M, Armillotta N, Pinto F. Differentiation of hepatocellular adenoma and focal nodular hyperplasia of the liver: comparison of power Doppler imaging and conventional color Doppler sonography. Eur Radiol. 1997; 7: 1410–5.

Becker D, Strobel D, Hahn EG. Tissue Harmonic Imaging und Contrast Harmonic Imaging. Verbesserung der Diagnose von Lebermetastasen? Internist. 2000; 41: 17–23.

Beissert M, Jenett M, Keberle M, et al. Vergleich von Contrast Harmonic Imaging im H-Mode mit stimulierter akustischer Emission, konventionellem H-Mode US and Spiral-CT in der Detektion fokaler Leberläsionen. Röfo Fortschr Geb Rontgenstr Neuen Bildgeb Verfahr. 2000; 172: 361–6.

Bezzi M, Silecchia G, De Leo A, Carbone I, Pepino D, Rossi P. Laparoscopic and intraoperative ultrasound. Eur J Radiol. 1998; 27 (Suppl. 2): S207–14.

Bin W, Jianguo L, Baowei D. The sonographic appearances of small bowel tumours. Clin Radiol. 1992; 46: 30–3.

Blanc JF, Bernard PH, Carles J, Le Bail B, Balabaud C, Bioulac-Sage P. Cholangiocarcinoma arising in Von Meyenburg complex associated with hepatocellular carcinoma in genetic haemochromatosis. Eur J Gastroenterol Hepatol. 2000; 12: 233–7.

Blum U, Rössle M, Haag K, et al. Budd–Chiari syndrome: technical, hemodynamic, and clinical results of treatment with transjugular intrahepatic portosystemic shunt. Radiology. 1995; 197: 805–11.

Boland GW, Slater G, Lu DS, Eisenberg P, Lee MJ, Mueller PR. Prevalence and significance of gallbladder abnormalities seen on sonography in intensive care unit patients. Am J Roentgenol. 2000; 174: 973–7.

Bowie JD. What is the upper limit of normal for the common bile duct on ultrasound: How much do you want it to be? Am J Gastroenterol. 2000; 95: 897–900.

Bozkurt T, Lux G. Transabdominelle Ultraschalldiagnostik bei entzündlichen und tumorösen Darmerkrankungen. Dtsch Med Wochenschr 1998; 123: 128–34.

Brambs HJ, Claussen CD. Pancreatic and ampullary carcinoma: ultrasound, computed tomography, magnetic resonance imaging and angiography. Endoscopy. 1993; 25: 58–68.

Busse HJ, Drescher T, Kroner M, Heine R, Schlee H, Dietrich R. Stellenwert der Ultraschalldiagnostik in Differential-Diagnose der Cholestase. Z Gastroenterol. 1993; 31 (Suppl. 2): 39–41.

Carson BW, Brown JA, Cooperberg PL. Ultrasonographically guided percutaneous biopsy of gastric, small bowel, and colonic abnormalities: efficacy and safety. J Ultrasound Med. 1998; 17: 739–42.

Caselmann WH, Blum HE, Fleig WE, et al. Leitlinien der Deutschen Gesellschaft fur Verdauung. Z Gastroenterol. 1999; 37: 353–65.

Caturelli E, Squillante MM, Andriulli A, et al. Hypoechoic lesions in the "bright liver": a reliable indicator of fatty change. A prospective study. J Gastroenterol Hepatol. 1992; 7: 469–72.

Chalasani N, Horlander JC, Said A, et al. Screening for hepatocellular carcinoma in patients with advanced cirrhosis. Am J Gastroenterol. 1999; 94: 2988–93.

Cherqui D, Rahmouni A, Charlotte F, et al. Management of focal nodular hyperplasia and hepatocellular adenoma in young women: a series of 41 patients with clinical, radiological, and pathological correlations. Hepatology. 1995; 22: 1674–81.

Chiche L, Dao T, Salame E, et al. Liver adenomatosis: reappraisal, diagnosis, and surgical management: eight new cases and review of the literature. Ann Surg. 2000; 231: 74–81.

Chintapalli KN, Ghiatas AA, Chopra S, Escobar B, Esola CC, Dodd GD III. Sonographic findings in cases of missed gallstones. J Clin Ultrasound. 1999; 27: 117–21.

Cottone M, D'Amico G, Maringhini A, et al. Predictive value of ultrasonography in the screening of non-ascitic cirrhotic patients with large varices. J Ultrasound Med. 1986; 5: 189–92.

Curley SA, Izzo F, Ellis LM, Nicolas VJ, Vallone P. Radiofrequency ablation of hepatocellular cancer in 110 patients with cirrhosis. Ann Surg. 2000; 232: 381–91.

Daldrup HE, Reimer P, RummenyEJ, Fischer H, Bocker W, Peters PE.Regression eines hepatozellulären Adenoms nach Absetzen hormonaler Kontrazeption. Röfo Fortschr Geb Rontgenstr Neuen Bildgeb Verfahr. 1995; 163: 449–51.

Danneels F, Steyaert L, Cappelle G, et al. Ultrasonographic findings in peptic ulcer: a report on 24 cases proven endoscopically. J Belge Radiol. 1990; 73: 253–6.

Di Lelio A, Cestari C, Lomazzi A, Beretta L. Cirrhosis: diagnosis with sonographic study of the liver surface. Radiology. 1989; 172: 389–92.

Di Stasi M, Caturelli E, De SI, Salmi A, Buscarini E, Buscarini L. Natural history of focal nodular hyperplasia of the liver: an ultrasound study. J Clin Ultrasound. 1996; 24: 345–50.

Dietrich CF, Brunner V, Lembcke B. Intestinale Sonographie bei seltenen Dünn- und Dickdarmerkrankungen. Z Gastroenterol. 1998a; 36: 955–70.

Dietrich CF, Zeuzem S, Caspary WF, Wehrmann T. Sonographische Lymphknotendarstellung im Abdomen und Retroperitoneum bei gesunden Probanden. Ultraschall Med. 1998 b; 19: 265–9.

Domland M, Gebel M, Caselitz M, Bleck J, Manns MP. Comparison of portal venous flow in cirrhotic patients with and without paraumbilical vein patency using duplex-sonography. Ultraschall Med. 2000; 21: 165–9.

Fanney DR, Castillo M, Casillas J, Montalvo B. Sonographic anatomy of the caudate lobe veins. J Clin Ultrasound. 1990; 18: 27–30.

Foster JH, Berman MM. The malignant transformation of liver cell adenomas. Arch Surg. 1994; 129: 712–7.

Fugazzola C, Procacci C, Bergamo Andreis IA, et al. The contribution of ultrasonography and computed tomography in the diagnosis of nonfunctioning islet cell tumors of the pancreas. Gastrointest Radiol. 1990; 15(2): 139–44.

Fujita N, Noda Y, Kobayashi G, Kimura K, Yago A. Diagnosis of the depth of invasion of gallbladder carcinoma by EUS. Gastrointest Endosc. 1999; 50: 659–63.

Gaiani S, Bolondi L, Li BS, Zironi G, Siringo S, Barbara L. Prevalence of spontaneous hepatofugal portal flow in liver cirrhosis. Clinical and endoscopic correlation in 228 patients. Gastroenterology. 1991; 100: 160–7.

Gaiani S, Casali A, Serra C, et al. Assessment of vascular patterns of small liver mass lesions: value and limitation of the different Doppler ultrasound modalities. Am J Gastroentero1. 2000; 95: 3537–46.

Gandolfi L, Fukuda M. Current Trends in Digestive Ultrasonography. Basel: Karger; 1997.

Gandolfi L, Leo P, Solmi L, Vitelli E, Verros G, Colecchia A. Natural history of hepatic haemangiomas: clinical and ultrasound study. Gut. 1991; 32: 677–80.

Garcia SJ. Direct sonographic signs of acute duodenal ulcer. Abdom Imaging. 1999; 24: 226–7.

Gasche C, Moser G, Turetschek K, Schober E, Moeschl P, Oberhuber G. Transabdominal bowel sonography for the detection of intestinal complications in Crohn's disease. Gut. 1999; 44: 112–7.

Gebel M, Caselitz M, Manns MP. Sonographische Diagnostik von Raumforderungen der Leber. Internist. 1997; 38: 901–7.

Giorgio A, Tarantino L, de Stefano G, et al. U1trasound-guided percutaneous ethanol injection under general anesthesia for the treatment of hepatocellular carcinoma on cirrhosis: long-term results in 268 patients. Eur J Ultrasound. 2000; 12: 145–54.

Görg C, Weide R, Schwerk WB. Lymphominfiltration der Leber: Spektrum sonographischer Erscheinungsformen bei 47 Patienten. Z Gastroenterol. 1994; 32: 597–602.

Goyal AK, Pokharna DS, Sharma SK. Ultrasonic diagnosis of cirrhosis: reference to quantitative measurements of hepatic dimensions. Gastrointest Radiol. 1990; 15: 32–4.

Grazioli L, Federle MP, Ichikawa T, Balzano E, Nalesnik M, Madariaga J. Liver adenomatosis: clinical, histopathological, and imaging findings in 15 patients. Radiology. 2000; 216: 395–402.

Hargreaves GM, Adam R, Bismuth H. Results after nonsurgical local treatment of primary liver malignancies. Langenbecks Arch Surg. 2000; 385: 185–93.

Harvey CJ, Blomley MJ, Eckersley RJ, et al. Hepatic malignancies: improved detection with pulse-inversion US in late phase of enhancement with SH U 508 A-early experience. Radiology. 2000; 216: 903–8.

Hashimoto L, Walsh RM, Vogt D, Henderson JM, Mayes J, Hermann R. Presentation and management of cystic neoplasms of the pancreas. J Gastrointest Surg. 1998; 2(6): 504–8.

Heyder N, Gunter E, Giedl J, Obenauf A, Hahn EG. Polypoide Läsionen der Gallenblase. Dtsch Med Wochenschr. 1990; 115: 243–7.

Hiatt JR, Phillips EH, Morgenstern L. Surgical diseases of the spleen. Berlin, Heidelberg, New York: Springer; 1997.

Holtkamp W, Müller W. Sonographisch gesteuerte perkutane Hochfrequenzthermotherapie von Lebertumoren mit perfundierten Nadelelektroden. Z Gastroenterol. 2000; 38: 221–7.

Hresson-Hadni S, Vuitton DA, Hartholomot B, et al. A twenty-year history of alveolar echinococcosis: analysis of a series of 117 patients from eastern France. Eur J Gastroenterol Hepatol. 2000; 12: 327–36.

Hwang JI, Chou YH, Tsay SH, et al. Radiological and pathological correlation of adenomyomatosis of the gallbladder. Abdom Imaging. 1998; 23: 73–7.

Jain D, Sarode VR, Abdul-Karim FW, HomerR, Robert ME. Evidence for the neoplastic transformation of Von-Meyenburg complexes. Am J Surg Pathol. 2000; 24: 1131–9.

Joseph AE, Saverymuttu SH, Al Sam S, Cook MG, Maxwell M. Comparison of liver histology with ultrasonography in assessing diffuse parenchymal liver disease. Clin Radiol. 1991; 43: 26–31.

Kane R, Eustace S. Diagnosis of Budd-Chiari syndrome: comparison between sonography and MR angiography. Radiology. 1995; 195: 117–21.

Kane RA, Jacobs R, Katz J, Costello P. Porcelain gallbladder: ultrasound and CT appearance. Radiology. 1984; 152: 137–41.

Kern P, Reuter S, Buttenschoen K, Kratzer W. Diagnostik der zystischen Echinokokkose. Dtsch Med Wochenschr. 2001 b; 126: 20–3.

Kimmey MB, Martin RW, Haggitt RC, Wang KY, Franklin DW, Silverstein FE. Histological correlates of gastrointestinal ultrasound images. Gastroenterology. 1989; 96: 433–41.

Kimura W, Makuuchi M. Operative indications for cystic lesions of the pancreas with malignant potential - our experience. Hepatogastroenterology 1999; 46(25): 483-91.

Kratzer W, Kachele V, Mason RA, et al. Gallstone prevalence in Germany: the Ulm Gallbladder Stone Study. Dig Dis Sci. 1998; 43: 1285–91.

Kubicka S, Rudolph L, Manns MP. Hepatozelluläres Karzinom: Diagnostik und multimodale Therapie. Intemist. 1997; 38: 954–62.

Kubicka S, Rudolph KL, Hanke M, et al. Hepatocellular carcinoma in Germany: a retrospective epidemiological study from a low-endemic area. Liver. 2000; 20: 312–8.

Lafortune M, Madore F, Patriquin H, Breton G. Segmental anatomy of the liver: a sonographic approach to the Couinaud nomenclature. Radiology. 1991; 181: 443–8.

LeBorgne J, deCalan L, Partensky C. Cystadenomas and cystadenocarcinomas of the pancreas: a multinstitutional retrospective study of 390 cases. French Surgical Association. Ann Surg. 1999; 8: 230(2): 152–61.

Lee SP, Nicholls JF, Park HZ. Biliary sludge as a cause of acute pancreatitis [see comments]. N Engl J Med. 1992; 326: 589–93.

Leifer DM, Middleton WD, Teefey SA, Menias CO, Leahy JR. Follow-up of patients at low risk for hepatic malignancy with a characteristic hemangioma at US. Radiology. 2000; 214: 167–72.

Limberg B. Sonographie des Gastrointestinaltraktes. Berlin, Heidelberg: Springer; 1998.

Lippert H. Praxis der Chirurgie. Stuttgart: Thieme; 1998.

Livraghi T, Benedini V, Lazzaroni S, Meloni F, Torzilli G, Vettori C. Long term results of single session percutaneous ethanol injection in patients with large hepatocellular carcinoma. Cancer. 1998; 83: 48–57.

Livraghi T, Goldberg SN, Lazzaroni S, et al. Hepatocellular carcinoma: radio-frequency ablation of medium and large lesions. Radiology. 2000; 214: 761–8.

Lock G, Schölmerich J. Vorgehen bei sonographisch nachgewiesener Raumforderung der Leber. Internist. 1997; 38: 924–7.

Mainprize KS, Gould SW, Gilbert JM. Surgical management of polypoid lesions of the gallbladder. Br J Surg. 2000; 87: 414–7.

Majeed AW, Ross B, Johnson AG, Reed MW. Common duct diameter as an independent predictor of choledocholithiasis: is it useful? Clin Radiol. 1999; 54: 170–2.

Martinoli C, Cittadini G, Conzi R, et al. Sonographic characterization of an accessory fissure of the left hepatic lobe determined by omental infolding. J Ultrasound Med. 1992; 11: 103–7.

Meckler U, Herzog P. Sonographischer Darmwandaufbau – Bedeutung für die Diagnose entzündlicher Darmerkrankungen. Ultraschall Med. 1989; 10: 152–7.

Meyer W, Kohler J, Gebhardt C. Cystic neoplasms of the pancreas – cystadenomas and cystadenomas. Langenbecks Arch Surg. 1999, 384: 44–9.

Misra SP, Dwivedi M. Pancreaticobiliary ductal union. Gut 1990; 31: 1144–9.

Mohr HH, Godderz W, Meyer zum Buschenfelde KH. Die Duplexsonographie der Leber und des Pfortadersystems. Med Klin. 1998; 93: 669–77.

Naganuma S, Ishida H, Konno K, et al. Sonographic findings of anomalous position of the gallbladder. Abdom Imaging. 1998; 23: 67–72.

Neubrand M, Sackmann M, Caspary WF, et al. Leitlinien der Deutschen Gesellschaft für Verdauungs- und Stoffwechselkrankheiten zur Behandlung von Gallensteinen. Gastroenterol. 2000; 38: 449–68.

Nicolau C, Torra R, Hianchi L, et al. Abdominal sonographic study of autosomal dominant polycystic kidney disease. J Clin Ultrasound. 2000; 28: 277–82.

Niederau C, Grendell JH. Diagnosis of pancreatic carcinoma: imaging techniques and tumor markers. Pancreas. 1992; 7: 66–86.

Niederau C, Sonnenberg A. Liver size eva1uated by ultrasound: ROC curves for hepatitis and alcoholism. Radiology. 1984; 153: 503–5.

Niederau C, Sonnenberg A, Mueller J. Comparison of the extrahepatic bile duct size measured by ultrasound and by different radiographic methods. Gastroenterology. 1984; 87: 615–21.

Oosterveld BJ, Thijssen JM, Hartman PC, Rosenbusch GJ. Detection of diffuse liver disease by quantitative echography: depen-

dence on a priori choice of parameters. Ultrasound Med Biol. 1993; 19: 21–5.
Orlando A, D'Antoni A, Camma C, et al. Treatment of small hepatocellular carcinoma with percutaneous ethanol injection: a validated prognostic model. Am J Gastroenterol. 2000; 95: 2921–7.
Pandey M, Sood BP, Shukla RC, Aryya NC, Singh S, Shukla VK. Carcinoma of the gallbladder: role of sonography in diagnosis and staging. J Clin Ultrasound. 2000; 28: 227–32.
Parulekar SG. Ultrasound evaluation of common bile duct size. Radiology. 1979; 133: 703–7.
Rickes S, Ocran K, Schulze S, Wermke W. Evaluation of Doppler sonographic criteria for the differentiation of hepatocellular carcinomas and regenerative nodules in patients with liver cirrhosis. Ultraschall Med. 2002; 23(2): 83–90.
Rieker O, Mildenberger P, Hintze C, Schunk K, Otto G, Thelen M. Segmentanatomie der Leber in der Computertomographie: Lokalisieren wir die Läsionen richtig? Röfo Fortschr Geb Rontgenstr Neuen Bildgeb Verfahr. 2000; 172: 147–52.
Ringe B, Lang H, Oldhafer KJ, et al. Which is the best surgery for Budd-Chiari syndrome: venous decompression or liver transplantation? A single-center experience with 50 patients. Hepatology. 1995; 21: 1337–44.
Rösch T, Lorenz R, Braig C, Classen M. Endoscopic ultrasonography in diagnosis and staging of pancreatic and biliary tumors. Endoscopy. 1992, 24: 304–8.
Sabba C, Merkel C, Zoli M, et al. Interobserver and interequipment variability of echo-Doppler examination of the portal vein: effect of a cooperative training program. Hepatology. 1995; 21: 428–33.
Sacerdoti D, Bolognesi M, Bombonato G, Gatta A. Paraumbilical vein patency in cirrhosis: effects on hepatic hemodynamics evaluated by Doppler sonography. Hepatology. 1995; 22: 1689–94.
Sanford NL, Walsh P, Matis C, Baddeley H, Powell LW. Is ultrasonography useful in the assessment of diffuse parenchymal liver disease? Gastroenterology. 1985; 89: 186–91.
Schepke M, Raab P, Hoppe A, Schiedermaier P, Brensing KA, Sauerbruch T. Comparison of portal vein velocity and the hepatic venous pressure gradient in assessing the acute portal hemodynamic response to propranolol in patients with cirrhosis. Am J Gastroenterol. 2000; 95: 2905–9.
Schlottmann K, Baer A, Lock G, Scholmerich J, Palitzsch KD. Der sonographische Befund einer echogenen Leber ist ein Indikator einer pathologischen Glukosetoleranz. Dtsch Med Wochenschr. 2000; 125: 517–22.
Schwerk WB, Gorg C, Görg K, Richter G, Heckh K. Perkutane Drainagen von Leber- und Milzabszessen. Z Gastroenterol. 1991; 29: 146–52.
Schwerk WB, Schwarz S, Rothmund M, Arnold R. Kolondivertikulitis: Bildgebende Diagnostik mit Ultraschall – eine prospektive Studie. Z Gastroenterol. 1993; 31: 294–300.
Seitz K, Wermke W. Portale Hypertension-derzeitiger Stand der sonographischen Diagnostik. Z Gastroenterol. 1995; 33: 349–61.
Shamsi K, Deckers F, De Schepper A. Is it a haemangioma? Röfo Fortschr Geb Rontgenstr Neuen Bildgeb Verfahr. 1993; 159: 22–7.
Sheth S, Bedford A, Chopra S. Primary gallbladder cancer: recognition of risk factors and the role of prophylactic cholecystectomy. Am J Gastroenterol. 2000; 95: 1402–10.
Shimizu M, Miura J, Tanaka T, Itoh H, Saitoh Y. Porcelain gallbladder: relation between its type by ultrasound and incidence of cancer. J Clin Gastroenterol. 1989; 11: 471–6.
Simonovsky V. The diagnosis of cirrhosis by high resolution ultrasound of the liver surface. Br J Radiol. 1999; 72: 29–34.
Stölzel U, Tannapfel A, Wittekind C, Hamm H, Schuppan D. Indikationen zur Leberbiopsie bei Lebertumoren. Dtsch Med Wochenschr. 2000; 125: 1041–4.
Strunk H, Stuckmann G, Fröhlich E, et al. Native und signalverstärkte Power-Doppler-Sonographie zur Charakterisierung von Leberherden. Röfo Fortschr Geb Rontgenstr Neuen Bildgeb Verfahr. 1998; 168: 344–51.
Sugiyama M, Hagi H, Atomi Y. Reappraisal of intraoperative ultrasonography for pancreatobiliary carcinomas: assessment of malignant portal venous invasion. Surgery. 1999; 125: 160–5.
Sugiyama M, Atomi Y, Yamato T. Endoscopic ultrasonography for differential diagnosis of polypoid gall bladder lesions: analysis in surgical and follow up series. Gut. 2000; 46: 250–4.
Tandon RK, Grewal H, Anand AC, Vashisht S. Caroli's syndrome: a heterogeneous entity. Am J Gastroenterol 1990; 85: 170–3.
Taourel P, Blanc P, Dauzat M, et al. Doppler study of mesenteric, hepatic, and portal circulation in alcoholic cirrhosis: relationship between quantitative Doppler measurements and the severity of portal hypertension and hepatic failure. Hepatology. 1998; 28: 932–6.
Teichgräber UK, Gebel M, Hecker H, Benter T, Manns MP. Importance of duplex velocity histograms in the diagnosis of liver cirrhosis. Röfo Fortschr Geb Rontgenstr Neuen Bildgeb Verfahr. 1996; 164: 401–5.
Terzi C, Sokmen S, Seckin S, Albayrak L, Ugurlu M. Polypoid lesions of the gallbladder: report of 100 cases with special reference to operative indications. Surgery. 2000; 127: 622–7.
Tous F, Busto M. Assessment of abdominal sonography in the diagnosis of tumors of the gastroduodenal tract. J Clin Ultrasound. 1997; 25: 243–7.
Truong M, Atri M, Bret PM, et al. Sonographic appearance of benign and malignant conditions of the colon. Am J Roentgenol. 1998; 170: 1451–5.
Uggowitzer MM, Kugler C, Mischinger HJ, et al. Echoenhanced Doppler sonography of focal nodular hyperplasia of the liver. J Ultrasound Med. 1999; 18: 445–51.
Van Bodegraven AA, Bohmer CJ, Manoliu RA, et al. Gallbladder contents and fasting gallbladder volumes during and after pregnancy. Scand J Gastroenterol. 1998; 33: 993–7.
Vilgrain V, Lewin M, Vons C, et al. Hepatic nodules in Budd-Chiari syndrome: imaging features. Radiology. 1999; 210: 443–50.
Von Herbay A, Frieling T, Niederau C, Häussinger D. Solitary hepatic lesions with a hypoechoic rim: value of color Doppler sonography. Am J Roentgenol.1997; 169: 1539–41.
Wagner HJ, Hoppe M, Klose KJ. Perkutane intraluminale Ultraschalluntersuchung der Gallenwege in der Diagnostik maligner biliärer Obstruktionen. Dtsch Med Wochenschr. 1995; 120: 472–7.
Weishorn HD, Seitz K. Sonographische Diagnostik bei Choledochuszysten. Ultraschall Med 1989; 10: 132–5.
Weiss H, Brockmann W, Bersch W, Fiedler L. Die Schichten der Gallenblasenwand: eine sonographisch-anatomische Vergleichsuntersuchung. Bildgebung. 1993; 60: 125–30.
Wernecke K, Henke L, Vassallo P, et al. Pathological explanation for hypoechoic halo seen on sonograms of malignant liver tumors: an in vitro correlative study. Am J Roentgenol. 1992a; 159: 1011–6.
Wernecke K, Vassallo P, Bick U, Diederich S, Peters PE. The distinction between benign and malignant liver tumors on sonography: value of a hypoechoic halo. Am J Roentgenol. 1992 b; 159: 1005–9.
Weyant MJ, Maluccio MA, Bertagnolli MM, Daly JM. Choledochal cysts in adults: a report of two cases and review of the literature. Am J Gastroenterol 1998; 93: 2580–3.
Wilkinson LS, Levine TS, Smith D, Chadwick SJ. Biliary sludge: can ultrasound reliably detect the presence of crystals in bile? Eur J Gastroenterol Hepatol. 1996; 8: 999–1001.
Wohlgemuth WA, Bottger J, Bohndorf K. MRI, CT, US and ERCP in the evaluation of bile duct hamartomas (von Meyenburg complex): a case report. Eur Radiol. 1998; 8: 1623–6.
Worlicek H, Dunz D, Engelhard K. Ultrasonic examination of the wall of the fluid-filled stomach. J Clin Ultrasound. 1989; 17: 5–14.
Wu CC, Ho YH, Chen CY. Effect of aging on common bile duct diameter: a real-time ultrasonographic study. J Clin Ultrasound. 1984; 12: 473–8.
Yassa NA, Yang J, Stein S, Johnson M, Ralls P. Gray-scale and color flow sonography of pancreatic ductal adenocarcinoma. J Clin Ultrasound 1997; 25(9): 473–80.

8 The Chest

Ch. Görg

Basic Facts

- Indications for thoracic sonography: Table 8.**1**.
- Sonographic assessment of the thorax is guided by the findings.
- Two scanning planes: intercostal and subcostal views (Fig. 8.**1**) (Mathis, 1996, 1997; Reuß, 1996; Schwerk and Görg, 1993).

Tabel 8.**1** Indications for thoracic sonography (based on Schwerk and Görg, 1993).

- Differentiation of masses in the chest wall
- Supplementary modality in extensive shadowing on chest films
- Suspected pulmonary embolism
- Ultrasound guidance for
  - Thoracentesis/catheter drainage/pleural biopsy
  - Percutaneous transthoracic FNA
- Assessment of diaphragmatic motion

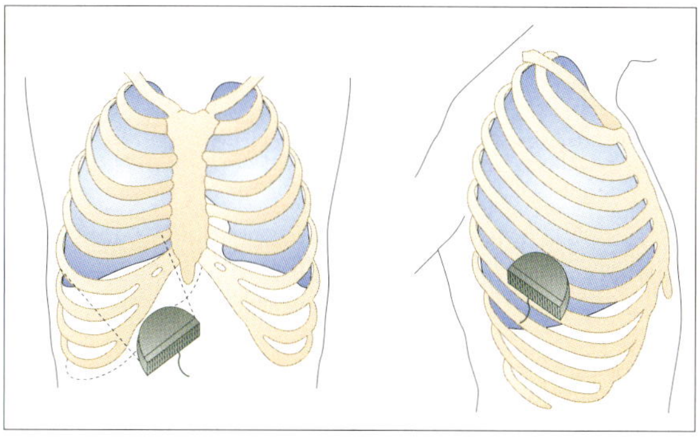

Fig. 8.**1** Schematic illustration of the probe movement in thoracic sonography.
Left image: subcostal transhepatic view of the inferior parts of the lung.
Right image: intercostal view paralleling the ribs.

Chest Wall Masses

Basic Facts

- Indications for sonography of the thorax are guided by clinical picture (e.g., localized pain in rib fracture) or palpable finding on physical examination.
- For purposes of differential diagnosis, masses of the chest wall fall into two groups–common and uncommon (Table 8.**2**).
- One major benefit of thoracic sonography is its ability for precise three-dimensional localization of masses (intracutaneous, subcutaneous, intramuscular, osseous, and pleural).
- Definitive histopathology samples can be obtained almost without complications by ultrasound-guided FNA or large-bore needle aspiration (Bitschnau et al., 1997; Wernecke, 1997).

Table 8.**2** Common and uncommon lesions of the thoracic wall

Common	Uncommon
- Rib/sternal fracture	- Skin metastasis
- Rib metastasis	- Lipoma
- Thoracic wall cancer	- Benign bone tumor
- Abscess	- Malignant lymphoma
- Hematoma	- Sarcoma
	- Malignant mesothelioma

Sonographic Criteria

- **Rib and sternal fractures:** Thoracic sonography cannot differentiate between traumatic and pathological fractures; callus formation during the healing phase can be visualized sonographically; the diagnostic accuracy of sonography in skeletal fractures of the thorax surpasses that of standard radiography. (Fig. 8.**2**, 8.**3**, Table 8.**3**)
- **Rib metastases:** Sonography is of limited use in the diagnostic workup of bony metastases and only complements standard imaging; it is helpful in treatment follow-up or for outlining a potential radiotherapy field (Fig. 8.**4**, Table 8.**4**).
- **Cancer/metastases of the thoracic wall:** Malignancies of the chest wall almost always are due to peripheral lung cancer or locally recurrent breast cancer (Figs. 8.**5**, 8.**6**, Table 8.**5**).
- **Hematoma:** Hyperechoic in the acute phase, they become progressively hypoechoic in their later course. Sonography benefits diagnostic workup and estimation of the blood volume sequestered (Fig. 8.**7**, Table 8.**6**).
- **Abscess:** Sonography benefits diagnostic workup and imaging for catheter drainage (Fig. 8.**8**, Table 8.**7**).

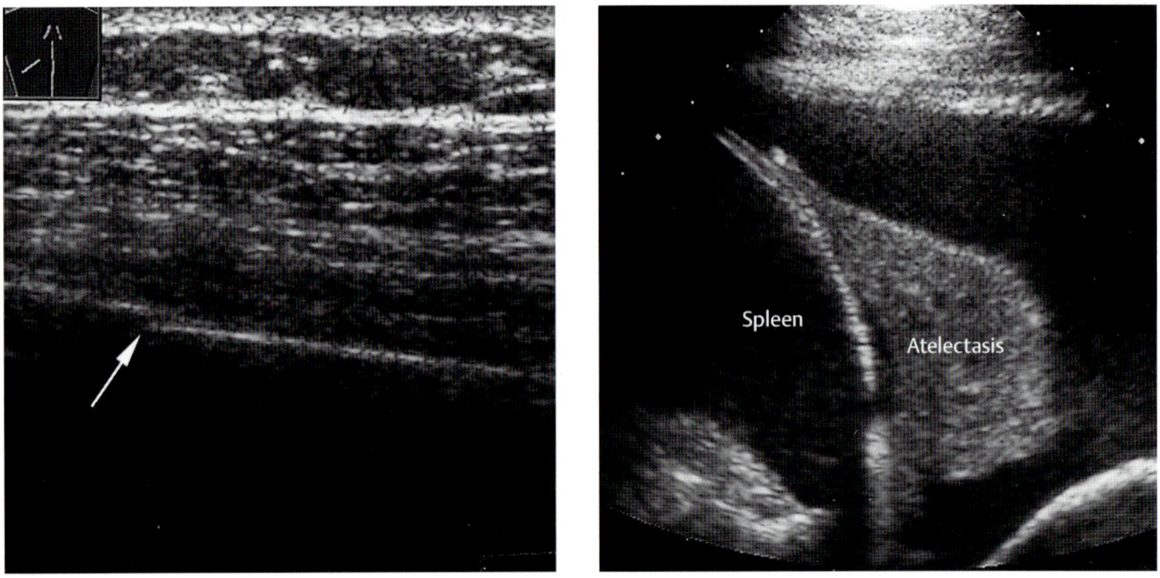

Fig. 8.**2** **a** A 43-year-old man with left-sided chest pain after falling from a horse.
Left image: The arrow marks a step-off, signaling a rib fracture.
Right image: Supradiaphragmatic pleural effusion with atelectasis of the lower lobe.

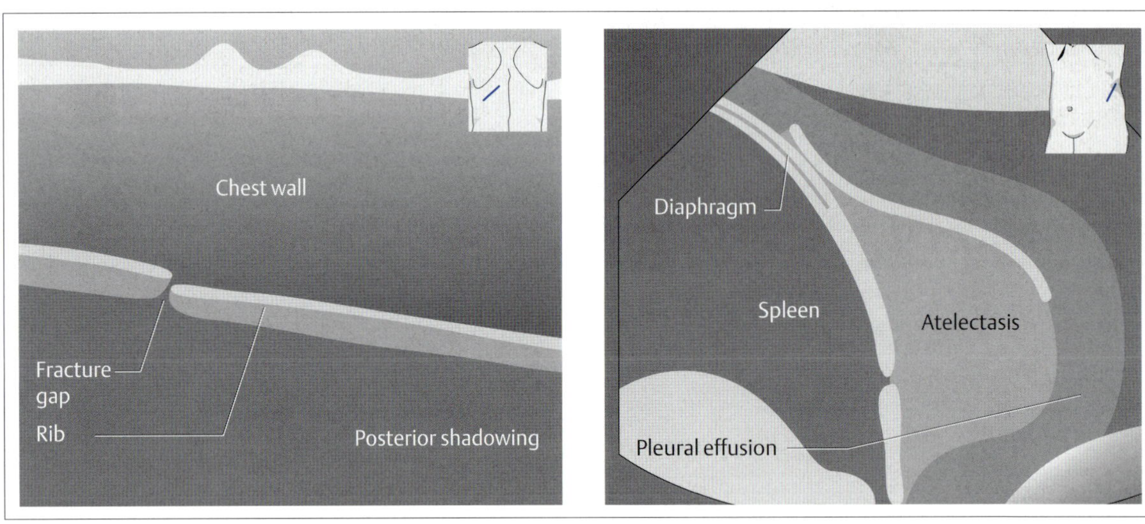

Fig. 8.**2** **b** Line drawings corresponding to left and right images of Fig. 8.**2** **a**.

Table 8.**3** Possible sonographic fracture signs

Direct Signs	**Indirect Signs**
– Break in the cortical echo – Fracture gap (step)	– Local hematoma – Pleural effusion – Pneumothorax – Hemothorax

Table 8.**4** Sonographic findings in rib metastasis

- Break in the cortical echo
- Local (in)complete ultrasound transmission
- Hypoechoic periosseous tumor
- Demonstration of flow signals in the tumor on color-flow Doppler ultrasound

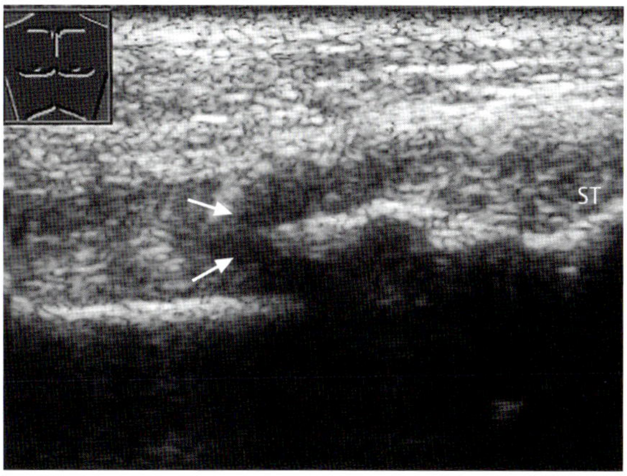

Fig. 8.**3 a** A 36-year-old woman with known breast cancer, complaining of pain over the sternum (ST). The arrows mark a step-off, signaling a fracture of the sternum. The cortical echo of the inferior sternal fragment is ill defined and surrounded by hypoechoic tissue. The finding is compatible with a pathological fracture of the sternum.

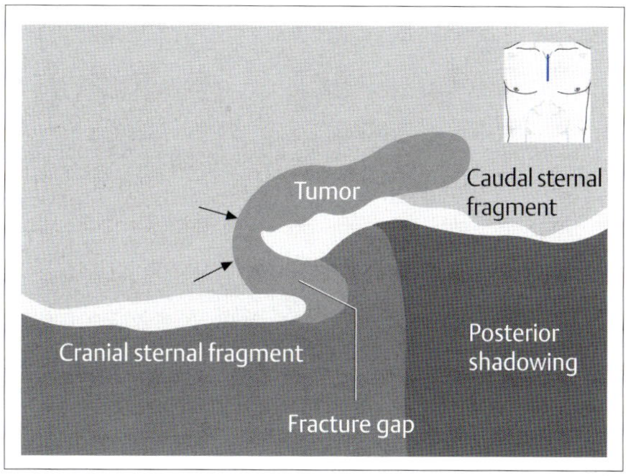

Fig. 8.**3 b** Line drawing.

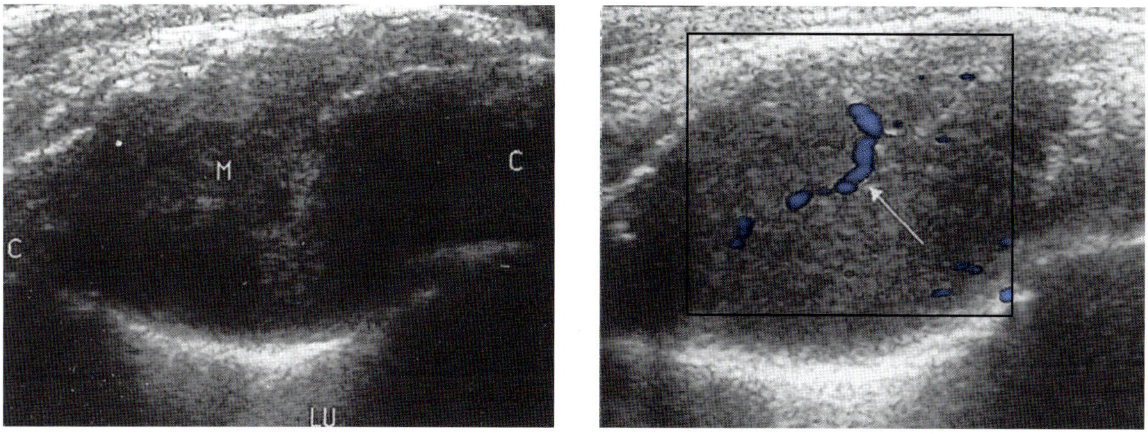

Fig. 8.**4 a** A 64-year old man with bronchial carcinoma and right parasternal pain.
Left image: The cortical echo of the rib (C) is disrupted and demonstrates complete through-transmission. A hypoechoic mass (M) can be seen. The lung (LU) is gliding over the mass.
Right image: On power Doppler sonography, flow signals in vessels can be demonstrated (arrow). The finding is compatible with rib metastasis.

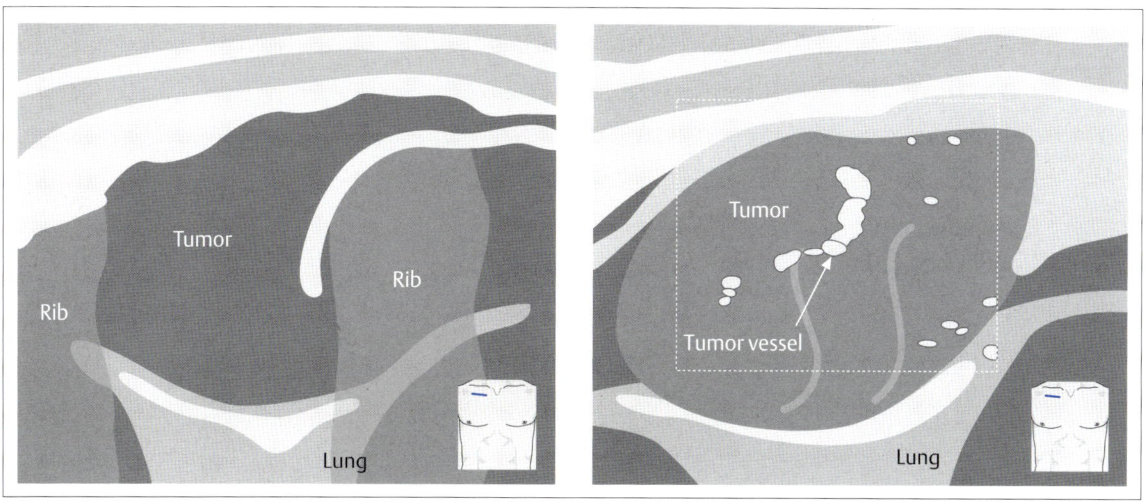

Fig. 8.**4 b** Line drawing corresponding to the left and right images of Fig. 8.**4 a**.

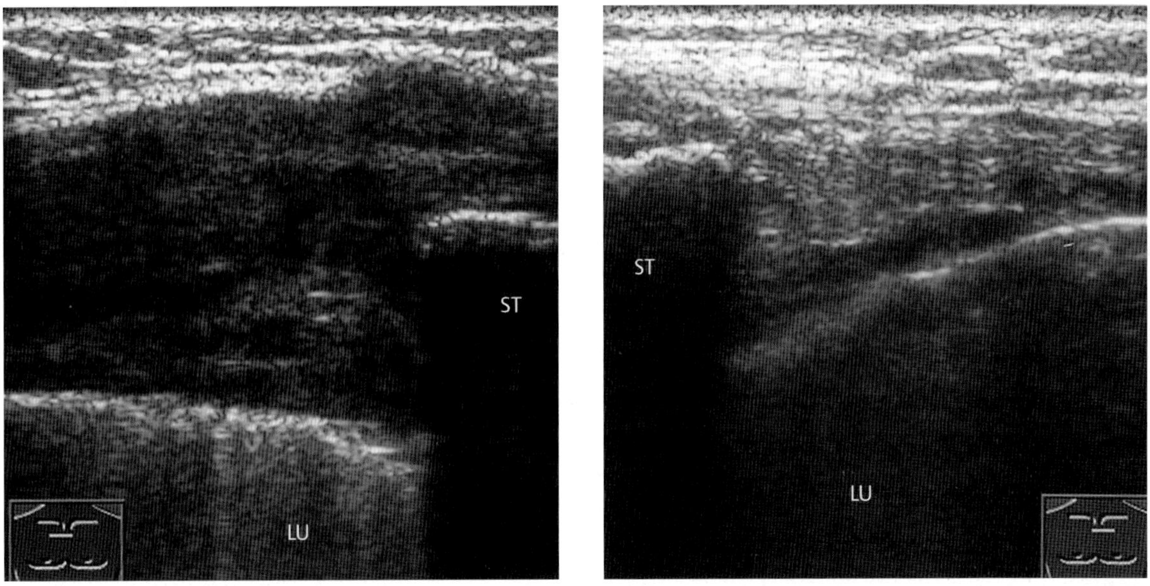

Fig. 8.**5 a** A 38-year old woman with known breast cancer and palpable mass to the right of the sternum.
Left image: Hypoechoic mass anterior and lateral to the sternum (ST). The lung (LU) is gliding over the malignancy. The finding is compatible with local recurrence in the chest wall.
Right image: Sonography of the left parasternal region demonstrates normal anatomical conditions.

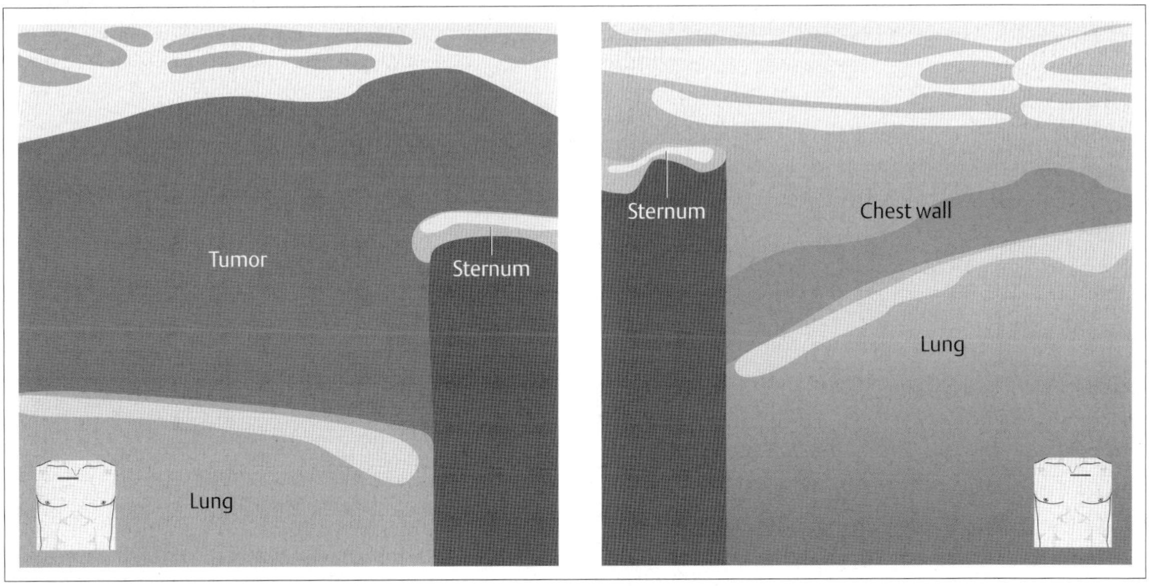

Fig. 8.**5 b** Line drawings corresponding to left and right images of Fig. 8.**5 a**.

Table 8.**5** Sonographic findings in thoracic wall cancer

- Complex hypoechoic lesion
- Irregular outline
- Invasive growth
- Demonstration of reduced flow signals in the tumor on color-flow Doppler ultrasound

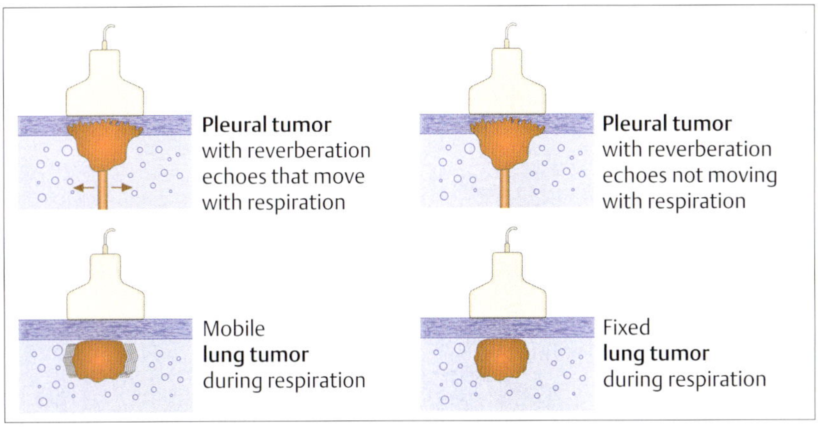

Fig. 8.**6** Schematic illustration of how to differentiate mobile from fixed pleural and pulmonary tumors. (Based on Wernecke, 1997.)

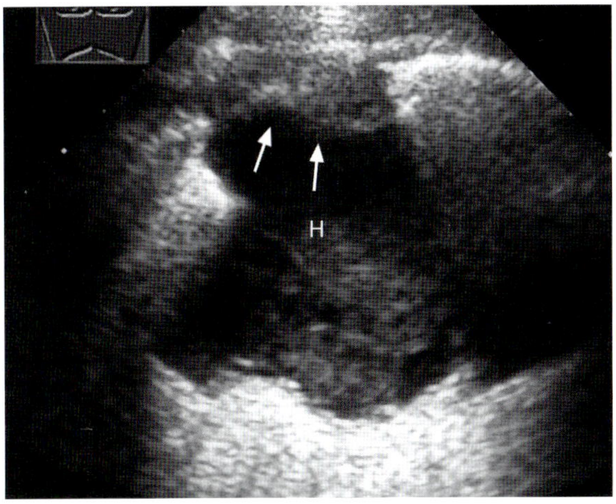

Fig. 8.**7a** A 44-year-old woman with metastatic sarcoma in the thoracic wall, hemoptysis, and a significant drop in hemoglobin. The arrows mark an area of tumorous thickening of the parietal pleura. Posterior to this lesion an echogenic area was demonstrated that exhibited motion artifacts on real-time sonography. Diagnostic thoracentesis yielded a hematoma in the pleural space.

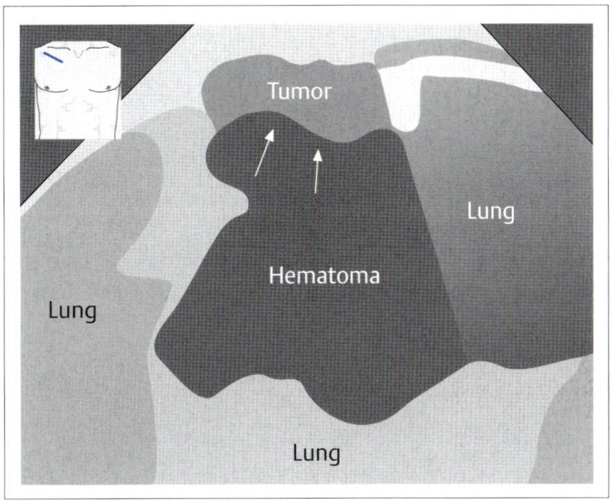

Fig. 8.**7b** Line drawing.

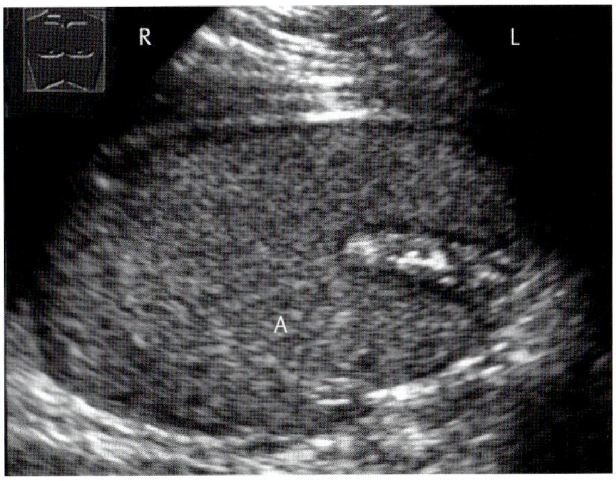

Fig. 8.**8a** A 36-year old woman with a right subclavian mass after venipuncture for a central venous line. An echogenic, smoothly delimited fluctuating mass was seen. Diagnostic aspiration yielding purulent matter identified this as an abscess (A).

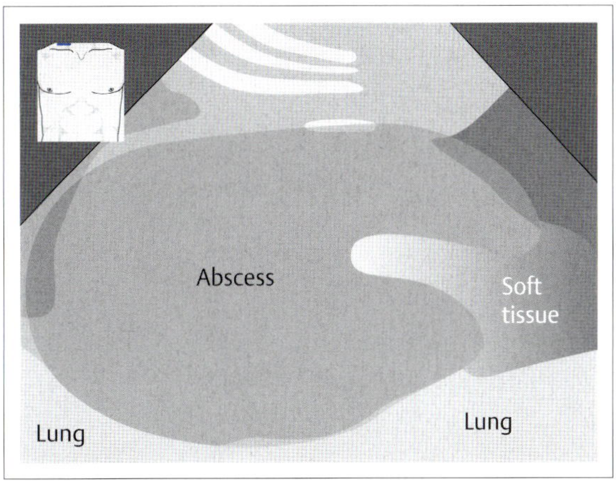

Fig. 8.**8b** Line drawing.

Table 8.**6** Sonographic findings in thoracic wall hematoma

Varied echogenicity
Smoothly delimited in most cases
Varied shape
Occasionally motile internal echoes
No flow signals on color-flow Doppler ultrasound

Table 8.**7** Sonographic findings in thoracic wall abscess

Varied echogenicity (sometimes with gas inclusions)
Varied delimitation (with hyperechoic capsule)
Varied shape
Displacement of internal echoes on compression
No flow signals on color-flow Doppler ultrasound

Consequences for Surgical Treatment

Diagnosis	Characteristic Findings	Management
Rib/sternal fracture	Circumscribed pain Stable thoracic wall Fracture gap	Nonsurgical management
Rib metastasis	Varied presentation Break in the cortical echo	Surgical resection Palliative radiotherapy
Thoracic wall cancer	Varied shape Hypoechoic lesion Invasive growth	Surgical resection Palliative radiotherapy Possibly chemotherapy
Hematoma	Rather varied presentation Smoothly delimited in most cases No symptomatic displacement No infection	Nonsurgical management
Abscess	Varied shape Fluctuating internal echoes Localized process	Ultrasound-guided drainage Surgical incision

Pleural Effusion

Basic Facts

- Sonography is the simplest and safest diagnostic modality for this most common pathology of the chest.
- The physical findings or extensive pulmonary shadowing on plain chest films set the indication for sonographic workup of the chest.
- Causes: Table 8.**8**.
- Pleural effusions are classified according to their protein contents (3 g/dl exudate, < 3 g/dl transudate). See Table 8.**9**.
- Knowledge of the result of the chest film is a prerequisite for full appraisal of the sonographic findings in pleural effusion. Etiology may be clarified by ultrasound-guided aspiration, pleural biopsy, and selective thoracentesis of any pleural thickening or tumor visualized, and/or by thoracoscopy (Fig. 8.**9**) (Gehmacher et al., 1997; Goecke and Schwerk, 1990; Görg et al., 1988, 1991).

Sonographic Criteria

- Differential diagnosis of pleural effusion: Table 8.**9**, Figs. 8.**10**–8.**15**.
- Estimation of the volume in pleural effusion by volumetry according to Goecke et al. (1990) (Fig. 8.**16**).

Table 8.**8** Potential causes of pleural effusion

Metastatic/hemodynamic (usually transudate)
- Cardiac failure
- Cirrhosis
- Uremia
- Hypercalcemia

Inflammatory (usually exudate)	**Neoplastic (usually exudate)**
- Pleurisy	- Pleural carcinomatosis
- Pneumonia	- Malignant mesothelioma
- Pulmonary infarction	- Malignant lymphoma
- Collagen disease	- Sarcoma
- Pancreatitis	

Table 8.9 Clinical and sonographic findings in pleural effusion

Transudate	Exudate				
	Inflammatory effusion	Hemorrhagic effusion	Chylous effusion	Purulent effusion	Malignant effusion
Aspirate analysis					
– Protein < 3 g/dl – Hypocellular – LDH < 200 U/l	– Protein > 3 g/dl – Hypercellular – Cholesterol > 60 g/dl	– Protein 3 g/dl – Hemorrhagic	– Protein > 3 g/dl – Milky/cloudy – Triglycerides > 110 g/dl	– Protein > 3 g/dl – Cell debris	– Protein > 3 g/dl – Possibly tumor cells
Examples					
– Cardiac failure – Cirrhosis – Hypoalbuminemia	– Pleuropneumonia – Pulmonary infarction – Collagen disease	– Hemothorax – Tumor bleeding	– Chest trauma – Malignant lymphoma	– Pleural empyema – Pyothorax	– Pleural carcinomatosis – Malignant mesothelioma – Malignant lymphoma
Characteristic ultrasound findings					
– Anechoic – Delicate pleural lines – Often bilateral	– Anechoic or with internal echoes – Septation – Fibrin strands – Marked pleural lines – Parenchymal lesions	– Hypoechogenic with internal echoes – Possibly sedimenting echoes ("snow storm")	– Hyperechoic with high-amplitude internal echoes ("snow storm")	– Varied – Possibly intense reflections – No pleural motion	– Anechoic or with internal echoes – Septation – Fibrin strands – Pleural tumors – Parenchymal lesions

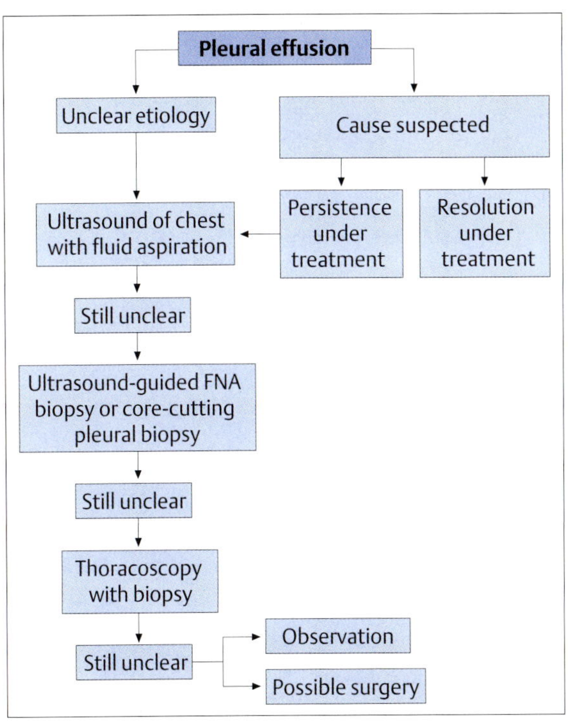

Fig. 8.9 Algorithm for diagnostic management in pleural effusion.

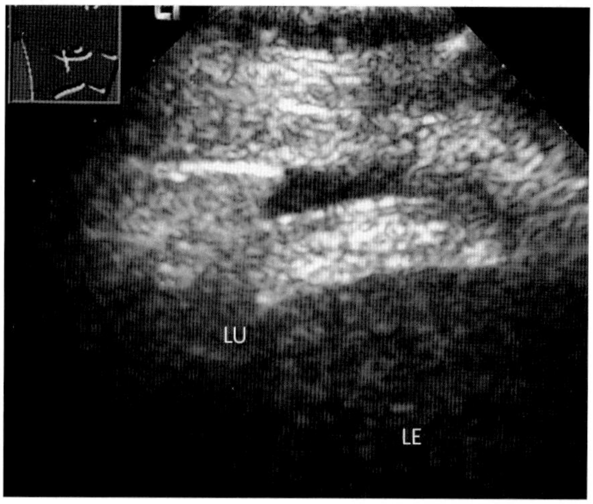

Fig. 8.**10a** The small anechoic triangle demonstrated in a sitting patient in the costodiaphragmatic recess is compatible with a minute pleural effusion (LU = lung, LE = liver).

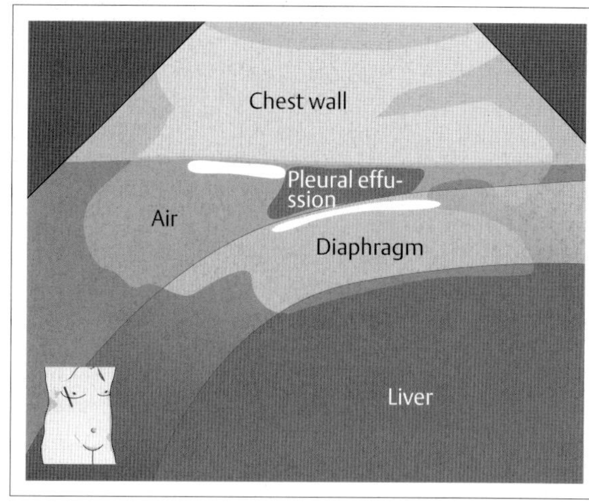

Fig. 8.**10b** Line drawing.

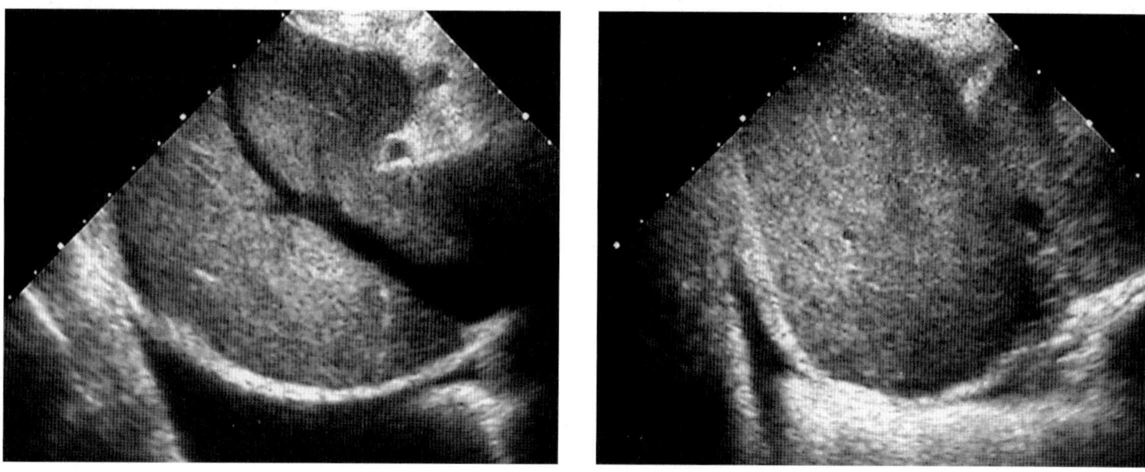

Fig. 8.**11a** With the patient supine, pleural effusion can be demonstrated on subcostal scanning with the probe oriented posteriorly (**left image**), while the rather reflective aerated lung is visualized when the probe is swept into the more anterior direction (**right image**).

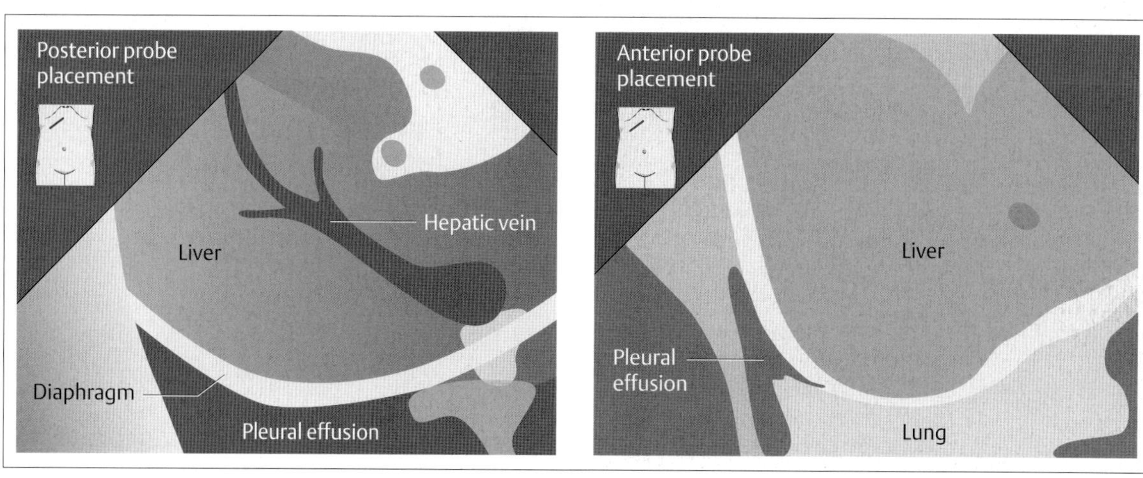

Fig. 8.**11b** Line drawings corresponding to left and right images in Fig. 8.**11a**.

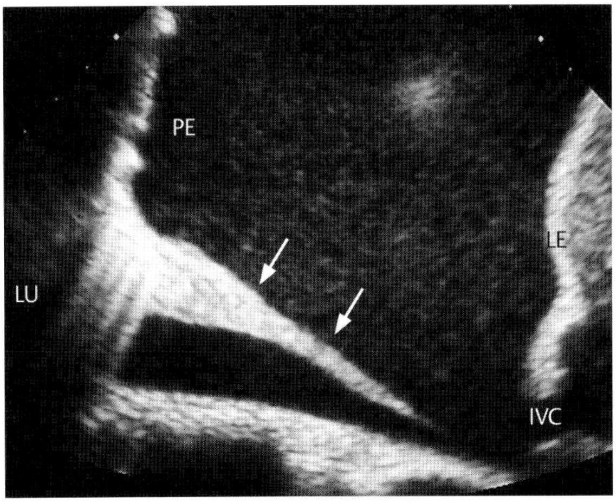

Fig. 8.**12 a** A 44-year old woman with breast cancer. A slightly echogenic pleural effusion (PE) was demonstrated. The arrows mark the compression atelectasis of the inferior lobe (LU = lung; IVC = inferior vena cava; LE = liver).

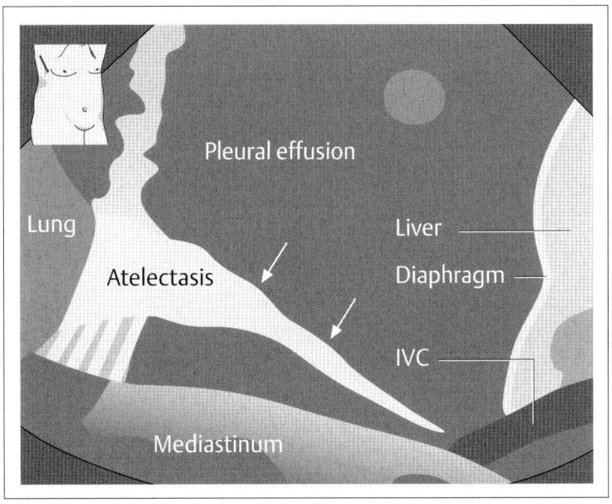

Fig. 8.**12 b** Line drawing.

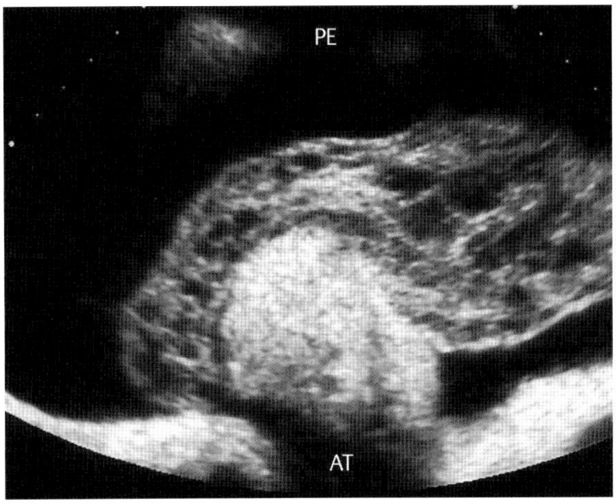

Fig. 8.**13 a** A 73-year old patient with bronchial carcinoma. An anechoic pleural effusion (PE) was seen. The atelectasis (AT) is hyperechoic and overlaid with matter rich in fibrin (assembled into a "fibrin structure") along the lines of an exudative effusion.

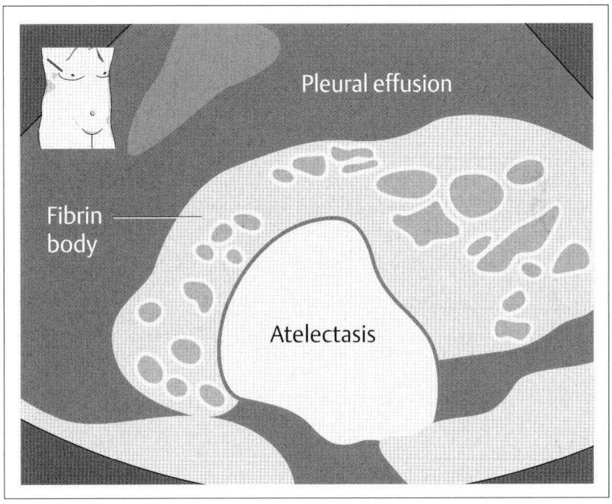

Fig. 8.**13 b** Line drawing.

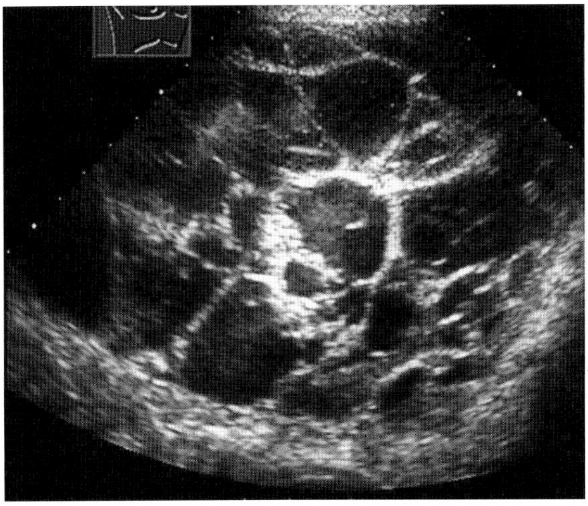

Fig. 8.**14 a** A 75-year old patient with pneumonia and exudative pleural effusion. The pleural effusion is riddled with fibrin strands. In such a case, relief by thoracentesis will not be successful.

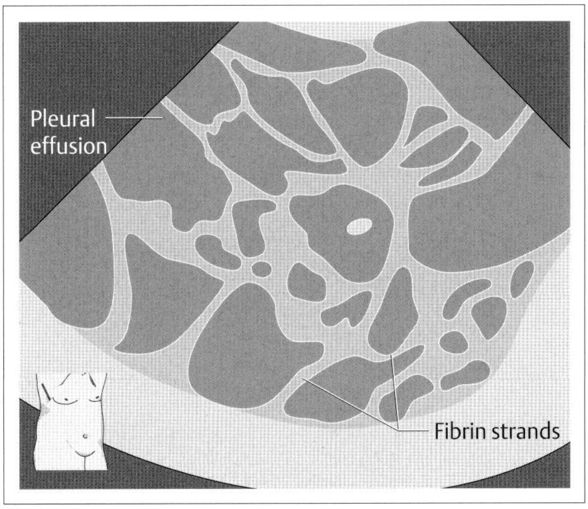

Fig. 8.**14 b** Line drawing.

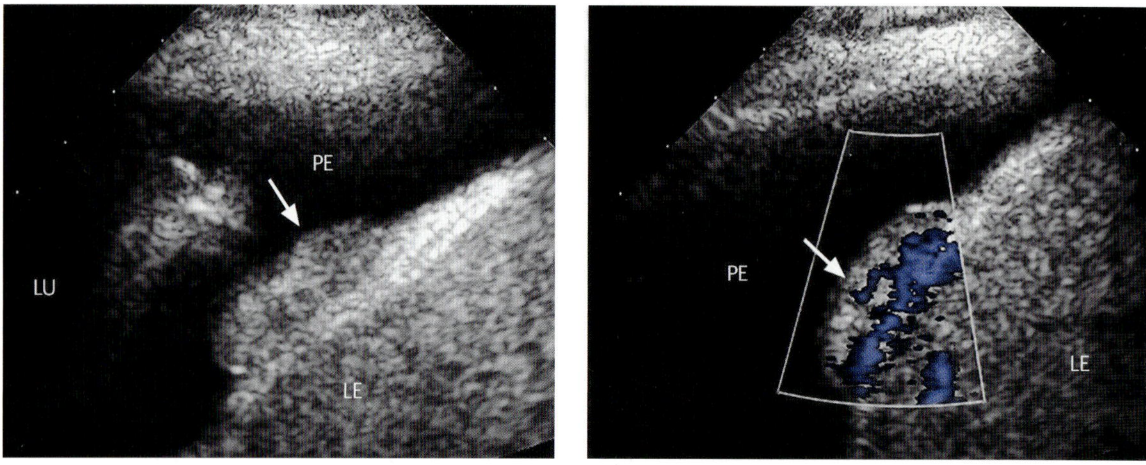

Fig. 8.**15 a** A 64-year old patient with metastatic renal cell carcinoma.
Left image: An anechoic pleural effusion (PE) was seen. A hypoechoic tumor formation (arrow) is readily identifiable immediately superior to the diaphragm (LU = lung, LE = liver).
Right image: Power Doppler sonography demonstrates tumor vessels originating from the diaphragm. This finding is compatible with pleural carcinomatosis.

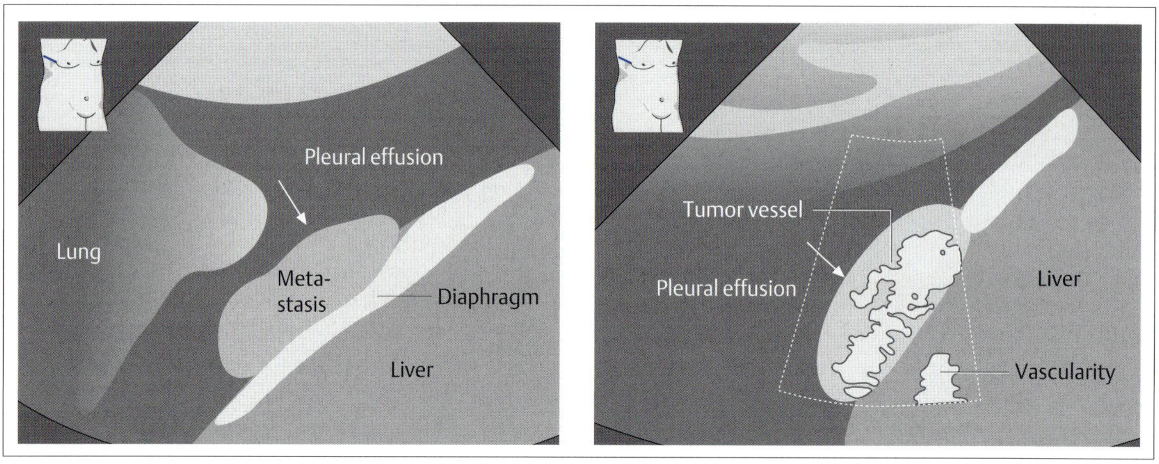

Fig. 8.**15 b** Line drawing.

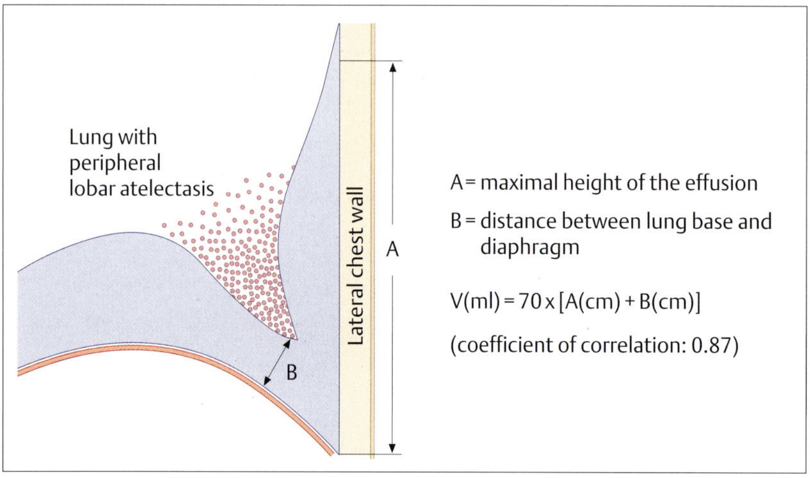

Fig. 8.**16** Schematic illustration of pleural effusion volumetry. (Based on Goecke et al., 1990.)

Consequences for Surgical Treatment

Diagnosis	Characteristic Findings	Management
Pleural effusion, transudative	Most often anechoic Next steps depend on etiology; physical findings are indicative	Ultrasound-guided drainage Nonsurgical treatment
Pleural effusion, exudative	Varied sonographic findings Next steps depend on etiology; physical findings are indicative	Ultrasound-guided drainage Nonsurgical treatment pleurodesis with suction drainage

Pulmonary Consolidation

Basic Facts

- Clinical and/or radiological suspicion of consolidated lung may mandate further evaluation by thoracic sonography.
- Consolidated lung is hypoechoic compared with the normal, highly reflective aerated lung.
- The diagnostic value of sonography is limited, as only peripheral lesions close to the pleura can be visualized. Diagnostic "dead spaces" (shadowing posterior to bony structures, central, and mediastinal lesions) restrict sonography to only a handful of indications, and even then only to answering specific questions.
- The anatomical relations of the pulmonary lobes: Fig. 8.**17**.
- Standard diagnostic modalities when extensive consolidated lung is seen on plain chest films are spiral CT and MRI.
- If a lesion can be mapped sonographically, ultrasound-guided fine-needle or large-bore needle aspiration biopsies are suitable for histopathological assessment and differentiation (e.g., of Pancoast tumors) (Blank, 1994; Gehmacher, 1996; Kroschel et al., 1991; Mathis and Dirschmid, 1993; Yang, 1996; Yang et al., 1988).

Sonographic Criteria

- Sonographic signs in extensive consolidated lung: Table 8.**10**.
- **Pneumonia:** The value of ultrasound is limited, as the majority of inflammatory (in particular interstitial and central) pulmonary changes cannot be visualized; however, peripheral pneumonia may be demonstrated. Possible sonographic findings: Table 8.**11**, Fig. 8.**18**. If sonographic signs are present, sonography may prove helpful on follow-up, in revealing complications (e.g., abscess formation), and in differential diagnosis.
- **Lung abscess:** Possible sonographic findings: Table 8.**12**. Differentiation from pleural empyema may prove difficult in individual cases. Inflammatory reaction in the tissue surrounding a pulmonary abscess close to the pleura commonly leads to local accretions between visceral and parietal pleura, thus fixing the mass to the thoracic wall. Ultrasound-guided thoracentesis lends itself to diagnostic confirmation, obtaining biopsies, and drainage (Fig. 8.**19**).
- **Pulmonary embolism:** A prerequisite for sonographic confirmation of pulmonary embolism is the presence of alveolar hypoventilation resulting from impaired perfusion. Due to effective collateralization usually via branches of the bronchial arteries, and since the more extensive pulmonary embolisms (occluding the pulmonary, lobar, and segmental arteries) do not necessarily result in infarction (Fig. 8.**20**), these pulmonary embolisms can hardly ever be directly demonstrated. In the hands of experienced sonographers, the diagnosis of pulmonary embolism has a sensitivity and specificity of around 90%. Possible sonographic findings in pulmonary embolism: Table 8.**13**, Fig. 8.**21**
- **Atelectasis:** Characterized by a lack of ventilation of pulmonary segments, lobes, or an entire lung, and classified according to its underlying cause (Figs. 8.**22**, 8.**23**). Compression atelectasis is caused by voluminous pleural effusions, the hydrostatic pressure of which exceeds intra-alveolar and airway pressure; obturation atelectasis secondary to complete bronchial obstruction results from gradual absorption of the air downstream of the blockage (Fig. 8. **24**).
  Possible sonographic findings: Tables 8.**14**, 8.**15**
- **Tumor/metastasis of the lungs:** Visualized sonographically as solid hypoechoic masses, if reaching up the visceral or parietal pleura. Tumor invasion of the chest wall results in a fixed lesion, which on respiration will be sessile with the chest wall rather than mobile. Possible sonographic findings: Table 8.**16**, Fig. 8.**26**.

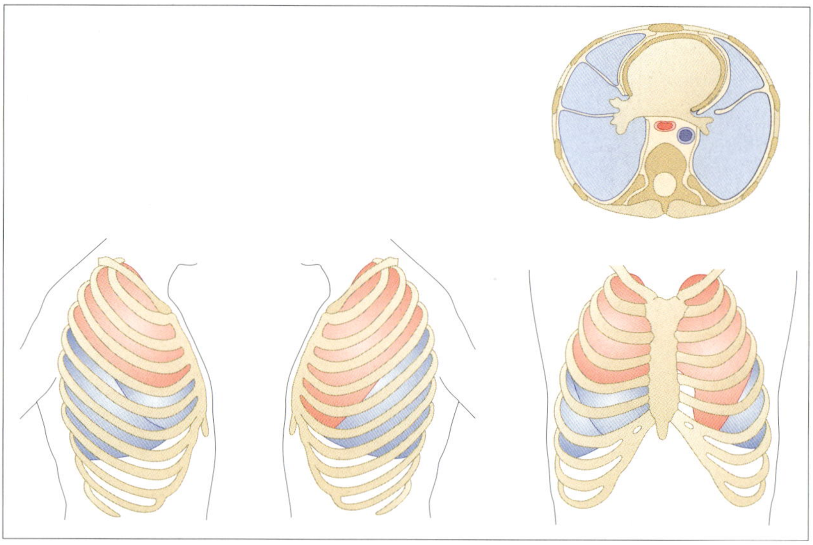

Fig. 8.**17** The anatomical relations of the pulmonary lobes.

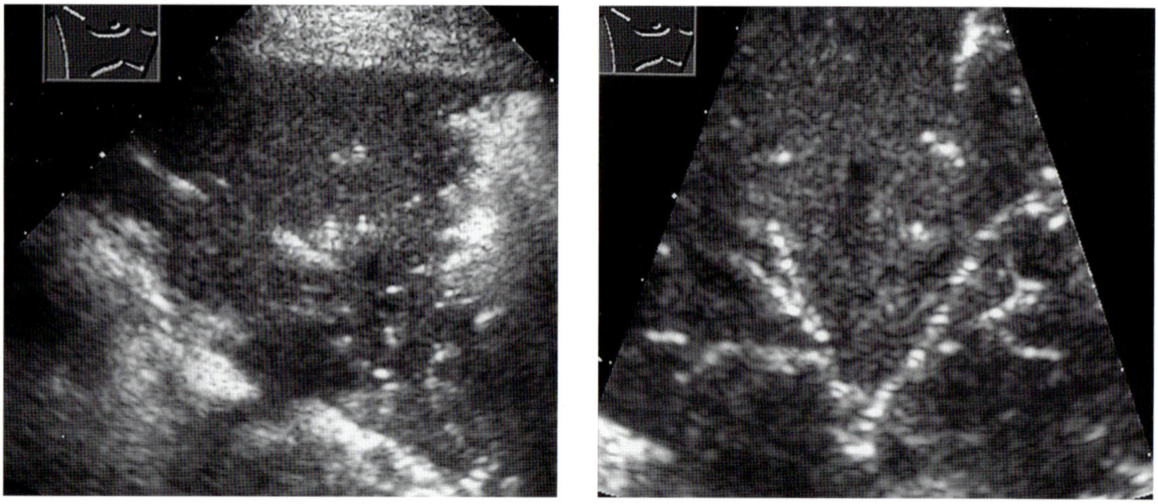

Fig. 8.**18 a** A 73-year-old patient with fever.
Left image: An echogenic, irregularly defined structure with discrete gas echoes was seen.

Right image: On inspiration, the treelike sonographic air bronchogram characteristic of pneumonia is visualized.

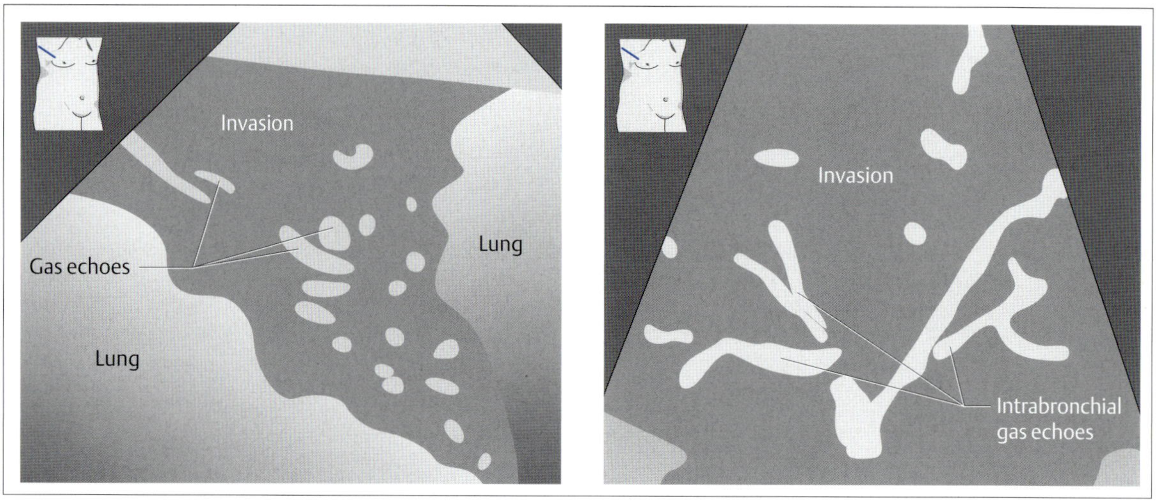

Fig. 8.**18 b** Line drawings corresponding to left and right images in Fig. 8.**18 a.**

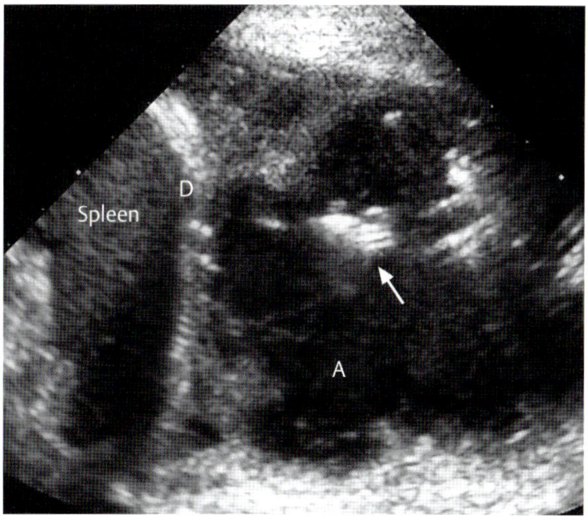

Fig. 8.**19 a** A 78-year-old alcoholic with fever. Sonography reveals a complex transformation of the left lung. In the center of an anechoic area, numerous hyperechoic gas echoes are demonstrated (arrow). This finding is compatible with a lung abscess (A). Ultrasound-guided thoracentesis with catheter drainage was performed.

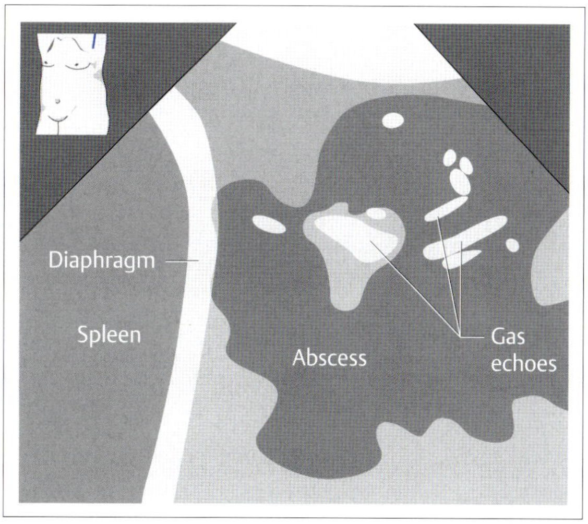

Fig. 8.**19 b** Line drawing.

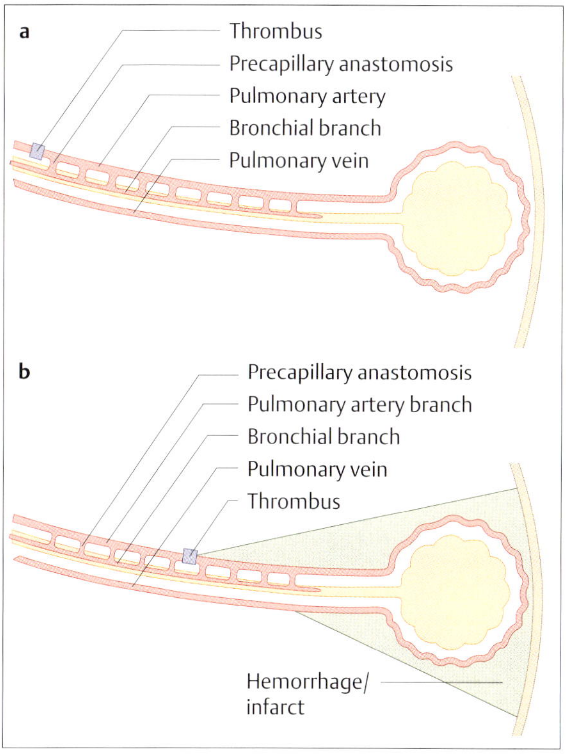

Fig. 8.**20 a, b** Schematic illustration of central versus peripheral occlusion of the pulmonary artery. Pulmonary infarction ensues only from peripheral occlusion of a branch of the pulmonary artery.

Table 8.**10** Sonographic criteria in extensive consolidated lung

B-mode imaging
- Echogenicity (hypoechoic, hyperechoic, complex)
- Echotexture (homogeneous, heterogeneous)
- Outline (smooth, irregular)
- Shape (round, ovoid, focal)
- Mobile internal echoes on real-time imaging

Color-flow Doppler imaging
- Flow signals (absent, present, enhanced)
- Flow waveforms (venous, arterial)

Table 8.**11** Possible sonographic findings in pneumonia

B-mode imaging
- Often hypoechoic transformation of lung tissue
- Most likely ill-defined against the aerated lung tissue
- Frequently identification of sonographic air bronchograms
- Often increased aeration on inspiration
- Frequently concomitant pleural effusion

Color-flow Doppler imaging
- Increased flow signals on intraindividual comparison with hepatic perfusion
- Triphasic spectrum of the arterial waveform on color-flow Doppler imaging of the pulmonary arteries (limb artery type)

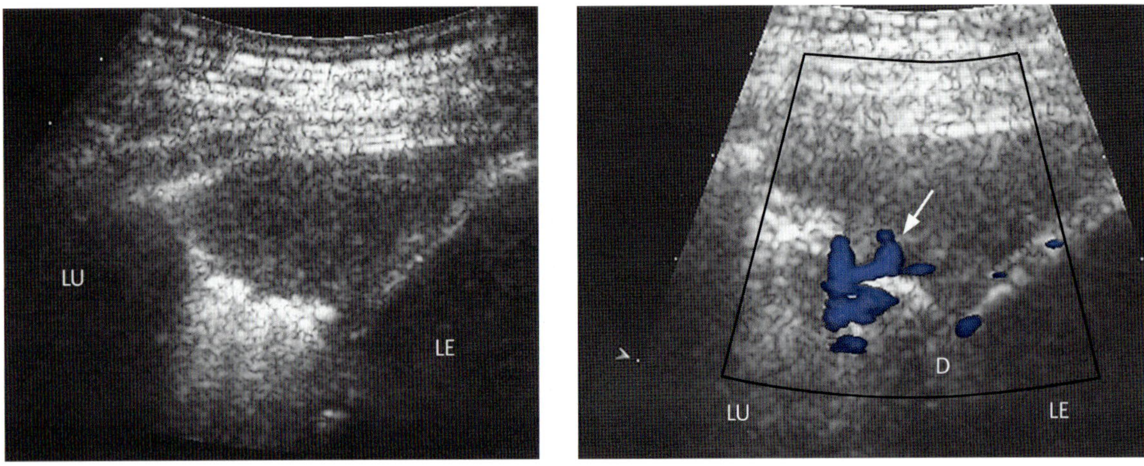

Fig. 8.**21 a** A 33-year-old woman with respiration-related chest pain and dyspnea.
Left image: Triangular homogeneous hypoechoic transformation of the lung tissue (LU = normal lung tissue; LE = liver).

Right image: On power Doppler sonography, no flow signals can be demonstrated in the transformed hypoechoic tissue. The arrow marks the site of the vascular occlusion. These findings are highly suspicious for postinfarction pneumonia secondary to pulmonary embolism (D = diaphragm; LU = lung; LE = liver).

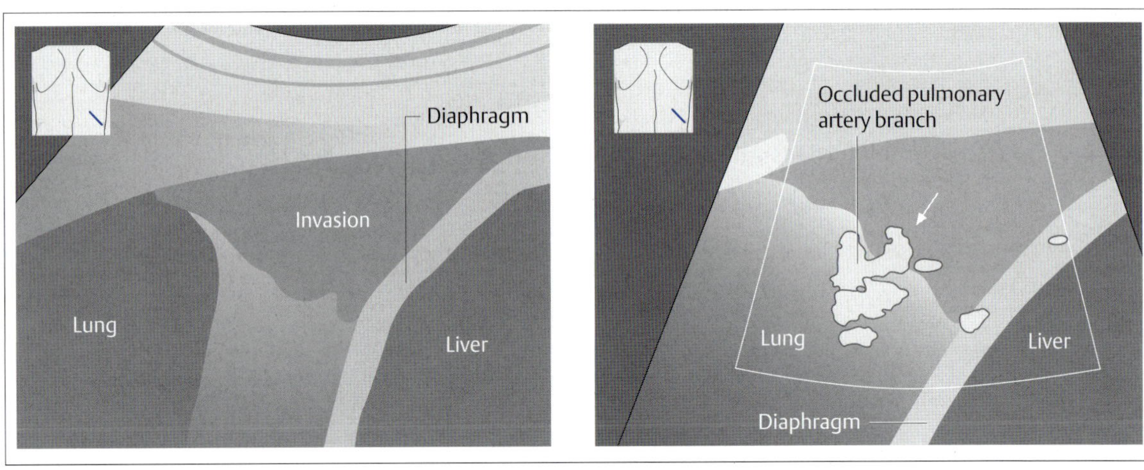

Fig. 8.**21 b** Line drawings corresponding to left and right images in Fig. 8.**21 a**.

Table 8.**12** Possible sonographic findings in lung abscess/empyema

B-mode imaging
- Complex transformation
- Sharply defined against the aerated lung tissue
- Echogenic margin of the mass
- Possibly gas inclusions and floating echoes within the lesion (liquefaction)

Color-flow Doppler imaging
- Lack of flow signals

Table 8.**13** Possible sonographic findings in pulmonary embolism

B-mode imaging
- Irregular localized entry echoes
- Striplike disrupted entry echo
- Wedge-shaped lesion
- Large extensive structural transformation

Color-flow Doppler imaging
- In most cases lack of flow signals in the infarct zone
- Rarely demonstration of an afferent vessel

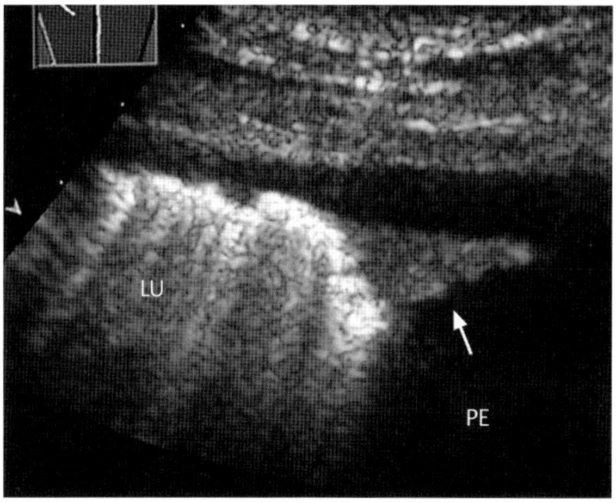

Fig. 8.**22a** A 62-year old patient with heart failure.
Left image: A moderately large pleural effusion (PE) is seen. A triangular hypoechoic area of transformation (arrow) is defined against the normal tissue of the lung (LU).

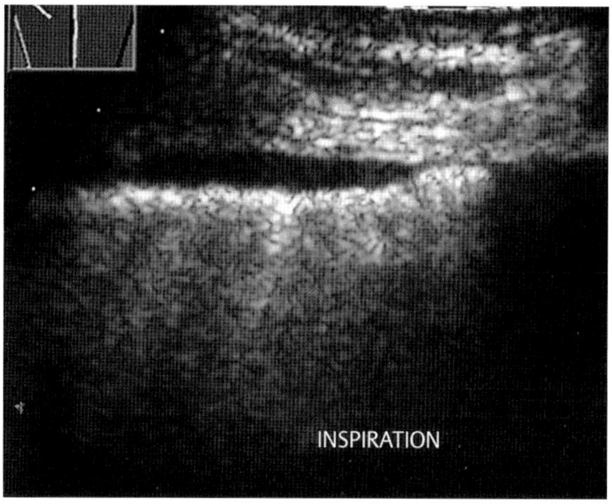

Right image: On inspiration, the hypoechoic transformed area is re-aerated. The finding is compatible with a compression atelectasis.

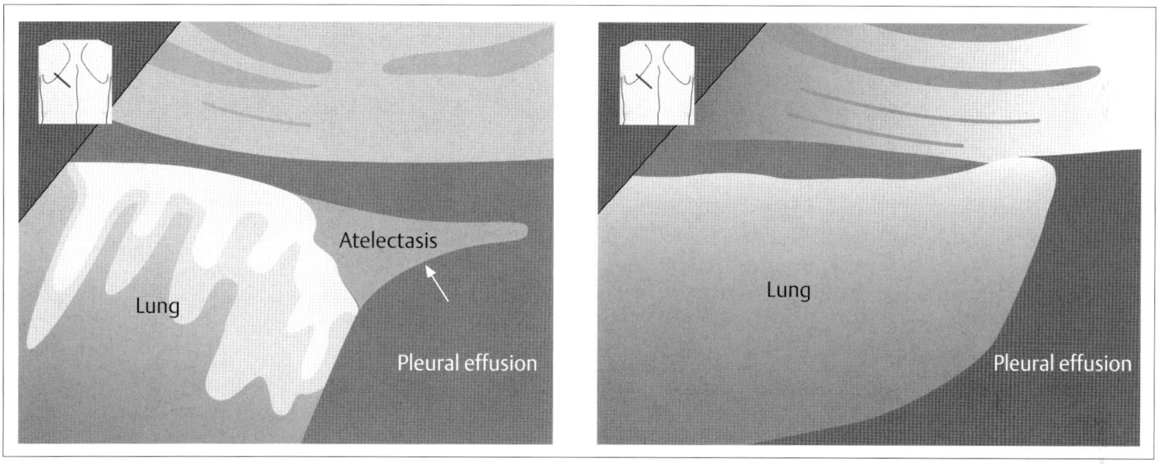

Fig. 8.**22b** Line drawings corresponding to left and right images in Fig. 8.**22a**.

Table 8.**14** Possible sonographic findings in compression atelectasis

B-mode imaging

- Moderate to marked pleural effusion
- Triangular hypoechoic transformation of lung parenchyma resembling a conical dunce's cap
- Ill-defined against the aerated lung tissue
- Partial re-aeration on inspiration (sonographic air bronchogram)
- Partial re-aeration after aspiration of the pleural effusion

Color-flow Doppler imaging

- Increased flow signals on intraindividual comparison with hepatic perfusion

Table 8.**15** Possible sonographic findings in obturation atelectasis

B-mode imaging

- Small or no pleural effusion
- Homogeneous hypoechoic transformation of lung parenchyma
- Possibly demonstration of echogenic bands of reflection (sonographic fluid bronchograms)
- Possibly demonstration of intraparenchymal foci
  - Parenchymal liquefaction
  - Micro-/macro-abscesses
  - Metastases
- Possibly demonstration of a central mass
- No re-aeration on inspiration

Color-flow Doppler imaging

- Increased flow signals on intraindividual comparison with hepatic perfusion
- Triphasic spectrum of the arterial waveform on color-flow Doppler imaging of the pulmonary arteries (limb artery type)

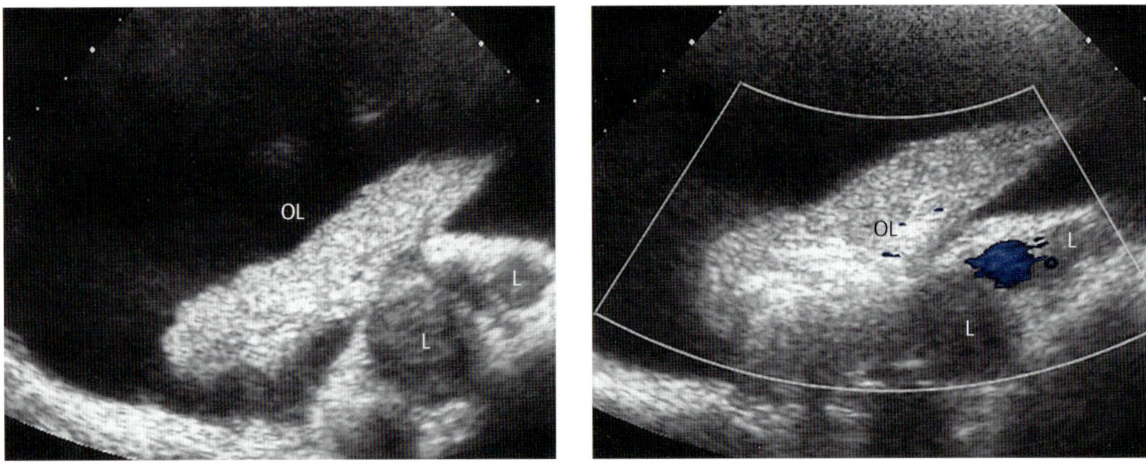

Fig. 8.**23 a** A 73-year old patient with CUP syndrome.
Left image: A marked pleural effusion is seen. The superior lobe (OL) has undergone echogenic transformation. Central hypoechoic lymphadenopathy (L) can be demonstrated.
Right image: After pleural aspiration partial re-aeration of the upper lobe (OL). The sonographic finding is compatible with a compression atelectasis.

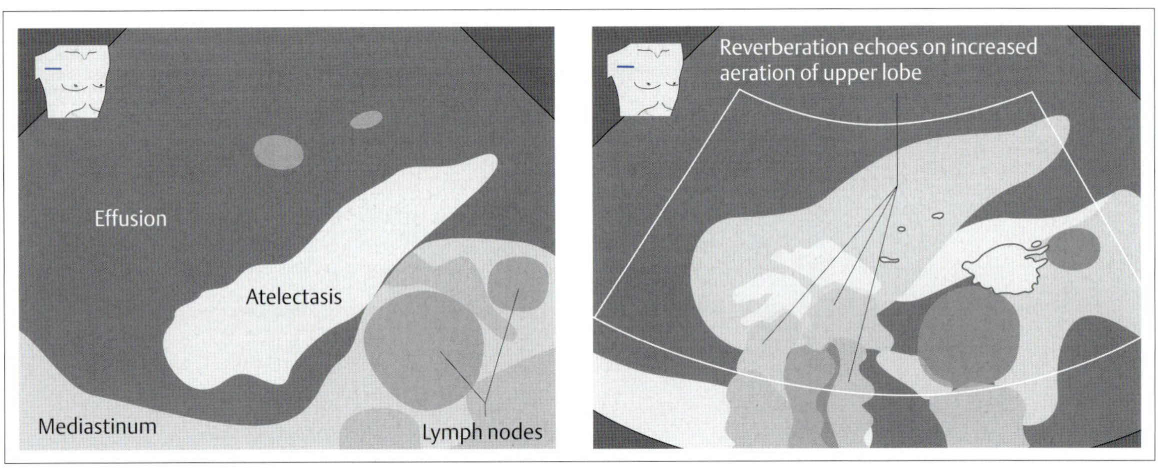

Fig. 8.**23 b** Line drawings corresponding to left and right images in Fig. 8.**23 a**.

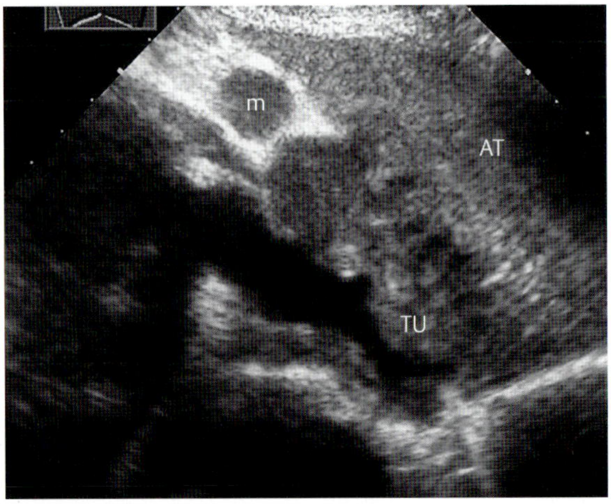

Fig. 8.**24 a** A 61-year-old woman with bronchial carcinoma. A central tumor (TU) with regional lymphadenopathy (M) is depicted. The lung tissue downstream has undergone hypoechoic transformation. The sonographic finding is compatible with an obstruction atelectasis (AT).

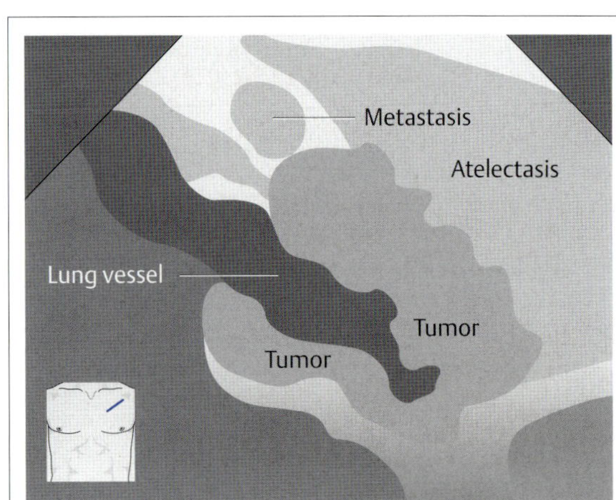

Fig. 8.**24 b** Line drawing.

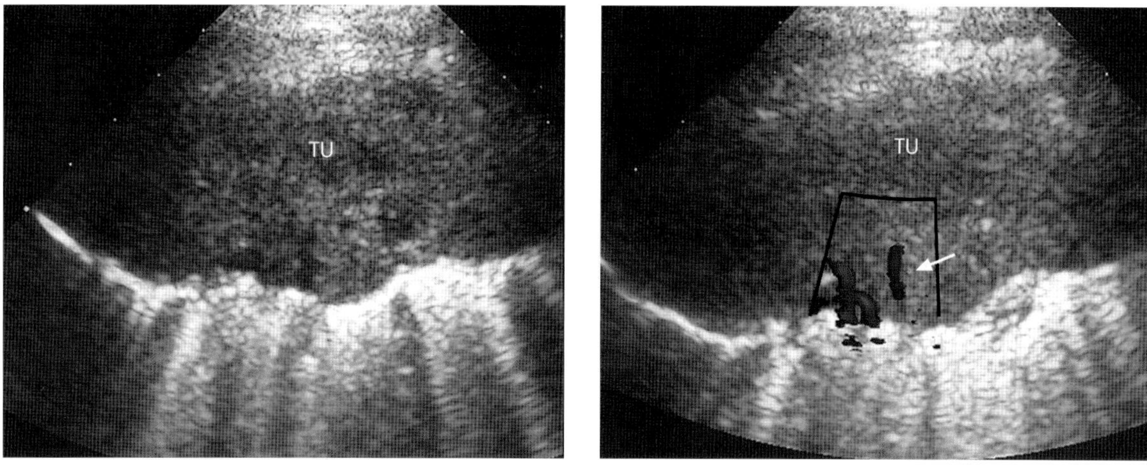

Fig. 8.**25a** A 72-year-old man with bronchial carcinoma.
Left image: The lung tissue has undergone hypoechoic transformation (TU).
Right image: Power Doppler sonography delineates delicate vascular echoes (arrow). The sonographic finding is compatible with a tumor fixed to the chest wall.

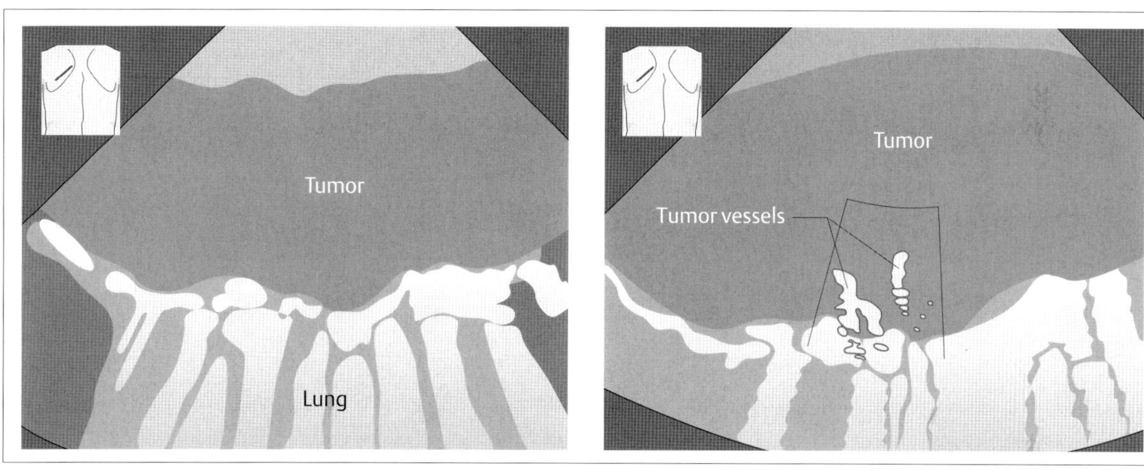

Fig. 8.**25b** Line drawings corresponding to left and right images in Fig. 8.**25a**.

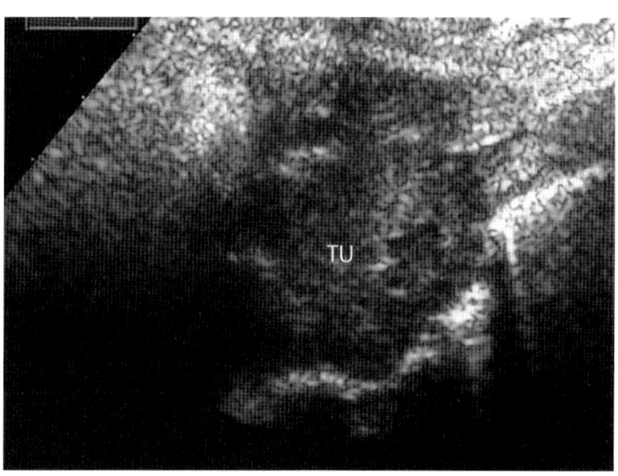

Fig. 8.**26a** Horner syndrome in a 50-year old man. A tumor (TU) is found in the right supraclavicular fossa, invading the thoracic wall. The lung no longer glides with respiration. The sonographic finding is compatible with a Pancoast tumor.

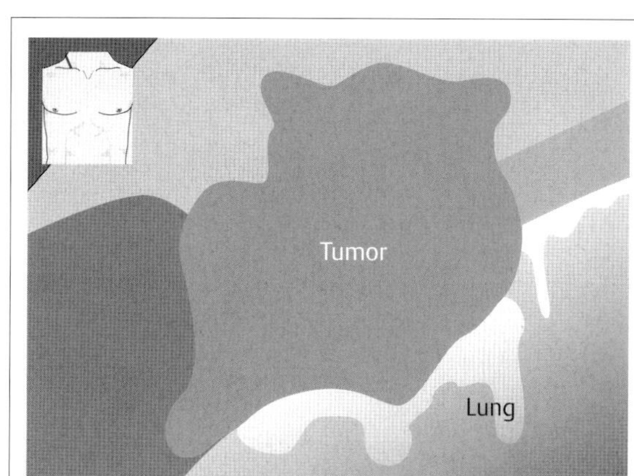

Fig. 8.**26b** Line drawing.

Table 8.16 Possible sonographic findings in peripheral lung tumors

B-mode imaging	Color-flow Doppler imaging
– Usually homogeneous hypoechoic transformation of lung tissue – Sharply defined against the aerated lung tissue – No sonographic air bronchogram – Occasionally central necrosis	– Decreased flow signals on intraindividual comparison with hepatic perfusion – Tumor vessels tend to show high diastolic flow velocities (parenchymal artery type)

Consequences for Surgical Treatment

Diagnosis	Characteristic Findings	Management
Pneumonia	Clinical diagnosis Hypoechoic lesion Positive sonographic air bronchogram	In case of abscess, conservative treatment Possibly drainage and surgical management
Abscess	Varied shape Fluctuating internal echoes Echogenic margin	Physical drainage; if not sufficient, then ultrasound-guided catheter insertion and possible surgical debridement
Pulmonary embolism	Clinical symptoms Hypoechoic lesion No flow signals on color-flow Doppler imaging	Nonsurgical treatment Surgical management dependent on the clinical situation
Atelectasis, compression	Smoothly defined hypoechoic lesion Pleural effusion	Nonsurgical management
Atelectasis, obturation	Smoothly defined hypoechoic lesion Central mass	Invasive diagnostic workup Bronchoscopy Thoracentesis Mediastinoscopy
Tumor/metastasis of the lungs	Hypoechoic lesion Possibly invasive growth	Ultrasound-guided biopsy Surgical resection

Bibliography

Bitschnau R, Gehmacher O, Kopf A, Scheier M, Mathis G. Ultrasonography in the diagnosis of rib and sternal fracture. Ultraschall Med. 1997; 18: 158–61.

Blank W. Sonographisch gesteuerte Punktionen und Drainagen. In: Braun G, Schwerk WB, eds. Ultraschalldiagnostik. Landsberg: ECO-Med; 1994: III.II: 5–12.

Gehmacher O, Kopf A, Scheier M, Bitschnau R, Wertgen T, Mathis G. Ist die Pleuritis sonographisch darstellbar? Ultraschall Med. 1997; 18: 214–9.

Gehmacher O. Ultrasound pictures of pneumonia. Eur J Radiol. 1996; 3: 161–7.

Goecke W, Schwerk WB. Die Real-Time-Sonographie in der Diagnostik von Pleuraergüssen. In: Gebhardt J, et al, eds. Ultraschalldiagnostik 89. Berlin, Heidelberg, New York, Tokyo: Springer; 1990: 385–7.

Görg C, Görg K, Schwerk WB, Kleinsorge F. Sonographie der Pleura diaphragmatica bei Tumorpatienten. Ultraschall Med. 1988; 9: 274–8.

Görg C, Schwerk WB, Görg K, Walters E. Pleural effusion: an "acoustic window" for sonography of pleural metastases. JCU. 1991; 19: 93–7.

Kroschel U, Seitz K, Reuß J, Rettenmeier G. Sonographische Darstellung von Lungenembolien. Ergebnisse einer prospektiven Studie. Ultraschall Med. 1991; 12: 263–8.

Mathis G. Lungen- und Pleurasonographie. 2nd ed. Berlin, Heidelberg, New York: Springer; 1996.

Mathis G. Thoraxsonography–part 1: Chest Wall and Pleura. Ultrasound Med Biol. 1997; 23: 1131–9.

Mathis G, Dirschmid K. Pulmonary infarction: sonographic appearance with pathological correlation. Eur J Radiol. 1993; 17: 170–4.

Reuß J. Sonographic imaging of the pleura: nearly 30 years experience. Eur J Ultrasound. 1996; 3: 125–39.

Schwerk WB, Görg C. Pleura und Lunge. In: Braun G, Schwerk WB, eds. Ultraschalldiagnostik. Landsberg: ECO-Med; 1993: 12. Supplementary issue. III 2.2: 1–43.

Wernecke K. Sonographic features of pleural disease. Am J Roentgenol. 1997; 168: 1061–6.

Yang PC. Color Doppler ultrasound of pulmonary consolidation. Eur J Radiol. 1996; 3: 169–78.

Yang PC, Lee LN, Luh KT, et al. Ultrasonography of Pancoast tumor. Chest. 1988; 94: 124–8.

9 Sonography of the Thyroid Gland and the Endocrine System

K. Reschke, H. Lehnert

Sonography of the Thyroid Gland

Indications for Sonography

Of high diagnostic yield and easy to perform, ultrasonography has, over recent years, become the most important imaging modality in the diagnostic workup of thyroid pathology. Accurate volumetry is possible, and nodular lesions can be confidently differentiated. In addition, changes in parenchymal echogenicity facilitate differential diagnosis of thyroid disease.

While ultrasonography assesses morphological features, scintigraphy with Tc-99m pertechnetate or iodine-125 provides functional information on endocrine activity. Ultrasound and scintigraphy should thus be combined as complementary diagnostic modalities of the thyroid gland.

Normal Thyroid Gland

Basic Facts

- Linear transducers (5–7.5 MHz) currently provide both deep ultrasound penetration and a wide near field of view.
- A standoff device (gel pad) placed between the probe and the skin improves coupling and increases image width; there are commercial linear transducers with built-in or removable standoff devices made of, e.g., Proxon® (Sonogel, Bad Camberg, Germany).
- Larger linear probes may present problems in longitudinal scanning of short necks or when the neck cannot be hyperextended.
- The patient is typically examined in the supine position, with the neck extended; a small roll under the neck or a pad or pillow under the shoulders provides better exposure.
- During the examination always adhere to the same sequence of steps:
  - Transverse views from cranial to caudal comparing both lobes: The probe is applied in a horizontal plane, orthogonal to the thyroid cartilage, and slowly moved in a cranial as well as a caudal direction.
  - Longitudinal views paralleling the longitudinal lobar axis, starting laterally and moving medially: Paralleling the sternocleidomastoid muscle, the probe is applied at the maximum longitudinal diameter of the lobe and then slowly moved laterally and medially.
- On transverse views, the normal thyroid gland resembles a butterfly, confined anteriorly to the superficial neck muscles, laterally to the large vessels of the neck, and medially to the trachea (Fig. 9.**1**).
- On longitudinal views, the thyroid is related laterally to the large vessels of the neck (carotid artery and jugular vein) and medially to the tracheal rings (Fig. 9.**2**).
- In thyroid lobes extending far caudad or retrosternally (anterior mediastinum), the lower poles may be impossible to visualize, and the volume cannot be measured precisely but only estimated (if needed, combine images and document this in the report).
- On occasion, retrosternal parts of the thyroid may shift into the real-time image by having the patient swallow.
- Normal variants comprise asymmetries in size (in most cases the left lobe is smaller; Fig. 9.**3**), up to aplasia of an entire lobe.
- For comparison of findings during follow-up, uniform ultrasound machine settings (output and gain) are recommended.
- Image documentation should include maximum transverse and longitudinal diameter of each lobe as well as any pathology.
- The report should include:
  - Location and size of each thyroid lobe (volume in ml)
  - Echotexture
  - Nodules and any irregular findings, including their location, extension, and echogenicity
- Volume is calculated according to the rotational ellipsoid method:
  - The total volume of the thyroid is the sum of both lobar volumes; in case of enlarged isthmus this should be mentioned in the report.
  - The volume of each lobe (in ml) is computed according to the following formula commonly used in clinical practice: **volume (ml) = maximum length × width × depth (each in cm) × correction factor 0.52**
  - When this method is used by experienced sonographers, the mean estimated error is approximately 10%, being larger for larger goiters or in thyroids extending below the sternum.
- The echotexture depends on the size of the thyroid follicles: Echogenicity increases with increasing thyroid follicular volume.

- Upper normal limits for sonographic measurement of total thyroid volume (Gutekunst et al., 1988):
  - 6–10 years: < 8 ml
  - 11–14 years: < 10 ml
  - 15–18 years: < 15 ml
  - Women: < 18 ml
  - Men: < 25 ml

Sonographic Criteria

- Normal-sized follicles of the healthy thyroid result in a homogeneous echotexture with fine internal echoes, thus being hyperechoic to the low-echogenicity strap muscles (Fig. 9.**1**–9.**3**).

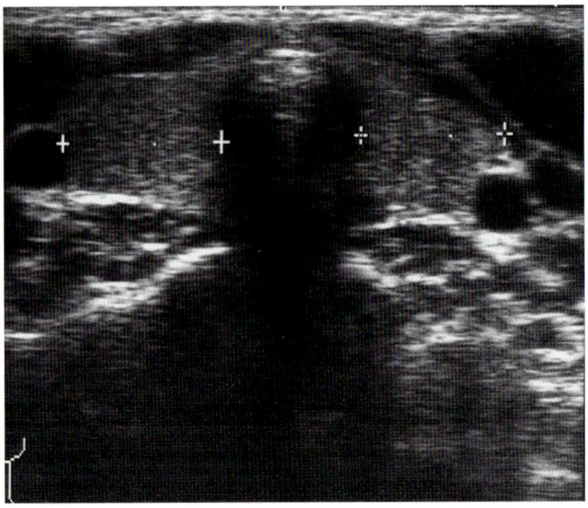

Fig. 9.**1 a** Transverse view of normal thyroid gland.

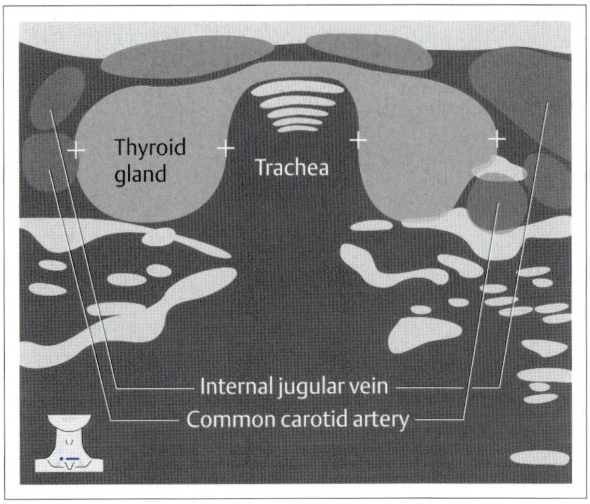

Fig. 9.**1 b** Line drawing.

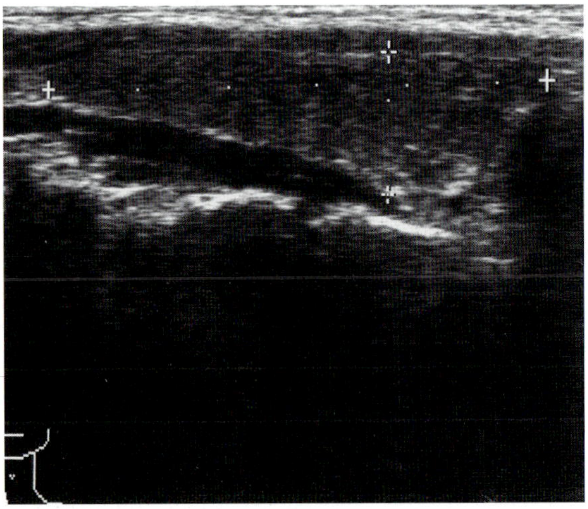

Fig. 9.**2 a** Longitudinal view of normal thyroid gland.

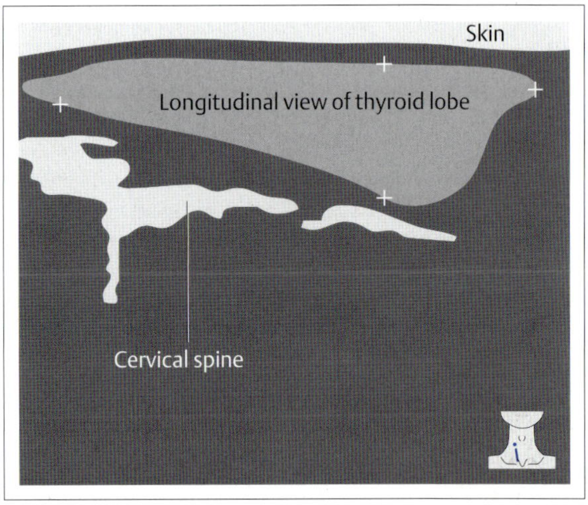

Fig. 9.**2 b** Line drawing.

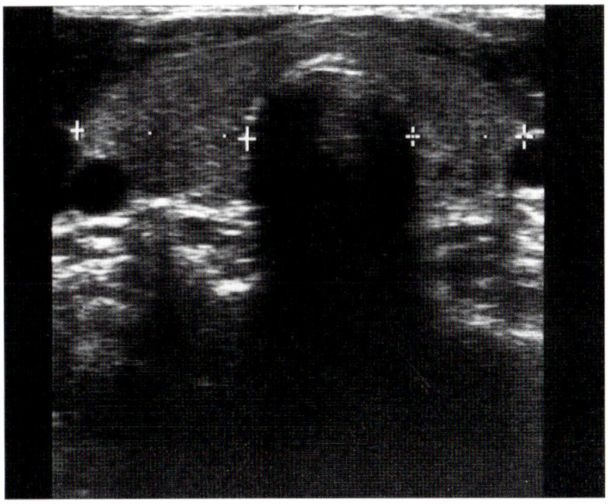

Fig. 9.3 **a** Asymmetrical thyroid gland with smaller left lobe (normal variant, transverse view).

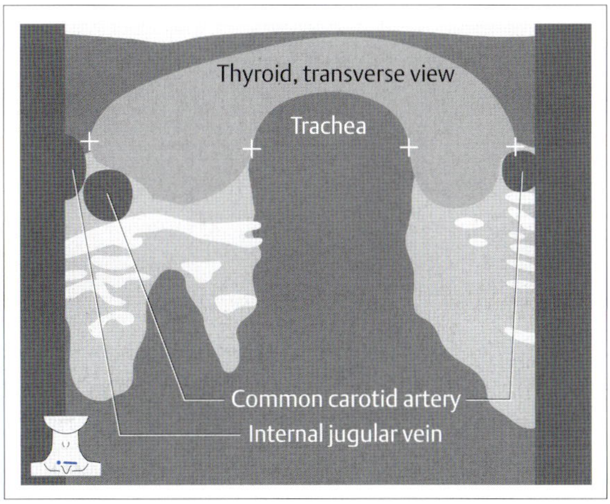

Fig. 9.3 **b** Line drawing.

Goiter

Basic Facts

- The incidence of endemic euthyroid goiter approximates 50% in iodine-deficient subjects in Germany (Hampel et al., 1995).
- Intrathyroidal iodine deficiency induces TSH-mediated cellular hypertrophy, while local growth factors (IGF, bFGF, EGF) promote proliferation of thyrocytes (Eggo and Sheppard, 1994).
- Sonographic volumetry is indispensable in the diagnosis of goiter and has replaced the WHO classification based solely on palpatory findings.
- On medical therapy with iodine and/or levothyroxine, goiter size reduces by around 30% within 6–12 months (Hintze et al., 1989).
- Iodine increases the rate of thyrocyte apoptosis (Sachse et al., 1997).
- Regressive changes (calcifications, postinflammatory scarring, or hemorrhage) and formation of nodules are increasingly encountered with advancing age; these are often also seen in recurrent goiter, e.g., following surgery.
- *Additional workup:* TSH for confirmation of normal thyroid function.

Sonographic Criteria

- Normal echotexture in the first years of manifest goiter.
- Organ enlargement (Figs. 9.**4**, 9.**5**).
- Regressive changes:
  - Heterogeneous, partly consolidated echotexture due to **scarring** and proliferated connective tissue.
  - **Cysts** (e.g., as sequelae of hemorrhage) appearing as anechoic areas with posterior acoustic enhancement.
  - **Calcifications** appearing as hyperechoic areas with posterior shadowing (Figs. 9.**6**, 9.**7**).

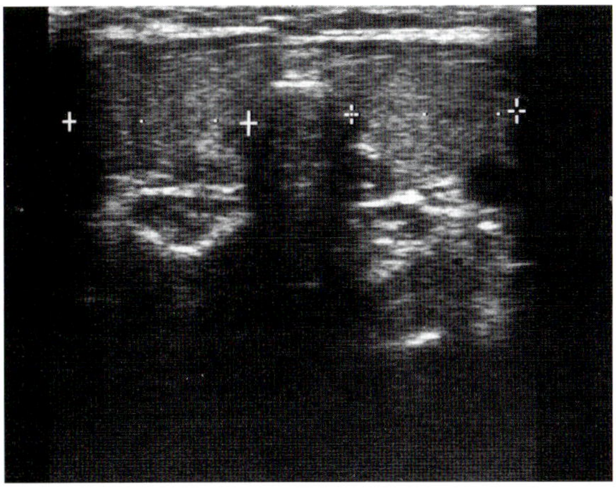

Fig. 9.4 **a** Transverse view of diffuse goiter, 29 ml total volume, homogeneous, and of normal echogenicity.

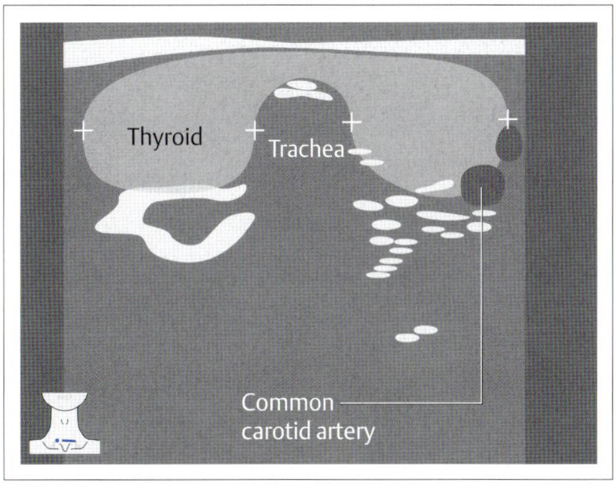

Fig. 9.4 **b** Line drawing.

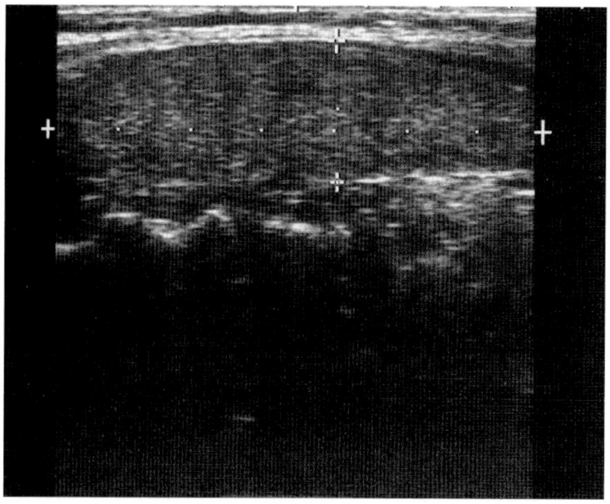

Fig. 9.**5 a** Same patient as in Fig. 9.**4**; longitudinal view.

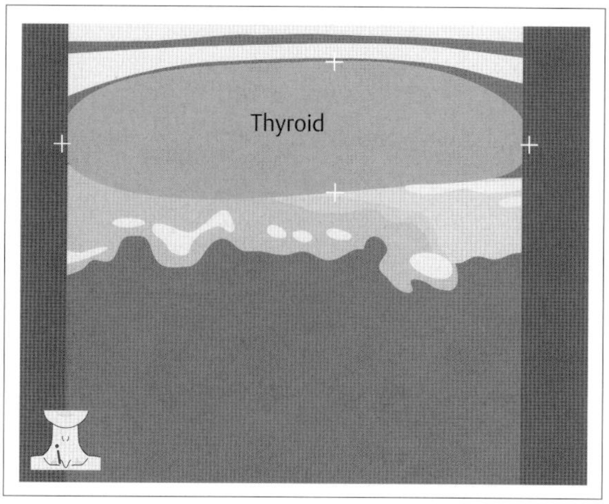

Fig. 9.**5 b** Line drawing.

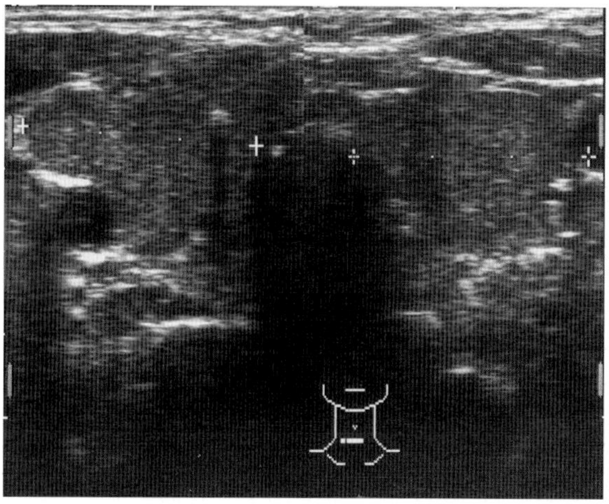

Fig. 9.**6 a** Transverse view of a goiter with regressive changes: Calcification (posterior shadowing) in the right thyroid lobe, heterogeneous echotexture.

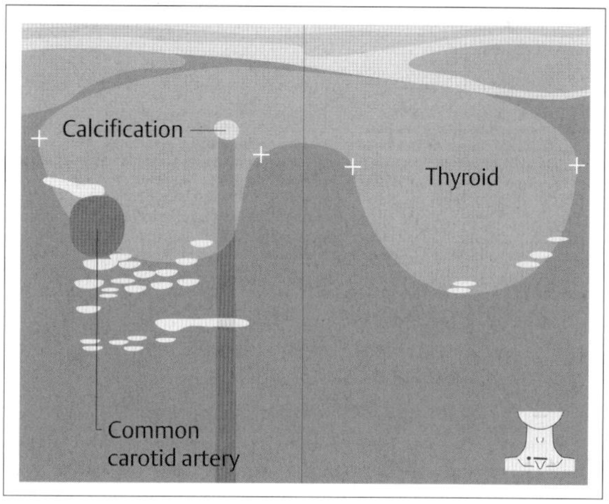

Fig. 9.**6 b** Line drawing.

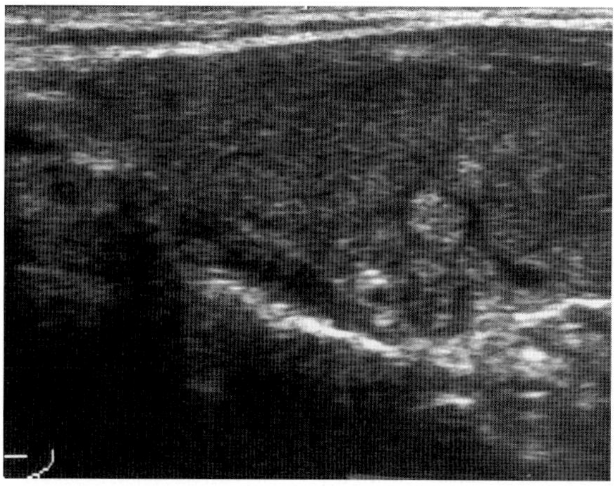

Fig. 9.**7 a** Longitudinal view with heterogeneities and small hyperechoic masses (regressive changes).

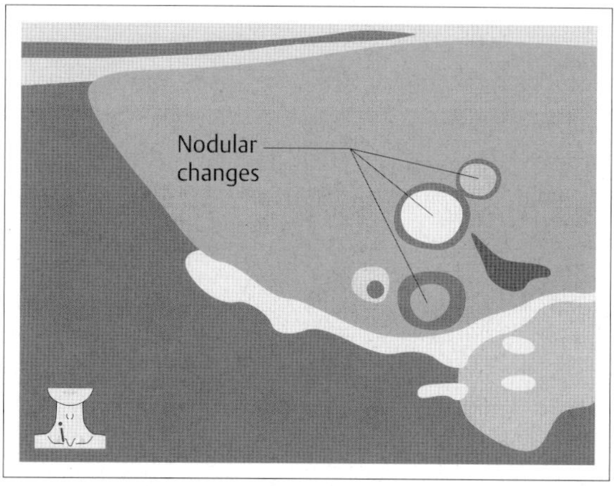

Fig. 9.**7 b** Line drawing.

Consequences for Surgical Treatment

Diagnosis	Characteristic Findings	Management
Goiter	Enlarged volume, normal echotexture	One year of medical therapy (e.g., 100–150 μg iodide + 50–125 μg levothyroxine/day (maintaining TSH at a low normal level), US follow-up after 6–12 months; surgery in refractory cases and in case of mechanical interference
Goiter with regressive changes, recurrent goiter	Heterogeneous echotexture, calcifications	Trial with levothyroxine over six months only in recurrent cases or volume increase confirmed by sonography; refractory cases and those with mechanical interference require reoperation or radioiodine ablation
Prophylaxis of recurrence after medical goiter treatment	Increase in the volume documented by sonography	Iodide 200 μg/day
Prophylaxis of recurrence after goiter surgery	(a) Volume > 8 ml (b) Volume < 8 ml (c) Very small residual volume	(a) Iodide 200 μg/day (b) Plus levothyroxine 50–150 μg/day (c) Levothyroxine alone 50–150 (max. 200) μg/day

Graves Disease

Basic Facts

- The pathogenesis of autoimmune hyperthyroidism (Graves disease) is not yet elucidated in every detail. It is multifactorial, with incidence in Germany estimated at 550 per 100 000 population per year.
- An autoimmune process with activation of T-lymphocytes is triggered by the influence of particular environmental factors (e.g., stress) in patients with corresponding genetic predisposition (Volpe, 1991).
- TSH receptor-stimulating antibodies (TRAbs) cause uncontrolled thyroid hormone synthesis.
- The typical clinical presentation of hyperthyroidism includes tachycardia, weight loss, sweating, and nervousness.
- Rate of recurrence is about 50%; higher for large goiters and in cases with high initial T_3 levels.
- As there are no definite predictors for lasting remission, long-term follow-up is mandatory; redevelopment of hypoechogenicity on ultrasound is suspicious for recurrent hyperthyroidism (Vitti et al., 1992).
- *Additional workup:* The diagnosis is established by laboratory parameters (e.g., TSH, fT_3, fT_4,), positive TRAbs; endocrine orbitopathy is pathognomonic of Graves' disease; the more severe orbitopathy requires ophthalmological co-treatment.

Sonographic Criteria

- In about 75% of patients, hypoechoic transformation (diffuse or small-focal) of the thyroid gland (Raue et al., 1992) and an increased A–P diameter are observed.
- Echogenicity frequently normalizes on remission.

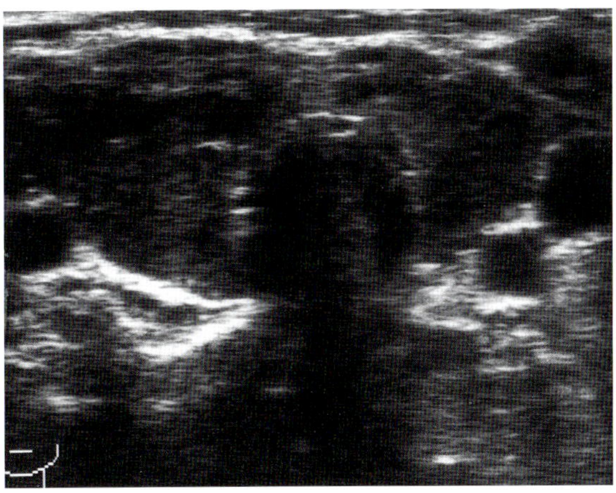

Fig. 9.**8a** Graves disease. Diffuse hypoechogenicity, increased A–P diameter (transverse view).

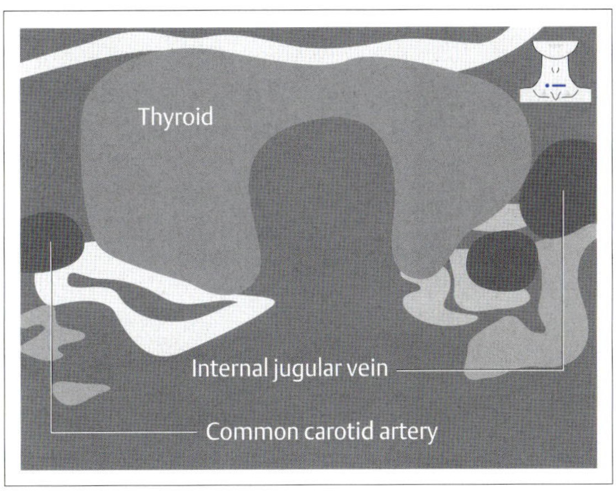

Fig. 9.**8b** Line drawing.

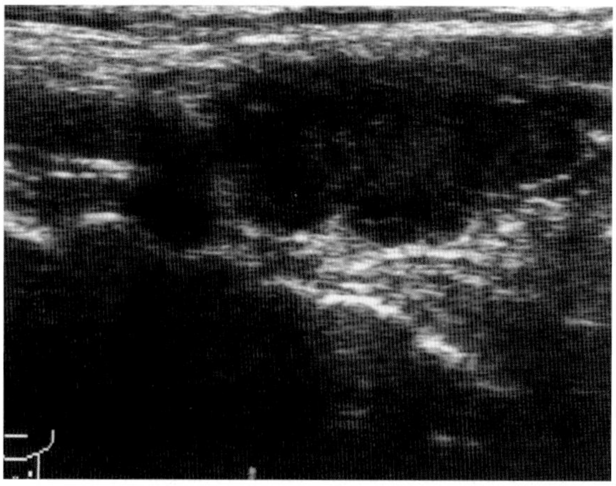

Fig. 9.**9 a** Graves disease. Longitudinal view of the thyroid gland with diffuse hypoechogenicity and irregular posterior surface.

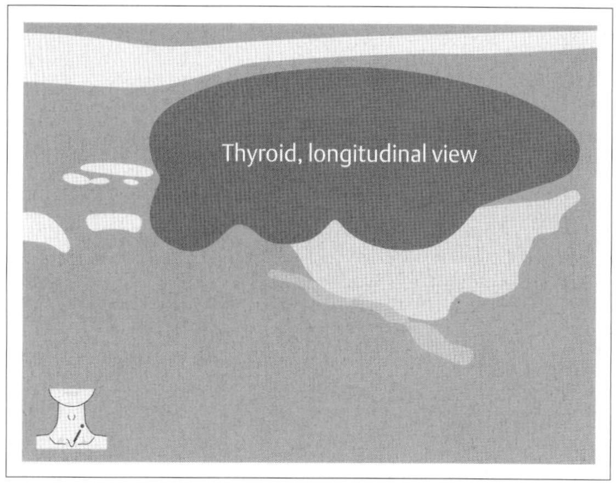

Fig. 9.**9 b** Line drawing.

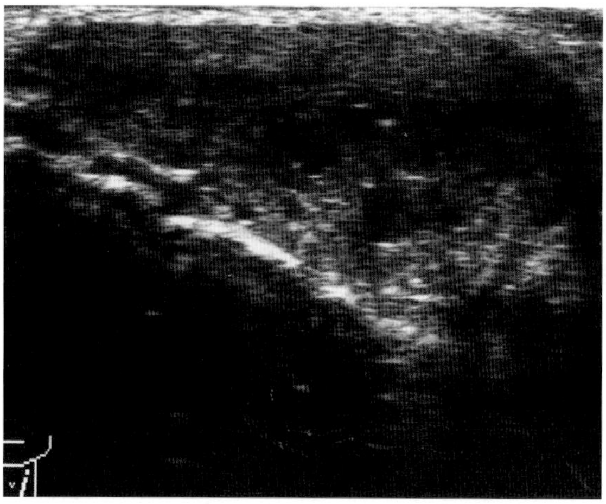

Fig. 9.**10 a** Longitudinal view of the thyroid gland with multiple small hypoechoic areas in a patient with Graves disease.

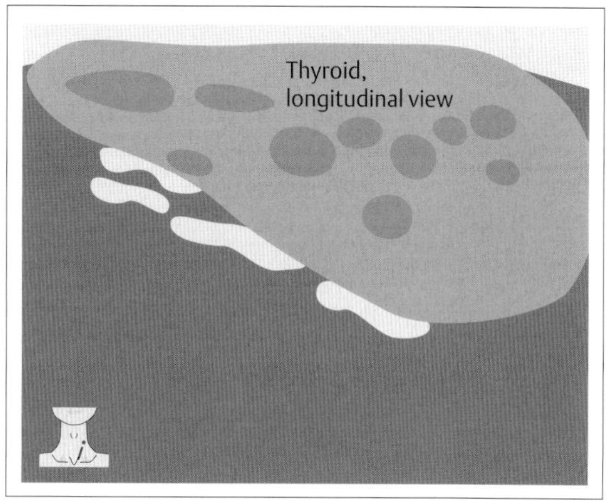

Fig. 9.**10 b** Line drawing.

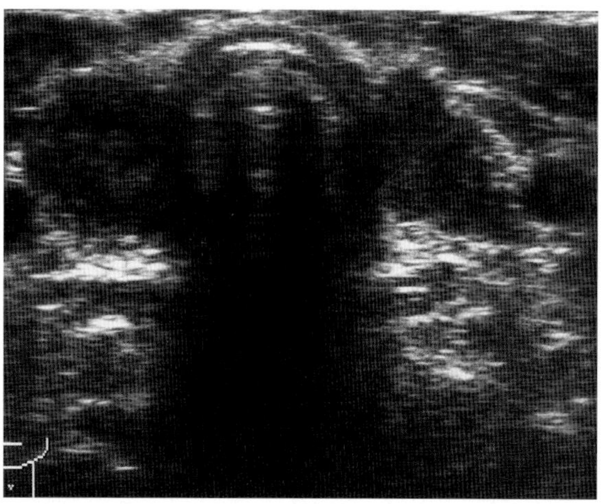

Fig. 9.**11 a** Recurrent Graves disease 25 years after thyroid surgery. Transverse view with predominantly right-sided hypoechoic recurrent goiter.

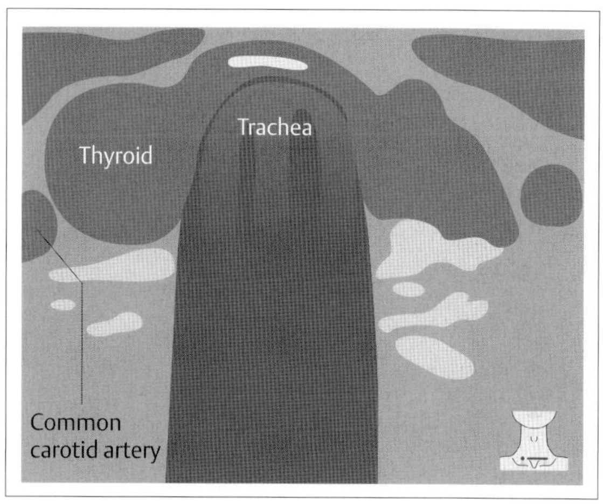

Fig. 9.**11 b** Line drawing.

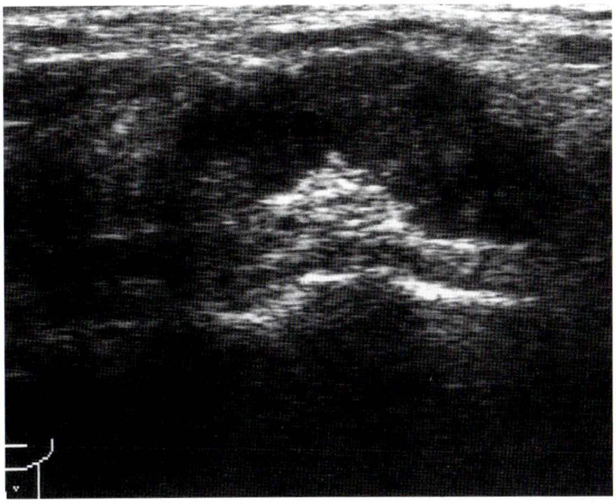

Fig. 9.**12a** Longitudinal view of the thyroid gland with recurrent goiter in a patient with Graves disease, lacking any normal lobar texture.

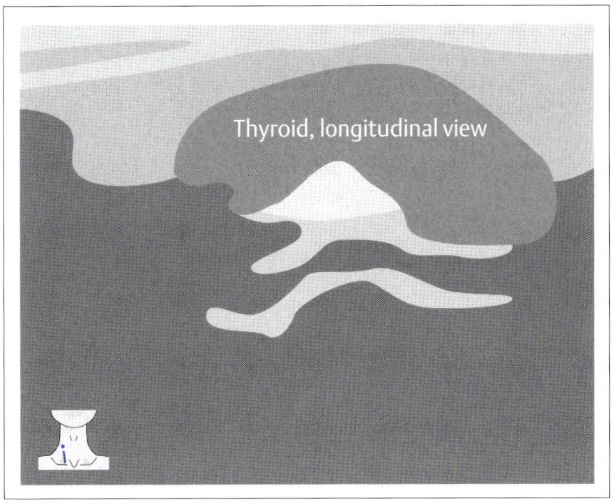

Fig. 9.**12b** Line drawing.

Consequences for Surgical Treatment

Diagnosis	Characteristic Findings	Management
Graves disease	Hypoechoic thyroid gland, increased A–P diameter	Primarily antithyroidal drug regimen (1–1.5 years), early surgical resection in case of side effects/large goiter with high initial T_3-levels In case of recurrence bilateral subtotal thyroid resection (residual volume below 3 ml) or radioiodine ablation, with 90% of patients requiring levothyroxine substitution (50–200 µg/day); a TSH level of 0.5–1.5 mU/l is recommended

Autoimmune Thyroiditis, Autoimmune Hypothyroidism, Postpartum Thyroiditis

Basic Facts

- Important features in the pathogenesis of autoimmune thyroiditis are infiltration of the thyroid gland with lymphocytes (Davies et al., 1991), liberation of cytokines, and cytotoxic antibody synthesis by autoreactive B-lymphocytes.
- In 90% of the patients, the level of thyroid peroxidase antibodies (TPO-Abs) is elevated.
- Increased thyrocyte apoptosis has been demonstrated (Hammond et al., 1997).
- The chronic inflammatory process remains clinically silent.
- Progressive destruction of thyrocytes eventually results in hypothyroidism with corresponding clinical signs and symptoms (weight gain, fatigue, impaired physical and mental performance, etc.)
- Concomitant goiter indicates Hashimoto thyroiditis, which must be differentiated from a primary chronic atrophic type with low thyroid gland volume.
- Postpartum thyroiditis is a syndrome of transient or permanent thyroid dysfunction within the first six months after delivery, leading to permanent hypothyroidism in 30% of affected women.
- Sonographic differential diagnosis has to consider diffuse thyroid hypoechogenicity commonly found after irradiation of the neck or radioiodine ablation; atrophy of the gland may be another sequela of radiation induced thyroiditis.
- *Additional workup:* blood chemistry–hypothyroidism is confirmed by elevated TSH levels; measurement of TPO-Abs and peripheral hormone levels is also recommended.

Sonographic Criteria

- Parenchymal hypoechogenicity (diffuse or small-focal), ill-defined against the surrounding structures of the neck; depending on the nature of the disease, **thyroid gland enlargement** or progressive atrophy is seen (Figs. 9.**13**, 9.**14**).
- In **autoimmune hypothyroidism** the hypoechoic echotexture of the gland does not normalize over the course of the disease.
- Focal (hypoechoic) nodules within the thyroid gland in confirmed **autoimmune thyroiditis** must undergo FNA and long-term follow-up, as there is an association with lymphoma and thyroid carcinoma (McKee et al., 1993).

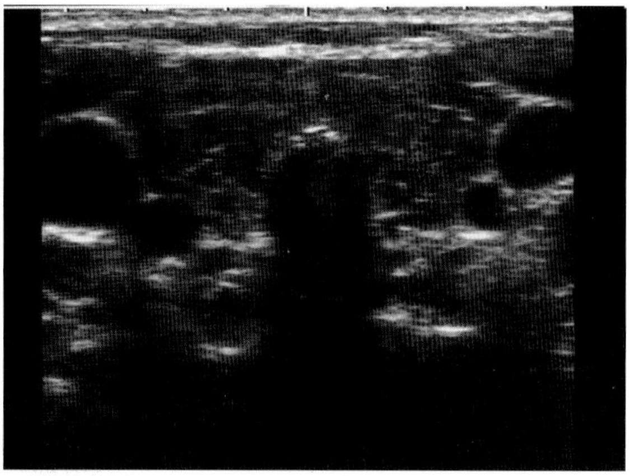

Fig. 9.**13 a** Autoimmune hypothyroidism. Transverse view of a low-volume thyroid gland with small hyperechoic areas of fibrosis.

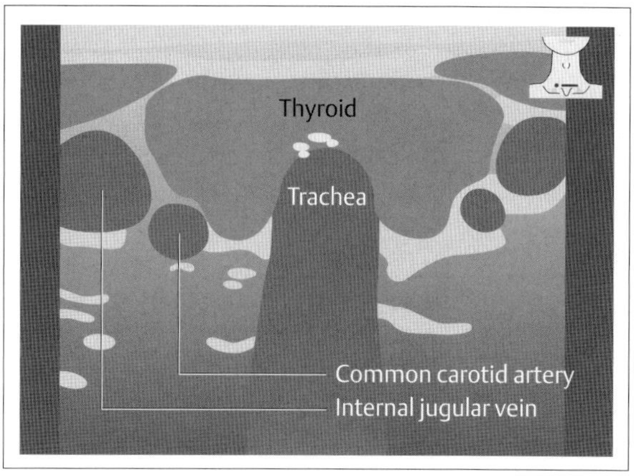

Fig. 9.**13 b** Line drawing.

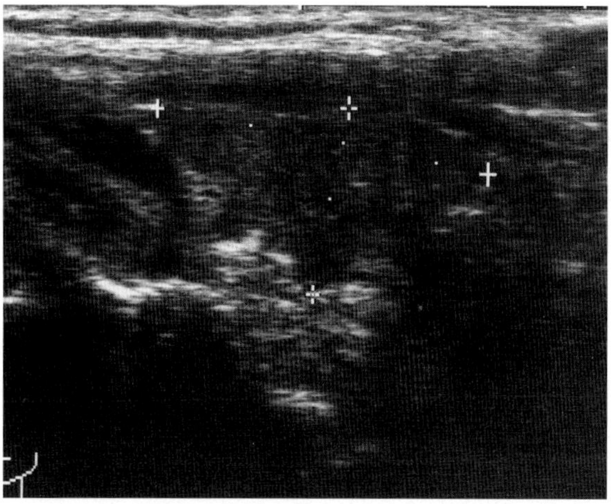

Fig. 9.**14 a** Longitudinal view of a thyroid gland with autoimmune hypothyroidism, poorly delimited against the surroundings; hypoechoic basic echotexture.

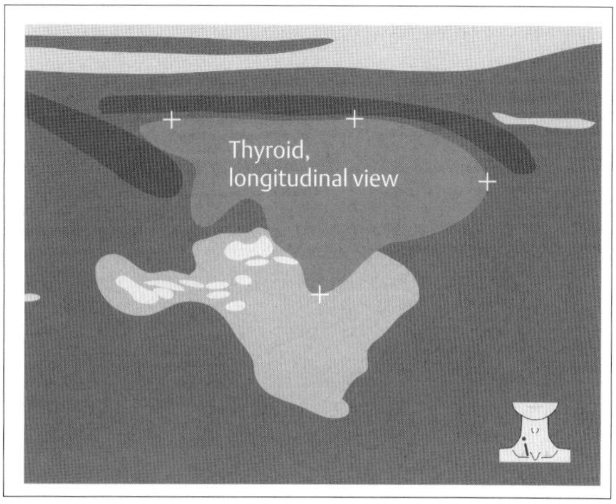

Fig. 9.**14 b** Line drawing.

Consequences for Surgical Treatment

Diagnosis	Characteristic Findings	Management
Autoimmune thyroiditis	Hypoechoic thyroid gland, atrophy (chronic-atrophic course) or goiter (Hashimoto thyroiditis) possible	In hypothyroidism, levothyroxine supplementation; TSH should be in the normal range (0.5–1.5 mU/l)
Postpartum thyroiditis	Hypoechoic thyroid gland	Possibly (transient) levothyroxine supplementation
Post irradiation/radioiodine ablation	Hypoechoic thyroid gland, small volume	Annual TSH check; in hypothyroidism, levothyroxine supplementation

Nodular Goiter

- In the general (German) population, nodular goiter has an incidence of approximately 30%.
- Sonographic classification is based on the echogenicity of the nodule, but this only permits morphological classification and not diagnosis (Table 9.**1**, Fig. 9.**15**)

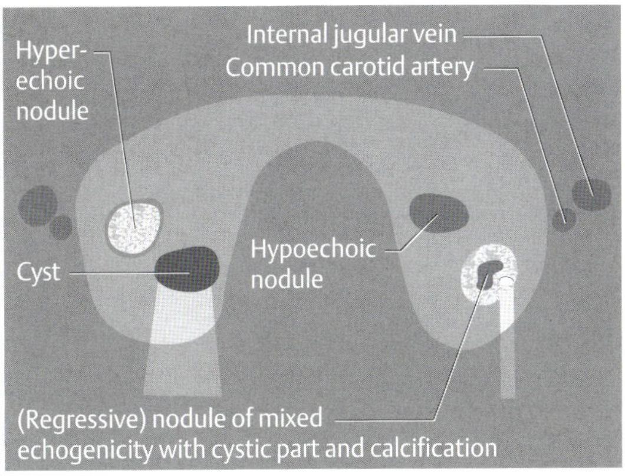

Fig. 9.**15** Nodular goiter. Line drawing.

Table 9.**1** Differentiation of thyroid nodules according to echogenicity

Echogenicity of the Nodule	Most Likely Diagnosis
Hyperechoic, isoechoic	Adenomatous (colloid) nodule
Hypoechoic	Follicular adenoma Malignoma Metastasis
Mixed echogenicity	Large nodules (follicular adenomas as well as colloid nodules) with regressive changes
Anechoic	Cyst

Adenomatous (Colloid) Nodule

Basic Facts

- Nodular areas, corresponding histologically to follicles rich in colloid, develop in the thyroid gland by proliferation and regressive parenchymal changes, especially in iodine-deficient regions.
- Mostly incidental sonographic findings; depending on their size they may become palpable or even visible.
- Scarring and connective tissue proliferation will increase echogenicity.
- About 15–25% of all focal autonomies are isoechoic or hyperechoic; hyperechogenicity is more likely to be observed in larger nodules with scarring and regressive changes (Becker et al., 1986).
- *Additional workup:* Assessment of metabolic situation (TSH); scintigraphy of large nodules (> 1.5–2 cm) in order to differentiate between functionally autonomous and nonfunctional tissue (cold nodules).

Sonographic Criteria

- **Colloid nodules** are isoechoic (Figs. 9.**16**, 9.**17**) or hyperechoic (Figs. 9.**18**, 9.**19**), frequently surrounded by a hypoechoic margin (halo, possibly fibrous or hyaline capsule), delimiting them against the remaining thyroid tissue (Fig. 9.**20**).
- **Malignancy** is unlikely if a hyperechoic nodule is completely surrounded by a halo (Daniels, 1996).
- **Calcifications** and cystic changes may be found within the nodule (cf. Fig. 9.**17**).

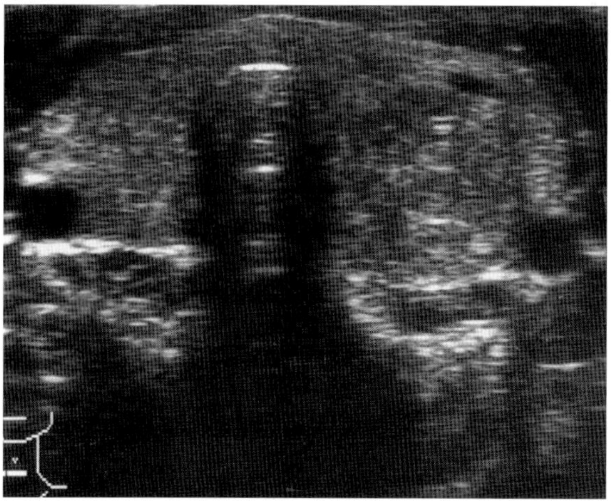

Fig. 9.**16 a** Isoechoic nodule in the left thyroid lobe (transverse view); scintigraphically cold; faint hypoechoic margin (halo).

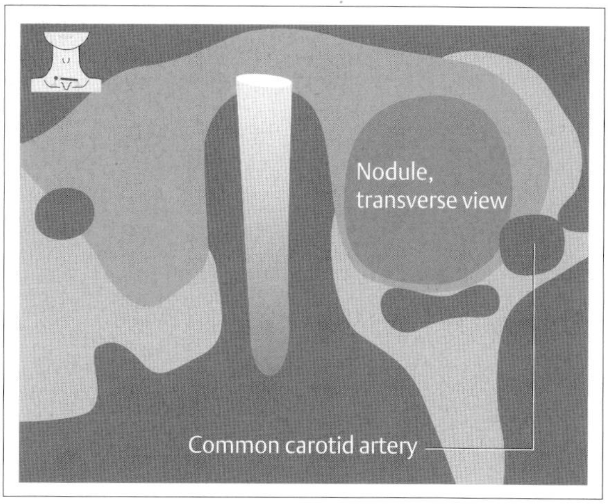

Fig. 9.**16 b** Line drawing.

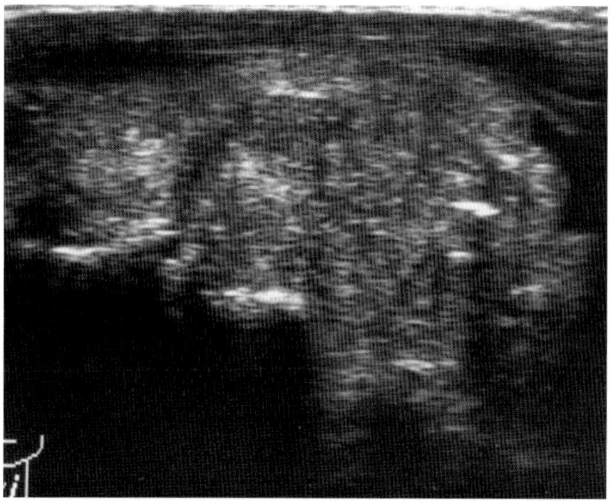

Fig. 9.**17 a** Longitudinal view through an isoechoic nodule with heterogeneous texture and calcification at its inferior margin.

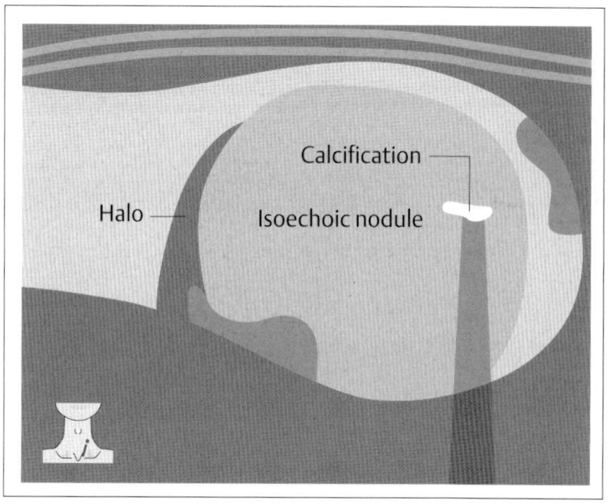

Fig. 9.**17 b** Line drawing.

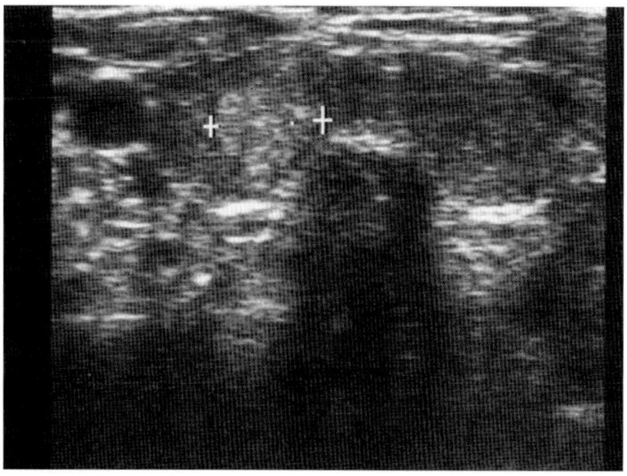

Fig. 9.**18 a** Hyperechoic nodule in the right thyroid lobe with a faint halo (transverse view).

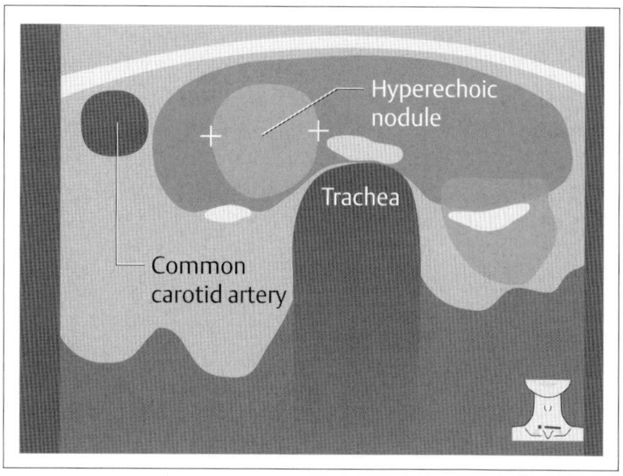

Fig. 9.**18 b** Line drawing.

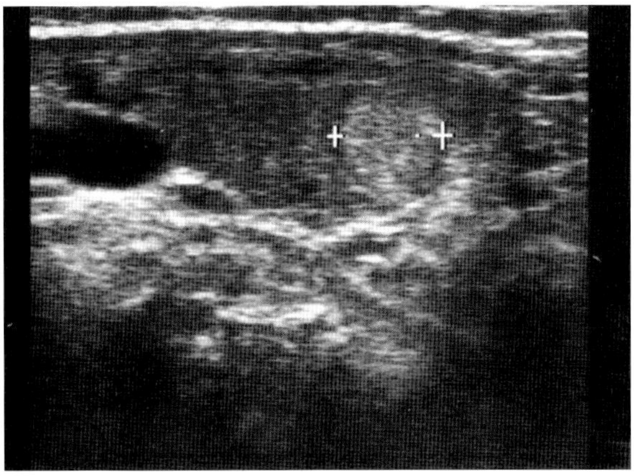

Fig. 9.**19 a** Hyperechoic nodule with a faint halo (longitudinal view).

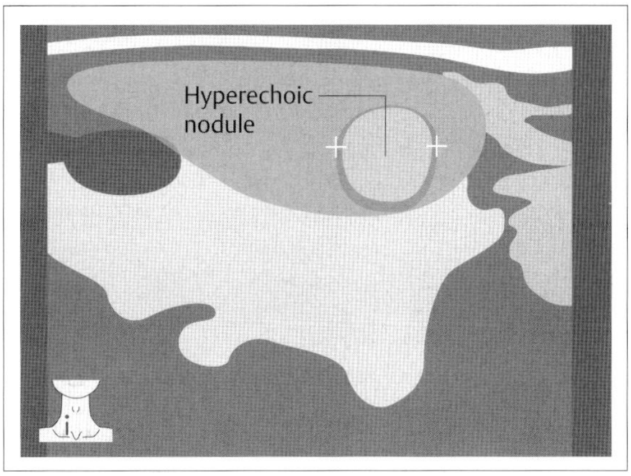

Fig. 9.**19 b** Line drawing.

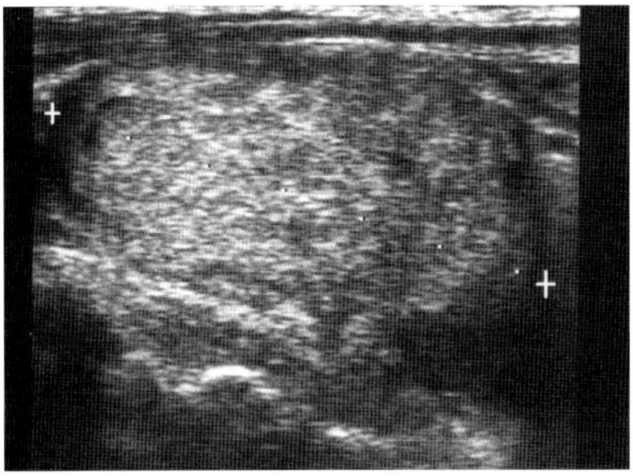

Fig. 9.**20 a** Large isoechoic heterogeneous nodule with halo, occupying almost all of the left thyroid lobe (longitudinal view).

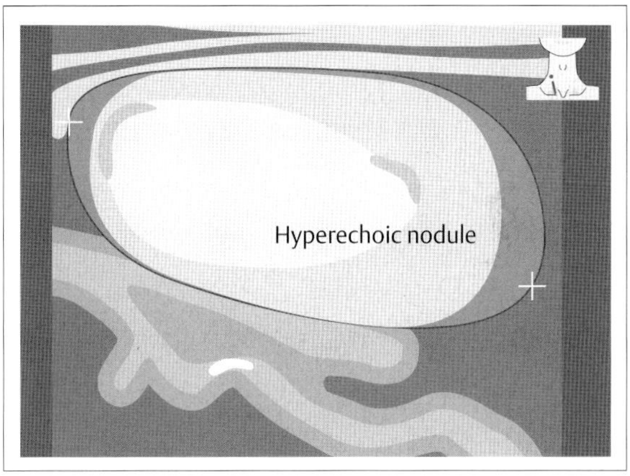

Fig. 9.**20 b** Line drawing.

Consequences for Surgical Treatment

Diagnosis	Characteristic Findings	Management
Adenomatous or colloid nodule	Isoechoic or hyperechoic nodule	Normal thyroid function: most probably benign → sonographic follow-up in 6–12 months; attempt at medical management only recommended for nodules < 2 cm; (functional) surgery in case of growth or symptoms

Follicular Adenomas

Basic Facts

- Intrathyroidal iodine deficiency is also relevant in the pathogenesis of thyroid adenoma.
- Thyrocyte populations can be characterized by different growth and functional qualities ("thyroid heterogeneity").
- Focal hyperplasia of cells with increased growth potential results in nodule formation by monoclonal or polyclonal proliferation (Berghout et al., 1990).
- In addition, somatic mutations in the TSH receptor gene or G-protein may also trigger formation of thyroid nodules (Russo et al., 1996).
- In Germany, the frequency of somatic mutations has been estimated at 40–50% (Hamacher et al., 1995).
- Follicular adenomas may appear as hyperfunctional as well as hypofunctional nodules.
- Sonographic echogenicity varies greatly and thus does not permit any inferences regarding either cellular morphology or metabolic activity, or sonographic differentiation from adenomatous-hyperplastic parenchymal lesions.
- About 70% of all autonomous adenomas correspond with hypoechoic thyroid nodules (Becker et al., 1986), 50% of which display a heterogeneous texture with hypoechoic and anechoic areas (Wiedemann et al., 1993).
- On scintigraphy, regressive/cystic changes are seen in hyperfunctional as well as hypofunctional adenomas.
- Determination of malignancy is not possible on the basis of sonomorphology alone, since adenomas, thyroid malignancy, and colloid nodules with small-cystic transformation may all appear as hypoechoic nodules.
- For a hypoechoic thyroid nodule, cytological and histological assessment must always be considered.
- Cytological findings of follicular neoplasia always require histopathological clarification, as follicular carcinoma cannot be ruled out.
- *Additional workup:* assessment of thyroid function (TSH, possibly fT_4); scintigraphy in euthyroid patients with nodules > 1.5 cm and in hyperthyroidism; FNA of solitary hypoechoic or otherwise suspect nodules.

Sonographic Criteria

- Typically hypoechoic nodules (Figs. 9.**21**, 9.**22**), sometimes mixed echogenicity with cystic changes (Fig. 9.**23**) or calcification.
- About one-third of all follicular adenomas present as isoechoic or hyperechoic nodules.

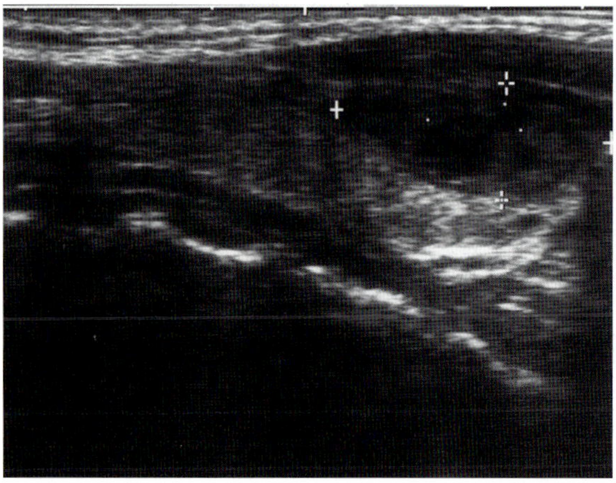

Fig. 9.**21 a** Longitudinal view of a hypoechoic nodule (small adenoma) with posterior enhancement.

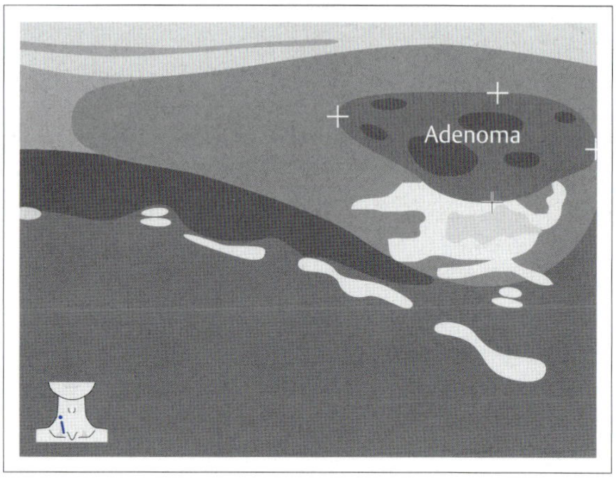

Fig. 9.**21 b** Line drawing.

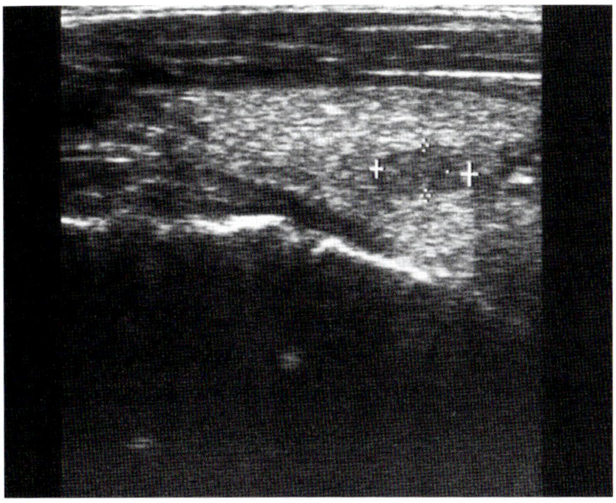

Fig. 9.22 a Longitudinal view of a hypoechoic nodule with anechoic areas and faint halo (follicular adenoma).

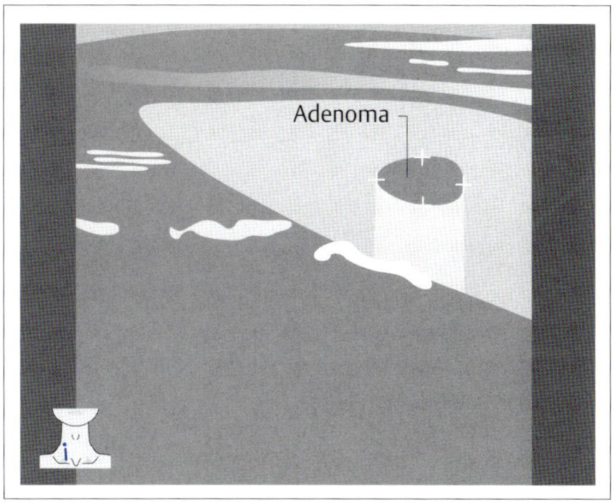

Fig. 9.22 b Line drawing.

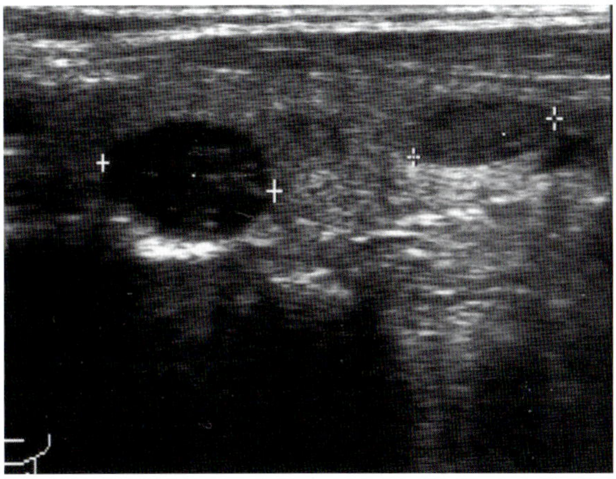

Fig. 9.23 a Two hypoechoic nodules: cranial nodule with anechoic (i.e., cystic) parts; small hypoechoic nodule caudal with posterior enhancement.

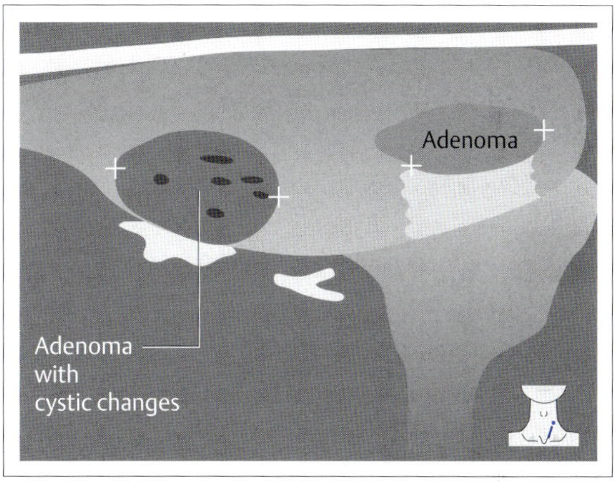

Fig. 9.23 b Line drawing.

Consequences for Surgical Treatment

Diagnosis	Characteristic Findings	Management
Adenoma	Primarily hypoechoic nodules (70%), the remainder hyperechoic; often isoechoic/hyperechoic plus cysts, calcification	*Hypofunctional nodule:* FNA–depending on outcome (malignancy or follicular neoplasia) or on mechanical symptoms the nodule should be excised; otherwise six-month follow-up *Hyperfunctional nodule:* Follow-up in case of normal thyroid function. Caveat: Iodine contamination at low TSH levels. In hyperthyroidism, antithyroid drug regimen until euthyroidism is obtained, then excision of the nodule or radioiodine ablation.

Thyroid Cysts

Basic Facts

- Between 15% and 25% of all thyroid nodules are cysts (Rojeski and Gharib, 1985).
- Contents may be serous, colloidal, or hemorrhagic fluid.
- Clinically, palpable nodules seem to arise "out of the blue," causing local symptoms depending on their size.
- Sonographic diagnosis confirmed by FNA.
- Purely serous cysts are benign.
- Hemorrhagic or "chocolate" cysts arise from hemorrhage into existing nodules and only rarely as sequelae to cervical trauma.
- Here, too, definitive diagnosis requires FNA.
- Cysts with solid wall areas are more likely to be malignant.
- After aspiration of the liquid contents, biopsies must be taken from the solid parts for cytological evaluation.
- Recurrence rates are high after simple aspiration of liquid cyst contents.
- *Additional workup:* None required if sonography provides unequivocal findings of a simple cyst in a clinically euthyroid patient; otherwise, TSH level and possibly scintigraphy (cysts appear as cold nodules on scintigraphy).

Sonographic Criteria

- **Serous or colloid cysts** can be reliably diagnosed sonographically by their appearance as anechoic masses with a smooth wall and posterior enhancement (Fig. 9.**24**)
- **Hemorrhagic cysts** display solitary internal echoes in most cases.
- With progressive absorption of blood constituents, the texture becomes heterogeneous, particularly along the margins; weblike, sometimes septated, hyperechoic structures (Fig. 9.**25**) and polypoid structures protruding into the lumen may be present (so-called **complicated cyst**; Fig. 9.**26**).

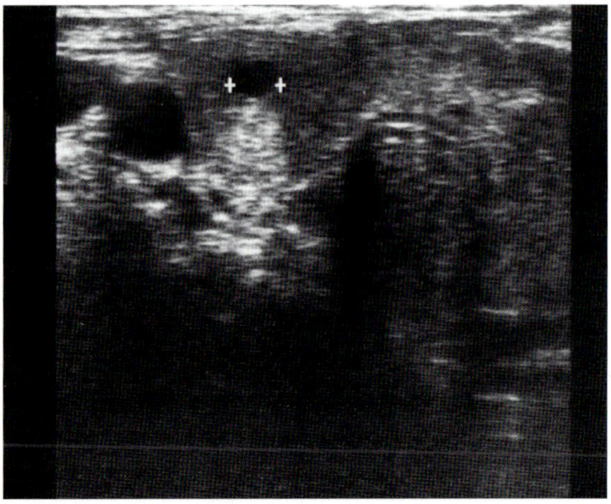

Fig. 9.**24 a** Transverse view of a small cyst (anechoic with posterior enhancement) in the right lobe of the thyroid gland.

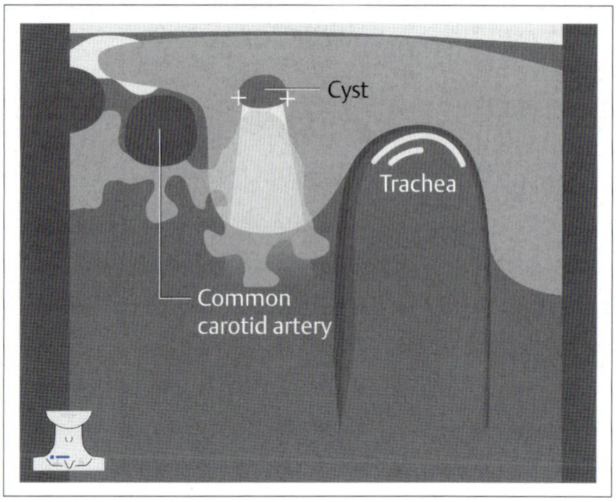

Fig. 9.**24 b** Line drawing.

Consequences for Surgical Treatment

Diagnosis	Characteristic Findings	Management
Serous cyst	Anechoic lesion, posterior enhancement	FNA evacuating the cyst; excision of recurrent cysts
Hemorrhagic cyst	Internal echoes possible, margin hyperechoic, septation (hyperechoic formations)	FNA; surgical excision in case of recurrence/local symptoms/suspected malignancy

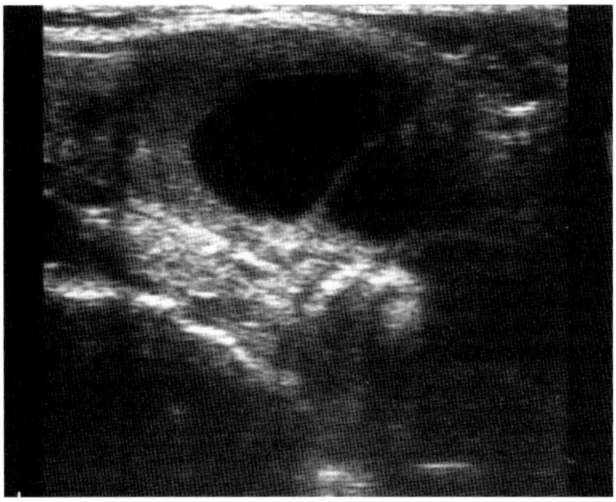

Fig. 9.25 a Large hemorrhagic cyst in the left lobe of the thyroid gland with hyperechoic margin and septation ("complicated cyst").

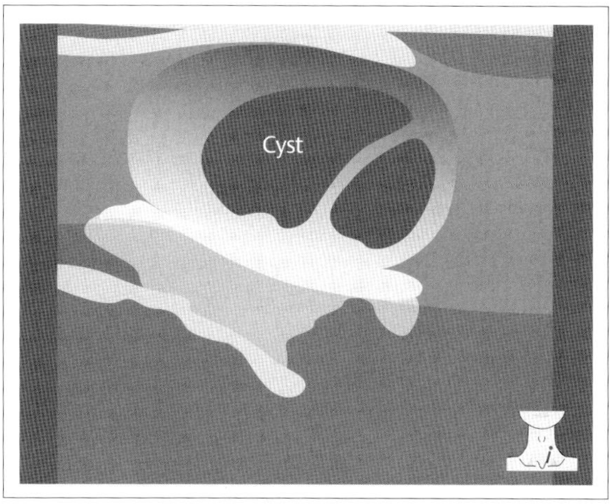

Fig. 9.25 b Line drawing.

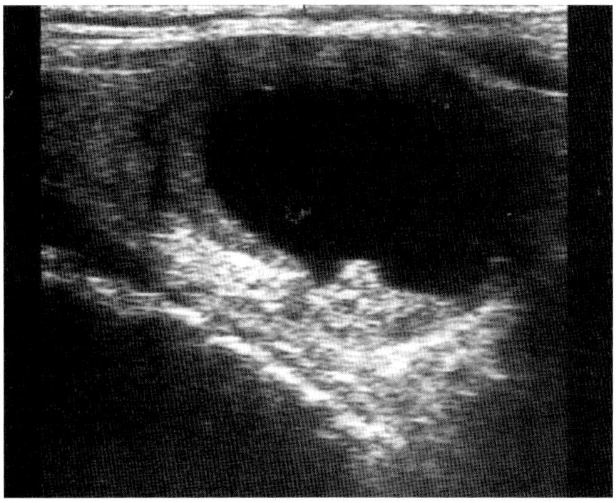

Fig. 9.26 a Large hemorrhagic cyst with hyperechoic margin and a polypoid structure protruding into the lumen.

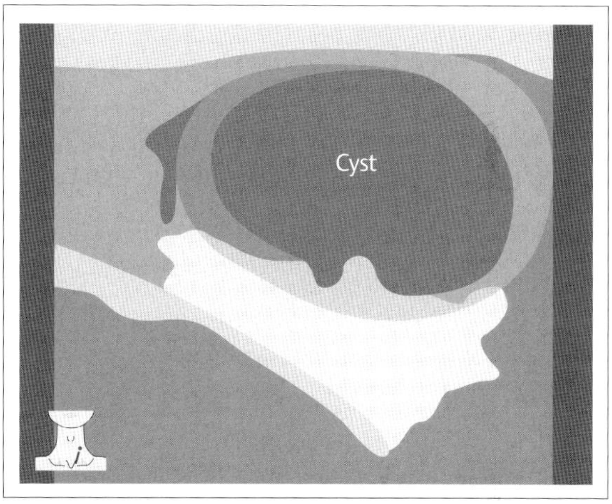

Fig. 9.26 b Line drawing.

Nodules with Cystic Changes

Basic Facts

- Rapid growth, hemorrhage, and regressive changes of nodules result in cystic lesions.
- Differentiation from a true cyst is difficult if a nodule exhibits large cystic parts.
- *Additional workup:* Thyroid function tests; in hyperthyroidism (including subclinical hyperthyroidism with TSH suppression) scintigraphy is needed to rule out focal autonomy.

Sonographic Criteria

- In **nodular goiter** with regressive changes, nodules of variable echogenicity are often intermixed with cystic formations (Fig. 9.**27**), calcifications, and a heterogeneous echotexture of the entire thyroid gland.
- A broad margin or intracystic remnants of solid thyroid tissue are characteristic of **former nodules**.

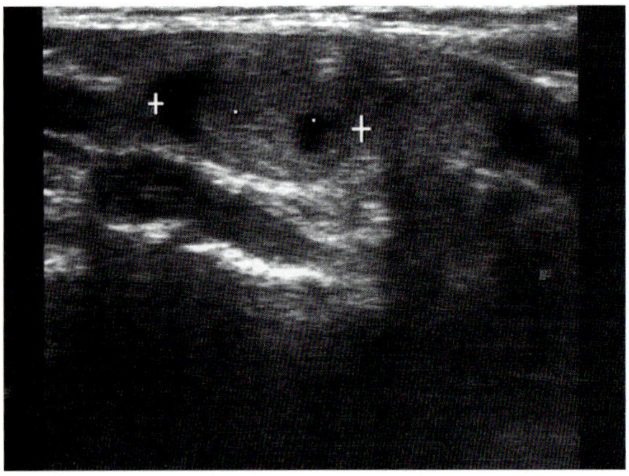

Fig. 9.**27 a** Longitudinal view of a small cystic hypoechoic nodule in the right lobe of the thyroid gland.

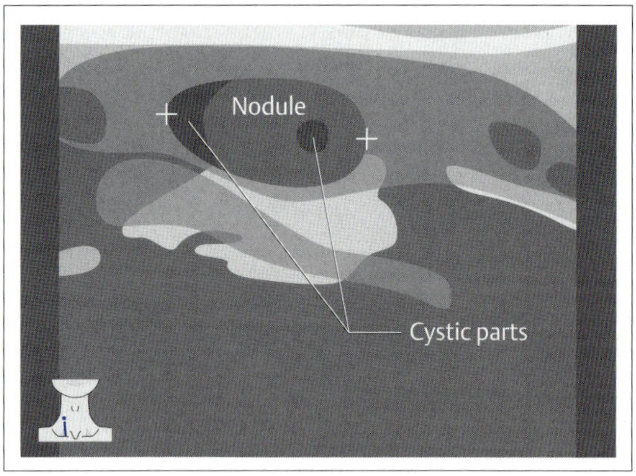

Fig. 9.**27 b** Line drawing.

Consequences for Surgical Treatment

Diagnosis	Characteristic Findings	Management
Solitary cystic nodule	Nodules with varying degrees of echogenicity and anechoic areas	Confirmation of diagnosis! (TSH, perhaps fT_3/T_4), possibly scintigraphy. Autonomous adenoma: in hyperthyroidism antithyroid medication and enucleation of nodule or radioiodine ablation. Cold nodule/mechanical symptoms: FNA, surgical resection
Cystic nodule in thyroid gland with nodular and/or regressive changes	Nodule with cystic areas, heterogeneous thyroid texture, possibly calcifications	Normal thyroid function: possibly FNA. Suspicious nodule: TSH, possibly scintigraphy. In hyperthyroidism/mechanical symptoms: function-oriented resection sparing normal tissue

Malignancy

Basic Facts

- With an incidence of 2–5 cases per 100 000 population per year, thyroid carcinoma is rare, comprising 0.5% of all malignant tumors (Raue, 1995); there is a female preponderance of 2–3 to 1 (Foitzik, 1996; Mann, 1994).
- About 5% of all hypoechoic thyroid nodules (Gharib, 1994; Giuffrida and Gharib, 1995) and 5–15% of all hypofunctional nodules are thyroid malignancies (Rojeski and Gharib, 1985).
- 60–90% of all thyroid malignancies are hypoechoic nodules, sometimes of irregular shape.
- Histologically, differentiated (papillary, follicular) and undifferentiated (anaplastic) tumors originate from the thyrocytes, while medullary carcinomas are derived from the calcitonin-producing C-cells; squamous cell carcinoma, sarcoma, and lymphoma are uncommon entities.
- Excellent 10-year survival rate for differentiated thyroid carcinoma (70–90%), with a significantly poorer prognosis for anaplastic carcinoma (3% after 2 years).
- At surgery, > 80% of papillary carcinomas have already metastasized to the regional lymph nodes (particularly into the central compartment), multilocular growth is possible.
- Microcarcinomas (nodules < 10 mm) are frequent incidental findings in surgical or postmortem gland specimens (10–13%) (Martinez-Tello et al., 1993); their biological significance is unknown to date.
- Work-up of medullary carcinomas must include molecular genetic screening for multiple endocrine neoplasia (MEN) and familial variants.
- *Additional workup:* TSH to confirm normal thyroid function; in case of clinical evidence of medullary carcinoma (e.g., diarrhea) or a positive family history, calcitonin level; possibly scintigraphy (cold nodule), FNA.
- **Caveat:** In males or after irradiation of the neck, workup of every hypoechoic nodule, particularly if solitary, must include the differential diagnosis of a carcinoma.

Sonographic Criteria

- Primarily hypoechoic nodules (Fig. 9.**28**)
- Finely dispersed microcalcifications or clumped calcifications have been described in papillary (Fig. 9.**29**) and medullary carcinomas (Wheeler, 1996).
- Sonographic signs of malignancy:
  - Irregular shape (Fig. 9.**28**)
  - Heterogeneous hypoechoic and anechoic areas
  - Intranodular calcification
  - Advanced tumor stage: spread beyond the thyroid gland with diffuse or absent demarcation against the surroundings (capsular break) (Fig. 9.**30**)
  - Lymphadenopathy
- Posterior attenuation despite an almost anechoic echotexture of the nodule, owing to fibrotic changes and calcifications (Wiedemann, 1993).
- Liquefaction is possible in tumor necrosis.

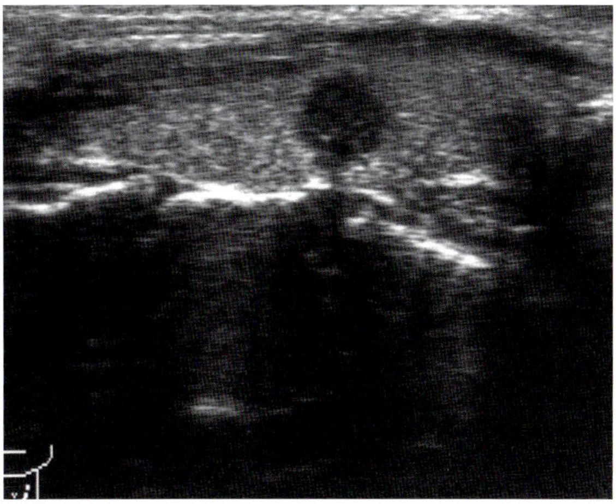

Fig. 9.**28a** Small hypoechoic nodule with polycyclic margin in the left lobe of the thyroid gland. Medullary carcinoma.

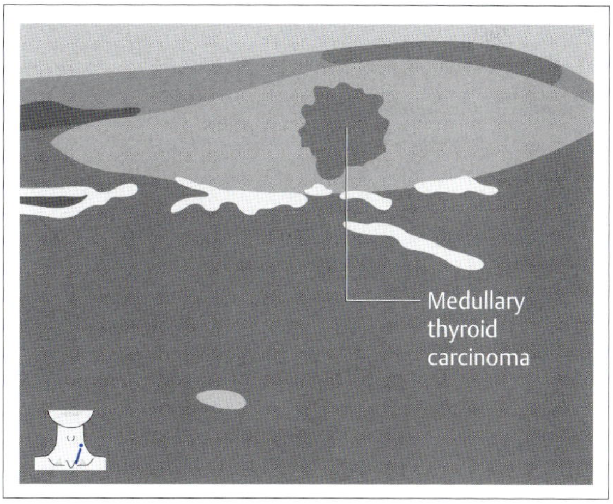

Fig. 9.**28b** Line drawing.

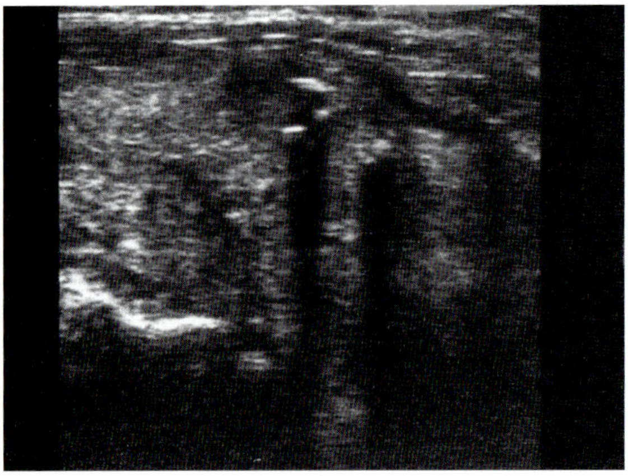

Fig. 9.**29 a** Papillary thyroid carcinoma. Small hypoechoic nodule with numerous intranodular and marginal microcalcifications.

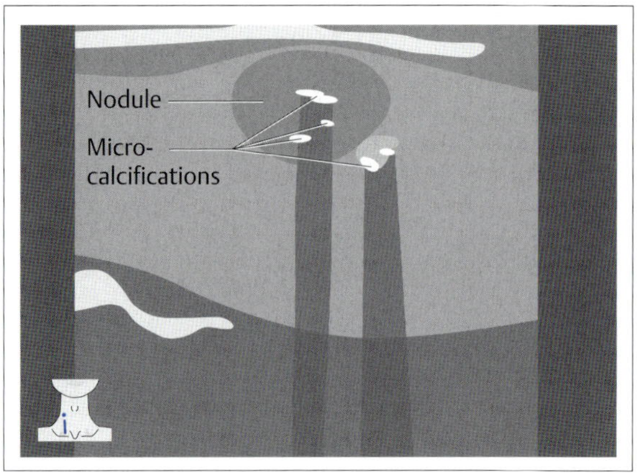

Fig. 9.**29 b** Line drawing.

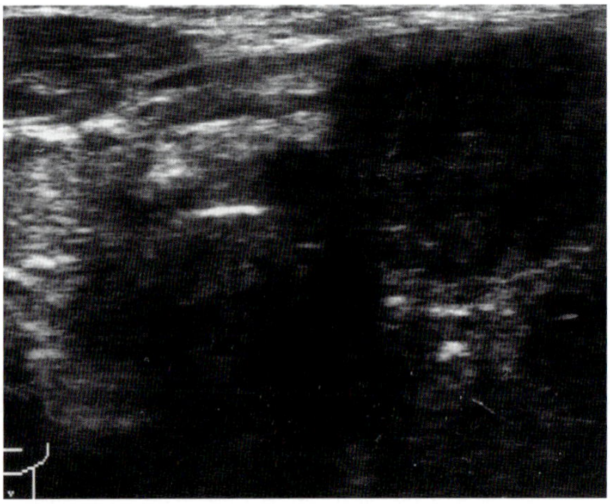

Fig. 9.**30 a** Large hypoechoic, almost anechoic mass completely filling the left lobe and not defined against the adjacent tissue. Anaplastic carcinoma.

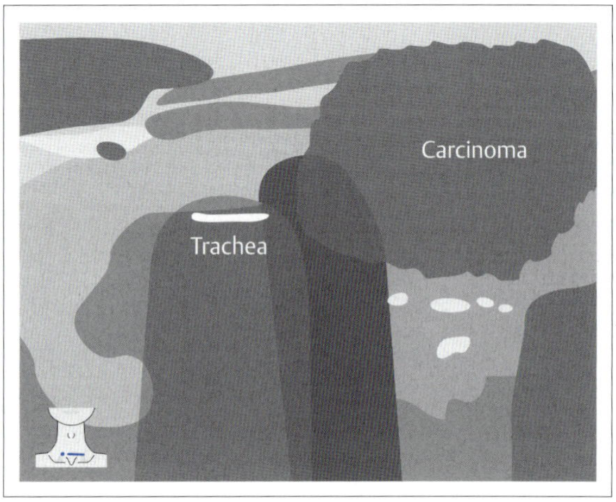

Fig. 9.**30 b** Line drawing.

Consequences for Surgical Treatment

Diagnosis	Characteristic Findings	Management
Malignancy	Hypoechoic nodule, irregular margin, microcalcifications, lymphadenopathy	Diagnostic confirmation by FNA; thyroidectomy, lymphadenectomy depending on histopathology (papillary/medullary carcinoma); in differentiated carcinomas subsequent radioiodine ablation followed by TSH suppressive drug therapy; in medullary carcinoma calcitonin level serves as tumor marker. Hemithyroidectomy is sufficient in papillary and follicular microcarcinomas up to 1 cm

Thyroiditis

Basic Facts

- Those parts of the gland affected by thyroiditis can be differentiated from normal thyroid tissue as hypoechoic or almost anechoic areas.
- Apart from resulting in sharply defined nodular lesions, the inflammation can invade entire thyroid lobes in a heterogeneous pattern.
- Both acute and subacute thyroiditis (except for "silent" thyroiditis) is characterized clinically by a painful gland; fever and elevated markers of inflammation are typical for the acute type.

Subacute De Quervain Thyroiditis

- Severe illness with a painful thyroid gland and flulike general symptoms.
- The pain can involve both lobes in succession and radiate to the angle of the mandible.
- A viral infection superimposed on a genetic predisposition probably plays a role in the pathogenesis.
- Disintegration of thyroid tissue affected by the inflammation liberates thyroid hormones, resulting in transient hyperthyroidism.
- Evident hypothyroidism later in the course develops only in a small percentage of patients.
- *Additional workup:* FNA (granulomatous inflammation with epithelioid and giant cells) confirms the diagnosis; blood tests: TSH, fT_4, markers of inflammation.

"Silent" Thyroiditis

- Up to 25% of subacute thyroiditis cases are clinically silent and only manifest when hyperthyroidism develops.
- Cytology reveals dense infiltration of the thyroid gland with lymphocytes; frequently precipitated by iodine exposure.
- *Additional workup:* TSH, TPO-Abs; missing Technetium uptake in scintigraphy permits differentiation from autoimmune hyperthyroidism.

Acute Thyroiditis

- Purulent inflammation of the thyroid gland is rare.
- Fever, significantly elevated markers of inflammation, and local tender swelling of the thyroid gland are pathognomonic.
- *Additional workup:* Possibly FNA to obtain specimens for microbiology (consider rare infections such as actinomycosis).

Sonographic Criteria

- **De Quervain thyroiditis** and **"silent thyroiditis"**: ill-defined, partially confluent hypoechoic areas within the thyroid gland between unaffected thyroid tissue of normal echogenicity (Fig. 9.**31**).
- The involved parts of the thyroid gland become hyperechoic the more fibrosis progresses.
- **Acute thyroiditis:** hypoechoic mass with coarse echotexture; in case of abscess also with hypoechoic or anechoic areas interspersed within an otherwise normal thyroid gland (Fig. 9.**32**).

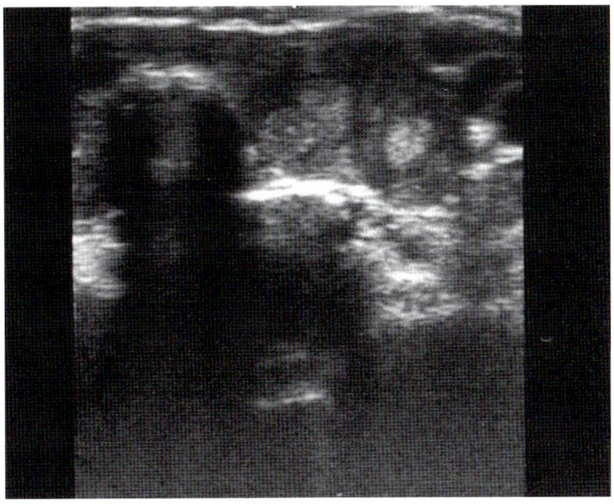

Fig. 9.**31 a** De Quervain thyroiditis affecting the left lobe of the thyroid gland, characterized partially by nodule-like confluent formations of mixed echogenicity.

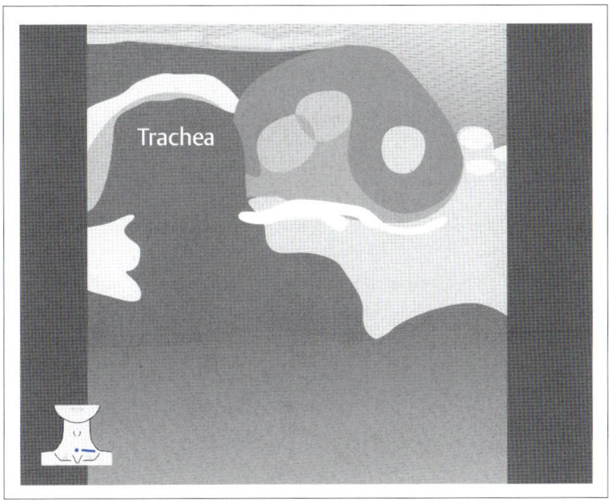

Fig. 9.**31 b** Line drawing.

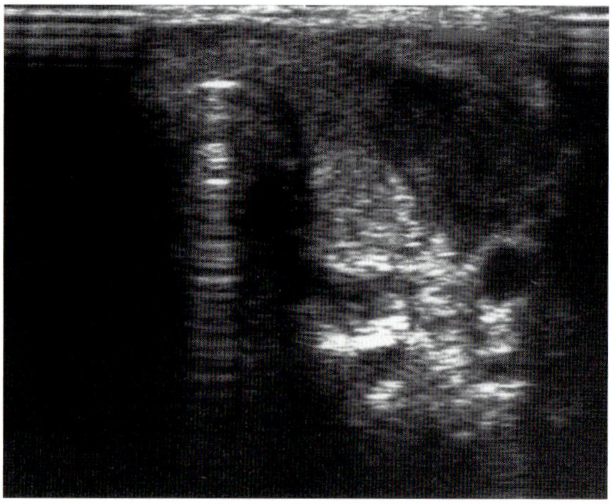

Fig. 9.**32a** Heterogeneous hypoechoic, irregularly defined structure in the left lobe of the thyroid gland in acute thyroiditis, compressing the normal thyroid tissue.

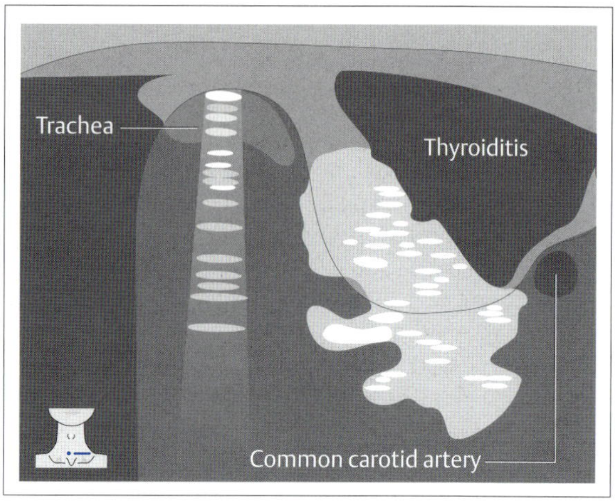

Fig. 9.**32b** Line drawing.

Consequences for Surgical Treatment

Diagnosis	Characteristic Findings	Management
De Quervain thyroiditis and "**silent thyroiditis**"	Hypoechogenic areas, either focal or involving larger parts of the thyroid lobes; hyperechoic or complex echogenicity changes in chronic stage or transition to fibrosis	Nonsurgical. Depending on the metabolic state: beta-blockers for hyperthyroidism due to cellular necrosis, NSAIDs, glucocorticosteroids (rapid clinical relief); levothyroxine in hypothyroidism
Acute thyroiditis	Hypoechoic masses depending on the degree of affection; in progressive inflammation ill-defined against the cervical soft tissues	FNA for MCS, antibiotics, possibly surgical resection

Riedel Thyroiditis

Basic Facts

- Chronic invasive fibrous thyroiditis, also called Riedel struma, is a rare disease with severe local discomfort and pain, characterized by the physical sign of an absolutely rigid goiter.
- Pathogenesis is assumed to be a cytokine-mediated excessive fibrotic reaction triggered by an autoimmune process (Heufelder and Hay, 1994).
- Association with fibrosis at other sites (e.g., retroperitoneum, orbit) has been demonstrated.
- *Additional workup:* In any firm infiltration of the thyroid gland malignancy must definitely be ruled out (FNA or surgery); TSH level to rule out hypothyroidism.

Sonographic Criteria

- Thyroid areas affected by the inflammation demonstrate a hypoechoic echotexture (Fig. 9.**33**).
- Fibrosis ill-defined against the surrounding tissue.

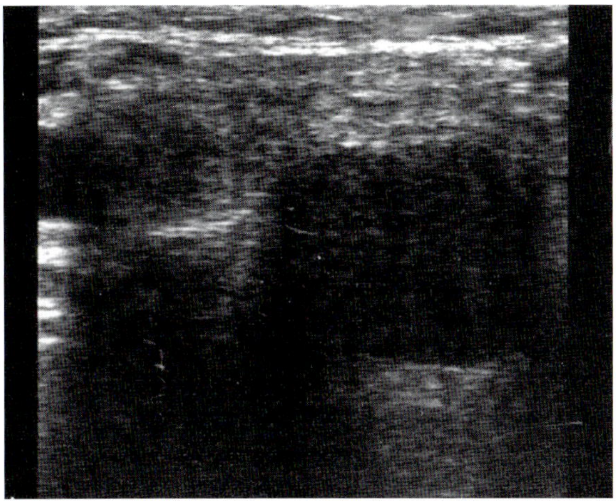

Fig. 9.**33 a** Large hypoechoic structure in the left thyroid lobe, not defined against the surroundings and toward caudal in Riedel struma.

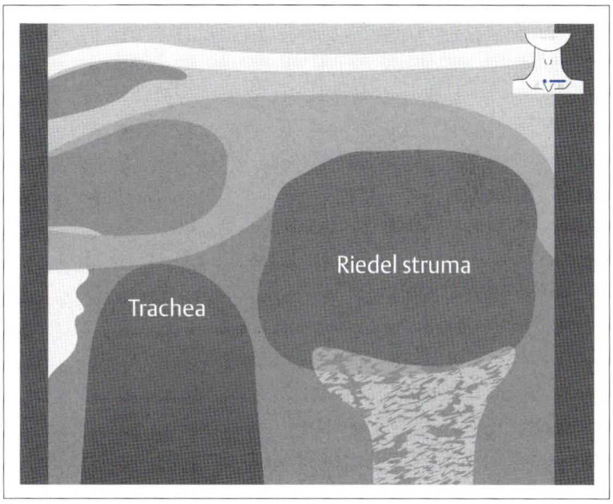

Fig. 9.**33 b** Line drawing.

Consequences for Surgical Treatment

Diagnosis	Characteristic Findings	Management
Riedel struma	Hypoechoic areas ill-defined against and invading/displacing the surrounding structures of the neck	Histopathological confirmation; complete surgical resection often not possible due to invasive changes, glucocorticoisteroids

Thyroid Metastases

Basic Facts

- The incidence of metastases in the thyroid gland on postmortem series can reach 24% (Nakhjavani et al., 1997).
- With decreasing frequency, these metastases originate from renal, breast, esophageal, and uterine carcinoma, often many years after diagnosis of the primary tumor (2 months to 22 years).
- *Additional workup:* Correct diagnosis can be established by FNA, better by histopathological assessment.

Sonographic Criteria

- Hypoechoic unifocal or multifocal intrathyroidal masses (Fig. 9.**34**).

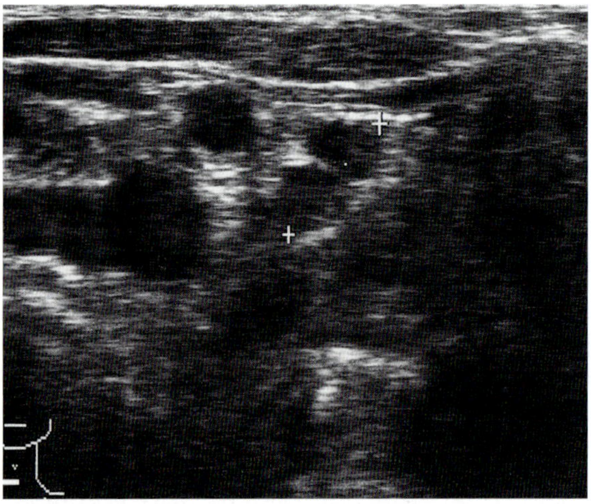

Fig. 9.**34a** Several small, partially confluent, hypoechoic masses in the right thyroid lobe in metastasis of renal cell carcinoma.

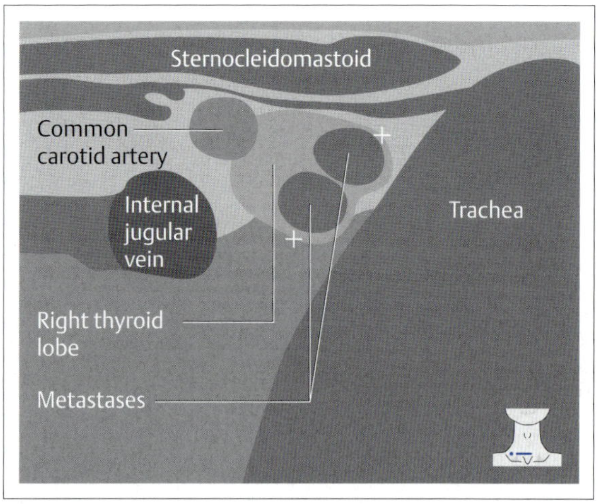

Fig. 9.**34b** Line drawing.

Consequences for Surgical Treatment

Diagnosis	Characteristic Findings	Management
Metastasis of solid tumors	Unifocal or multifocal hypoechoic mass	Possibly FNA, surgery, and histological confirmation

Parathyroid Glands

Basic Facts

- Normal parathyroid glands (diameter about 5 mm) cannot be visualized sonographically.
- The incidence of parathyroid adenomas averages about 25 cases per 100 000 population per year, 15% of the patients display multiple adenomas.
- Parathyroid carcinoma is rare, comprising < 1% of all parathyroid tumors.
- Monoclonal growth of parathyroid cells results in autonomous parathyroid hormone synthesis.
- Parathyroid adenomas may arise in the context of multiple endocrine neoplasia (MEN 1 or 2).
- 3% of all parathyroid adenomas are intrathyroidal and thus cannot be differentiated sonographically from thyroid nodules.
- Sonography cannot demonstrate any adenomas in the mediastinum.
- Lymphadenopathy at the superior or inferior poles of the thyroid gland cannot be differentiated sonographically from parathyroid masses.
- Elevated parathyroid hormone and calcium levels confirm the diagnosis.
- Only symptomatic hyperthyroidism (confirmed osteoporosis, renal calculi) requires surgical exploration of the parathyroid glands.
- Irregular margins and heterogeneous echotexture must raise the suspicion of parathyroid carcinoma.
- *Additional workup:* For primary diagnosis, cervical sonography suffices as the sole imaging modality; in recurrent hyperparathyroidism, MRI of the neck and mediastinum and Tc-99m-MIBI-scintigraphy should be added, possibly complemented by selective venous sampling.

Sonographic Criteria

- Extracapsular, hypoechoic smoothly delimited masses at the superior or inferior pole of the thyroid gland; in some cases, the parathyroid capsule is visible as a hyperechoic rim (Figs. 9.**35**, 9.**36**).

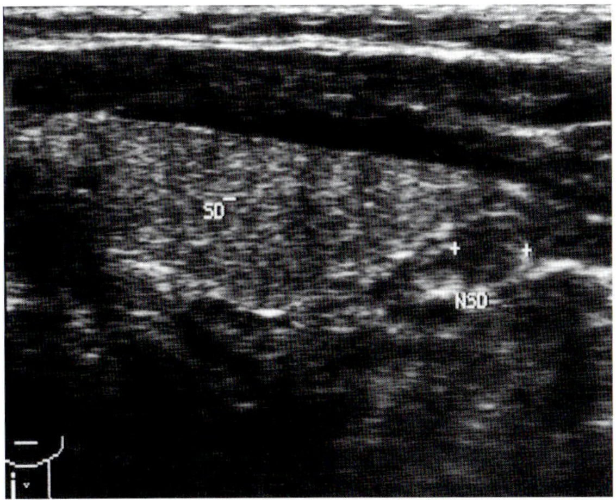

Fig. 9.**35a** Small hypoechoic extracapsular mass at the inferior pole of the right thyroid lobe. Parathyroid adenoma (NSD). SD = thyroid.

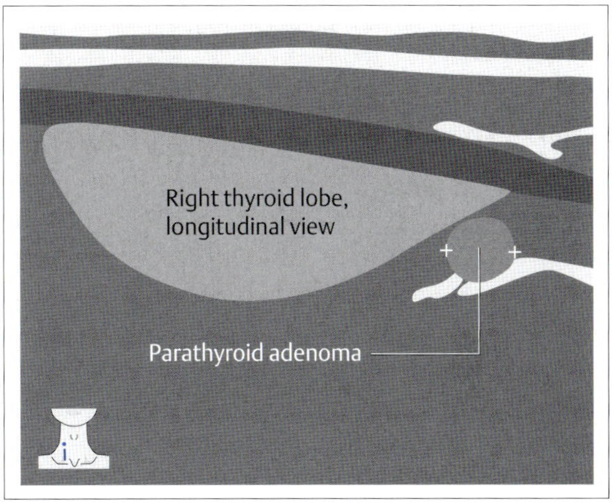

Fig. 9.**35b** Line drawing.

Consequences for Surgical Treatment

Diagnosis	Characteristic Findings	Management
Parathyroid adenoma	Hypoechoic mass at the superior or inferior pole of the thyroid lobe	Surgical resection of symptomatic parathyroid adenomas with exploration of all four parathyroid glands to rule out concurrent hyperplasia of the healthy-appearing glands, intraoperative measurement of PTH to confirm removal of adenoma

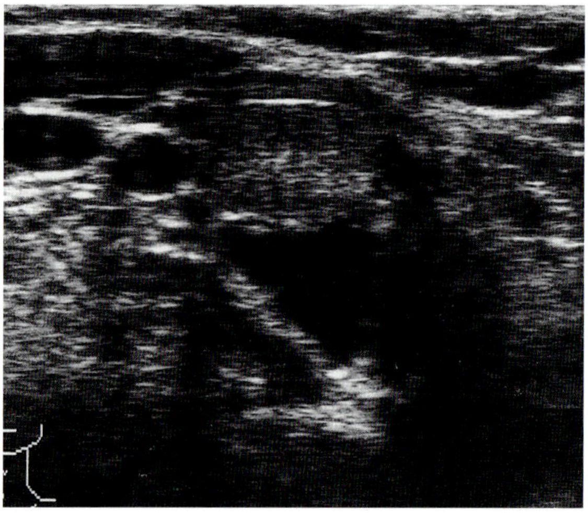

Fig. 9.36a Large parathyroid adenoma at the inferior pole of the right thyroid lobe, presenting as a triangular hypoechoic structure.

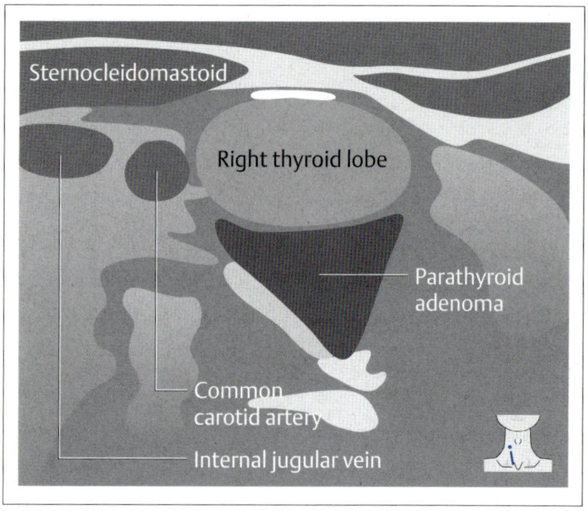

Fig. 9.36b Line drawing.

Adrenal Glands

Basic Facts

- Adrenal glands of normal size usually cannot be seen on ultrasound, suprarenal masses can be delineated upward of 1.5–2 cm in diameter.
- The region of the right adrenal gland can be visualized either by a subcostal approach through the liver, medial and anterior to the superior pole of the kidney, or through the kidney, demonstrating its superior pole.
- The left adrenal region is between superior pole of the kidney and the aorta.
- Adrenal adenoma and carcinoma are rare tumors that must be evaluated for hormonal activity.
- Often belated diagnosis of adrenal carcinoma; usually by then the large heterogeneous tumors have invaded neighboring structures (liver, kidney, spleen, vessels).
- Metastases in the adrenal glands derive predominantly from bronchial and breast cancer as well as melanoma, lymphoma, and renal cell carcinoma.
- Adrenal tuberculosis, rare nowadays, resulting in adrenal calcifications may lead to Addison disease.
- *Additional workup:* Thin-section CT or MRI of the suprarenal area is mandatory; note and evaluate any clinical signs of excessive hormone levels (hyperadrenocorticism, hyperandrogenism, hypertension).
- **Caveat:** Never operate on an adrenal mass without having ruled out pheochromocytoma.

Sonographic Criteria

- **Adrenal hyperplasia and adenoma**
  - Nodular adrenal hyperplasia or adenoma upward of 1.5 cm in diameter can be detected, usually as a hypoechoic mass (Fig. 9.**37**); hyperplasia also may appear as a homogeneous hyperechoic mass.
- **Adrenal carcinoma**
  - Large hypoechoic mass (Figs. 9.**38**, 9.**39**), possible invasion of adjacent organs
- **Pheochromocytoma**
  - Small pheochromocytomas are visualized as hypoechoic masses; in larger ones, there are regressive changes of mixed echogenicity with hyperechoic parts and cysts
- **Lipoma and myelipoma**
  - Hyperechoic adrenocortical tumors with small hypoechoic areas and a smooth margin (Fig. 9.**40**)
- **Adrenal metastases, adrenal involvement in non-Hodgkin lymphoma**
  - In most cases hypoechoic masses; depending on their size, their margin may be polycyclic; in hemorrhage there may be hypoechoic or anechoic areas
- **Hemorrhage, hematoma, cysts**
  - Hypoechoic masses; in case of cysts also anechoic structure in the adrenal region
  - Possibly older hematomas with calcifications
- **Adrenal tuberculosis**
  - Calcifications (posterior shadowing) in the adrenal fossa typical of adrenal tuberculosis

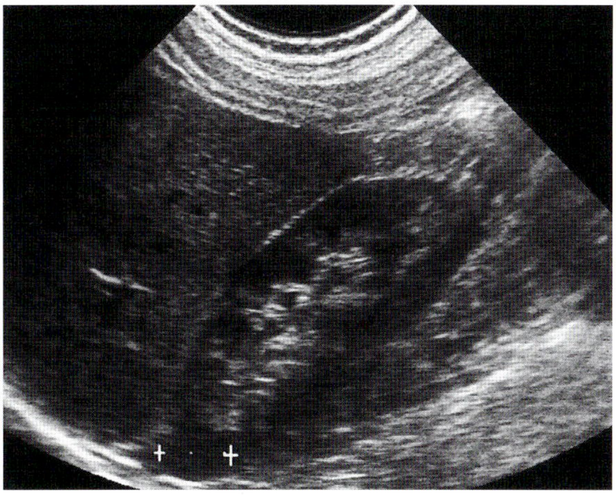

Fig. 9.**37 a** Hypoechoic round mass at the superior pole of the right kidney. Adrenal adenoma.

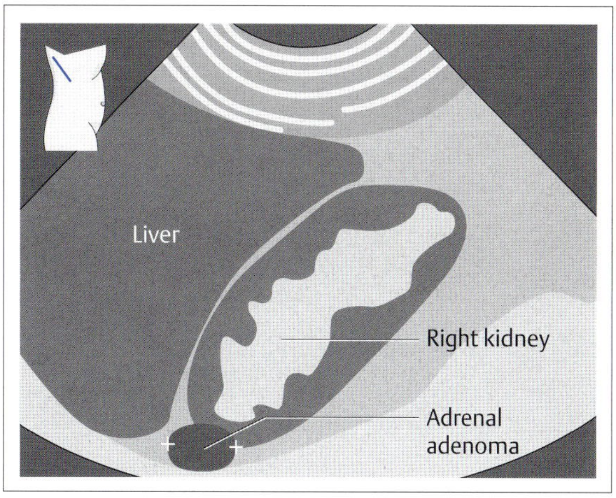

Fig. 9.**37 b** Line drawing.

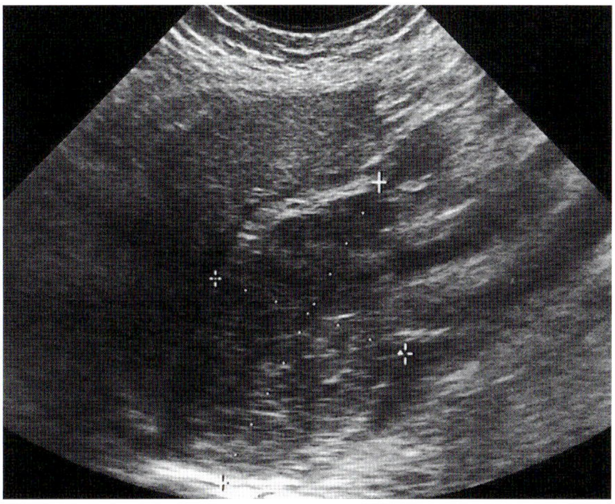

Fig. 9.**38 a** Large heterogeneous tumor in the right adrenal fossa indenting the liver. Adrenal carcinoma.

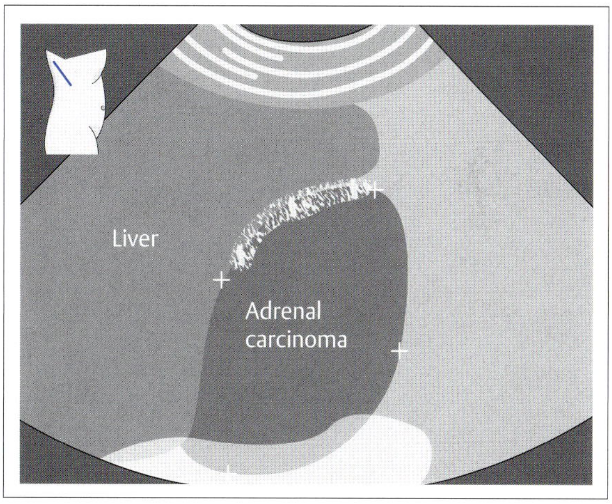

Fig. 9.**38 b** Line drawing.

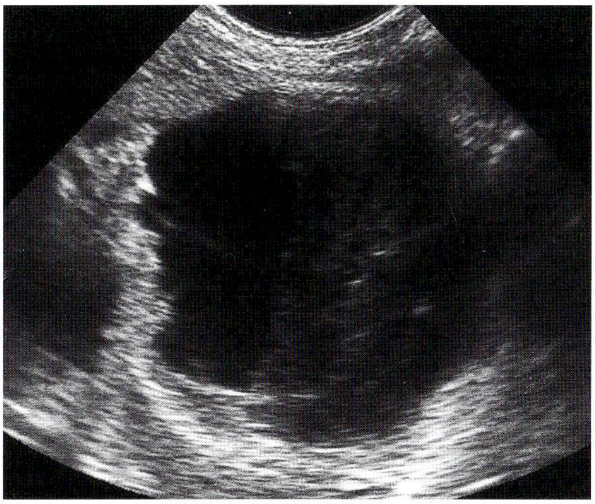

Fig. 9.**39 a** Carcinoma of the right adrenal gland with irregular margin and mixed hyperechoic as well as hypoechoic areas.

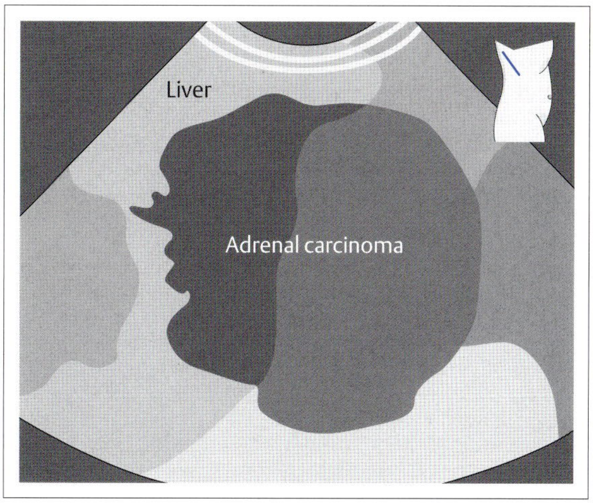

Fig. 9.**39 b** Line drawing.

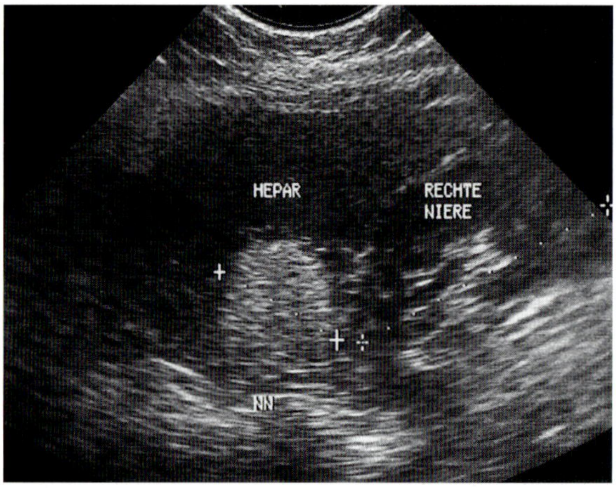

Fig. 9.**40 a** Hyperechoic tumor at the right adrenal gland. Myelolipoma.

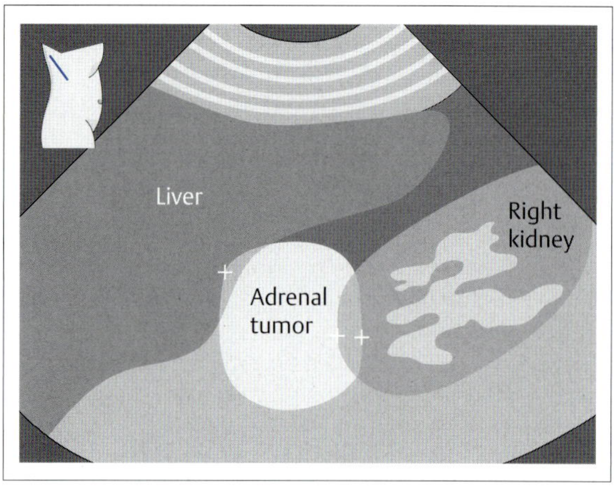

Fig. 9.**40 b** Line drawing.

Consequences for Surgical Treatment

Diagnosis	Characteristic Findings	Management
Adrenal mass	Tumor of varied echogenicity, calcifications possible	Additional diagnostic workup: CT or MRI, hormone levels Hormone producing tumors: adrenal resection (rule out pheochromocytoma; before pheochromocytoma surgery anti-α-adrenergic treatment is mandatory) Tumors without hormone activity: surgical resection only if tumor size > 5 cm (possible malignancy)

Bibliography

Becker W, Börner W, Gruber G. Szintigraphie und Sonographie bei der Diagnostik der Schilddrüsenautonomie. Dtsch Med Wschr. 1986; 111: 1630–5.

Berghout A, Wiersinga W M, Smits N J, et al. Interrelationships between age, thyroid volume, thyroid nodularity and thyroid function in patients with sporadic nontoxic goiter. Am J Med. 1990; 89: 602–8.

Daniels GH. Thyroid nodules and nodular thyroids: a clinical overview. Comprehens Ther. 1996; 22(4): 239–50.

Davies TF, Martin A, Concepcion ES, Graves P, Cohen L, Ben-Nun A. Evidence of limited variability of antigen receptors on intrathyreoidal T cells in autoimmune thyroid disease. N Engl J Med. 1991; 325: 238–44.

Eggo MC, Sheppard MC. Autocrine growth factors produced in the thyroid. Mol Cell Endocrinol. 1994; 100(1–2): 97–102.

Foitzik T. Systematik und Epidemiologie benigner und maligner Schilddrüsenerkrankungen. In: Buhr HJ, Runkel N, eds. Operationskurs Schilddrüse. Berlin: Blackwell; 1996: 1–15.

Gharib H. Current evaluation of thyroid nodules. Trends Endocrinol Metab. 1994; 5: 365–9.

Giuffrida D, Gharib H. Controversies in the management of cold, hot, and occult thyroid nodules. Am J Med. 1995; 99: 642–50.

Gutekunst R, Becker W, Hehrmann R, Olbricht T, Pfannenstiel P. Ultraschalldiagnostik der Schilddrüse. Dtsch Med Wschr. 1988; 113: 1009–12.

Hamacher C, Studer H, Zbaeren J, Schatz H, Derwahl M. Expression of functional stimulatory guanine nucleotide binding protein in nonfunctioning thyroid adenomas is not correlated to adenylate cyclase activity and growth of these tumors. J Clin Endocrinol Metab. 1995; 80: 1724–32.

Hammond LJ, Lowdell MW, Cerrano PG, Goode AW, Bottazzo GF, Mirakian R. Analysis of apoptosis in relation to tissue destruction associated with Hashimoto's autoimmune thyroiditis. J Pathol. 1997; 182: 138–44.

Hampel R, Kühlberg T, Klein K, et al. Strumaprävalenz in Deutschland größer als bisher angenommen. Med Klinik. 1995; 90: 342–9.

Heufelder AE, Hay ID. Evidence for autoimmune mechanisms in the evolution of invasive fibrous thyroiditis (Riedel' s struma). Clin Invest. 1994; 72: 788–93.

Hintze G, Emrich D, Köbberling J. Treatment of endemic goitre due to iodine deficiency with iodine, levothyroxine, or both: results of a multicentre trial. Eur J Clin Invest. 1989; 19: 527–34.

Mann K. Schilddrüsenkarzinome. In: Wilmanns W, ed. Internistische Onkologie. Stuttgart: Thieme; 1994: 600–10.

Martinez-Tello F, Martinez-Cabruja R, Fernandez-Martin J, Lasso-Oria C, Ballestin-Carcavilla C. Occult carcinoma of the thyroid. Cancer. 1993; 71: 4022–9.

Mc Kee RF, Krukoski ZH, Matheson NA. Thyroid neoplasia coexistent with chronic lymphocytic thyroiditis. Br J Surg. 1993; 80: 1303–4.

Nakhjavani MK, Gharib H, Goellner JR, van Heerden JA. Metastasis to the thyroid gland. Cancer. 1997; 79: 574–8.

Raue F. Struma maligna. Nuklearmediziner. 1995; 18: 147–52.

Raue F, Kohlwagen R, Ziegler R. Immunthyreopathie–Morbus Basedow. Diffuse Echoarmut in der Schilddrüsensonographie als diagnostisches Kriterium. Inn Med. 1992; 19: 76–9.

Rojeski MT, Gharib H. Nodular thyroid disease: evaluation and management. N Engl J Med. 1985; 313: 428–36.

Russo D, Arturi F, Suarez HG, et al. Thyrotropin receptor gene alterations in thyroid hyperfunctioning adenomas. J Clin Endocrinol Metab. 1996; 81: 1548–51.

Sachse A, Burzler C, Schopohl D, Gärtner R. Effect of iodine in comparison to *d*-iodolactone on apoptosis in porcine thyroid follicles in vitro. Endocrine Society. 1997; Abstr 97: P2–16.

Vitti P, Rago T, Mancusi F, et al. Thyroid hypoechogenic pattern at ultrasonography as a tool for predicting recurrence of hyperthyroidism after medical treatment in patients with Graves' disease. Acta Endocrinol. 1992; 126: 128–31.

Volpe R. Autoimmunity causing thyroid dysfunction. Endocrin Metab Clin North Am. 1991; 20(3): 565–87.

Wheeler MH. Investigation of the solitary thyroid nodule. Clin Endocrinol. 1996; 44: 245–7.

Wiedemann W. Sonographie und Szintigraphie der Schilddrüse. Stuttgart; Thieme; 1993: 61.

10 Endosonography (EUS)

U. Will

Indications and Technique

- **General aspects:** Endosonography (synonym: endoscopic ultrasound or EUS) employs high-frequency ultrasound probes mounted on the tip of fiberoptic endoscopes or probes; acoustic coupling with the surrounding tissue is achieved via a water-filled balloon standoff device and/or distension of the intestinal lumen with water.
- **Scanners:** Mechanical sector scanner (7.5/12 MHz; 360° panoramic cross-sectional image perpendicular to long axis of instrument; depth of penetration 6–8 cm); curved linear array (5/7.5 MHz; 105° sector image perpendicular to long axis of instrument; allows spectral analysis, color-flow and power Doppler sonography, and EUS-guided FNA). Mini-ultrasound probes are inserted through the biopsy channels of the endoscope (diameter 1.9–2.4 mm; 10–20 MHz; 360° panoramic image perpendicular to long axis of instrument; limited depth of penetration of 2–3 cm); applications in intraductal ultrasound (IDUS) of the bile duct and pancreatic duct. *Non-endoscopic probes* are rigid instruments: radial, linear, multiplanar (3D) probes, 15–20 cm long, mainly used in endorectal sonography.
- **Resolution:** Structures and lesions down to 2–3 mm in diameter.
- **Procedure:** Patient in left lateral decubitus, light sedation preferred (5–15 mg midazolam), length of examination 5–20 minutes depending on clinical question and experience of sonographer
- **Technique:**
- 1. Endoscopically oriented examination (coupling at endoscopically evident pathological or equivocal findings in the esophagus, stomach, duodenum, duodenal papilla, and rectum).
- 2. Sonomorphologically oriented examination (diagnostic assessment of GI tract tumors; tumors/lymphadenopathy (LN) in the posterior mediastinum; pathological findings of the biliary tree and pancreas).
- **Special techniques:** EUS-guided FNA with 19G or 22G needles for histological/cytological confirmation of tumors and suspicious lymph nodes; intravenous administration of US contrast agents (mixture with microbubbles for signal enhancement (Sono-Vue–Altana) combined with EUS color-flow Doppler or spectral Doppler sonography for visualizing vessels in GI tumors (mesenchymal stromal tumors, neuroendocrine, and cystic tumors of the pancreas) and for more precise assessment of the vascular involvement of adjacent tumors.
- **Complication rate:** Overall 0.05%; mortality 0.003%.
- **Benefit:** This is the only modality permitting systematic assessment of the gastrointestinal wall and its surroundings.
- There is a clear relationship between the histological layering and the five sonographic layers of the gut signature (Table 10.**1**; Fig. 10.**3**).
- This allows preoperative tumor staging.
- **Main indications:** T/N staging and assessment of tumor resectability within the GI tract (esophagus, stomach including lymphoma, pancreas, duodenal papilla, biliary tree, rectum); basis for multimodal treatment regimens.
- EUS helps to reduce the rate of exploratory surgery and risky, highly expensive procedures in 55% of cases (Nickl, 1996); it also has a significant impact on treatment strategy in 74% of patients (Nickl, 1996).
- EUS is used in preoperative prognostic assessment for estimation of survival time, which, for patients with tumors of the GI tract, depends on tumor size, presence of nodal and distant metastases, and resection status; EUS accuracy in tumor staging is 80–90%; for nodal staging 70–80%; for assessment of resectability 80–90%, compa-

Table 10.**1** Correlation of endosonographic wall layers, histological findings, and tumor stage T (uT) in tumors of the GI tract

EUS Layer	Echogenicity	Histological Correlation	T stage
1st layer	Hyperechoic	Entrance echo/mucosa	
2nd layer	Hypoechoic	Mucosa	uT1m
3rd layer	Hyperechoic	Submucosa	uT1sm
4th layer	Hypoechoic	Muscularis propria	uT2
5th layer	Hyperechoic	Exit echo and subserosa, serosa (stomach, duodenum), adventitia (esophagus), perirectal fat (rectum)	uT3

rable in all GI tumors. Staging by EUS clearly superior to all other imaging modalities.
- *Before EUS distant metastasis must always be ruled out (US, CT) since an EUS finding of metastasis probably will not change treatment strategy.*
- Without definitive signs of invasion, a structure regarded on EUS as a suspicious mass cannot be distinguished as benign or malignant (pancreatic carcinoma vs. chronic pancreatitis; malignant vs. benign gastric ulcer; adenoma vs. T1 carcinoma).
- Inflammatory changes around the tumor result in false-positive overstaging in 10–15% of cases, particularly in T1 and T2 carcinomas; cellular tumor spread into deeper layers cannot be detected and will lead to false-negative understaging (5–10%).

Esophageal Cancer

Basic Facts

- Comprises 7% of all malignant tumors of the GI tract (80–90% squamous cell carcinoma, 10–20% distal adenocarcinoma); if > 75% of tumor growth is within the tubular esophagus, this endoscopic finding is highly suggestive of primary esophageal carcinoma).
- Incidence: 2–5/100 000. Risk factors: chronic alcohol and nicotine abuse.
- Barrett's esophagus as precancerous condition in adenocarcinoma.
- If the tumor is > 5 cm, there is lymph node metastasis in 90% of cases; if the tumor is stenotic, tumor stage T3–T4 in 90% of patients.
- Lymph node metastasis in early cancer: mucosal type 1–3%; submucosal type 20–40%. For the mucosal type this justifies minimally invasive procedures, since perioperative mortality exceeds the incidence of lymph node metastasis.
- Five-year survival rate is 10–40%; perioperative mortality is 5–8%.
- EUS only after endoscopic and histological confirmation of the tumor; distant metastasis and mediastinal invasion is ruled out by US, CT, and possibly bronchoscopy. In suspicious endoscopic findings and negative histology, EUS helps clarify whether deep biopsy is required; whether EUS-guided FNA is required; and whether there is invasion from outside the esophagus.
- In order to ensure complete EUS, dilation of stenotic esophageal tumor before EUS should be reserved for special cases only, since these tumors can be staged as T3 or T4 in over 90% of cases. The issues that EUS can help settle (LN involvement at celiac trunk or hepatogastric ligament? uT3, uT4 tumor?) will aid in the decision on a palliative or a curative treatment regimen. **Caveat:** Increased risk of perforation (minimized by use of flexible endoscopic dilators or mini-probe EUS).
- EUS-guided FNA of intra-abdominal lymph nodes for optimum specificity of N staging and treatment protocol (R0 resection of esophageal cancer with lymph node metastasis at the celiac trunk is possible in only 10% of patients).
- The therapeutic effect of radiochemotherapy (RT/CT) can be monitored by EUS, including documentation of any reduction in tumor size, although the clinical usefulness of EUS follow-up after RT/CT has not been proven yet; possibly selection of those patients who might profit from surgery after initial RT/CT (downstaging).
- Clinical usefulness of postoperative EUS (local recurrence?) has not been demonstrated; there are frequent false-positive tumor findings due to fibrosis or inflammation.
- *Additional workup:* bronchoscopy; EUS-guided FNA of subdiaphragmatic lymph node metastasis; laparoscopy; FNA cytology of pleural effusion; thoracoscopy.

Sonographic Criteria

- Hypoechoic thickening of the wall with destruction of the lamellar layering, correlating with the depth of tumor invasion and thus the **tumor stage**.
  - *Early stages* (uT1): In most cases, focal wall thickening of layers 1–3, while the layering at the periphery of the tumor (muscularis propria, adventitia) remains intact (Fig. 10.**1**).
  - *Advanced stages* (uT3, uT4): Concentric or eccentric transmural wall thickening with complete loss of layering, irregular tumor margins (uT3), hypoechoic tumor offshoots invading bronchi and vessels (uT4) (Fig. 10.**2**).
- **Pleural effusions** with peritumorous hyperechoic thickening, demonstrating reticular invasion by hypoechoic tongues of tumor may indicate **pleural carcinomatosis**.
- Any lymphadenopathy demonstrated in the vicinity of a histologically confirmed carcinoma must be considered malignant, irrespective of its configuration. There are no definite criteria for **lymph node metastasis**. Signs of lymph node metastasis include diameter > 1 cm, round, homogeneous hypoechoic texture, smooth margin, and absent band-shaped hyperechoic central echo (accuracy 60–70%) (Fig. 10.**2**).
- EUS-guided FNA of lymph nodes can increase specificity to > 90%.

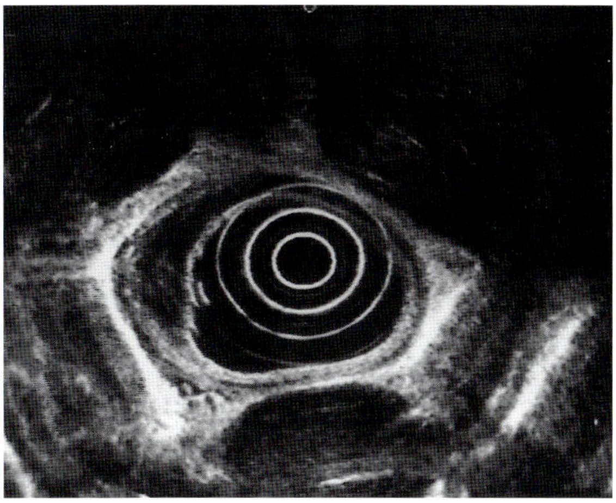

Fig. 10.**1 a** Early esophageal cancer; uT1 N0.

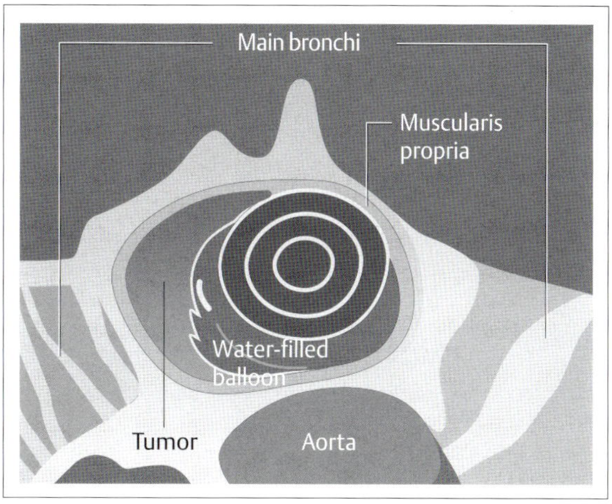

Fig. 10.**1 b** Line drawing.

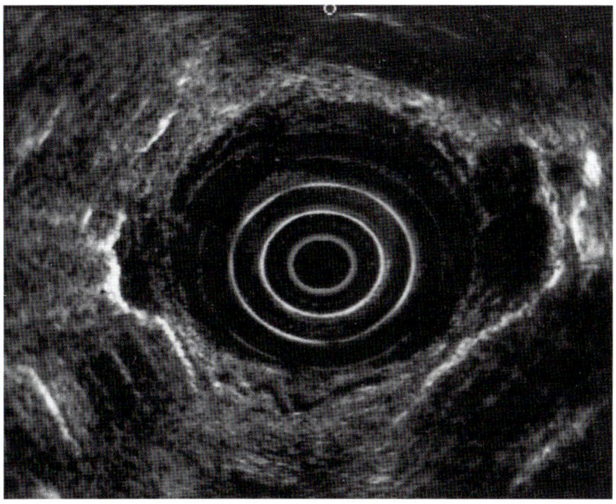

Fig. 10.**2 a** Esophageal cancer invading the right main bronchus; uT4 N1.

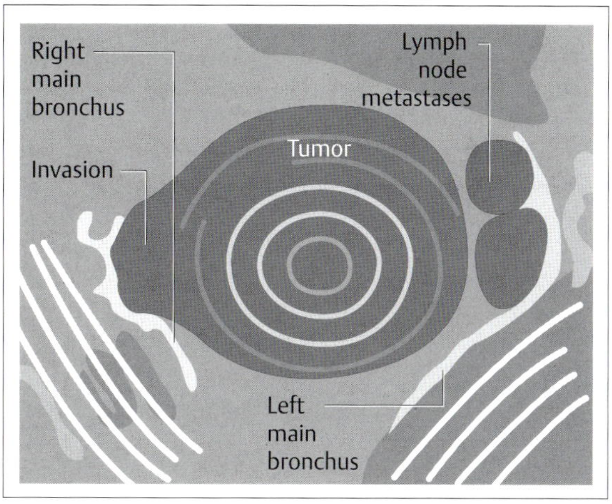

Fig. 10.**2 b** Line drawing.

Consequences for Surgical Treatment

Diagnosis	Other Relevant Factors	Management
Hypoechoic tumor limited to the mucosa (uT1m)	No ulcers < 3 cm No lymphadenopathy Submucosa intact	Endoscopic mucosectomy If R1 resection or submucosa invaded → surgery
Hypoechoic tumor limited to layers 1–4 above and below the tracheal bifurcation (uT1, uT2) and tumors below the bifurcation invading the adventitia (uT3) w/o lymph nodes	No co-morbidity No subdiaphragmatic lymph nodes (celiac trunk, hepatogastric ligament)	1. Primarily curative resection 2. Neoadjuvant RT/CT in clinical trials (positive lymph nodes, if below bifurcation uT3)
Hypoechoic tumors above the tracheal bifurcation with peri-esophageal invasion (uT3)	Positive locoregional lymph nodes No subdiaphragmatic lymph nodes	Neoadjuvant RT/CT with subsequent surgery after restaging
Invasion of adjacent organs (uT4)	Tumor spread into bronchi, left atrium, azygos vein, aorta Lymph node metastasis at celiac trunk	(Stent in case of stenosis, palliative RT/CT, brachytherapy)

Gastric Cancer and Lymphoma

Basic Facts

- Incidence 30–50/100 000; male preponderance of 2 : 1.
- Adenocarcinoma 90% (Lauren classification: intestinal type 9%, diffuse type 1%).
- Lymphomas 70–80%, and malignant and benign mesenchymal stromal tumors 20–30%.
- Risk factors: smoking, alcohol, *N*-nitroso compounds, chronic atrophic gastritis, intestinal metaplasia, infection with *H. pylori*, status post subtotal gastric resection, Ménétrier disease, adenomas, hyperplastic polyps.
- Five-year survival rate: 6–25% (early cancer > 90%). Perioperative mortality: 4–7%.
- Incidence of lymph node metastasis: mucosal type pT1m < 3%; submucosal type pT1sm 20%; pT2 40%; pT3 75%; minimally invasive surgery is justified in mucosal type.
- Gastric lymphoma: secondary involvement in 50–70% of cases; primary manifestation in 20–30%. Histopathology: high/low grade; 70–75% of the low-grade lymphomas staged as uT1 (IE1 in Musshoff's classification) can be healed by eradication of *H. pylori*.
- EUS is a secondary modality after endoscopic/histological confirmation of tumor and after distant metastasis has been ruled out (US, CT), or in case of suspicious endoscopic findings (coarse irregular mucosal folds, atypical ulcers, and negative histology). Issues to be addressed include: deep biopsy or EUS-guided FNA? Invasive/scirrhous tumor growth? Lymphoma? Ménétrier disease?
- EUS is highly sensitive in assessment of invasive intramural involvement of the esophagus in proximal gastric cancer–an important aspect in surgical decision making.
- After aspiration of the gas as the first step, coupling is achieved by use of a concentric water-filled balloon at the scanhead and filling the stomach with water. In case of inadequate coupling, reposition the patient (subcardiac region, angular incisure, fundus of stomach). **Caveat:** There may be artifacts due to oblique view, recognizable by their differences in width and by the blurred wall layering; they can be corrected by repositioning of the endoscope.
- EUS is sensitive for detecting local and anastomotic recurrence; however, specificity is compromised by fibrosis and inflammation, which often may mimic malignancy.
- EUS follow-up is mandatory after exclusive RT/CT in lymphoma; also in carcinoma after RT/CT or surgery but only if it results in any therapeutic consequences;
- *Additional workup:* EUS-guided FNA, snare biopsy; laparoscopy.

Sonographic Criteria

- Tumor of hypoechoic or mixed echogenic texture (polypoid, ulcerative, diffuse) with destruction of one or more wall layers.
  - *Early stages* (early cancer): mucosal type uT1m; submucosa (third layer) smoothly delineated against the tumor (Fig. 10.**3**).
  - *Submucosal type **uT1** sm:* hypoechoic tumor spread invading the submucosa. uT2: invasion of the muscularis propria/subserosa (Fig. 10.**4**).
  - *Advanced stages:* Destruction of the wall by the tumor with complete loss of layering, and irregular peripheral contour (uT3); demonstration of hypoechoic tumor spread into adjacent organs (uT4) (Fig. 10.**5**).
- In confirmed primary, any **regional lymphadenopathy** visualized in EUS must be regarded as malignant (see Esophageal Cancer, above).
- Diffuse gastric carcinoma exhibits a pathognomonic image: Concentric ballooning of the wall, mostly with a smooth peripheral contour; heterogeneous derangement of the wall layering ("pseudolamellation" with thickened submucosa and muscularis propria (Fig. 10.**6**).
- Demonstration of **ascites** with hyperechoic perigastric structures not floating with respiration and pulse, signaling peritoneal carcinomatosis.
- **Advanced lymphoma** is characterized by a heterogeneous EUS image: hypoechoic destruction of the wall with complete loss of layering next to concentric thickening of the wall with blurred layering, the latter displaying clearly thickened submucosa and muscularis propria (DD: scirrhous carcinoma).

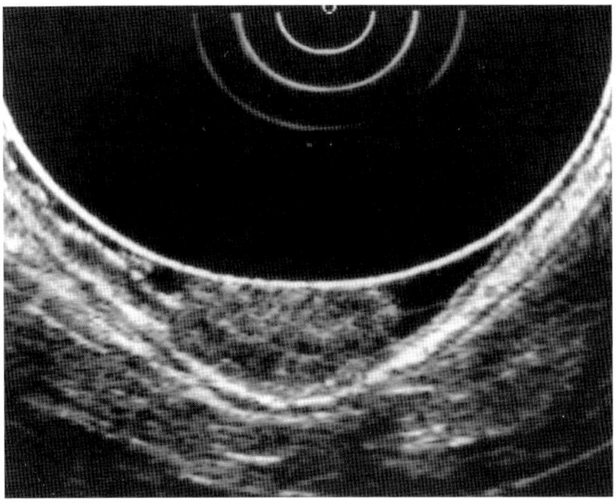

Fig. 10.**3 a** Polypoid early gastric cancer; uT1m.

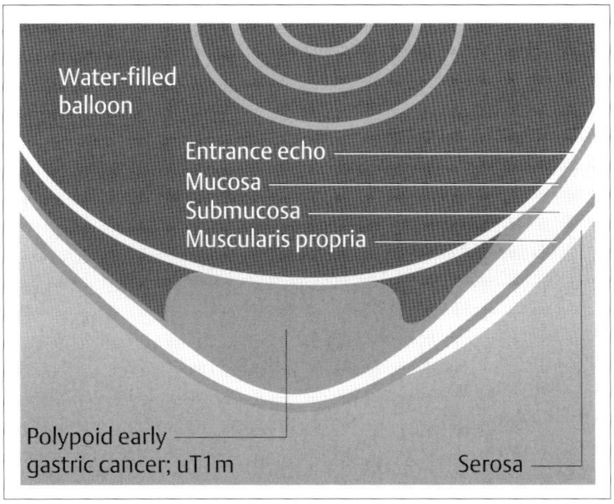

Fig. 10.**3 b** Line drawing.

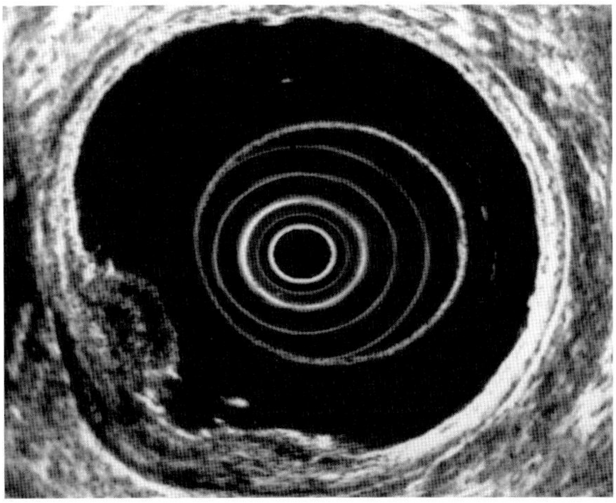

Fig. 10.**4 a** Ulcerative gastric cancer; uT2 N0.

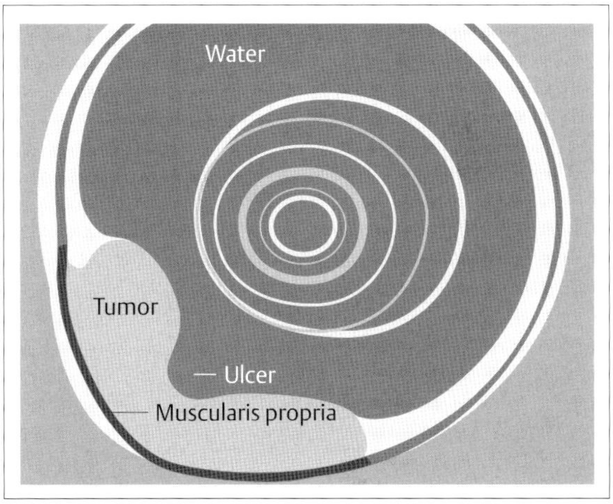

Fig. 10.**4 b** Line drawing.

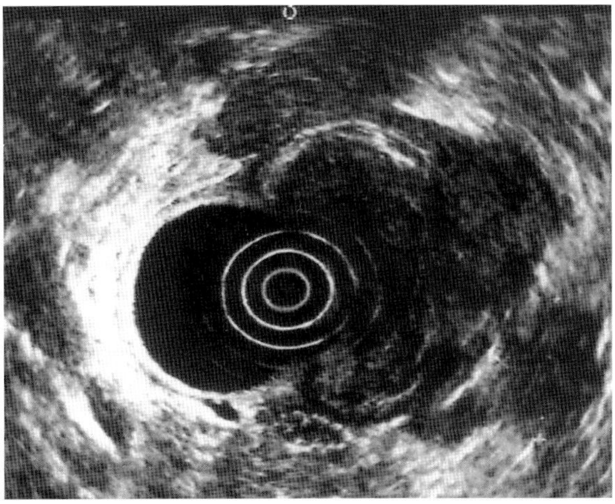

Fig. 10.**5 a** Advanced gastric carcinoma with satellite pancreatic metastasis; uT4 Nx.

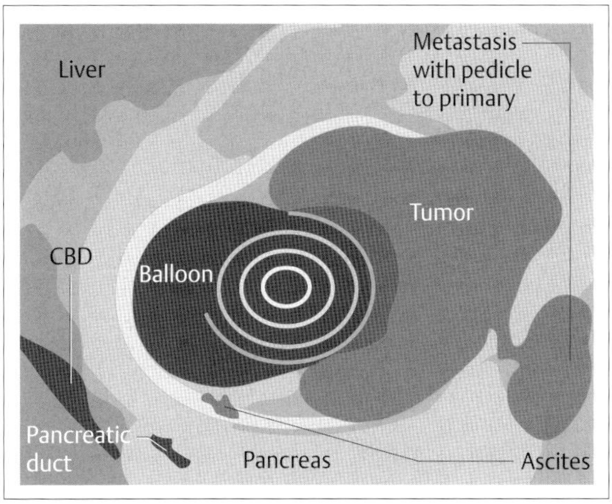

Fig. 10.**5 b** Line drawing.

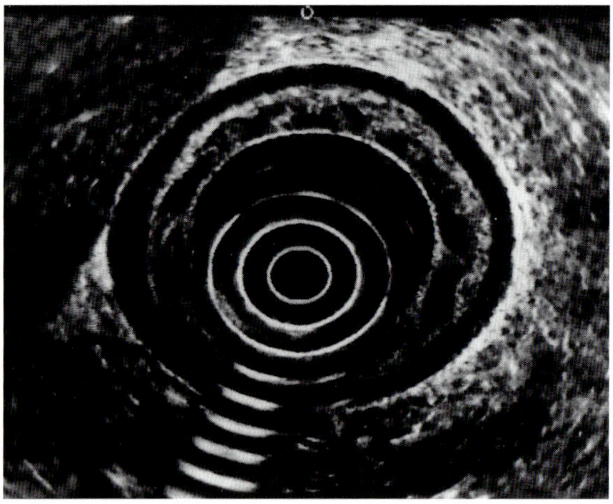

Fig. 10.**6a** Pathognomonic EUS finding in scirrhous gastric carcinoma; uT3 N0.

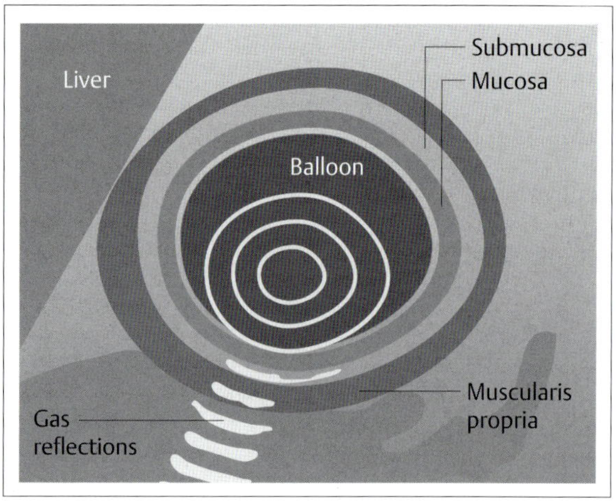

Fig. 10.**6b** Line drawing.

Consequences for Surgical Treatment

Diagnosis	Other Relevant Factors	Management
Tumor limited to the mucosa (uT1m)	Patient with co-morbidity and surgical risk; no lymphadenopathy; submucosa definitely intact	Endoscopic mucosectomy; laser ablation; APC; combined modalities
Lymphoma limited to the mucosa (IE1)	No lymphadenopathy Low-grade lymphoma, *H. pylori* positive	Medical *H. pylori* eradication (clinical trials)
Tumor or lymphoma limited to layers 1–4 (uT1, uT2/IE1–IIE1) w/o locoregional lymph node involvement	Patient with neither co-morbidity nor increased surgical risk	Primarily curative resection (lymphoma IIE1 with postoperative RT/CT) (chemotherapy of *high-grade* lymphomas IIE1 without surgery)
Tumor invading serosa and surrounding tissue (uT3) with locoregional lymph node involvement as well as at the celiac trunk/ hepatoduodenal ligament	Patient with neither co-morbidity nor increased surgical risk	1. Primary resection with extended lymphadenectomy (compartment I and II) or 2. Downstaging by neoadjuvant chemotherapy and subsequent surgery (in trials)
Lymphoma invading organs and lymph nodes N2 (IIE2, IV)		Chemotherapy, radiotherapy
Invasion of adjacent organs (uT4)	Tumor invading pancreatic tail, colon, left hepatic lobe Peritoneal carcinomatosis, diffuse hepatic metastasis	Primarily palliative management

Submucosal Tumors

Basic Facts

- Mesenchymal stromal tumors represent approximately 1% of all GI tumors; they can be classified immunohistologically according to their origin and grade of malignancy, e.g., benign leiomyomas vs. leiomyosarcomas, and schwannomas vs. malignant schwannomas. Next to leiomyomas, gastrointestinal stromal tumor (GIST) comprises the largest group with 30–40%.
- While leiomyomas do not become malignant, this supposedly is not true for GIST.
- GIST is characterized by the expression of the pathognomonic surface markers CD34 and CD117, absent in leiomyomas.
- Lipomas and cysts (including duplication cysts) are uncommon and hardly ever present with complications; lipomasarcoma is a rare entity.
- Diagnostic workup: incidental endoscopic finding (protrusion, bridging folds), manifested by dysphagia, obstruction or erosive hemorrhage from an ulcerative tumor (mesenchymal stromal tumors are profusely vascularized; Fig. 10.**7**).
- EUS can reliably differentiate between segmental GI tract compression by neighboring organs (aorta, ventricle, mediastinal lymph nodes, spleen, splenic artery and vein, liver, gallbladder) or a submucosal tumor.
- Layer of origin, size, contour, and echotexture permit inferences to be made regarding type and possible malignancy of the tumor.
- *Additional workup:* EUS-guided FNA, snare ablation (tumors in layers 1–3).

Sonographic Criteria

- **Leiomyomas, GIST:** Hypoechoic, round or spindle-shaped tumors in the muscularis propria, of homogeneous echotexture and smooth margin (Fig. 10.**8**).
- Less commonly tumors in the muscularis mucosae (layer 2) with intact peripheral wall layering; in EUS contrast-enhanced color flow and spectral Doppler sonography, larger tumors demonstrate flow signals (Fig. 10.**7**).
- **Lipoma:** Hyperechoic, round or spindle-shaped tumors of homogeneous echotexture and smooth margin in the submucosa (layer 3); adjacent muscularis propria and mucosa intact.
- **Carcinoid, ectopic pancreatic tissue:** Usually hypoechoic, submucosal, and frequently ill-defined against the muscularis propria (DD: leiomyoma? invasion?) Early deep biopsy or ablation for diagnostic confirmation, required particularly in patients displaying clinical symptoms
- Characteristics of **malignant mesenchymal stromal tumors:** heterogeneous echotexture of mixed echogenicity with anechoic cystoid or tubular structures and hyperechoic foci; irregular contour; ill-defined against adjacent wall layers (Fig. 10.**9**); on contrast-enhanced EUS and color-flow Doppler sonography there are irregular vascular formations within the tumor; measurable growth on EUS follow-up.

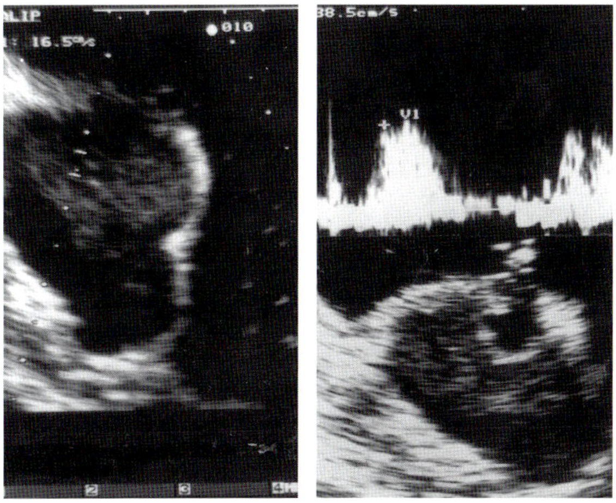

Fig. 10.**7 a** Ulcerative gastric leiomyoma with demonstration of arterial blood flow within the tumor.

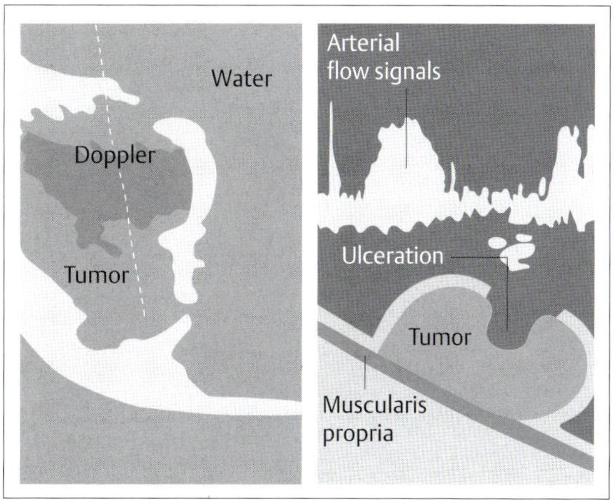

Fig. 10.**7 b** Line drawing.

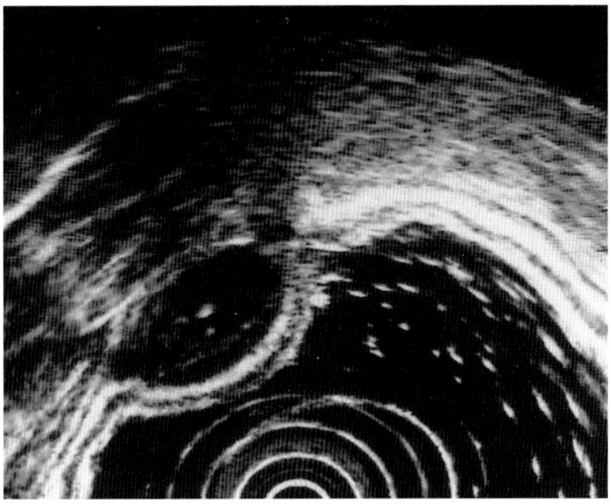

Fig. 10.**8 a** Leiomyoma of the stomach.

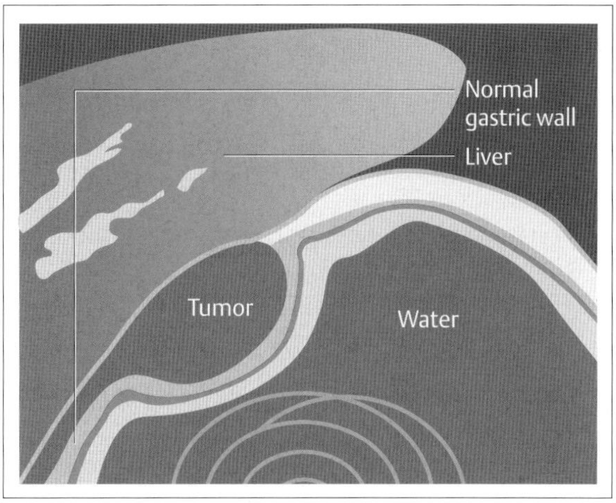

Fig. 10.**8 b** Line drawing.

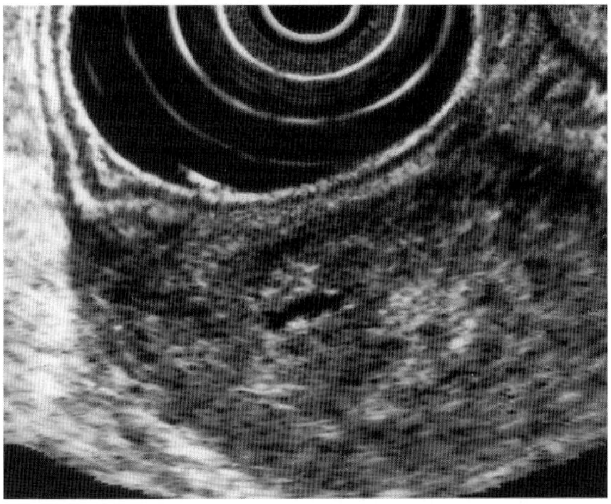

Fig. 10.**9 a** Gastric leiomyosarcoma, originating at the muscularis propria.

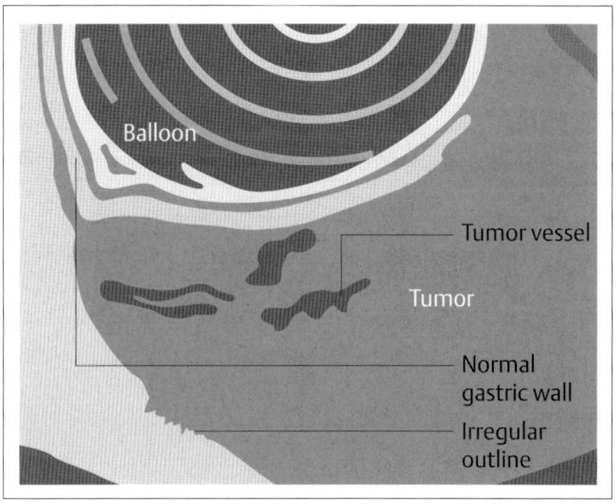

Fig. 10.**9 b** Line drawing.

Consequences for Surgical Treatment

Diagnosis	Other Relevant Factors	Management
Tumor < 3 cm, smooth contour, homogeneous texture, intact wall layering	Patient without symptoms Tumor without complications	Observation, follow-up every 6 months over 2 years; possibly EUS-guided FNA, endoscopic ablation (layers 1–3)
Tumor > 3–4 cm or (irrespective of size) with irregular contour and heterogeneous echotexture (cystoid, hyperechoic foci), complete loss of wall layering	Patient with symptoms Tumor with complications Suspicious locoregional lymph nodes Growth/change in echotexture on EUS follow-up Malignancy or CD117 on EUS-guided FNA	Immediate surgery

Tumors of the Pancreas

Basic Facts

- 80–85% ductal adenocarcinoma with poor prognosis, 5–10% cystic neoplasia including intraductal papillary mucinous tumor (IPMT), < 1% acinar cell carcinoma, lymphoma, etc.
- Incidence: 80–100/100 000.
- Resectability 20–40%; surgical mortality in high-caseload centers 5%, otherwise up to 40%.
- Median survival time 4–7 months; 5-year survival rate of all tumors < 5%, 5-year survival rate after R0 resection 17–37% (depending on lymph node metastasis and perineural invasion).
- Risk factors: nicotine and alcohol abuse, chronic pancreatitis (increased risk, 10- to 16-fold).
- Incidence of lymph node metastasis correlates with T stage (uT1 40%; uT2 60%, uT3 80%, uT4 100%).
- Neuroendocrine tumors (gastrinoma, insulinoma, somatostatinoma, carcinoid tumors) may display hormone activity (clinical symptoms) or–more commonly–will not; EUS sensitivity 80–90%.
- EUS is indicated whenever pancreatic pathology is suspected, after distant metastasis has been ruled out (particularly in a pancreas normal on US or CT), or if the ERCP ductogram is equivocal. It is the most sensitive modality for detection of "occult" cancer, for staging, and for assessment of resectability of pancreatic tumors.
- Excellent resolution due to direct coupling at the pancreas without troublesome gas artifacts.
- EUS objectives:
  1. Selection of patients amenable to curative resection (assessment of vascular invasion uT4, definite sign for incurable condition).
  2. Avoidance of unnecessary exploratory surgery.
  3. Increase in the rate of R0 resections.
  4. Cost savings.
- Differential diagnosis between segmental focal chronic pancreatitis and pancreatic cancer is difficult.
- Assessment of depth of invasion into the arterial tree is limited–if invasion is suspected, combined duplex sonography, EUS duplex imaging, and angiography may be helpful.
- If malignancy cannot be ruled out preoperatively and EUS demonstrates resectability, exploratory surgery with a view toward curative resection is mandatory (the rate of pseudotumors in chronic pancreatitis primarily operated on as suspected cancer is 5–8%).
- *Additional workup:* EUS-guided FNA (Fig. 10.**14**) (sensitivity 95%, specificity 88%), EUS contrast-enhanced color flow Doppler sonography (Fig. 10.**12**); duplex sonography; angiography; laparoscopy (peritoneal carcinomatosis); PET;

Sonographic Criteria

- **Carcinoma:** Hypoechoic tumors; homogeneous or heterogeneous echotexture (most often depending on size); irregular outline with hypoechoic spread in advanced tumor; loss of basic texture when compared with adjacent pancreas (no echoes of vascular wall and ducts, no lobulation); pancreatic duct upstream most often dilated (obstructed by tumor); common bile duct dilated if tumor is located in the prepapillary segment of the pancreatic head (leading symptom: jaundice) (Fig. 10.**10**); no flow signals on color-flow Doppler sonography.
- **Signs of nonresectable tumor:** Demonstration of tumor spread into the portal system, mostly with peripancreatic tubular anechoic structures (venous collaterals) (Fig. 10.**11**).
- Equivocal signs of **vascular invasion**: irregular periportal reinforcement, loss of the borderline echo.
- **Caveat:** Acoustic artifact.
- *Characteristics of **segmental focal chronic pancreatitis**–pseudotumor:* Hypoechoic lobulated honeycomb echotexture with hyperechoic septated structures in the adjacent pancreas; pancreatic duct with irregular course and marked hyperechoic borderline echo; tumor most often in head of pancreas with heterogeneous, predominantly hypoechoic echotexture, discernible tubular and ductal structures, hyperechoic broadened periportal reinforcement; multiple flow signals in the tumor on contrast-enhanced EUS color-flow Doppler imaging (inflammatory hyperemia).
- **Neuroendocrine tumors:** Usually smooth outline, heterogeneous echogenicity sometimes with tubular anechoic structures identified as vessels on EUS color-flow Doppler sonography (Fig. 10.**12**).
- **Cystic neoplasia:** Multiple small (serous cystadenoma) or larger cysts of irregular outline (mucinous cystadenoma, cystadenocarcinoma) accompanied by broadened hyperechoic septated, sometimes solid structures with flow signals on EUS color-flow Doppler sonography (Fig. 10.**13**); invasion of peripancreatic tissue indicating malignant transformation **(mucinous cystadenocarcinoma). Caveat:** Differential diagnosis: atypical pseudocyst in chronic pancreatitis. **Intraductal papillary mucinous tumors:** dilated sections of the pancreatic duct system, resembling cysts with sessile hyperechoic mural masses within the duct system.

Neuroendocrine tumors: somatostatin receptor scintigraphy; intraoperative sonography.

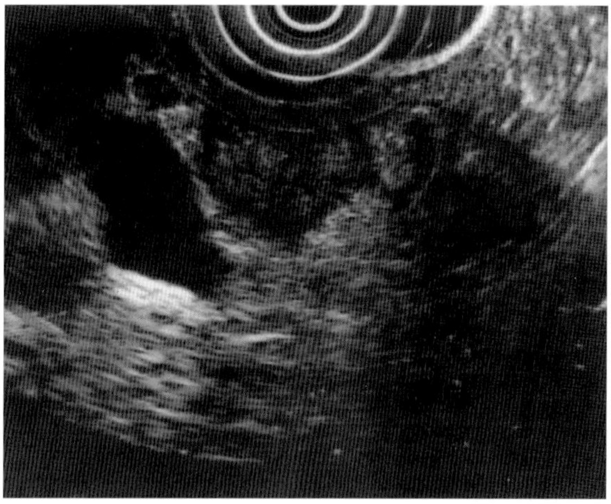

Fig. 10.**10 a** Small pancreatic carcinoma with locoregional lymph node metastasis; uT1 N1.

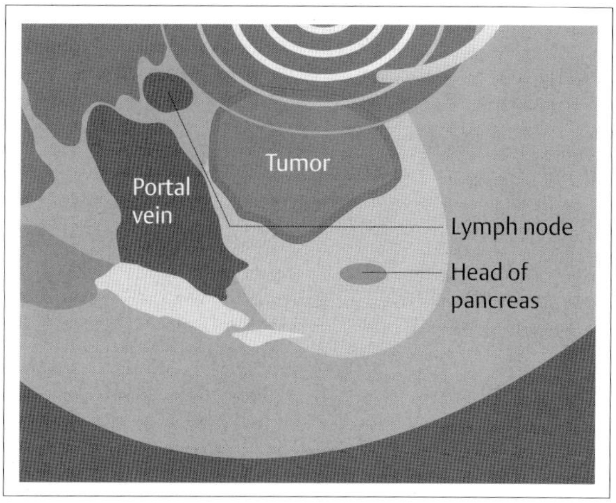

Fig. 10.**10 b** Line drawing.

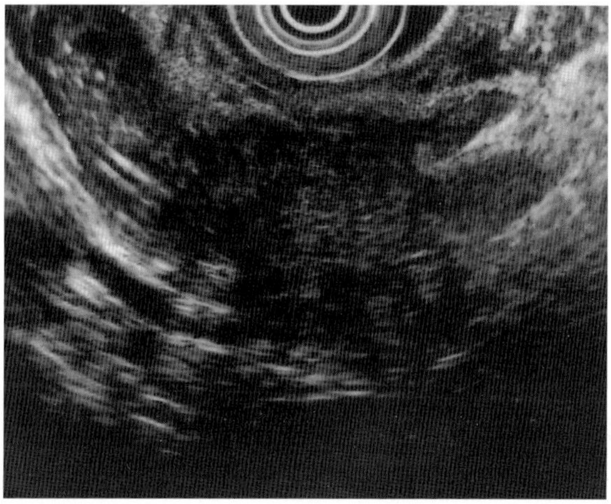

Fig. 10.**11 a** Pancreatic carcinoma invading the portal system; uT4 Nx.

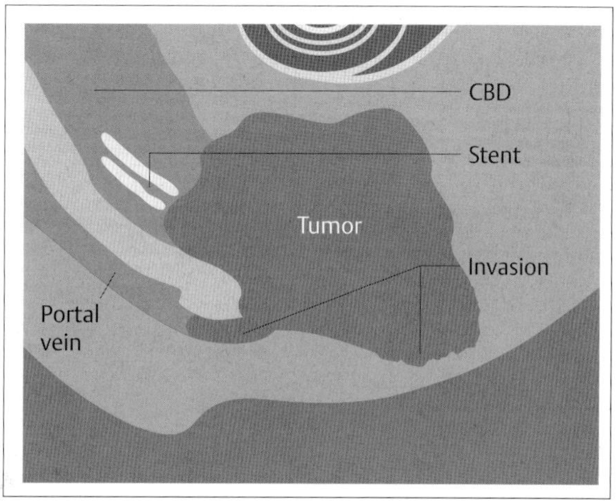

Fig. 10.**11 b** Line drawing.

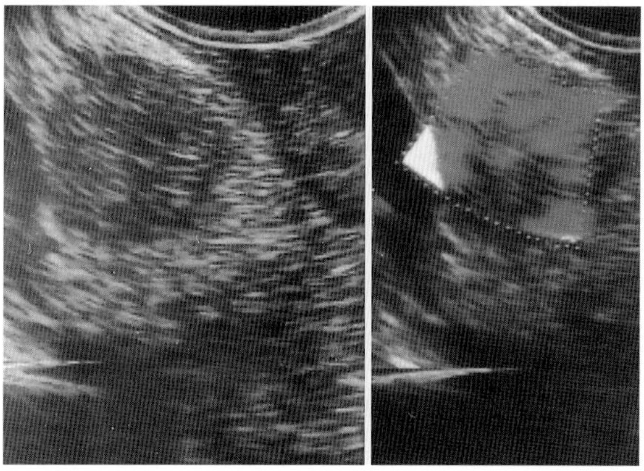

Fig. 10.**12 a** B-mode and contrast-enhanced color-flow Doppler sonogram (power mode) of a highly vascularized mass in the tail of the pancreas, histologically: insulinoma.

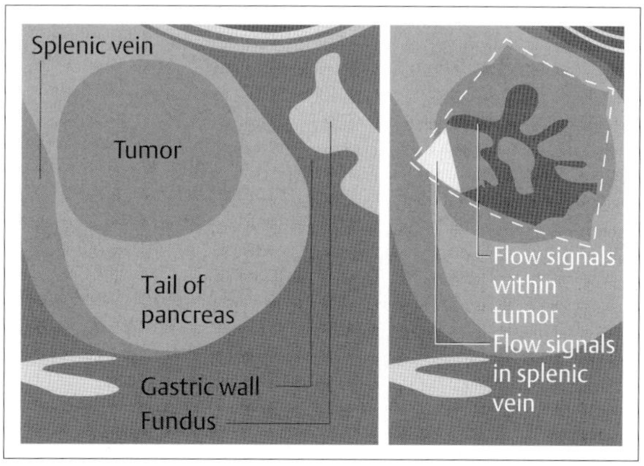

Fig. 10.**12 b** Line drawing.

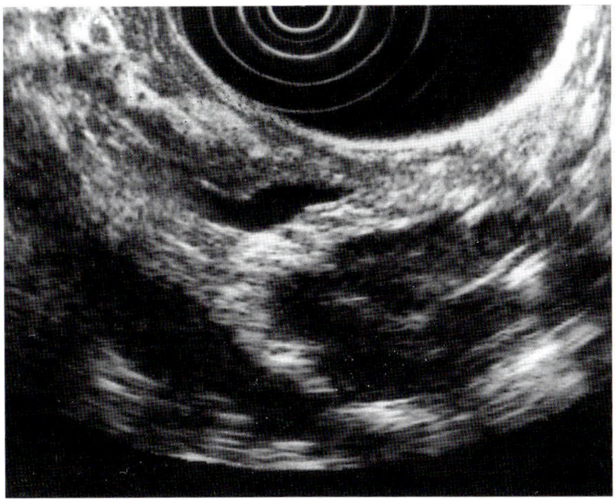

Fig. 10.**13 a** Polycystic mass in the head of the pancreas; histologically: mucinous cystadenoma.

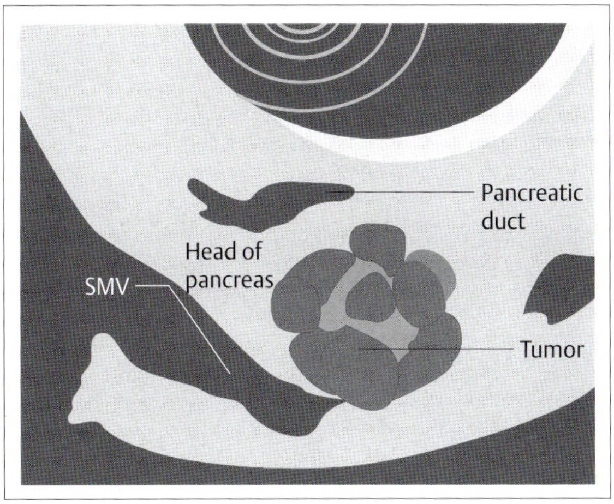

Fig. 10.**13 b** Line drawing.

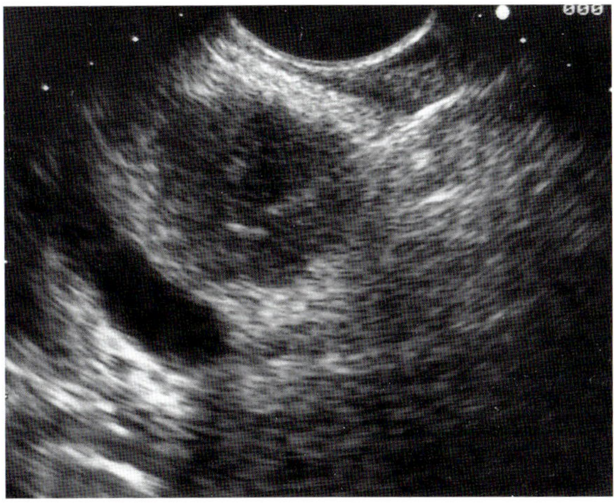

Fig. 10.**14 a** EUS-guided FNA of a small mass in the head in the pancreas: uT1 N0; histologically, adenocarcinoma.

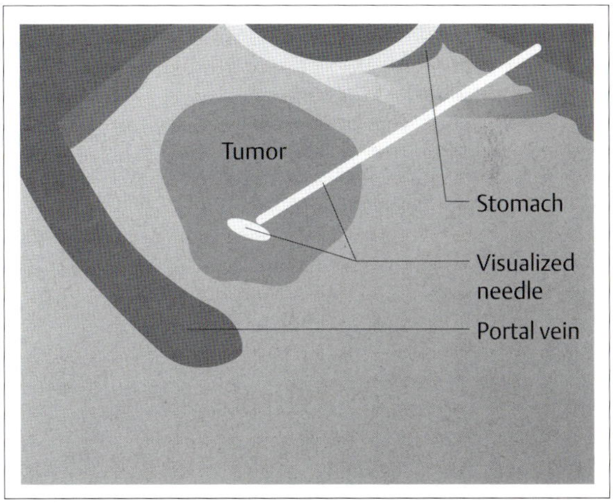

Fig. 10.**14 b** Line drawing.

Consequences for Surgical Treatment

Diagnosis	Other Relevant Factors	Management
Tumor limited to pancreas, <2 cm (uT1), > 2 cm (uT2) Tumor invading the CBD, duodenum, peripancreatic tissue (uT3)	Patient without co-morbidity No malignant lymph node at celiac trunk No peritoneal carcinomatosis No vascular invasion	Primary resection with curative intention, even without preoperative histology, if the tumor appears resectable
Tumor with signs of vascular invasion (uT4)	Independent of T stage: Distant spread Peritoneal carcinomatosis Malignant lymph node at celiac trunk (EUS-guided FNA) Patient with co-morbidity	Primarily palliative management (jaundice–endoscopic stenting or bilioenteric bypass; duodenal obstruction–gastroenterostomy)
Highly vascularized, round hypoechoic tumor (endocrine tumor suspected–DD: metastasis of renal cell carcinoma)	Patient without increased surgical risk Patient with endocrine symptoms	Primary operation (enucleation if benign, otherwise pancreatogastroduodenectomy)

Tumors of the Biliary Tree

Basic Facts

- Incidence 1–5/100000. Leading symptom: jaundice.
- Risk factors: sclerosing cholangitis, parasitic infection, ulcerative colitis, choledochal cysts, cholangiolithiasis, bile duct papillomatosis.
- 95% adenocarcinoma of the papillary or sclerosing type.
- Classification according to size and localization (Bismuth–Corlette types I–IV).
- Five-year survival rate 20–40%; perioperative mortality 5–27%, in high-caseload centers 5%.
- In confirmed tumor and after distant metastasis has been ruled out (US, CT), EUS is indicated for assessment of resectability (invasion of portal system) and in equivocal ERCP ductograms without confirmed tumor (obstructive jaundice of uncertain origin).
- EUS limitations: Since demonstration of the bile duct bifurcation is limited, tumors of type IIIa/IV (invasion of right hepatic duct/liver) are rather difficult to assess.
- Tumors localized in the distal segment of the CBD cannot be differentiated from carcinoma of the head of the pancreas (entity of the so-called peripapillary carcinomas).
- Differential diagnosis of inflammatory from malignant stenosis is unreliable unless specific criteria of tumor invasion are found; in negative transpapillary diagnosis EUS-guided FNA is indicated for possible confirmation (accuracy 80–90%).
- *Additional workup:* ERCP, MRC, duplex sonography, ductoscopy plus biopsy, IDUS, laparoscopy.

Sonographic Criteria

- Hypoechoic tumor projected onto the CBD within the hepatoduodenal ligament, upstream CBD (triple layering) distended with marked layering (due to the cholestasis). Loss of wall layering at the tumor (smooth outline–uT2; irregular outline, tumor spread into the pancreas–uT3; vascular invasion [most often the portal vein]–uT4) (Fig. 10.**15**).

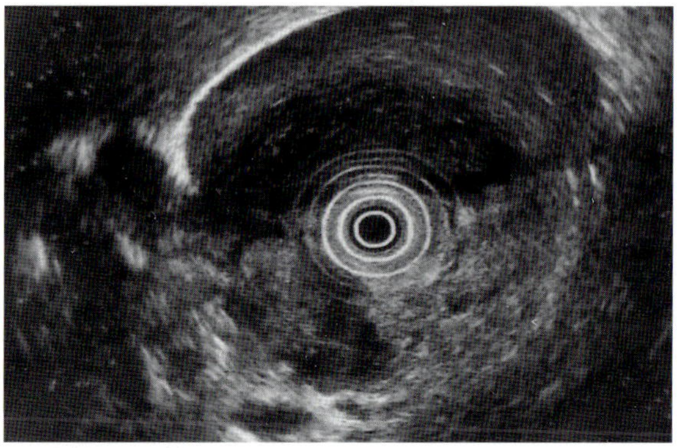

Fig. 10.**15 a** Cancer of the bile duct invading the portal vein; uT4 N1.

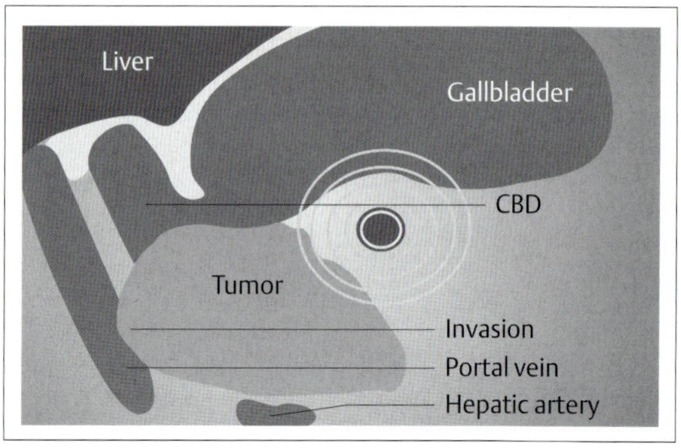

Fig. 10.**15 b** Line drawing.

Consequences for Surgical Treatment

Diagnosis	Other Relevant Factors	Management
Tumor of the middle/distal CBD (limited for the proximal CBD) restricted to the wall (uT1, uT2) or invading the surroundings (uT3)	Generally suitable for surgery No peritoneal carcinomatosis	Curative surgery (pancreatogastroduodenectomy)
Tumor of the proximal third of the CBD (Klatskin's tumor), up to uT3	Generally suitable for surgery No lymph node metastasis at celiac trunk No metastasis	Resection and hepaticojejunostomy; if R1 resection, possibly postoperative irradiation (afterloading); LTx
Tumor with definite vascular invasion (uT4)	Independent of T stage: Peritoneal carcinomatosis Lymph node metastasis at celiac trunk Co-morbidity	Palliative management (hepaticojejunostomy, endoscopic stenting, brachytherapy, PDT)

Tumors of the Major Duodenal Papilla

Basic Facts

- 5% of all neoplasias of the GI tract.
- Type of growth: ampullary, polypoid, ulcerative.
- Histopathology: adenomas, adenocarcinomas, neuroendocrine tumors, lymphomas.
- Entity of peripapillary tumors: localized at the ampullary region, the origin of the tumor being equivocal (papilla, pancreas, duodenum, distal CBD) (Fig. 10.**16**).
- Resectability 50–90%; 5-year survival rate 40–60% (pT1/2 70%; pT3/4 0–5%).
- Risk factors: familial adenomatous polyposis (FAP), Gardner syndrome, adenomas ("adenoma–carcinoma sequence")
- Incidence of lymph node metastasis: pT1 < 1%; pT2 40%; pT3 50%; pT4 100%; this justifies minimally invasive surgery in stage uT1.
- Indications for EUS:
  - 1. Obstructive jaundice of unknown origin (early symptom), after duodenoscopy possibly biopsy and ruling out of distant metastasis indicated.
  - 2. In negative biopsy but abnormal endoscopic finding at the papilla.
  - 3. Pathological ductogram and seemingly normal papilla (intramural tumor? deep biopsy after papillotomy appropriate?).
- In obstructive jaundice of unknown origin, EUS before ERCP is recommended because:
  - 1. It gives reliable demonstration of the cause of the obstruction.
  - 2. It defines treatment strategy (ERCP, operation; curative–palliative management).
  - 3. Compared with ERCP it gives comparable information but without complications.
- Without signs of invasion, papillary tumors cannot reliably be classified as benign/malignant. **Caveat:** Inflammatory papillary stenosis may mimic a tumor.

Sonographic Criteria

- **Adenoma:** Homogeneous echotexture of varying echogenicity, smooth outline, submucosa and muscularis propria intact, no locoregional lymphadenopathy (Figs. 10.**17** and 10.**18**).
- Signs of malignant transformation despite bioptic diagnosis of adenoma: Tumor of mixed echogenicity (e.g., hyperechoic on the luminal side, hypoechoic at the base), irregular outline, loss of demarcation of the submucosa, suspicious locoregional lymph nodes. *Caveat*: Inflammatory episode in cholestasis; pseudotumor on EUS after manipulation (papillotomy)–a further reason to perform EUS prior to ERCP.
- **Carcinoma:** Hypoechoic texture, smooth outline, submucosa intact, limited to the ampulla (uT1); hypoechoic irregular outline–transmural tumor spread to the duodenal wall (uT2); hypoechoic periduodenal tumor spread into the pancreas < 2 cm (uT3); tumor spread > 2 cm into pancreas or adjacent organs and vascular invasion (uT4)–at this stage differentiation from pancreatic cancer or carcinoma of the biliary tree is no longer possible.
- Signs of stenosis of benign organic origin (adenomyomatosis, stenosing papillitis): Ampullary segment of the CBD with bilateral hypodense masses protruding bilaterally into the lumen and entering the papilla. The lumen of the CBD is reduced to a filiform stenosis, the wall still being intact–no signs of deep invasion (Fig. 10.**19**).
- EUS findings as indication for papillotomy plus transpapillary biopsy to rule out intramural adenoma/carcinoma, since EUS cannot reliably differentiate benign from malignant lesions.

- *Additional workup, diagnostic papillectomy:* ERCP, IDUS, papillotomy followed by transpapillary biopsy, laparoscopy.

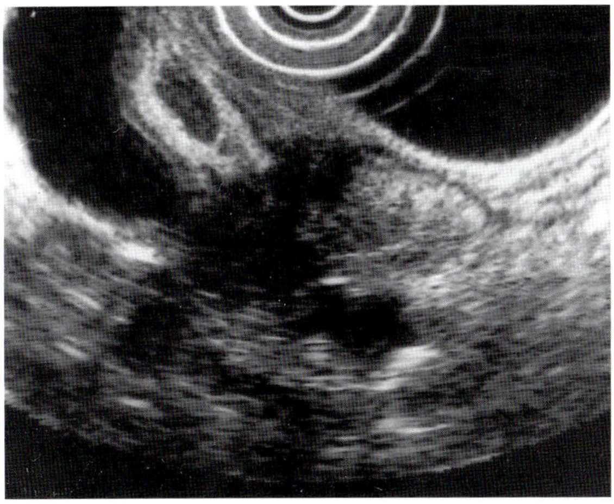

Fig. 10.**16a** Peripapillary carcinoma with locoregional lymph node metastasis; uT3 N1.

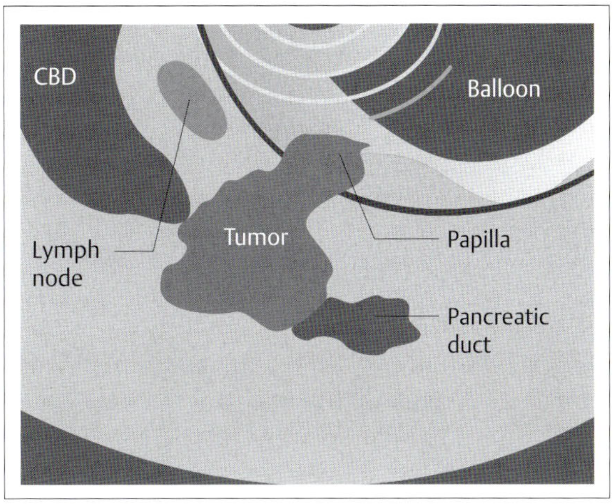

Fig. 10.**16b** Line drawing.

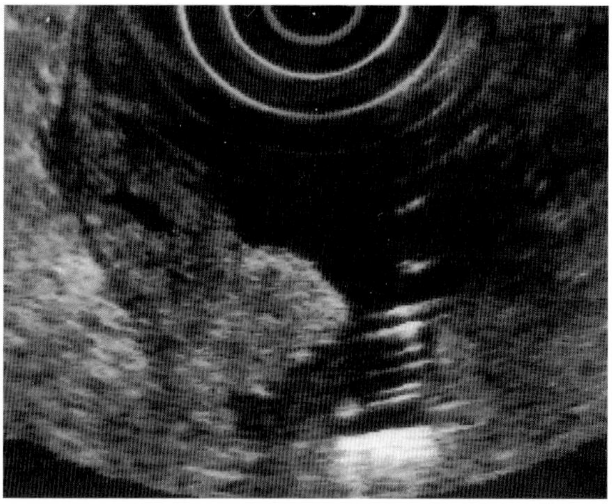

Fig. 10.**17 a** Adenoma of the major duodenal papilla.

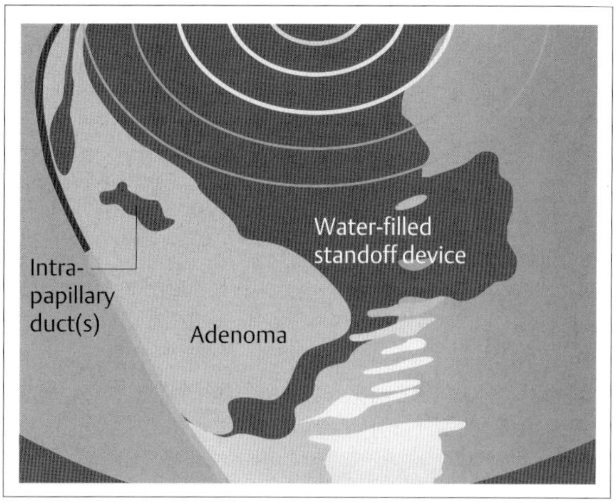

Fig. 10.**17 b** Line drawing.

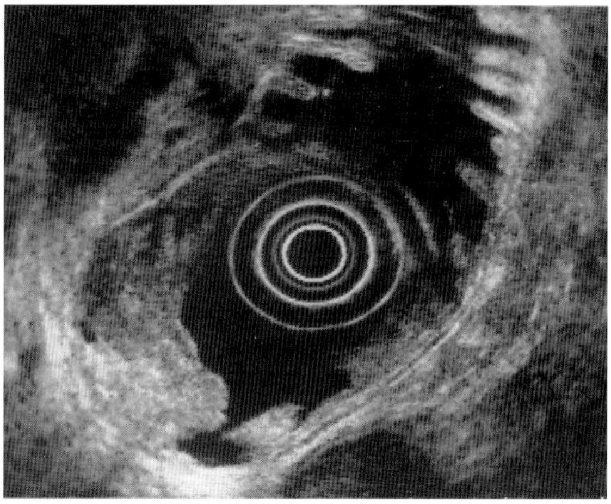

Fig. 10.**18 a** Sessile tubular adenoma of the major duodenal papilla.

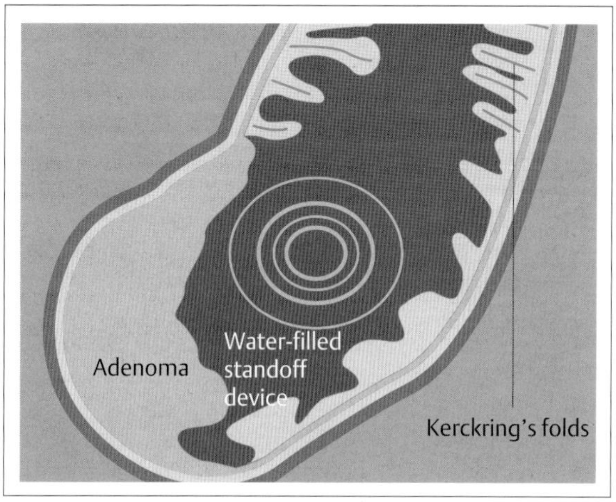

Fig. 10.**18 b** Line drawing.

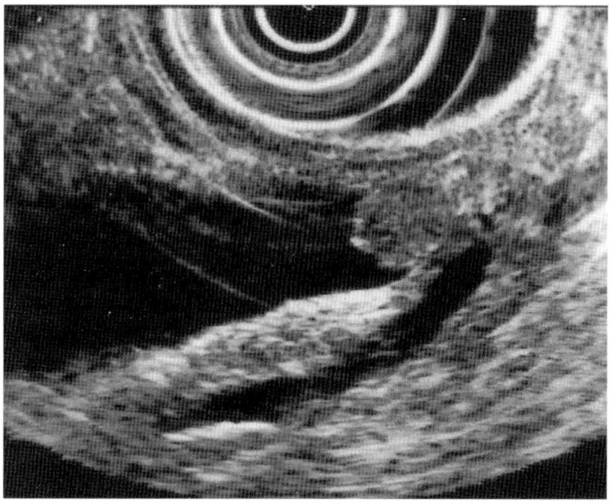

Fig. 10.**19 a** Adenomyomatosis of the major duodenal papilla.

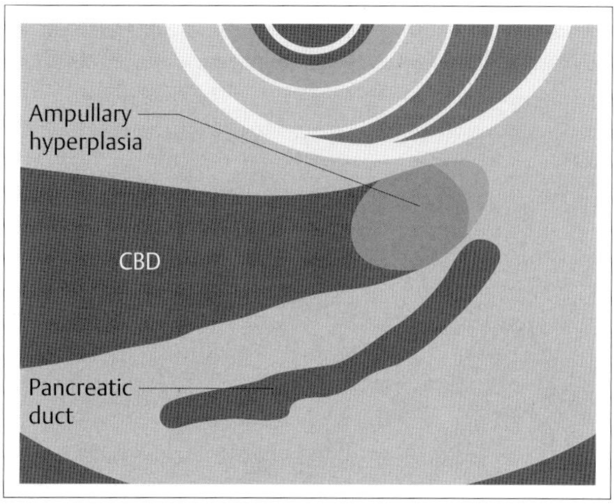

Fig. 10.**19 b** Line drawing.

Consequences for Surgical Treatment

Diagnosis	Other Relevant Factors	Management
Tumor limited to the papilla (uT1), histologically adenoma	No suspicion of malignant transformation No lymphadenopathy	Endoscopic papillectomy 1. R0 resection of adenoma → follow-up after 6 months 2. Adenoma with carcinoma → surgery
Tumor limited to the papilla–histologically adenoma or carcinoma uT1	Patient with co-morbidity No lymphadenopathy	Endoscopic papillectomy combined with APC; surgical resection of the papilla
Malignant tumor of the papilla without vascular invasion (uT1–uT3)	Low-risk patient No malignant lymph node at celiac trunk or hepatic portal (N2) No vascular invasion	Primary surgical resection Pancreatoduodenectomy
Extensive tumor with invasion of vessels and the hepatic portal (uT4)	Independent of T stage: Peritoneal carcinomatosis Patient with co-morbidity/ not suitable for surgery	Endoscopic papillotomy plus drainage of CBD

Colorectal Cancer

Basic Facts

- Etiology: 1% familial adenomatous polyposis (FAP), 5% hereditary nonpolyposis colorectal cancer (HNPCC), 4% de novo cancer, 90% adenoma–carcinoma sequence.
- Adenoma: 30–40% of patients > 60 years; 80% tubular, 15% tubulovillous, 5% villous; 20–50% of adenomas > 3–4 cm have undergone malignant transformation.
- Adenomas with malignant transformation (uT1) that underwent surgery after histological workup of the biopsy (endoscopic R0 ablation) revealed locoregional lymph node metastasis in only 0.3% (pediculated) and 1.5% (sessile) respectively–this justifies minimally invasive procedures.
- Resectability: 80–85%; mortality of colon resection 2–5%; 5-year survival rate dependent on stage (Dukes A 90%, B 70%, C (positive lymph nodes) 40%, D (metastasis) 1–3%).
- After distant metastasis has been ruled out, EUS is indicated in:
  1. Rectal adenomas (most often sessile) which cannot be resected endoscopically or only at increased risk.
  2. Staging of all histologically confirmed rectal cancer.
  3. Relative indications for EUS: EUS in adenoma/cancer of the colon (selection of T1 tumors) for planning of laparoscopic surgery.
- **Caveat:** Poor lymph node staging in colon cancer: sensitivity 40–60%.
- Differentiation between uT1 carcinoma and adenoma is not possible.
- EUS in follow-up: detection of anastomotic and extraluminal recurrence following minimally invasive rectal surgery (more sensitive than endoscopy plus CT; anastomositis yields false-positive findings, improved by EUS-guided FNA).
- Response to preoperative neoadjuvant treatment is not reliably validated by EUS: sensitivity about 50% (inflammation, fibrosis, necrosis mimicking residual tumor).
- *Additional workup:* MRI, EUS-guided FNA, PET.

Sonographic Criteria

- **Adenoma:** homogeneous echotexture of varying echogenicity, smooth outline, submucosa and muscularis propria intact, no locoregional lymphadenopathy.
- Signs of malignant transformation despite bioptic diagnosis of adenoma: tumor of heterogeneous echogenicity (*caveat:* status post biopsy!), irregular outline, submucosa no longer demarcated, suspicious locoregional lymph nodes.
- **Carcinoma:** hypoechoic heterogeneous echotexture, limited to mucosa and submucosa, smooth outline with defined muscularis propria (uT1) (Fig. 10.**20**).
- **Tumor with transmural spread** and smooth perirectal echo, muscularis propria no longer demarcated against the tumor (uT2); hypoechoic tumor spread into the perirectal fat (uT3); invasion of adjacent organs (uT4).

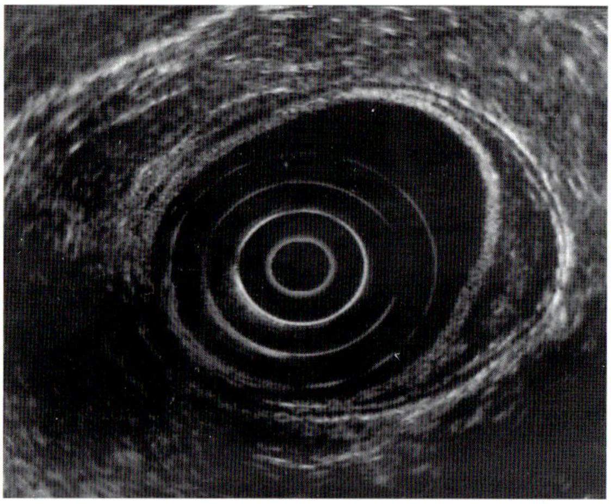

Fig. 10.**20 a** Rectal cancer; uT1 N0.

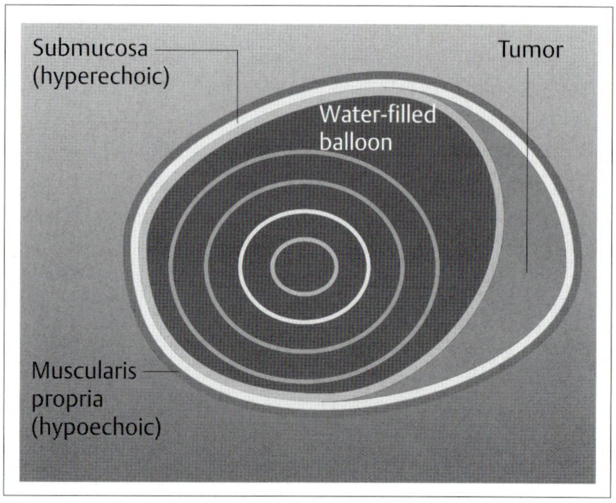

Fig. 10.**20 b** Line drawing.

Consequences for Surgical Treatment

Diagnosis	Other Relevant Factors	Management
Tumor (adenoma) limited to the mucosa; submucosa intact (uT1)	Resection technically possible; no lymphadenopathy on EUS	Endoscopic resection–if resection margin is not tumor-free or if carcinoma, then transanal endoscopic microsurgery (TEM) or surgery.
Carcinoma uT1; adenoma not respectable endoscopically	No lymph node metastasis on EUS uT2 N0 carcinoma and co-morbidity or high-risk	TEM
Carcinoma uT2, uT3	Perirectal lymphadenopathy	Curative resection; adjuvant RT/CT (for N+; T3)
Tumor with organ invasion (uT4)	Perirectal lymphadenopathy Liver metastases	Preoperative neoadjuvant RT/CT; surgery of metastases; palliative surgery

Additional Indications

- Achalasia: Concentric wall thickening at the level of the cardia, with thickened muscularis propria upstream. Signs of tumor-induced secondary achalasia: eccentric thickening of the cardia with spread cephalad and caudad, suspicious lymph nodes–EUS-guided FNA.
- Chronic pancreatitis: Stage I–Hypoechoic lobulated honeycomb structure with hyperechoic reticular septation; pancreatic duct of normal caliber but with marked mural echoes. Stages II and III–Calcification, cysts, ductal distension, irregular ductal course, pancreatic duct calculi, EUS-guided FNA (CEA, CA19–9, amylase, lipase, cytology) for differential diagnosis of cystic neoplasia vs. pseudocyst, drainage of pancreatic pseudocysts.
- Bile duct stones: Sensitivity 96%, specificity 95%; selective indication before cholecystectomy for treatment planning (ERCP, laparoscopy, surgical bile duct exploration).
- Gallbladder pathology with equivocal assessment by TAUS.
- Mediastinal tumors, lymph node metastasis in bronchial carcinoma–EUS-guided FNA.
- Workup of pararectal abscess; defects of the anal sphincter.
- EUS-guided FNA for celiac trunk neurolysis in pancreatic pathology.

Bibliography

Caletti G, Fusaroli P, Bocus P: Endoscopic Ultrasonography. Endoscopy. 1998; 30: 198–221.

Dancygier H.: Endoskopische Sonographie in der Gastroenterologie. Stuttgart: Thieme,; 1997.

Nickl NJ, Bhutani MS, Catalano M, et al. Clinical implications of endoscopic ultrasound: the American Endosonography Club Study. Gastrointest Endosc. 1996; 44: 371–377.

Rösch T, Classen M.: Gastroenterologicological Endosonography. Stuttgart: Thieme,; 1992.

Rösch T, Will U, Chang K.: Longitudinal Endosonography. Heidelberg, New York: Springer Verlag,; 2001.

Tio T.: Gastrointestinal TNM Cancer Staging by Endosonography. New York, Tokyio: Igaku-Shoin, New York – Tokio; 1995.

Van Dam J: · Endosonography 2000. Gastrointestinal Endoscopy 2000; 6 (Suppl.): 52.

Wiersema MJ, Vilmann P, Giovannini M, et al. Endosonography-guided fine-needle aspiration biopsy: diagnostic accuracy and complication assessment. Gastroenterology. 1997; 112: 1087–1095.

11 Sonography of the Urinary Tract and the Male Genital System

G. Kaiper

Indications for Sonography

- Sonography of the *k*idneys, *u*reters, *b*ladder (KUB), and scrotum is the basic imaging modality in diagnostic urological workup.
- The objective is a general evaluation of the organs based on the clinical symptoms.
- Palpable changes in the scrotum may be due to wide range of pathologies.
- Acute scrotal pain is mainly caused by epidydimitis, orchitis, abscess, strangulated inguinal hernia, trauma, or acute torsion of the spermatic cord, testis, or testicular appendage. On the other hand, testicular tumor, hydrocele, spermatocele, chronic epidydimitis, varicocele, uncomplicated hernia, and persistent torsion of the spermatic cord, testis, or testicular appendage tend to be painless conditions
- Normal ureters cannot be delineated, and thus evaluated, by sonography.
- Ureters can be visualized only if dilated, most clearly in their subpelvic and prevesical course.
- Sonography of the scrotum complements inspection, palpation, and transillumination and is particularly helpful in the differential diagnosis of pathologies with similar clinical manifestations.

Specific Technique and Diagnostic Evaluation

- 3.5–5.0 MHz probe for the abdominal views and a 7.5–10 MHz (small-parts) scanner for the scrotum
- Duplex and color-flow duplex scanning can help evaluate testicular blood flow when torsion is suspected
- Transrectal probe (6–7.5 MHz) for prostate and seminal vesicles
- Patient positioning – Table 11.**1**
- Assessment of position, shape, and size of the kidneys
- Assessment of position, shape, and filled volume of the bladder
- Assessment of size and echotexture of the testes
- In case of paired organs both must always be evaluated in longitudinal as well as in transverse views
- Abnormal findings must be considered within the clinical context, since a number of changes are clinically irrelevant.

Table 11.**1** Patient positioning in sonography of the urinary tract and scrotum

Supine	– Right kidney (employing the liver as acoustic window) – Left kidney (imaging frequently incomplete due to bowel gas interference) – Bladder (when filled) – Prostate/seminal vesicles (suprapubic view, with the filled bladder acting as acoustic window) – Scrotum (the penis should be pulled cephalad)
Left lateral decubitus	– Right kidney
Right lateral decubitus	– Left kidney
Sitting	– Both kidneys (posterior approach)

Normal Kidney

- Renal size (a) Adults: length 10–12 cm, width 5–6 cm, depth 4 cm
  (b) Children: depends on age
- Parenchymal thickness 13–18 mm.
- Sonographic anatomy of the kidney:
  - Parenchyma–hypoechoic, homogeneous, pyramids frequently even more hypoechoic.
  - Central echo complex (renal sinus)–hyperechoic (vessels, collecting system, fat).
  - Fibrous capsule–hyperechoic lining (Fig. 11.**1**)

Normal Urinary Bladder

- Sonography of the filled (> 200 ml) bladder via TAUS in the suprapubic region.
- Transverse view: ovoid to square shape.
- Longitudinal view: triangular, with rounded corners.
- Smooth inner surface.
- Wall thickness varying with degree of filling (5–10 mm at < 50 ml; 1–3 mm with maximum filling).

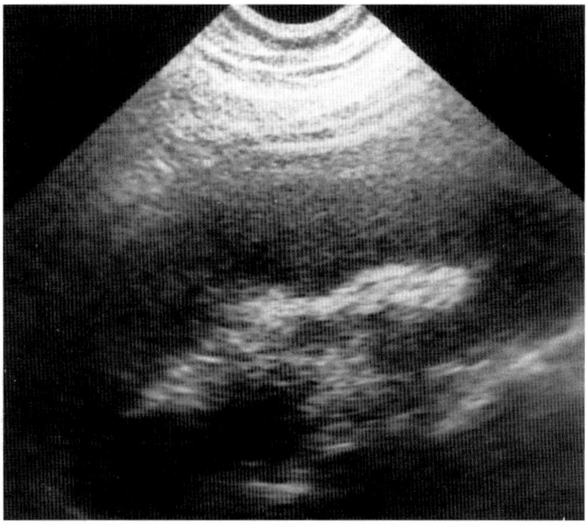

Fig. 11.**1 a** Sonogram of a normal kidney.

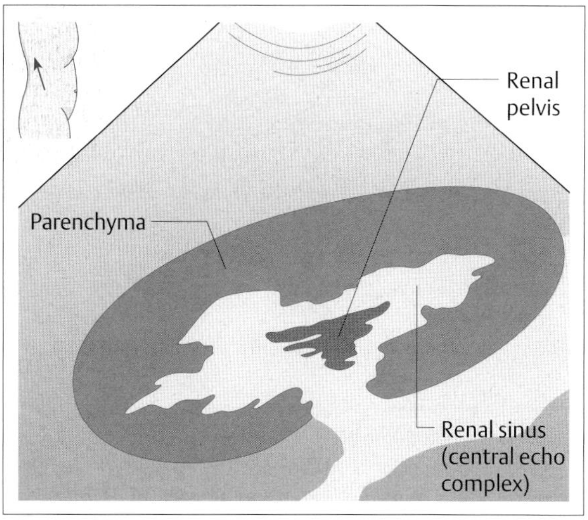

Fig. 11.**1 b** Line drawing.

Normal Prostate and Seminal Vesicles

- Suprapubic view (filled bladder)–triangular in transverse plane, harder to assess in longitudinal plane (Fig. 11.**2**).
- Homogeneous delicate echotexture (variable due to enhancement induced by the filled bladder).
- Transrectal ultrasonography (TRUS) with a special probe (6–7.5 MHz) better depicts details of the glandular anatomy.
- Seminal vesicles–posterolateral to the bladder and best viewed suprapubically (filled bladder). Better detailed assessment via TRUS (Fig. 11.**3**).

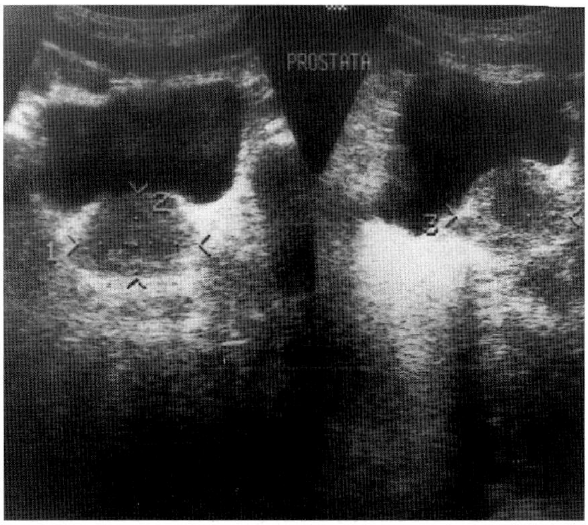

Fig. 11.**2 a** Suprapubic view of the prostate in two planes.

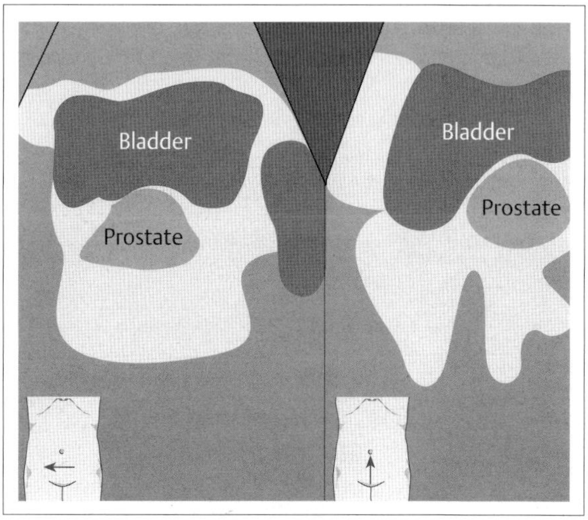

Fig. 11.**2 b** Line drawing.

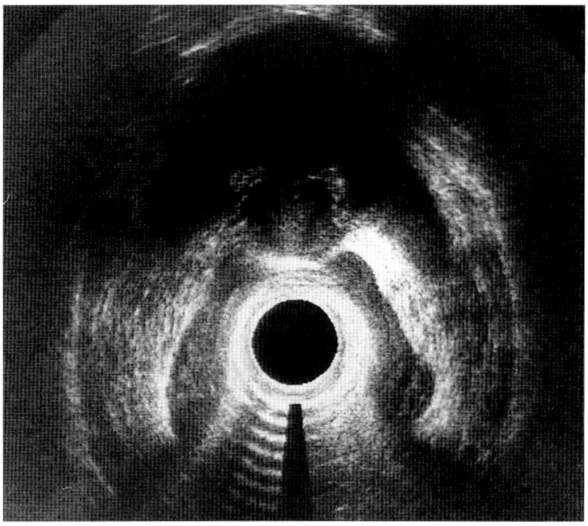

Fig. 11.**3 a** Transverse view of the seminal vesicles on transrectal ultrasound.

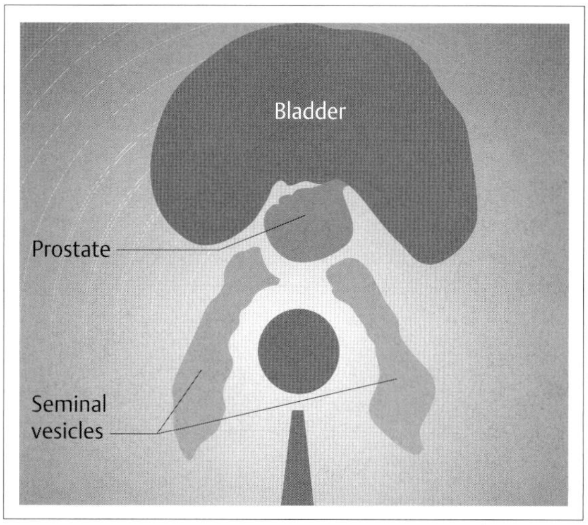

Fig. 11.**3 b** Line drawing.

Normal Testis and Epididymis

- Variable size.
- Homogeneous echotexture, intermediate echogenicity (resembling that of the thyroid gland).
- The head of the epididymis with its ovoid shape along the longitudinal axis caps the superior pole of the testis; it is slightly hyperechoic to the testicular parenchyma. Body and tail of the epididymis are more difficult to delineate.
- Frequently, the parietal and visceral layers of the tunica vaginalis are separated by a thin film of liquid (Fig. 11.**4**).

Post-Voiding Bladder Volume Estimation

- TAUS–longitudinal and transverse view (split image) for determination of the maximum size in each plane.
- Measurement of maximum length, depth, and width (in cm); the volume is approximated by the formula for a rotational ellipsoid: In practice a simplified equation is used:
  - Volume (ml) = length × depth × width × 0.52.
  - For volumes of 60–100 ml there is an error of ± 25 %.

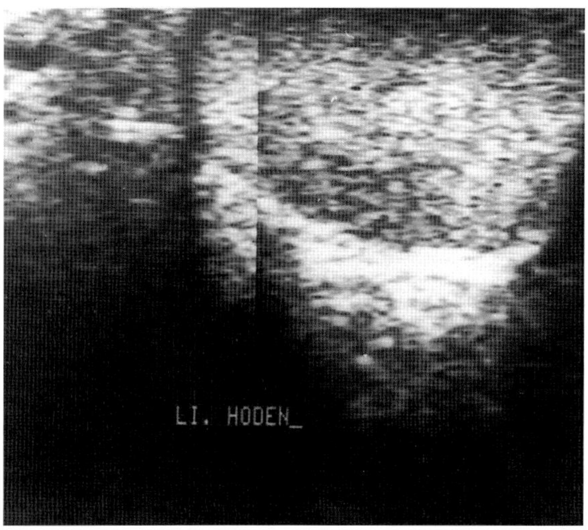

Fig. 11.**4 a** Sonogram of a normal testis and epididymis.

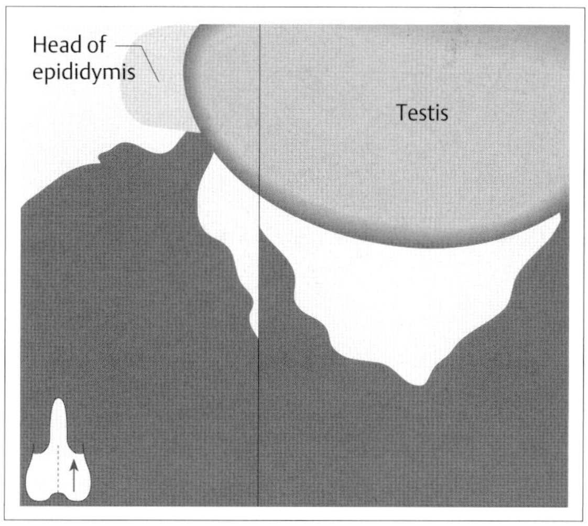

Fig. 11.**4 b** Line drawing.

Obstructive Hydronephrosis

Basic Facts

- Hydronephrosis is a rather common manifestation of variable etiology (stones, tumors of the ureter and bladder, non-urinary-tract conditions).
- Clinical symptoms include dull persistent flank pain, possibly accompanied by fever.
- Dilatation of the renal pelvis and calices leads to pressure atrophy of the papillae and later of the parenchyma, finally resulting in hydronephrosis.

Sonographic Criteria

- Central echo complex fanned out by anechoic confluent areas (corresponding to renal pelvis and calices) (Fig. 11.**5**).
- Hydronephrosis is classified into four degrees (Table 11.**2**).
- Echoes within the collecting system are indicative of purulent matter.

Table 11.**2** Classification criteria used in hydronephrosis

Degree I	Central fanning of the central echo complex extending into the calices Major calices dilated to 5–10 mm; parenchymal width normal
Degree II	Renal pelvis dilated and branching out into the calices Major calices dilated to 10–16 mm; parenchymal width normal
Degree III	Caliceal diameter > 16 mm; calices frequently only rudimentary in appearance Parenchymal width thinned
Degree IV	Septated liquid structures almost resembling cysts, classic picture of hydronephrosis; parenchymal width reduced to just a few millimeters

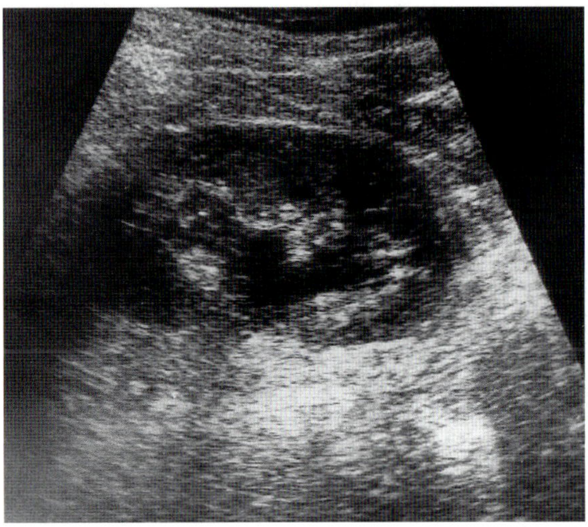

Fig. 11.**5 a** First/second degree hydronephrosis.

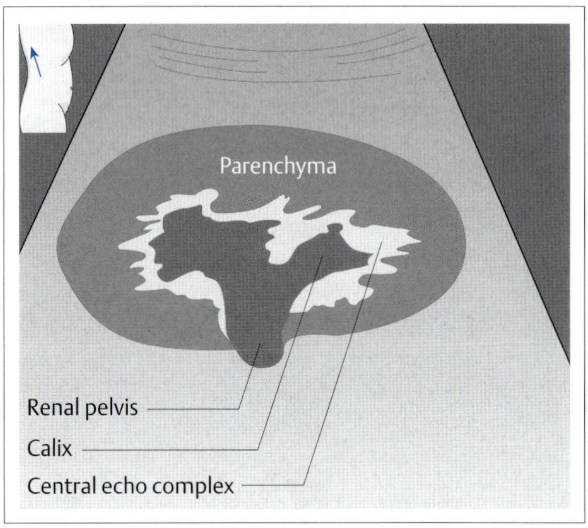

Fig. 11.**5 b** Line drawing.

Consequences for Surgical Treatment

Diagnosis	Characteristic Findings	Management
I°/II° hydronephrosis No clinical symptoms	Caliceal diameter < 16 mm	Further workup (i. v. urography, retrograde ureteropyelography, endoscopic urinary drainage)
II°/III° hydronephrosis With febrile temperature	Caliceal diameter > 16 mm; possibly sludge in the renal pelvis	Retrograde exploration (pigtail catheter insertion, percutaneous nephrostomy), additional treatment depending on the cause
IV° hydronephrosis (most often asymptomatic)	Kidney with cystic appearance; possibly with ureteral dilatation	Renal scintigraphy (residual function?), possibly nephrectomy

Nephrolithiasis

Basic Facts

- Incidence of nephrolithiasis in the general population is up to 5% and recurrence is common.
- Clinical presentation is characterized by colic and possibly hematuria.
- Quite often, renal calculi are completely asymptomatic.

Sonographic Criteria

- Due to the significant difference in impedance, calculi produce strong echoes with posterior shadowing (Fig. 11.**6**).
- In case of intracaliceal location or small size (< 4 mm), visualization becomes difficult (Fig. 11.**7**).
- Secondary changes due to obstructing stones (hydronephrosis) may also be demonstrated (Fig. 11.**8**).

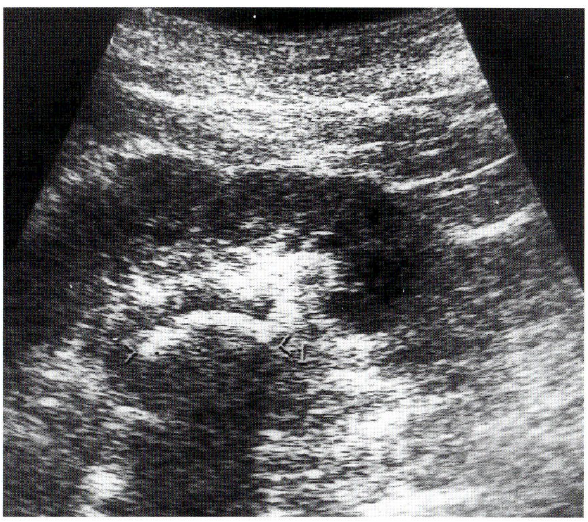

Fig. 11.**6a** Large nonobstructing pelvic stone.

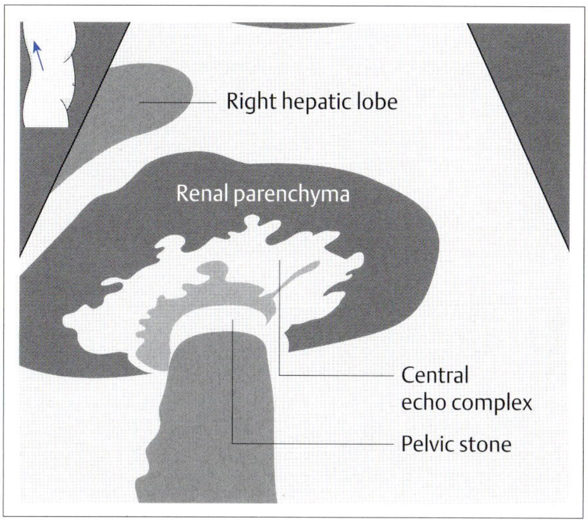

Fig. 11.**6b** Line drawing.

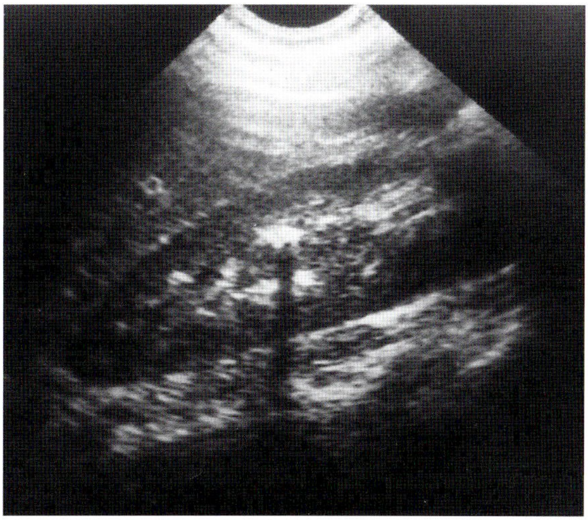

Fig. 11.**7a** Stone in the middle calix of the right kidney.

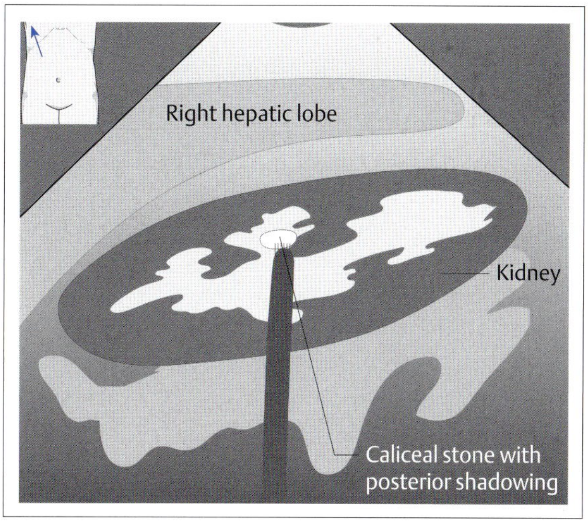

Fig. 11.**7b** Line drawing.

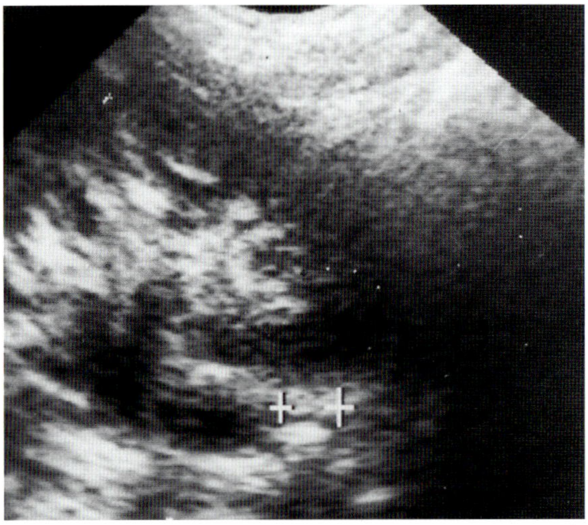

Fig. 11.8a Hydronephrosis secondary to a proximal ureteral stone.

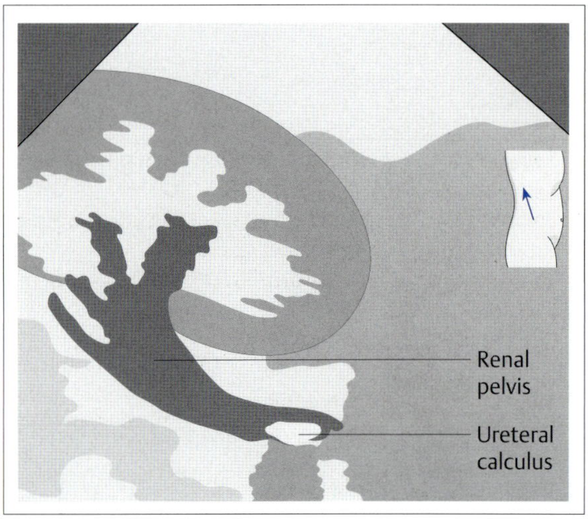

Fig. 11.8b Line drawing.

Consequences for Surgical Treatment

Diagnosis	Characteristic Findings	Management
Small asymptomatic nonobstructing caliceal stone	< 4–5 mm calculus demonstrated close to a papilla	Follow-up; ESWL if increase in size
Pelvic calculus, stone acting like a flap-valve, or proximal ureteral stone	Larger stone in renal pelvis or proximal ureter with urinary obstruction	ESWL in situ, possibly preceded by push-back of the stone and insertion of pigtail catheter; percutaneous nephrostomy (PCN)
Staghorn calculus	Adjacent cap-shaped echoes with summation of posterior shadowing	Depending on renal function (clearance!) percutaneous nephrolithotomy (PCNL) and ESWL (residual stones) or primarily open surgical approach

Renal Cysts

Basic Facts

- Renal cysts develop as part of genetically determined aging, possibly influenced by exogenous factors.
- They originate from Bowman's capsule and the proximal tubules, which become dilated and cystic.
- Parapelvic cysts probably arise from ectatic parts of the lymphatics.
- Cysts may be solitary, multilocular, unilateral, or bilateral.
- "Atypical cysts" are those differing from the normal appearance.

Sonographic Criteria

- Anechoic internal echotexture with a narrow rim of entry–exit echoes.
- Posterior enhancement.
- Larger cysts present edge shadowing.
- Cysts are classified according to their location: superficial, parenchymal, parapelvic, and central (Fig. 11.**9**).
- Chambered cysts, focal wall thickening, and internal echoes are characteristic of "atypical cysts."

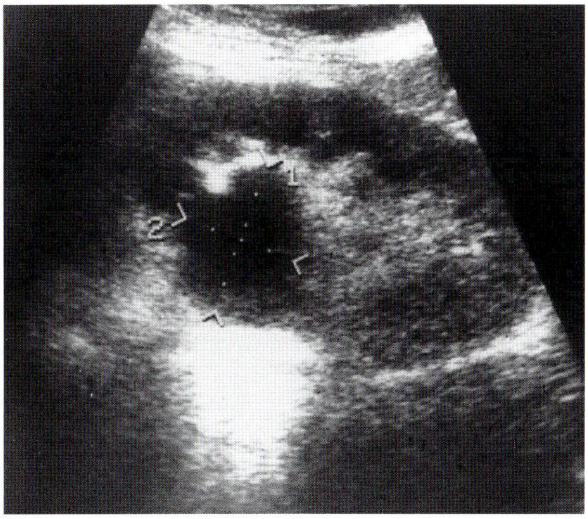

Fig. 11.**9a** Central renal cyst.

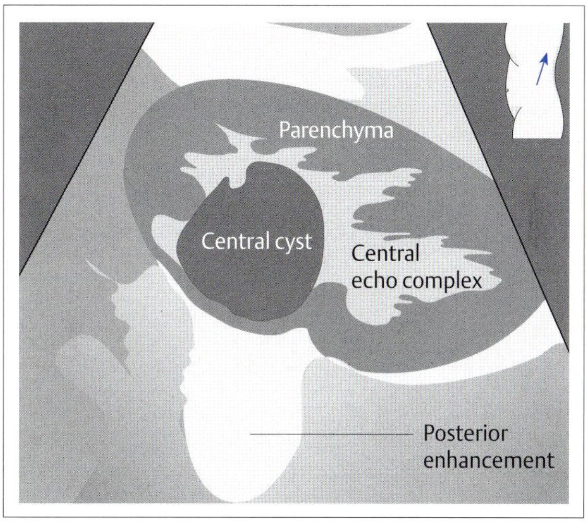

Fig. 11.**9b** Line drawing.

Consequences for Surgical Treatment

Diagnosis	Characteristic Findings	Management
Asymptomatic solitary or multiple cysts	Characteristic anechoic round areas without secondary sequelae	None; possibly follow-up
Cysts causing subjective discomfort and/or impaired urinary flow	Cysts at the pyeloureteral junction; secondary urinary retention	US-guided percutaneous aspiration (cytology, LDH level); possibly sclerotherapy or open surgery
Atypical cysts	Irregular wall, internal echoes	Further workup (CT, FNA cytology, LDH level); surgical exploration if malignancy is suspected

Polycystic Kidney Disease

Basic Facts

- Intermingling of normal nephrons and those with cystic dilatation (adult type Potter III) found diffusely throughout the kidney. Autosomal dominant. Incidence 1/1000.
- Cysts increase in size with age and thus may become painful.
- Pressure atrophy of the functioning nephrons gives rise to progressive renal failure and possibly hypertension.
- Becomes manifest with renal failure/hypertension at age 30–40 years.
- In 20–30% associated with cysts in other organs (liver, spleen, pancreas).

Sonographic Criteria

- Moderate to extreme increase in renal size.
- Multiple cysts of different size diffusely distributed throughout the entire organ.
- Solid parts (parenchyma) only visualized in the initial stages of the disease (Fig. 11.**10**).
- Central echo complex (renal sinus) cannot be delineated reliably.
- Polycyclic contour of the enlarged kidney(s), with internal echoes in some of the cysts (blood?).

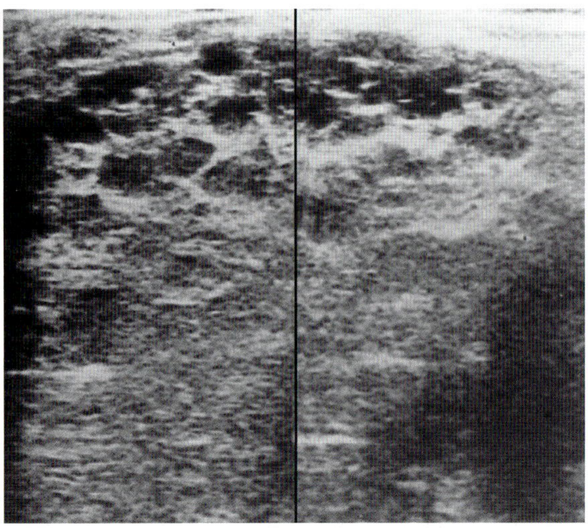

Fig. 11.**10 a** Polycystic kidney disease (Potter III).

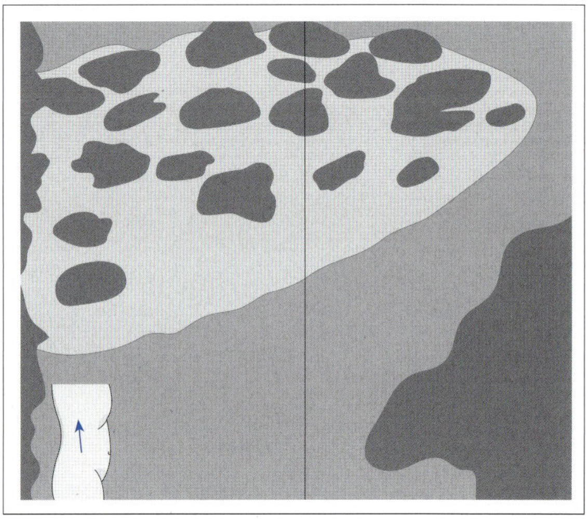

Fig. 11.**10 b** Line drawing.

Consequences for Surgical Treatment

Diagnosis	Characteristic Findings	Management
Asymptomatic bilateral kidney enlargement; renal failure	Multiple bilateral cysts of varying size; spots of parenchyma	Conservative
Subjective discomfort, possibly fever	Internal echoes in some cysts; urinary retention cannot be ruled out sonographically	Hydronephrosis ruled out by retrograde ureteropyelography; CT if hemorrhage is suspected; possibly indication for nephrectomy (particularly in the septic patient)

Parenchymal and Pelvic Tumors of the Kidney

Basic Facts

- Around 90% of all solid adult tumors are renal cell carcinomas; it is the most common malignancy affecting 5–8/100 000 with a female preponderance of 2 : 1; incidence and mortality are on the rise.
- The shape of the tumors is rather varied.
- Benign tumors (angiomyolipoma, adenoma, fibroma) are less common.
- Hematuria is regarded as proof that the tumor has breached the collecting system.
- Even giant tumors may remain asymptomatic for a long time and are discovered incidentally.
- Tumors of the collecting system present early with frank hematuria; although usually painless, clots may give rise to obstruction and thus discomfort.

Sonographic Criteria

- Sonographic morphology varies greatly and the tumors tend to be hypoechoic to or isoechoic with the renal parenchyma.
- Tumors < 2 cm are rarely detected.
- Bulging of the renal contour or destruction of structures of the central echo complex (Fig. 11.**11**).
- Irregular anechoic areas signal necrosis within the tumor.
- Sonography cannot differentiate between benign and malignant tumors, except for angiomyolipoma with its characteristic homogeneous hyperechoic appearance (Fig. 11.**12**).
- Irregular hypoechoic structures in the sinus or in a dilated renal pelvis raise the suspicion of a tumor within the collecting system (Fig. 11.**13**).

Consequences for Surgical Treatment

Diagnosis	Characteristic Findings	Management
Parenchymal mass	Homogeneous, hyperechoic; central structures hypoechoic, if visible at all	Suspected angiomyolipoma, CT with densitometry (fatty tissue). Follow-up for tumors < 3 cm; surgery, possibly subtotal nephrectomy, if increasing in size
Hematuria and/or pain, possibly palpable tumor	Heterogeneous, mostly hypoechoic texture, well defined to the parenchyma, bulging of the kidney contour	Suspected renal tumor, further workup (urography, CT, possibly DSA), radical or subtotal (small tumors, renal failure) nephrectomy
Hematuria, possibly pain on voiding of clots or in urinary retention	In the central echo complex, hypoechoic structures along the collecting system or mural irregularities	Suspected pelvic tumor, urography, urinary cytology, retrograde ureteropyelography, ureterorenoscopy with biopsy, CT, nephroureterectomy including bladder cuff

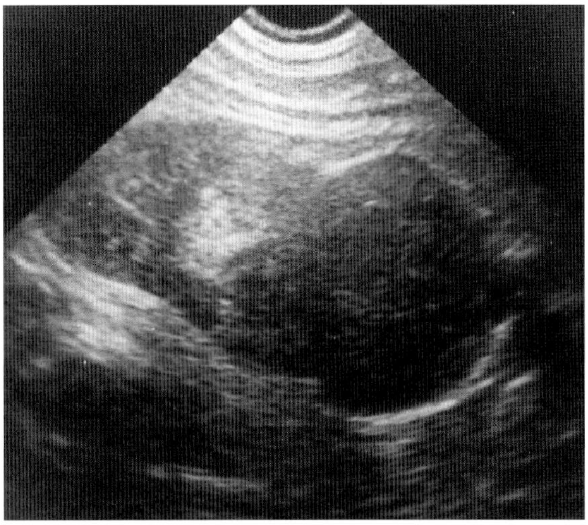

Fig. 11.**11 a** Solid tumor at the inferior pole of the kidney.

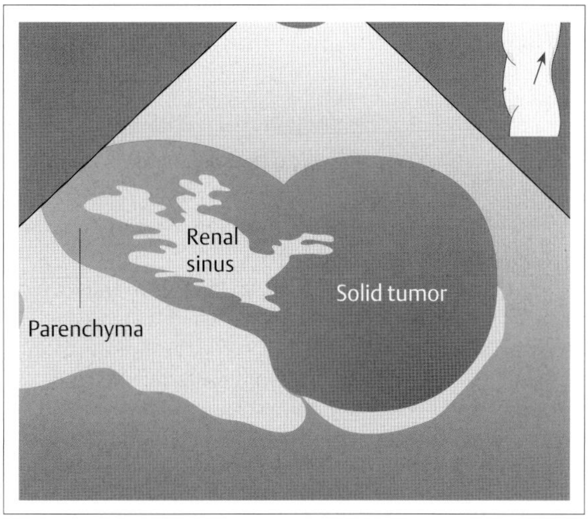

Fig. 11.**11 b** Line drawing.

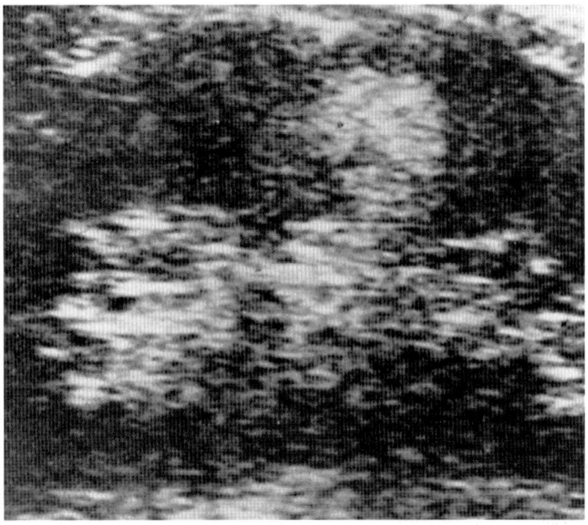

Fig. 11.**12 a** Mid-level angiomyolipoma of the kidney.

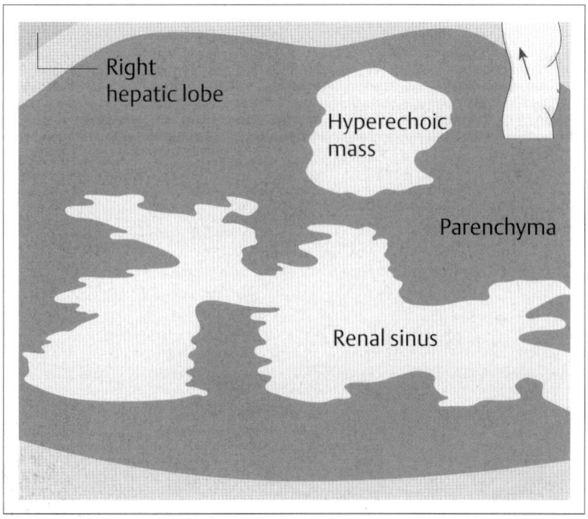

Fig. 11.**12 b** Line drawing.

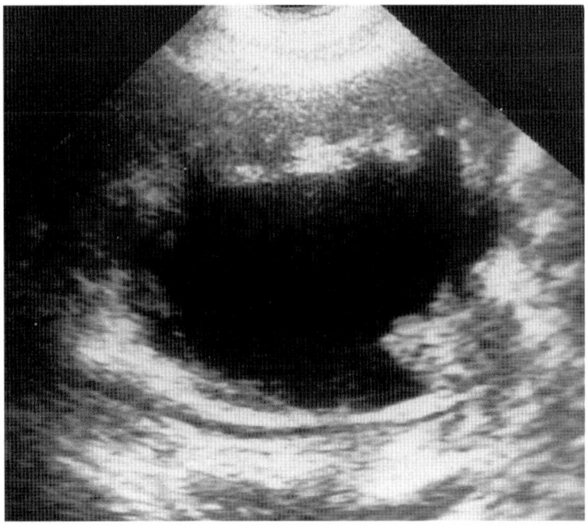

Fig. 11.**13 a** III° hydronephrosis secondary to a tumor in the renal pelvis.

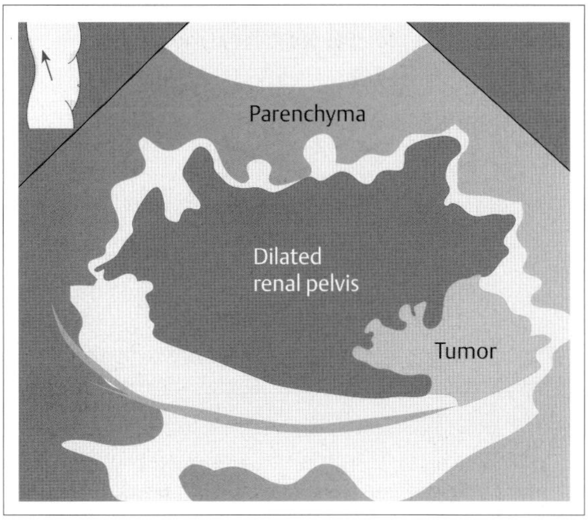

Fig. 11.**13 b** Line drawing.

Diffuse Renal Parenchymal Disease with Acute Presentation

Basic Facts

- Diffuse parenchymal disease of the kidneys includes:
  - Bacterial interstitial nephritis (pyelonephritis)
  - Acute nonbacterial interstitial nephritis
  - Acute glomerulonephritis
- Predominant clinical signs of bacterial kidney infections are pain (possibly unilateral) and fever.
- Acute glomerulonephritis is accompanied by hematuria, proteinuria, hypertension, and renal failure.
- Acute renal failure has mainly cardiovascular etiology.
- Sonographic assessment of acute diffuse renal disease is limited.

Sonographic Criteria

- A finding of both kidneys enlarged with a broadened hypoechoic parenchymal rim is rather characteristic of acute renal failure; indistinct narrowed renal sinus.
- The parenchyma becomes more hypoechoic and the pyramids are prominent (Fig. 11.**14**).
- In bacterial nephritis the affected kidney is enlarged, with broadened hypoechoic parenchymal rim but with a heterogeneous echotexture.
- In suppurative pyelonephritis with abscess formation the parenchyma becomes more heterogeneous, and the border between parenchyma and central echo complex becomes faded.

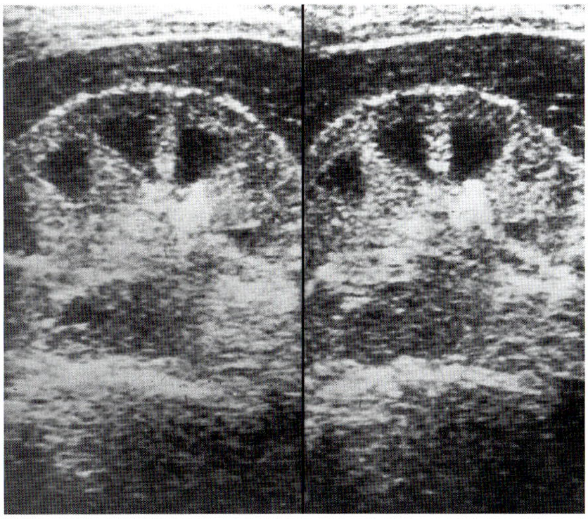

Fig. 11.**14 a** Renal changes in glomerulonephritis.

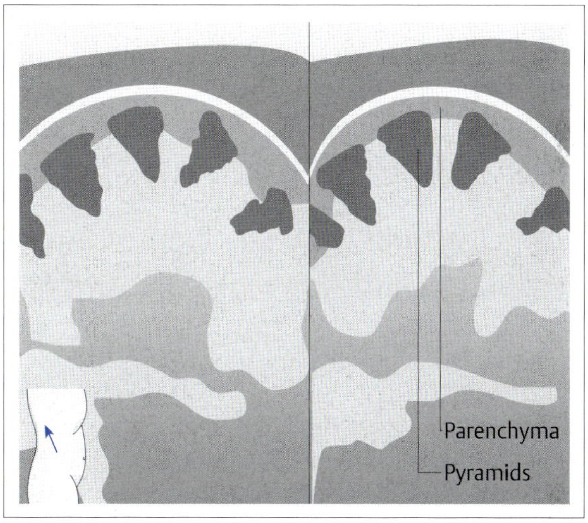

Fig. 11.**14 b** Line drawing.

Consequences for Surgical Treatment

Diagnosis	Characteristic Findings	Management
Painless microhematuria, proteinuria, hypertension, impaired renal function in glomerulonephritis	Parenchyma of more pronounced echogenicity with prominent pyramids	Nonsurgical treatment after confirmation by FNA biopsy
Acute renal failure	Both kidneys enlarged with hypoechoic parenchyma, narrowed indistinct renal sinus	Acute dialysis and treatment of the underlying disease
Unilateral or bilateral renal pain, fever, suspected pyelonephritis	Enlarged kidney, parenchyma more hypoechoic but heterogeneous	Broad-spectrum antibiotics (urine culture) followed by workup of underlying pathology
Unilateral renal pain, high fever, possibly diabetes, suspicion of pyelonephritis with abscess formation	Heterogeneous renal parenchyma, indistinct border between parenchyma and central echo complex	Rule out mechanical cause (urinary drainage in hydronephrosis)

Renal and Pararenal Abscess

Basic Facts

- Renal abscesses are confluent, embolizing suppurative lesions in the renal cortex (carbuncle).
- Cortical abscesses are blood-borne (*S. aureus* infection), less commonly arising from suppurative pyelonephritis (gram-negative bacteria); diabetes is a predisposing factor.
- Pararenal abscess = pus collection between the renal capsule and perirenal (Gerota's) fascia, usually secondary to a renal abscess. Predisposing factors: diabetes and urinary stones.
- Clinical symptoms include fever and a painful, possibly swollen, flank and/or reddening in perinephric and pararenal abscess.
- Abscess sonomorphology is variable.
- In pararenal abscess the kidney displays limited mobility on respiration.

Sonographic Criteria

- **Abscesses** may appear as partly cystic with internal echoes, often with a hyperechoic rim, but always indistinctly delineated from the parenchyma (Fig. 11.**15**).
- **Superficial abscesses** have indistinct delineation from the renal contour, while a heterogeneous echotexture of the surrounding tissue (intermingling of hypoechoic, anechoic, and hyperechoic structures) is characteristic of pararenal abscess.

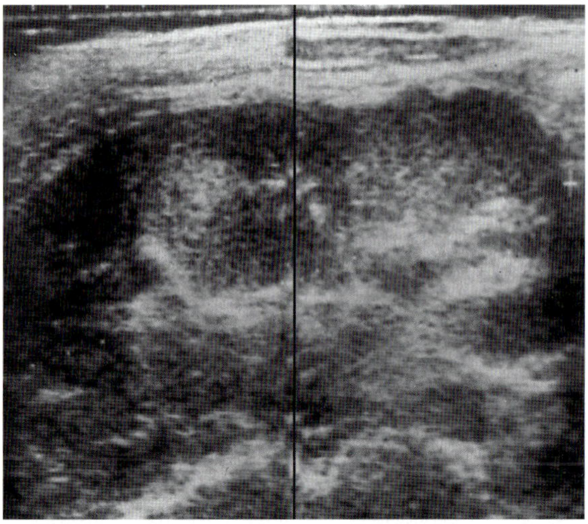

Fig. 11.**15a** Mid-level renal abscess (renal carbuncle).

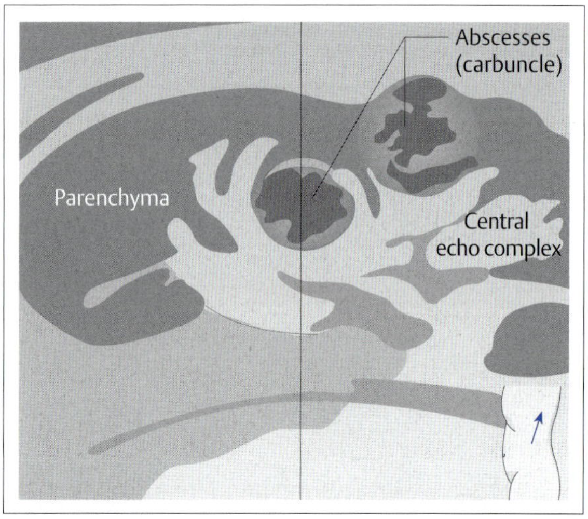

Fig. 11.**15b** Line drawing.

Consequences for Surgical Treatment

Diagnosis	Characteristic Findings	Management
Unilateral flank pain, high fever	Hypoechoic focal mass with internal echoes and a rim–suspicious for renal abscess	Further workup including CT, broad-spectrum antibiotics; possibly percutaneous drainage of the abscess
Flank pain, fever, possibly swelling and reddening of the flank	Indistinct renal contour with focal transition into heterogeneous perinephric tissue, loss of renal mobility on respiration	CT if pararenal abscess is suspected; percutaneous drainage or surgical exploration

Bladder Disease

Basic Facts

- Tumors of the bladder are the most common neoplasms of the collecting system, affecting men four times as often as women. They are mainly seen with advancing age (peak between 60 and 70 years); only 5% of the tumors arise during the first three decades of life.
- Leading symptom is hematuria (usually painless), possibly severe enough to fill the entire bladder with coagulated blood (tamponade).
- Sonographic visualization of bladder tumors depends on the filling volume of the bladder and location of the tumor. Predominant site: trigone and lateral wall; often multiple tumors.
- Bladder calculi mostly lead to vesical complaints, usually accompanied by subvesical obstruction (benign prostatic hyperplasia, cancer of the prostate, sclerosis of the neck, urethral stricture).
- Bladder diverticula, predominantly located posteriorly close to the ureteral orifice, comprise all layers of the wall, communicating with the lumen of the bladder via a neck of varying width; often they are clinically silent, and they carry the risk of malignant transformation.

Sonographic Criteria

- **Bladder carcinomas** present as pointed or polycyclic structures encroaching on the lumen; hypoechoic to the wall but heterogeneous; differentiation between benign/malignant not possible; possible invasion of the wall cannot be assessed by suprapubic sonography (Fig. 11.**16**).
- **Bladder calculi:** Characteristic bright echoes with posterior shadowing; on patient repositioning they display a definite change in position.
- **Bladder diverticula** are characterized by perivesical liquid areas; definite diagnosis requires demonstration of the diverticular neck; an irregular wall may herald the presence of diverticular cancer.
- Cystitis does not exhibit specific sonomorphological features.

- Acute cystitis is common. Diagnosis is mainly based on the clinical symptoms (dysuria, pollakisuria, possibly terminal hematuria) and laboratory results.

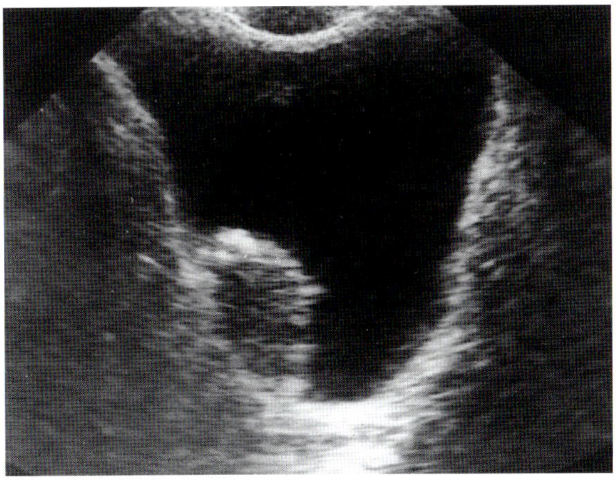

Fig. 11.**16 a** Solid tumor in the right wall of the bladder.

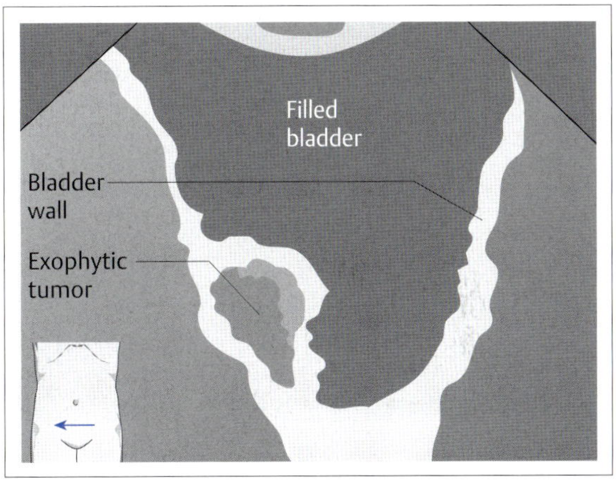

Fig. 11.**16 b** Line drawing.

Consequences for Surgical Treatment

Diagnosis	Characteristic Findings	Management
Severe dysuric complaints, suprapubic tenderness, possibly hematuria; suspicion of cystitis	On sonography, the bladder tends to be poorly filled without specific pathology	Conservative
Painful voiding and hematuria, particularly after physical activity; clinical suspicion of bladder calculi	Characteristic image of a stone within the vesical lumen, nonsessile on repositioning, possibly accompanied by an enlarged prostate	Urography, endoscopy, treatment of underlying infection, lithotripsy, possibly combined with prostatectomy
Macrohematuria (most often painless or intermittent)	Bladder with hyperechoic structures; vesical tamponade; suspected focal masses encroaching on the lumen	Bladder tamponade: evacuation, continuous irrigation; endoscopy, transurethral resection of confirmed tumor; further treatment guided by tumor stage (cystectomy, chemotherapy)

Prostate Disease

Basic Facts

- Prostatitis is an acute inflammation of the prostate gland. Symptoms include perineal pain and voiding problems possibly culminating in retention of urine; on palpation the prostate appears enlarged, of rubbery consistency, and tender.
- Prostatitis may result in prostate abscess; rather tender fluctuant swelling, fever.
- Benign prostatic hyperplasia (BPH) is the result of normal physiological aging; multiple fibroadenomatous nodules, probably originating within the periurethral glands (inner gland), with peripheral displacement of the prostate proper (outer gland). Clinical picture: incomplete emptying (postvoid residual) including urinary retention; secondary changes in the bladder (hypertrophic wall, trabeculation).
- Prostate cancer originates in the outer gland; symptoms resemble those of BPH. Clinical diagnosis is by palpation (firm to hard masses) and elevated levels of prostate-specific antigen (PSA).

Sonographic Criteria

- **Age-corrected** enlargement, hypoechogenicity, and homogeneity of the **prostate** imply inflammation.
- **Prostatic abscess:** irregular, mostly anechoic areas within the gland (Fig. 11.**17**).
- Embedded hyperechoic structures, partly plaque-shaped or with posterior shadowing (prostatic calcifications) in chronic prostatitis or inflammatory residual disease.
- **Benign prostatic hyperplasia:** enlarged gland of intermediate echogenicity with a homogeneous echotexture, possibly indenting the floor of the bladder (DD: bladder tumor) (Fig. 11.**18**).
- **Bladder wall hypertrophy** (trabeculated bladder): diffuse serrated or wavy appearance of the mucosa.
- **Prostate cancer:** hypoechoic focal changes. Suprapubic TAUS would be overtaxed here; if cancer is suspected, transrectal ultrasound (TRUS) with a special probe is preferred (Fig. 11.**19**).

Consequences for Surgical Treatment

Diagnosis	Characteristic Findings	Management
Perineal pain, dysuria. Prostate soft on palpation	Enlarged hypoechoic homogeneous prostate characteristic of prostatitis	Nonsurgical (antibiotics), in significant dysuria, suprapubic catheter placement may be warranted
Perineal pain, dysuria, pyrexia; rectal examination. With fluctuant swelling, suspect abscess	Enlarged prostate with anechoic, irregularly defined areas	Abscess drainage by transurethral electrocautery or perineal aspiration, suprapubic catheterization, broad-spectrum antibiotics
Voiding problems, nycturia, increased postvoid residual or urinary retention; firm elastic prostate on rectal examination	Enlarged prostate of intermediate echogenicity, possibly indenting the floor of the bladder. Secondary changes in the bladder (wall hypertrophy = trabeculated bladder)	Medical treatment if postvoid residual is low; in urinary retention, Foley or suprapubic catheterization, surgery (TURP or open surgery)
Voiding problems. Prostate with a firm mass on palpation is suspicious for cancer	Possibly asymmetric enlargement of the prostate with a hypoechoic mass. Preferably transrectal ultrasound (TRUS)	PSA level, TRUS, US-guided biopsy or, in diffuse changes, random biopsy. Stage-adjusted treatment after pathological confirmation

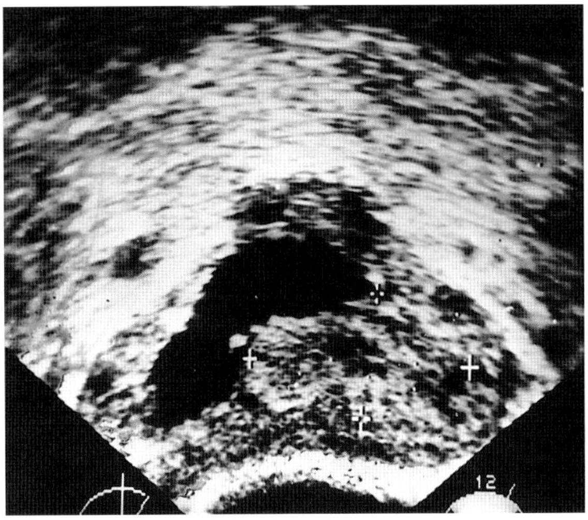

Fig. 11.**17 a** Transrectal ultrasound (TRUS) in a prostatic abscess.

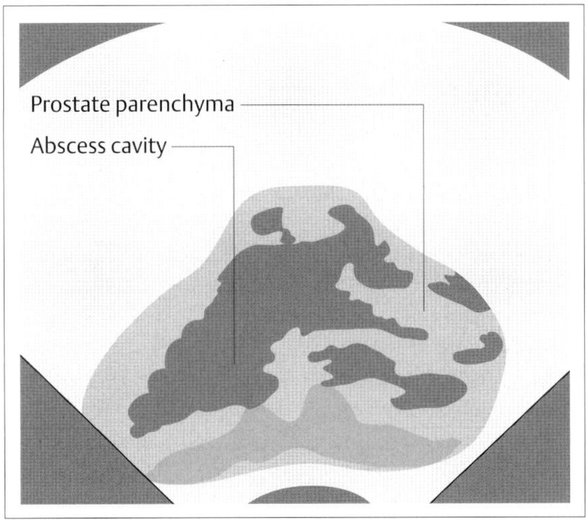

Fig. 11.**17 b** Line drawing.

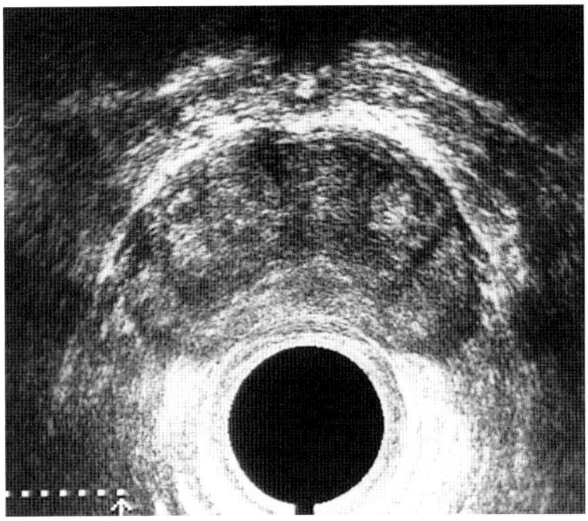

Fig. 11.**18 a** TRUS in benign prostatic hyperplasia (delineation of inner and outer gland).

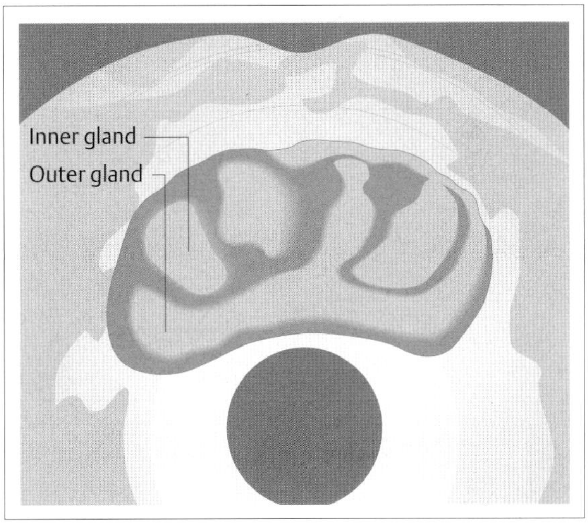

Fig. 11.**18 b** Line drawing.

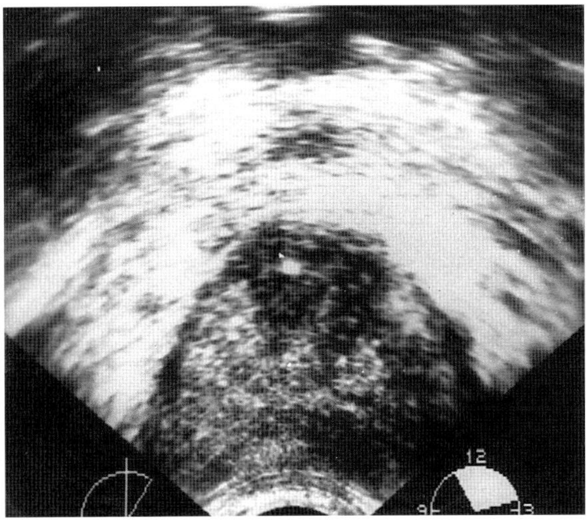

Fig. 11.**19 a** TRUS in prostate cancer, mainly affecting the left lobe.

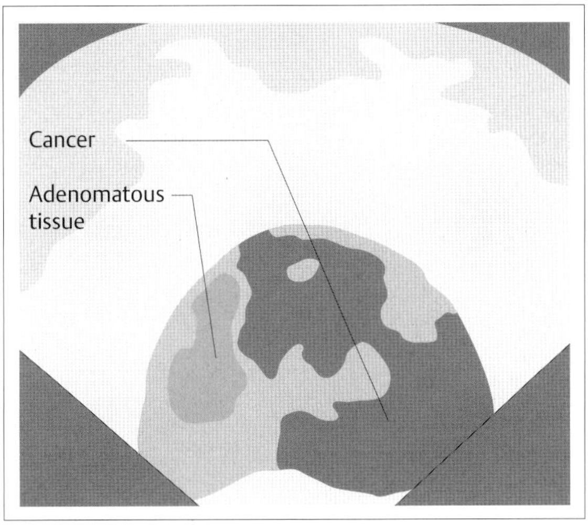

Fig. 11.**19 b** Line drawing.

Scrotal Disease

Basic Facts

- Scrotal swelling may have numerous causes.
- The most frequent cause is hydrocele, a tense-elastic and painless swelling, easily separated from the spermatic cord but ill-defined or not defined against the testis.
- Focal hard nodules at the epididymis may be indicative of spermatocele.
- Any painless induration of the testis with or without enlargement of the organ should always raise the suspicion of malignancy.
- Inflammation (orchitis, epididymitis) is accompanied by painful changes in the testis.
- Acute-onset pain with initial nausea, cutaneous edema, testicular retraction, loss of the cremasteric reflex, no fever; commonly seen in children and adolescents.
- Distinct scrotal swelling and hematoma in scrotal trauma.

Sonographic Criteria

- **Hydrocele** is characterized by an anechoic layer around the testis, while the latter appears normal. It is well defined from the spermatic cord (Fig. 11.**20**).
- **Spermatocele:** anechoic area in or adjacent to the epididymis (usually at the head) with posterior shadowing (Fig. 11.**21**).
- Hypoechoic or heterogeneous intratesticular masses are characteristic of **tumors**; sonography cannot differentiate between benign and malignant masses (Fig. 11.**22**).
- In orchitis, the testis is enlarged and hypoechoic (compare with contralateral testis); in abscess there are irregular, ill-defined anechoic areas within the testis.
- **Epididymitis** is characterized by an enlarged heterogeneous epididymis and possible **concomitant hydrocele** (Fig. 11.**23**).
- In B-mode imaging **testicular torsion** lacks any characteristic features (hypoechoic parenchyma, possibly demonstration of the twisted spermatic cord). Doppler or color-flow Doppler imaging preferred (impaired or absent testicular perfusion) (Fig. 11.**24**).
- **Testicular trauma:** demonstration of anechoic parenchymal structures, possibly defects in the tunica albuginea or simply changes consistent with hematocele or subcutaneous hematoma (Fig. 11.**25**).

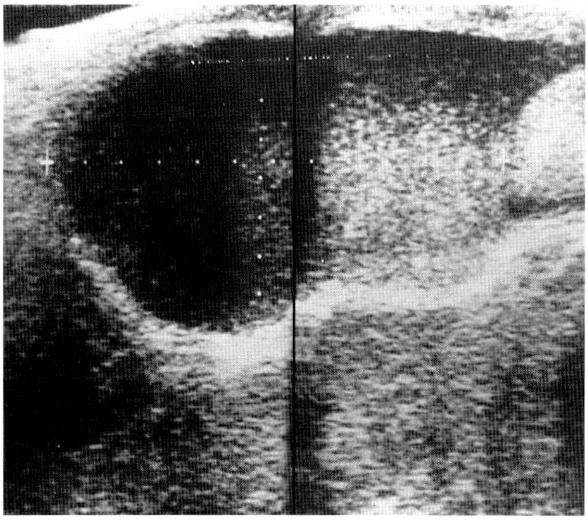

Fig. 11.20 a Large hydrocele with partial sludge phenomenon.

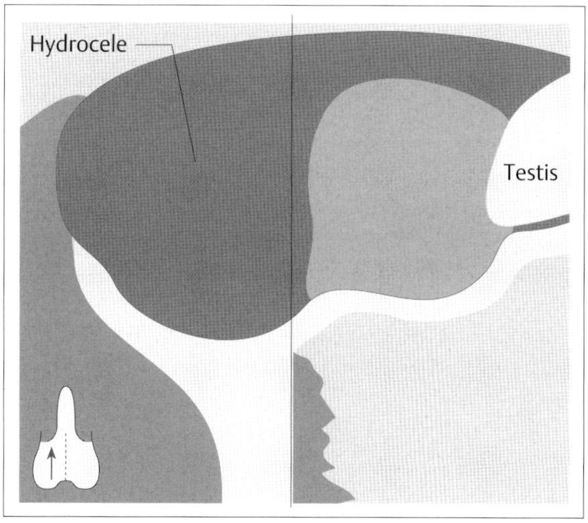

Fig. 11.20 b Line drawing.

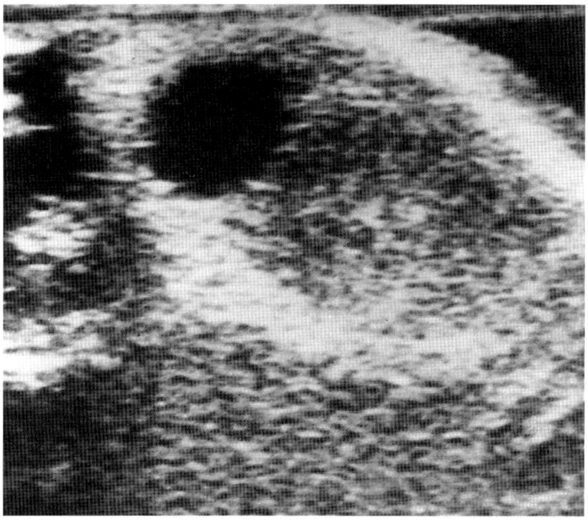

Fig. 11.21 a Cyst in the head of the epididymis (spermatocele).

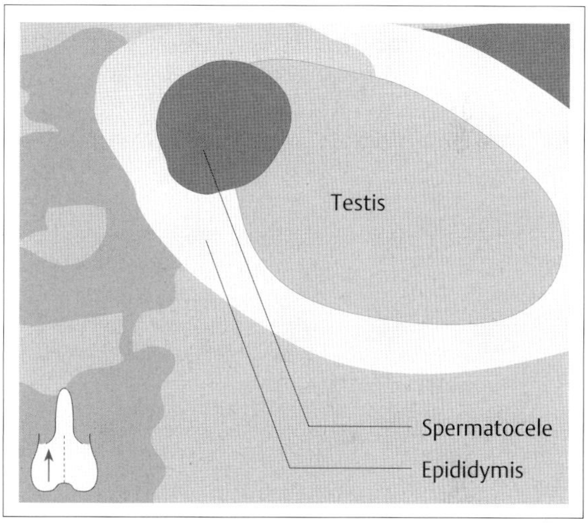

Fig. 11.21 b Line drawing.

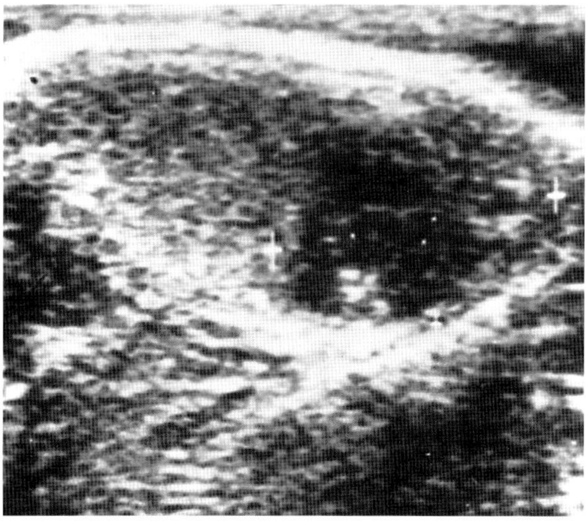

Fig. 11.22 a Intratesticular solid mass.

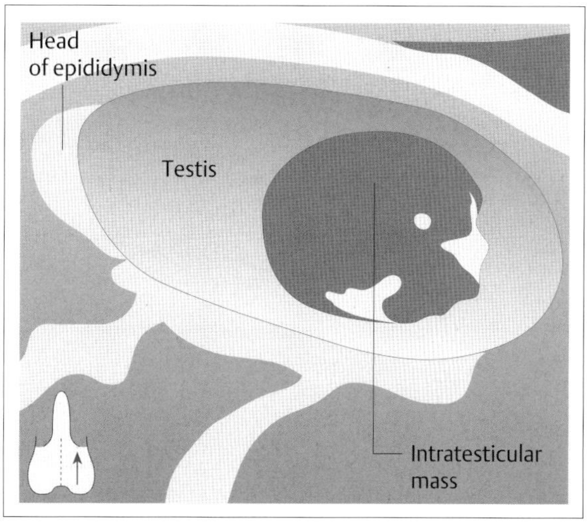

Fig. 11.22 b Line drawing.

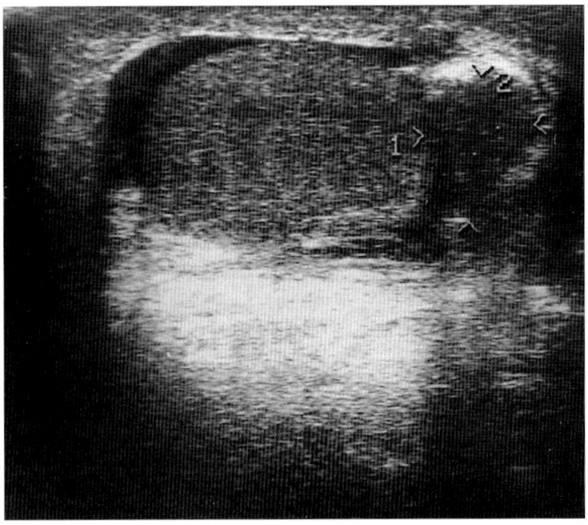

Fig. 11.23 a Epididymitis at the tail with concomitant hydrocele.

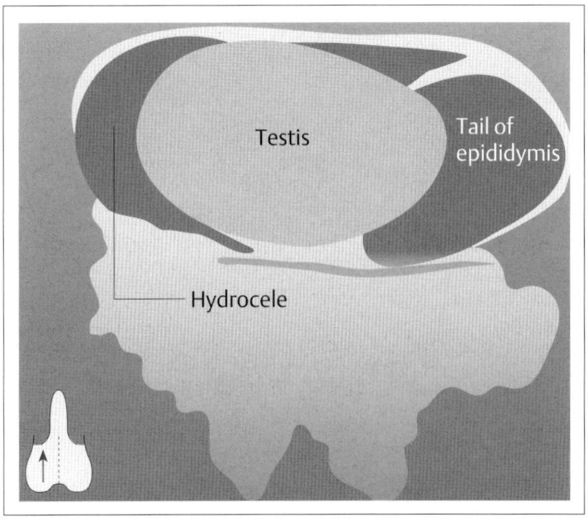

Fig. 11.23 b Line drawing.

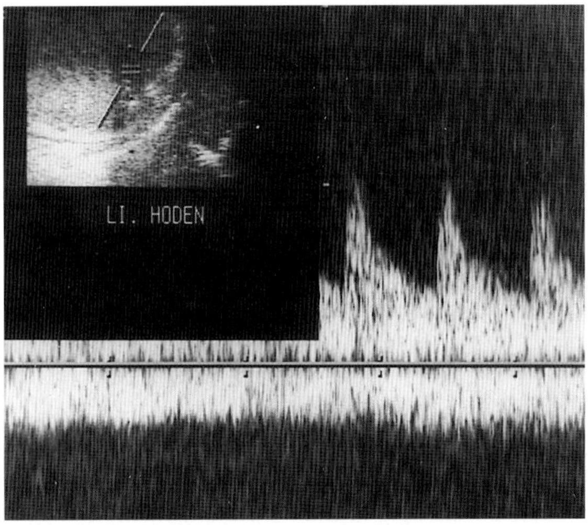

Fig. 11.24 a Doppler imaging of the left testis; normal blood flow.

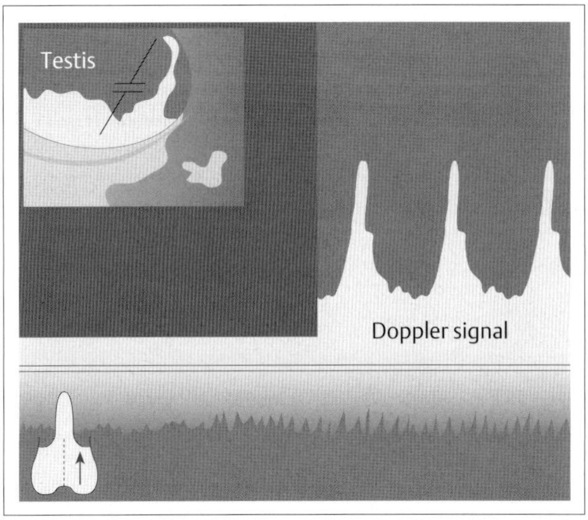

Fig. 11.24 b Line drawing.

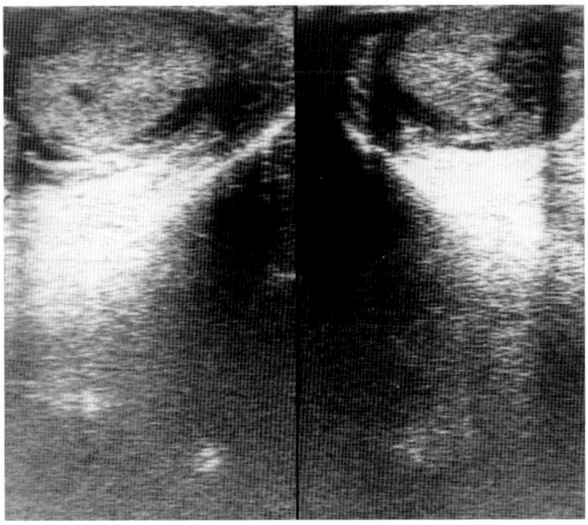

Fig. 11.25 a Traumatic ruptured testis.

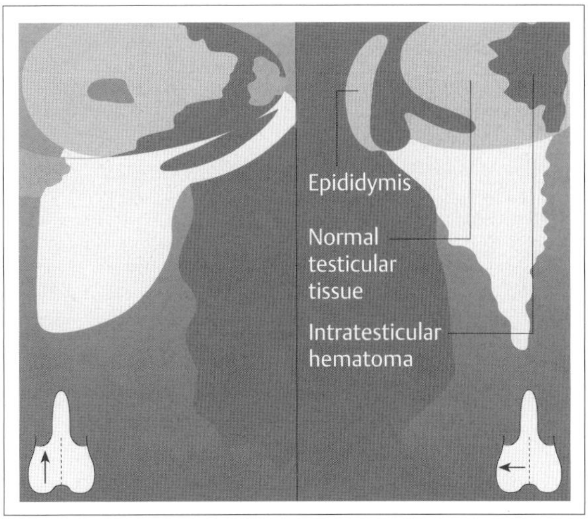

Fig. 11.25 b Line drawing.

Consequences for Surgical Treatment

Diagnosis	Characteristic Findings	Management
Painless tense-elastic swelling, testis not palpable, positive transillumination	Thick anechoic rim around the testis and epididymis, characteristic of hydrocele	Hydrocelectomy (numerous techniques)
Hard, round, and painless nodules at the superior pole of the testis	Normal testis; anechoic area in the head of the epididymis characteristic of spermatocele	Follow-up; resection if increasing in size
Painless enlargement of the testis, firm consistency	Demonstration of an anechoic or heterogeneous parenchymal mass raises suspicion of tumor	Surgical exploration for pathological confirmation; extended testicular resection followed by stage- and grade-adjusted treatment
Painful enlarged testis, fever. Possibly bilateral involvement; rule out mumps outbreak	Homogeneous hypoechoic enlarged testis = orchitis	Nonsurgical (broad-spectrum antibiotics)
Red swollen scrotum, fever, tender epididymis = epididymitis	Normal testis, epididymis (head or tail) enlarged, heterogeneous, and hypoechoic	Nonsurgical (broad-spectrum antibiotics and local anti-inflammatory measures); in case of abscess, testicular resection may become necessary
Swollen scrotum with hematoma. Testis/epididymis not clearly defined	Demonstration of fluid within the lumen of the scrotum (hematocele) or subcutaneous anechoic structures = hematoma. Rupture: testis with anechoic intratesticular areas and defects in the tunica albuginea	Nonsurgical for hematocele and subcutaneous hematoma. Surgical exploration in intratesticular hematoma and tunica defects
Acute testicular pain, possibly with initial nausea/vomiting. Reddened scrotum, testicular retraction, no fever	Mild hydrocele, hypoechoic testis, possibly hyperechoic twisted spermatic cord = suspicious of torsion Doppler imaging preferred	If torsion is confirmed or suspected, surgical exploration is mandatory (time to infarction 6 hours!). Untwisting of the cord, orchidopexy (plus prophylactic fixation of contralateral testis)
Acute painful scrotal swelling without palpable cranial border	Normal testis/epididymis, heterogeneous structures cephalad (possibly with gas inclusions) = suspicious of strangulated hernia	Surgery

Bibliography

Braun B, Günther R, Schwerk W. Ultraschalldiagnostik: Lehrbuch und Atlas. 7th ed.Landsberg, München, Zürich: ecomed Verlagsgesellschaft; 1990.

Gladisch R. Praxis der abdominellen Ultraschalldiagnostik. 2nd ed. Stuttgart, New York: Schattauer Verlag; 1992.

Jocham D, Miller K. Praxis der Urologie. (2 vols.). 2nd ed. Stuttgart: Georg Thieme Verlag; 2003.

Meckler U, Wermke W. Sonographische Differentialdiagnostik–systematischer Atlas. Köln: Deutscher Ärzteverlag; 1997.

Rassweiler J, Merkle W. Ultraschall in der Urologie. Stuttgart: Georg Thieme Verlag; 1997.

Walsh PC, Retik AB, Vaughan ED Jr, Wein AJ. Campbell's Urology, 8th ed. Vols. 1–4. Philadelphia: Saunders; 2002.

Hemodialysis Shunt Complications

Basic Facts

- Incidence of end-stage renal failure is rising steadily.
- Preferred vascular access for hemodialysis is via the Brescia–Cimino shunt in the forearm (Fig. 11.**26**): latero-terminal arteriovenous anastomosis. If this access cannot be fashioned in the forearm, one option is the upper arm with the brachial artery and cephalic vein (Fig. 11.**31**). Other shunts with autologous vessels should be reserved for special cases, and thus the next option would be straight (Fig. 11.**29**) or looped (Fig. 11.**30**) PTFE (Gore-Tex) grafts in the upper arm; however, this implies a lateroterminal plus terminolateral anastomosis susceptible to stenosis and thrombosis. Major shunt types: Figs. 11.**26**, 11.**29**, 11.**30**.
- For autologous shunts, primary patency after one year averages about 60%, dropping to only 30% after five years; for PTFE shunts the rates are significantly lower. Secondary patency, e.g., after percutaneous transarterial angioplasty (PTA), is also lower.
- Flow rates insufficient for hemodialysis may be due to stenosis or thrombosis.
- High-volume fistulas that are too large may induce circulatory failure and local steal phenomena (about 5% of all hemodialysis shunts).
- Circumscribed or diffuse local hematomas and thrombophlebitis are mostly transient problems.
- *Additional workup:* Radiological shunt imaging, preferably as intravenous DSA (especially valuable if details of the surgery are unknown or in intricate anatomy).

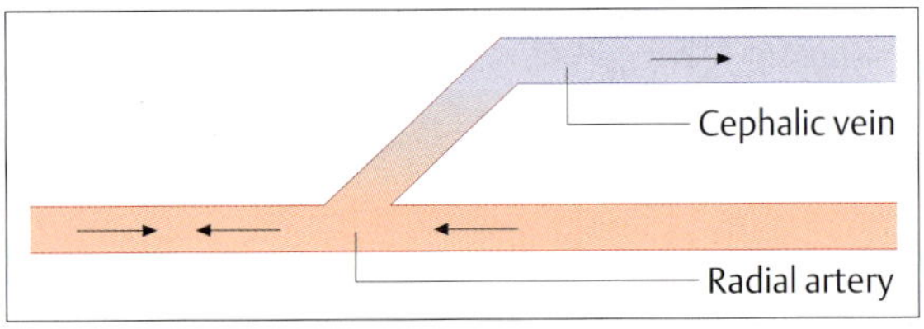

Fig. 11.**26** Schematic illustration of the principle of the Brescia–Cimino hemodialysis shunt in the forearm.

Sonographic Criteria

- **Vascular stenosis** is particularly common around the anastomosis (Fig. 11.**28**). Luminal narrowing can easily be demonstrated by color-flow duplex imaging. There is a turbulent color pattern with a coarse high-frequency PW and CW Doppler signal. Flow may also be impaired by external compression, e.g., by hematoma. Precise direct quantitative assessment of the stenosis is almost impossible.
- **Thrombosis**, especially in the venous limb (Fig. 11.**28**), is characterized by the absence of flow signals on color-flow Doppler imaging and by reduced compressibility of the affected vessel. Echogenicity increases with the duration of the thrombosis.
- **Perivascular hematomas** are circumscribed or diffuse masses of varying echogenicity, sometimes liquid/liquefied or thrombosed, usually with strong absorption of ultrasound.
- **Thrombophlebitis** results in irregular focal thickening of the vascular wall.
- Walls of shunt vessels often display significant hyperechoic calcifications.
- Extended excessive dilatation may arise primarily in the venous limb; circumscribed forms correspond to **aneurysms** (Fig. 11.**27**).
- Most modern ultrasound units for color-flow duplex imaging give the user the option of menu-guided **volume measurement** (Figs. 11.**32**–11.**35**). The examination is performed with the patient supine or sitting. It may be performed on the arterial as well as the venous limb. Correct measurement is improved by a slightly pulsatile blood flow, which allows for adjustment of the cardiac cycle. Blood flow should not be too turbulent. Partial volume effects of venous collaterals may be one source of potential error.
- The equation includes the vascular diameter (assuming circular geometry, the cross-sectional area and the angle-adjusted flow rate over the entire cross-section, most often averaged over two or three cardiac cycles): Vascular diameter × mean flow rate (in ml/min). Flow volume measurement should be repeated several times and the mean value used. Optimum shunt perfusion rates determined by color-flow duplex imaging are about 450 (± 200) ml/min for Brescia–Cimino fistulas, and 600–800 ml/min for PTFE shunts.

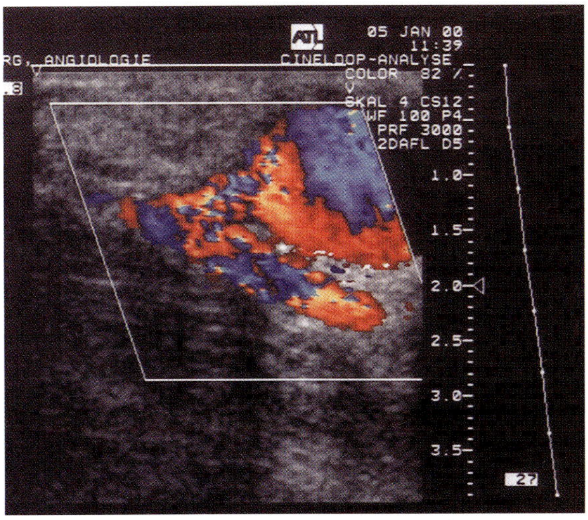

Fig. 11.**27 a** Brescia–Cimino shunt in the forearm with venous aneurysm and mural thrombosis in a stenosis secondary to the aneurysm.

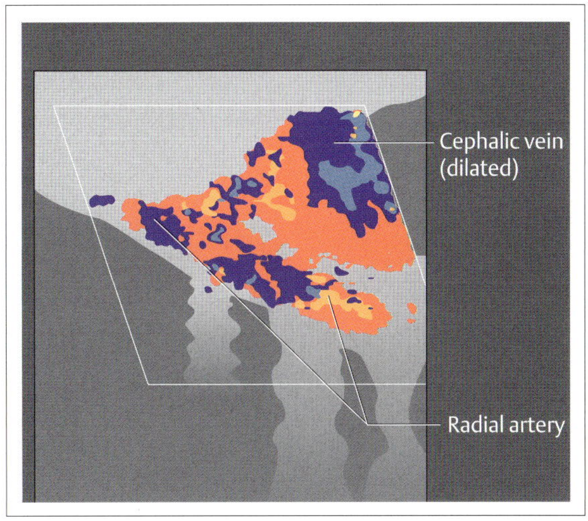

Fig. 11.**27 b** Line drawing.

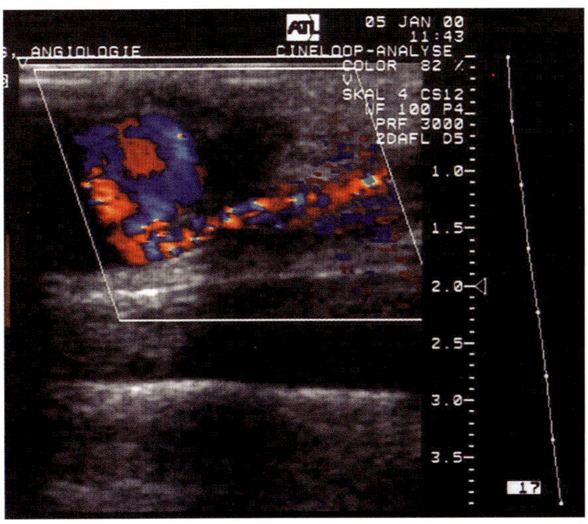

Fig. 11.**28 a** Brescia–Cimino shunt in the forearm with venous aneurysm and mural thrombosis in a stenosis secondary to the aneurysm. Fig. 11.**2** continued cephalad.

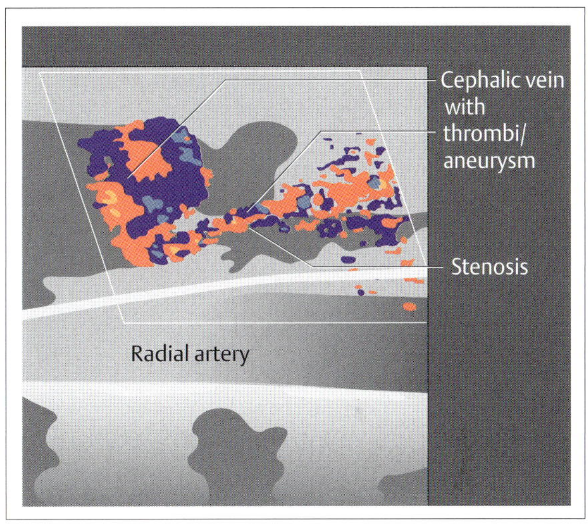

Fig. 11.**28 b** Line drawing.

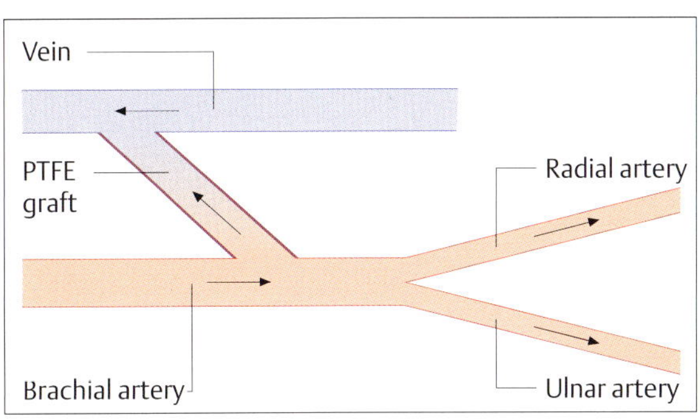

Fig. 11.**29** Schematic illustration of the principle of the straight PTFE shunt.

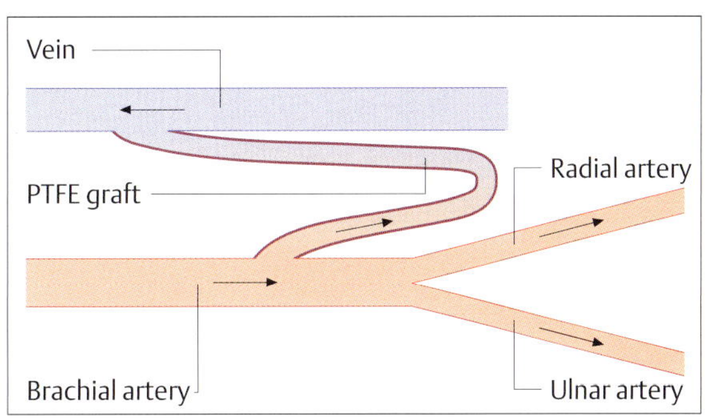

Fig. 11.**30** Schematic illustration of the principle of the looped PTFE shunt.

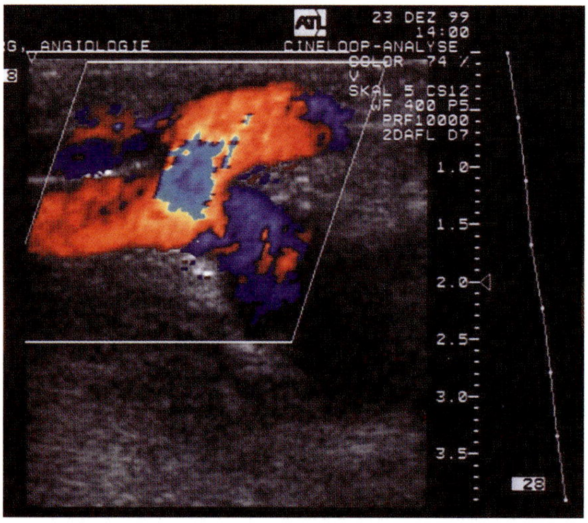

Fig. 11.**31 a** Brescia–Cimino shunt at the level of the elbow.

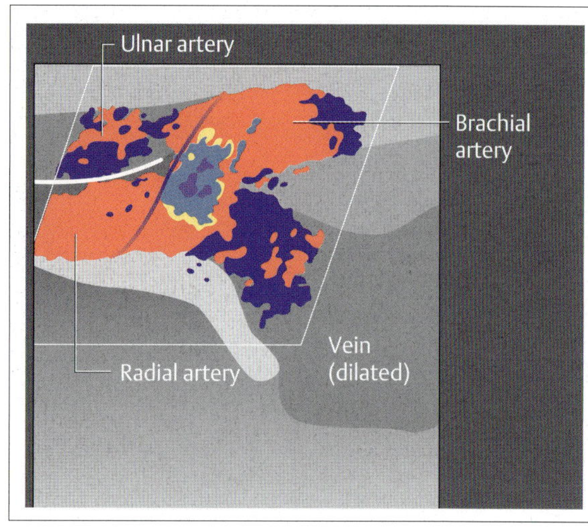

Fig. 11.**31 b** Line drawing.

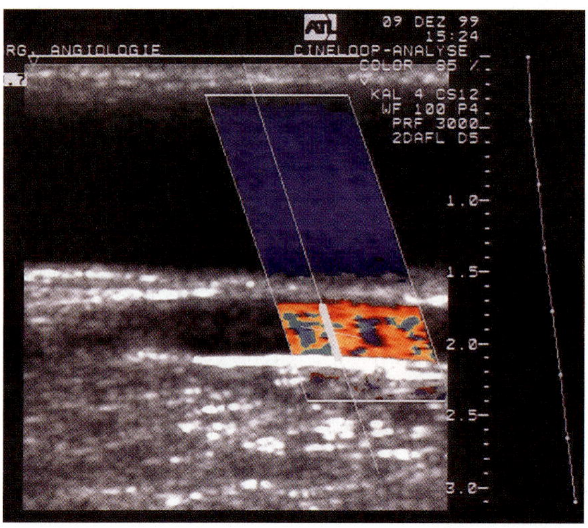

Fig. 11.**32 a** Flow volume measurement in the shunt artery.

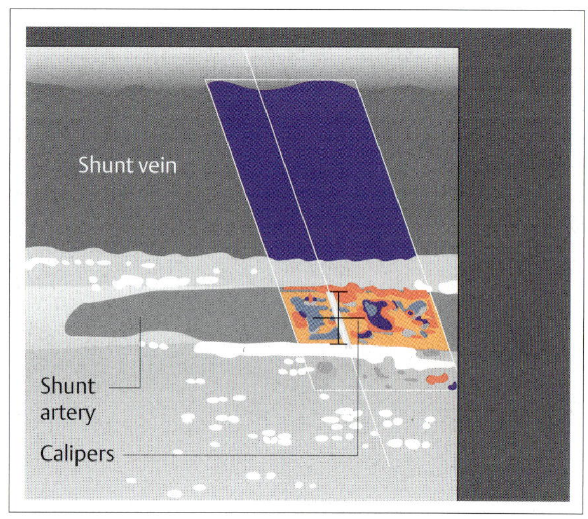

Fig. 11.**32 b** Line drawing.

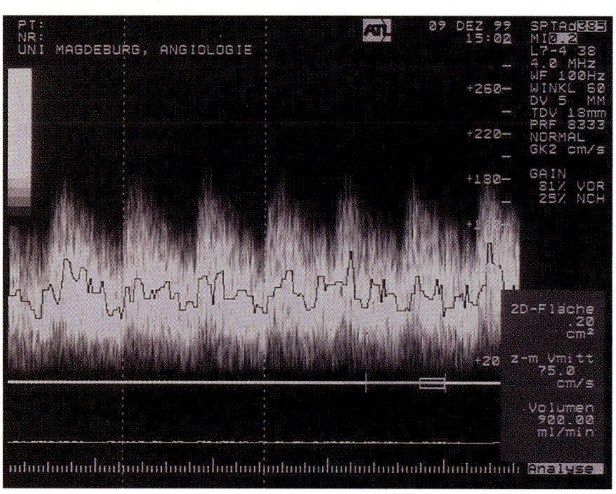

Fig. 11.**33 a** Flow volume measurement in the shunt artery (continued from Fig. 11.**32**).

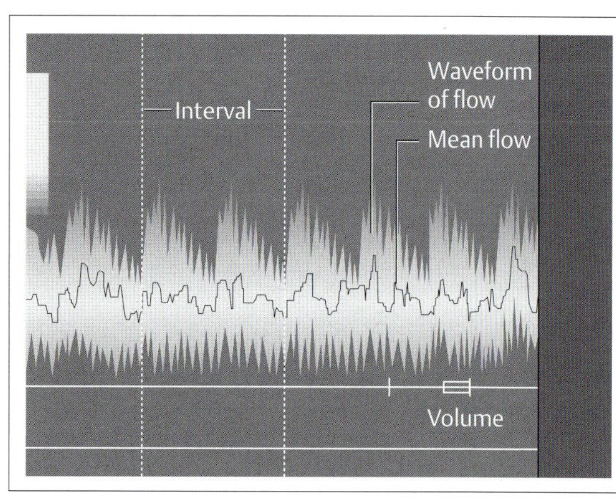

Fig. 11.**33 b** Line drawing.

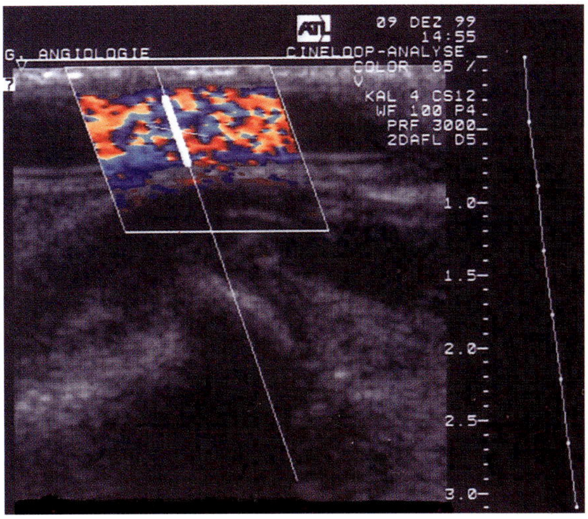

Fig. 11.**34a** Flow volume measurement in a PTFE shunt (rather turbulent flow).

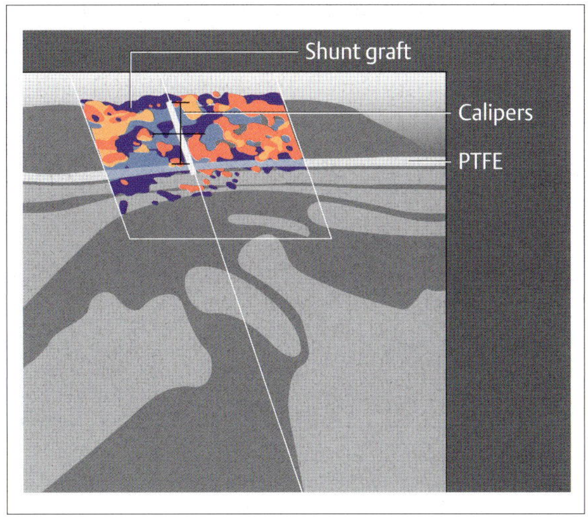

Fig. 11.**34b** Line drawing.

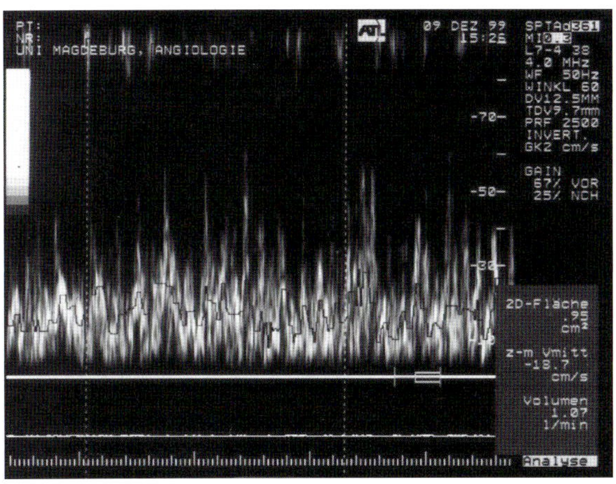

Fig. 11.**35a** Flow volume measurement in a PTFE shunt (continued from Fig. 11.**34**).

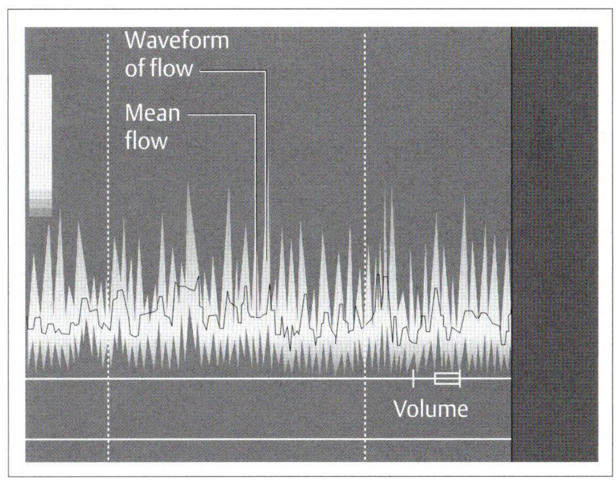

Fig. 11.**35b** Line drawing.

Consequences for Surgical Treatment

Diagnosis	Characteristic Findings	Management
Insufficient flow volume	< 200–300 ml/min	Thrombolysis PTA Stent Surgical shunt enlargement
Excessive flow volume	> 1000 ml/min	Surgical shunt restriction (e.g., banding)
Thrombophlebitis	Irregular wall thickening	Long-term subcutaneous application of low-molecular-weight heparin
Hematoma	Perivascular mass (for description see Sonographic Criteria)	Usually nonsurgical

Bibliography

Edwards JM, Zierler RE. Duplex ultrasound assessment of upper extremity arteries. In: Zwiebel WJ, ed. Introduction to Vascular Ultrasonography. 3rd ed. Philadelphia: WB Saunders; 1992: 223–35.

Kathrein H, König P, Weimann S, Judmaier G, Dittrich P. Nicht-invasive morphologische und funktionelle Beurteilung arteriovenöser Fisteln von Dialysepatienten mit der Duplexsonographie. Ultraschall. 1989; 10: 33–40.

Leapman SB, Boyle M, Pescovitz MD. The arteriovenous fistula for hemodialysis access: gold standard or archaic relic? Am Surg. 1996; 62: 652–6.

Morsy AR, Hulbasky M, Chen C. Incidence and characteristics of patients with hand ischemia after a hemodialysis procedure. J Surg Res. 1998; 74: 8–10.

Rosenfield K, Schainfeld R, Isner JM. Percutaneous revascularization in peripheral arterial disease. In: Loscalzo J, Creager MA, Dzau VJ, eds. Vascular Medicine. 2nd ed. Boston: Little, Brown; 1996: 717–64.

12 Sonography of the Breast

H. Madjar

Indications for Sonography

The most common carcinoma in Western industrialized countries is breast cancer, affecting around 10% of the female population. Particularly frightening is the fact that the incidence is increasing and that despite all progress to date no decisive breakthrough in treatment has been achieved. In asymptomatic women, mammography is the imaging modality of choice for primary screening. Worldwide studies have demonstrated that early diagnosis can help reduce mortality. Mammography is particularly accurate in postmenopausal women with involutional breast changes. However, the value of primary mammography is lower in dense breasts; accordingly, mammography frequently fails in younger women with dense breast tissue. One other significant factor limiting effective screening is the issue of quality assurance, since systematic audits are particularly difficult to implement in countries with decentralized health care systems.

Sonography is the most important secondary modality, since it permits assessment of dense parenchyma. With suitable equipment, soft-tissue changes can be better characterized than with mammography. Today, for a complete breast assessment, mammography should always be complemented by sonography unless advanced glandular involution renders mammographic misdiagnosis highly unlikely. Unfortunately, ultrasound performance greatly depends on equipment technology as well as operator experience. Since no generally accepted standards exist yet, the indication for sonography must be viewed critically. On the one hand, there is the standard diagnostic workup that any physician with accredited training in basic general sonography should be able to perform. This is to be distinguished from advanced assessment reserved for the specialist with first-rate skills and experience, and top-quality equipment.

Standard Diagnostic Workup

- Assessment of dense breasts in young women.
- Differentiation between cystic and solid masses.
- Ambivalent findings in pregnancy and lactation.
- Dense mammographic findings.
- Ambivalent palpatory findings.
- Mastitis.

Advanced Assessment

- Assessment of possible malignancy in solid tumors.
- Preoperative planning: preoperative staging; tumor size; multifocality and multicentricity; axillary, parasternal, infraclavicular, and supraclavicular lymph node metastasis.
- Follow-up for patients with silicone implants.
- Follow-up after mastectomy and breast-conserving surgery.
- Extended screening in patients at risk.
- Interventional sonography

Specific Technique and Diagnostic Evaluation

Basic facts

Many examiners focus exclusively on targeted sonography of palpable lesions. Since state-of-the art high-resolution ultrasound systems can detect even minute, clinically occult lesions, the examination should follow a standardized sequence to ensure a comprehensive evaluation of the entire breast.

Examination technique (Fig. 12.**1**):

- Supine position.
- Arms elevated and hands crossed behind the neck.
- In sagittal views the transducer is moved in serpentine fashion from cranial to caudal and in transverse views from lateral to medial.
- In case of mammary duct pathologies radial views should also be included.
- The probe should always be kept perpendicular to the surface of the breast.
- Mild pressure on the probe resulting in an even skin contact suffices for good acoustic coupling.
- Targeted compression with the probe may become necessary if deep penetration is insufficient or for evaluation of focal mass elasticity.

Image quality depends not only on transducer frequency but even more on signal processing within the system itself. Currently, objective data on the quality of an ultrasound system can only be based on a standardized phantom test. As no sufficient regulations for quality assurance exist so far, there is no uniform rating that allows reliable determination of the value of diagnostic breast sonography. Recommendations for equipment quality are given below.

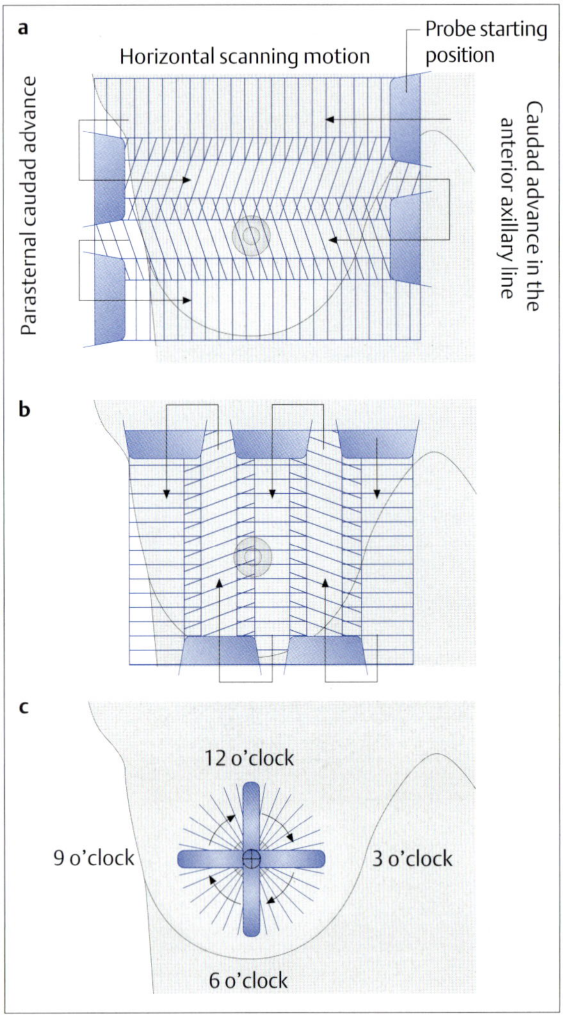

Fig. 12.**1** Standardized systematic examination of the breast.
a In sagittal views of the breast the probe is moved in serpentine fashion with overlapping planes from cranial to caudal.
b For transverse views the probe is moved horizontally.
c Radial views in sonographic breast examination.

Equipment

- High-frequency (7–13 MHz) probes with a penetration depth of at least 4 cm.
- High image contrast coupled with high spatial resolution.
- Axial resolution of at least 1 mm over the entire depth of the image.
- Dynamic focusing between 1 and 4 cm.
- Multifocusing–taking into account that with an increasing number of focal zones the image will be constructed much more slowly. Uniform focusing to a depth of up to 4 cm combined with a fast real-time image, permitting rapid transducer movements without streaking/ghosting on the monitor.
- Lateral (horizontal) resolution of 1 mm or less at maximum focus.
- Lateral (horizontal) resolution of 2 mm or less over the entire depth of penetration (4 cm).
- Numerous other aspects of equipment safety and technology are regarded as standard today, e.g., correct image geometry, ultrasound velocity calibration, calipers, > 64 gray levels, adjustable dynamic range, transmitter and receiver power, depth gain compensation, suitable annotation and documentation facilities.

Anatomy

Basic Facts

Every ultrasound assessment includes a complete examination of both breasts, together with a concise description. Any interpretation has to take into account the clinical and mammographic findings as well as the patient's age (Figs. 12.**2**, 12.**3**).

Sonographic Criteria of Assessment

- **Parenchymal texture** (normal, fibrosis, extensive fibrosis, small cystic changes).
- **Fatty tissue fraction** (percentage of total tissue or at least differentiation between involuted, partially involuted, moderately dense, and dense breast).
- **Limitations** (assessment reliability may be impaired in extensive fibrosis or breast hypertrophy).
- **Mammary ducts** (caliber, contour, ductal irregularities, conspicuous internal echoes).
- **Skin thickness** (usually 1–2 mm). Tumors, infections, and irradiation may result in cutaneous edema.
- **Lymphatic drainage.** Size, location, and echotexture (hyperechoic hilum, as in reactive changes, or heterogeneous/hypoechoic internal texture) of any axillary lymph nodes visualized. Any pathology detected mandates thorough screening of the parasternal, infraclavicular, and supraclavicular regions.

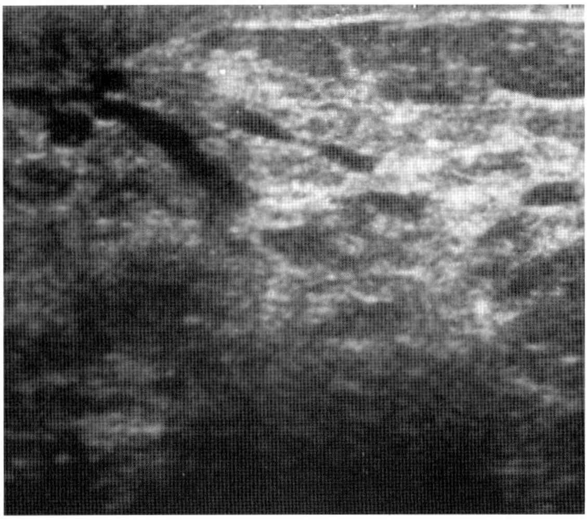

Fig. 12.**2a** Sagittal mid-breast view of normal breast anatomy. Premenopausal woman with dense parenchyma (hyperechoic), little subcutaneous fat (hypoechoic), and fluid-filled lactiferous ducts.

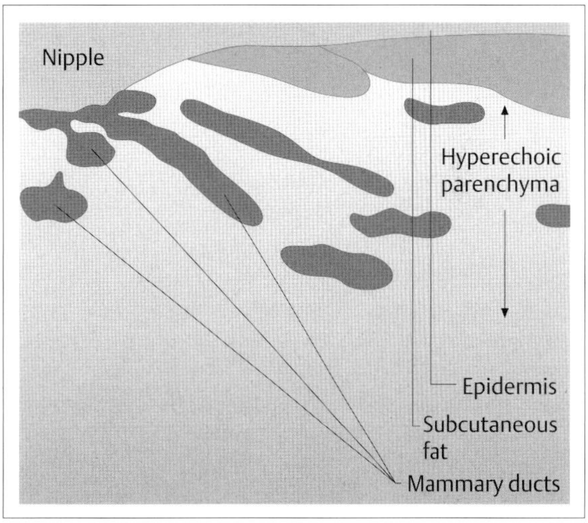

Fig. 12.**2b** Line drawing.

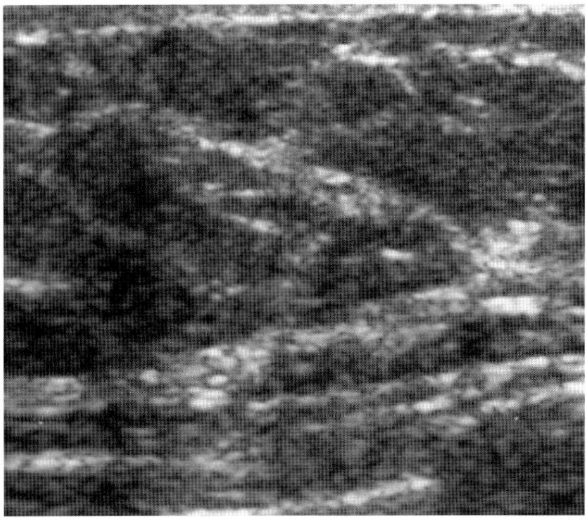

Fig. 12.**3a** Involuted breast. Islands of residual parenchyma and a high percentage of fat. Mammary ducts cannot be delineated.

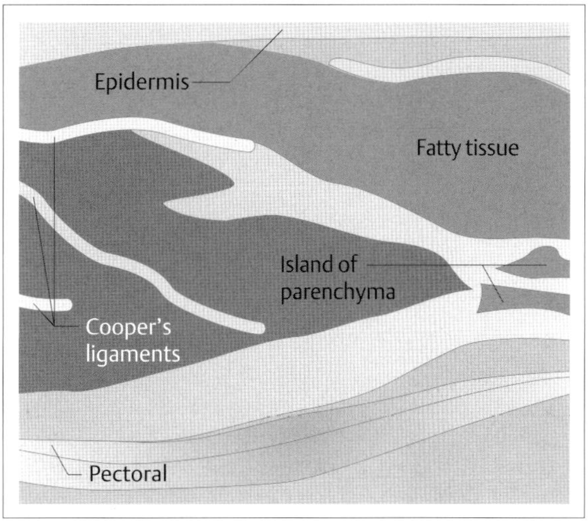

Fig. 12.**3b** Line drawing.

Focal Findings

Basic Facts

Any pathology must be measured in two orthogonal planes and be documented with an exact annotation of its location. The only exception permitted is in case of multiple cysts, where after conscientious examination of all cysts precise measurement and documentation of the largest cyst is sufficient. The location of each cyst should be marked on a diagram.

General Criteria for Assessment

- Tumor size.
- Location (clock face position, distance from the nipple, distance from the skin).
- Shape (round, oval, irregular).
- Long tumor axis (horizontal, indifferent, vertical).
- Margin (circumscribed, lobulated, microlobulated, indistinct).
- Boundary (abrupt interface, echogenic halo).
- Echo pattern (anechoic, hypoechoic, isoechoic, hyperechoic, complex).
- Sound transmission (shadowing, indifferent, enhancement).
- Elasticity (not compressible, moderately compressible, or easily compressible).
- Mobility (not mobile, moderately mobile, or easily mobile).
- Surrounding tissue (duct changes, Cooper's ligament changes, edema, architectural distortion, skin thickening, skin retraction/irregularity).

Cysts

Basic Facts

- Cysts are frequently accompanied by circumscribed or diffuse pain, often related to the menstrual cycle, and present as palpable nodules.
- Cysts are associated with menstrual disorders and hormonal imbalance.
- There is no increased risk of malignant transformation. However, cancer is easily overlooked in a cystic breast because cysts are more obvious, and because mammographic assessment may be limited by high parenchymal density.
- Cysts are a common finding, most typically encountered between ages 40 and 50 years; 50% of women of this age group are affected, albeit to a rather variable extent.

Problem cases:
- Cysts with viscous contents or hemosiderin deposits display homogeneous internal echoes and resemble fibroadenomas.
- Cystic conglomerates are occasionally associated with proliferative disease.
- Proliferation is signaled by focal wall thickening.
- Intracystic papillomas must be excised; however, innocuous bleeding may mimic papilloma or mural proliferation.
- Cysts harboring different fluids (serous and oily) display fluid levels. These must not be confused with solid internal structures.
- Juvenile cysts are common during puberty, presenting as painful nodules which should be managed in a strictly conservative fashion.

Sonographic Criteria for Assessment
(Figs. 12.**4**, 12.**5**)

- Shape (round oval).
- Long tumor axis (horizontal).
- Margin (circumscribed).
- Boundary (abrupt interface).
- Echo pattern (anechoic).
- Sound transmission (enhancement).
- Elasticity (moderately compressible).
- Mobility (easily mobile).
- Surrounding tissue changes (none).

Consequences for Surgical Treatment

Diagnosis	Characteristic Findings	Management
Simple cyst	Asymptomatic	None
Simple cyst	Painful nodules	US-guided aspiration
Papillomas	Most often asymptomatic	Surgery – no aspiration; otherwise preoperative localization is problematic. Possibly selective aspiration of the solid structure
Juvenile cyst	Asymptomatic	Conservative, usually spontaneous regression
Juvenile cyst	Pain, inflammation	Aspiration, since surgery risks partial excision of the mammary bud and should thus be avoided
Suspected proliferation	Ambivalent mammogram	Surgery in case of polymorphic clustered microcalcification

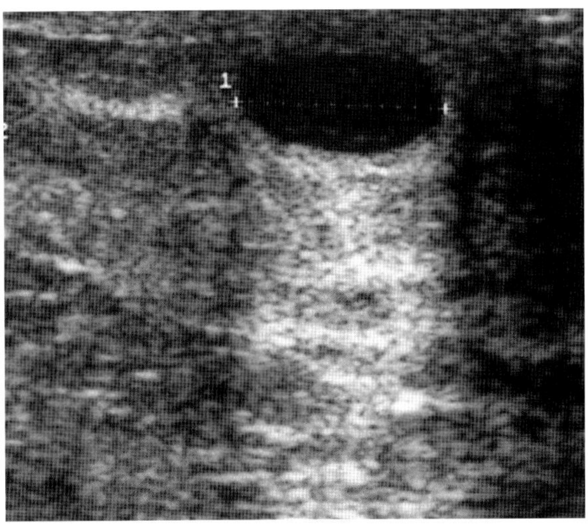

Fig. 12.**4a** Typical cyst.

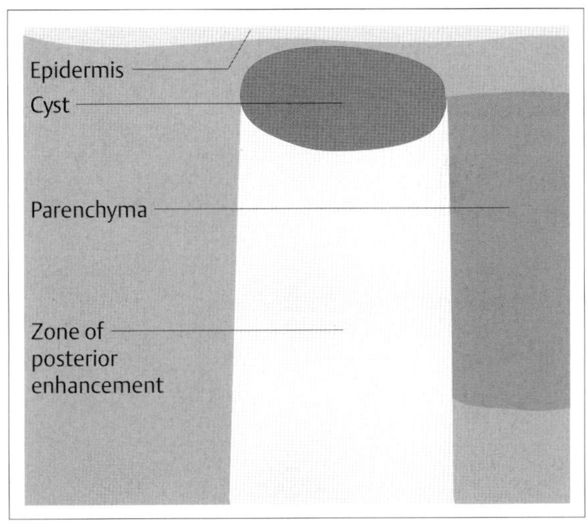

Fig. 12.**4b** Line drawing.

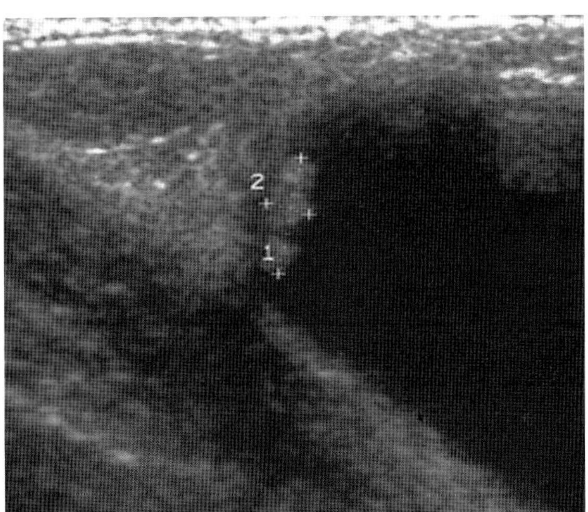

Fig. 12.**5a** Cyst with intracystic papilloma.

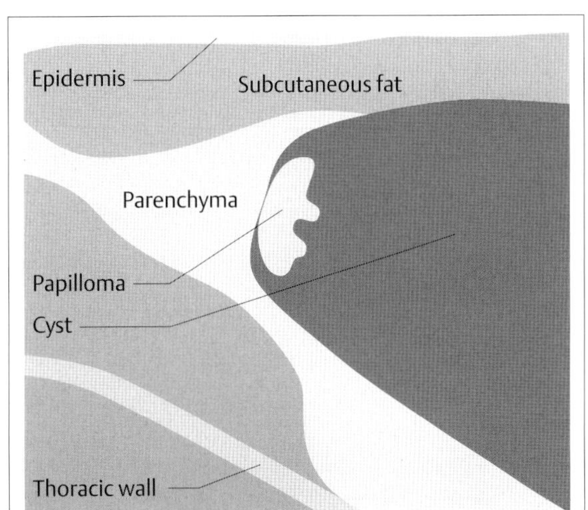

Fig. 12.**5b** Line drawing.

Fibroadenoma, Benign Tumor

Basic Facts

- The most common tumor in young women.
- Clinically, fibroadenoma presents as a smooth mobile mass.
- In the absence of proliferation, the risk of carcinoma increases only marginally.
- Sometimes multiple tumors arise in different regions of the breast. Some women suffer from repeated occurrence of fibroadenomas.
- Significant growth is frequently observed in periods of increased hormone activity, e.g., in pregnancy and lactation.
- Development in menopause is rare. Screening mammography at this age may, however, reveal long-standing but so far unnoticed tumors.

Problem cases:

- Proliferative or regressive fibroadenomas and those with intracanalicular growth are often heterogeneous and display somewhat indistinct borders.
- In about 2% of cases a presumed fibroadenoma will instead be a carcinoma with smooth borders.
- With aging, fibroadenomas tend to develop coarse calcifications. These produce a suspicious ultrasound image with posterior shadowing.
- Differentiation from viscous cysts may be difficult.

Sonographic Criteria for Assessment (Figs. 12.**6**, 12.**7**)

- Shape (ovoid).
- Long tumor axis (horizontal).
- Margin (circumscribed, lobulated).
- Echo pattern (hypoechoic).
- Sound transmission (indifferent to enhanced).
- Elasticity (not compressible).
- Mobility (easily mobile).
- Surrounding tissue changes (none).

Consequences for Surgical Treatment

Diagnosis	Characteristic Findings	Management
Typical finding	Homogeneous structure	Excision not required, but FNAB or core biopsy for histological confirmation
Atypical finding	Suspected proliferation, heterogeneous structure	Surgery
Atypical sonogram with posterior shadowing	Mammography: characteristic coarse calcification	Follow-up

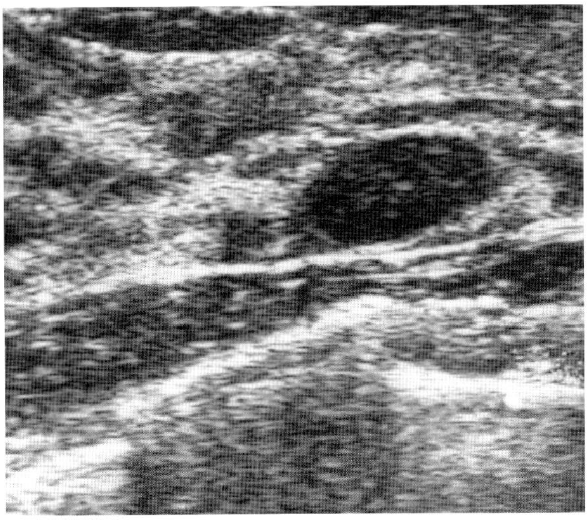

Fig. 12.**6 a** Typical fibroadenoma.

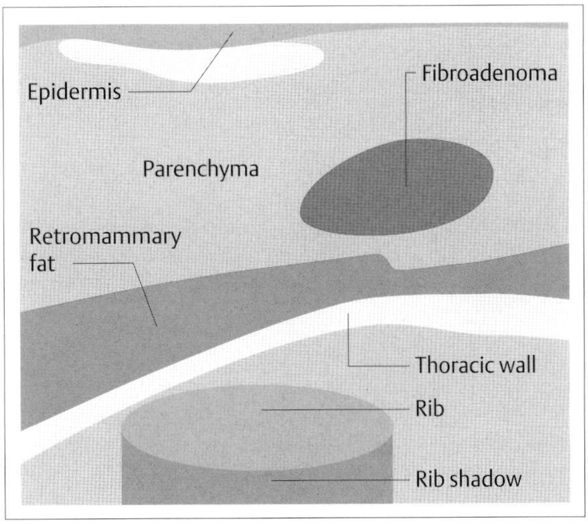

Fig. 12.**6 b** Line drawing.

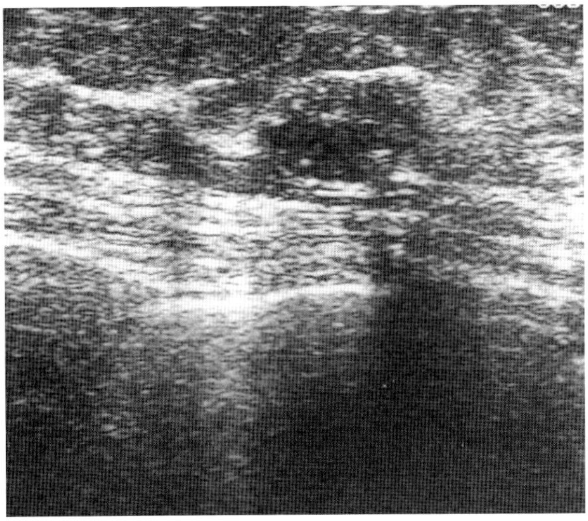

Fig. 12.**7 a** Fibroadenoma with regressive changes.

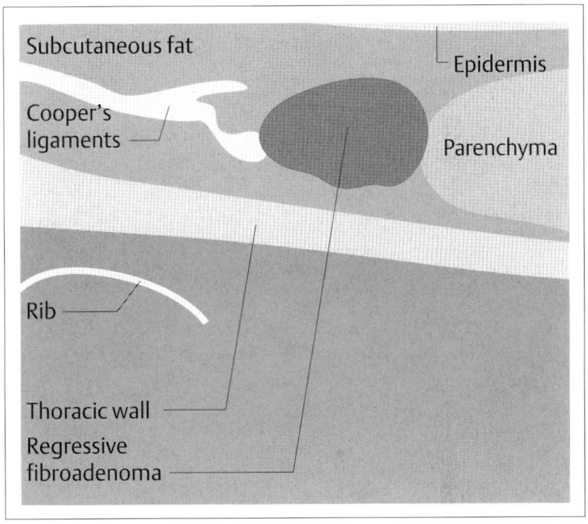

Fig. 12.**7 b** Line drawing.

■ Other Benign Tumors

Basic Facts

- Differential diagnosis has to include other benign tumors as well as fibroadenomas.
- Fibroma, adenofibroma, fibrolipoma, nodular benign breast disease (mastopathy): the sonomorphology usually corresponds with that of the fibroadenomas (see above).
- Lipomas can be distinguished clinically by their compressibility and soft consistency.
- Benign phyllodes tumors–as well as their malignant counterpart cystosarcoma phyllodes–are characterized by cystic internal structures.

Mastitis

Basic Facts

- There are two forms of mastitis: puerperal and nonpuerperal.
- Both typically present with fever and painful erythema of the breast. Diffuse induration of the breast follows; in case of colliquation there will be fluctuation.
- Important differential diagnosis: inflammatory carcinoma.

Problem cases:
- Cancer may mimic mastitis.
- Mammography is of little diagnostic value during the acute stage.
- As long as there is no colliquation, follow-up after basic documentation will be sufficient. Once the acute inflammation has subsided, bilateral mammography is recommended.

Sonographic Criteria for Assessment
(Figs. 12.**8**, 12.**9**)

- Shape (diffuse or circumscribed tissue edema in florid inflammation; irregular focal lesion in colliquation).
- Long tumor axis (usually horizontal).
- Margin (indistinct in diffuse colliquation, smooth or lobulated in focal colliquation).
- Echo pattern (hypoechoic to complex).
- Sound transmission (enhancement).
- Elasticity (moderately compressible).
- Mobility (moderately mobile).
- Surrounding tissue (possibly perifocal edema).

Consequences for Surgical Treatment

Diagnosis	Characteristic Findings	Management
Diffuse inflammation	Tissue edema	No surgery, antibiotics; after inflammation has settled, mammography to rule out carcinoma
Abscess formation	Sonographic mass	Incisional drainage. In infected cysts, US-guided aspiration may suffice

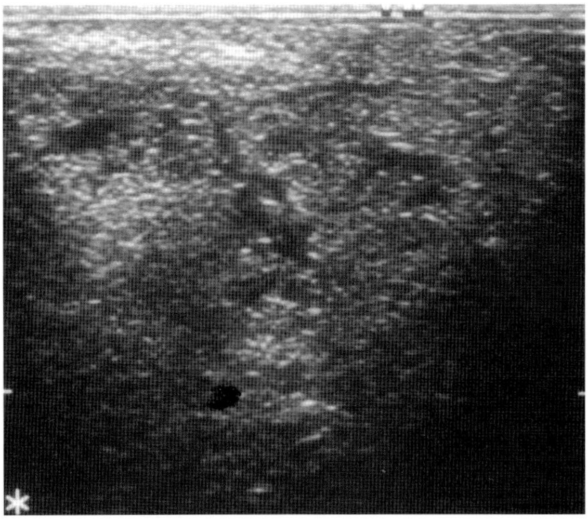

Fig. 12.**8 a** Mastitis. Early inflammatory stage with tissue edema.

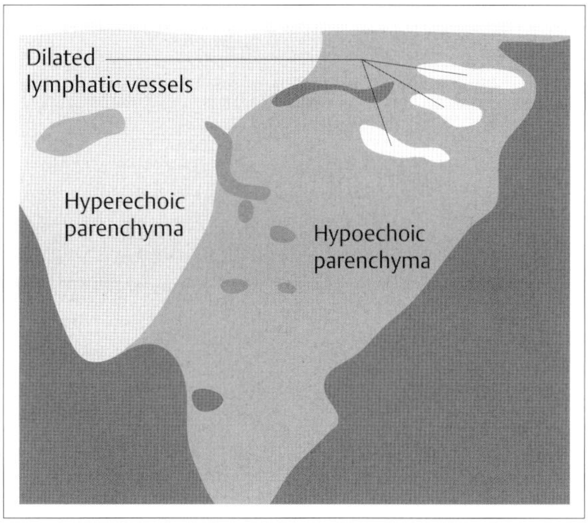

Fig. 12.**8 b** Line drawing.

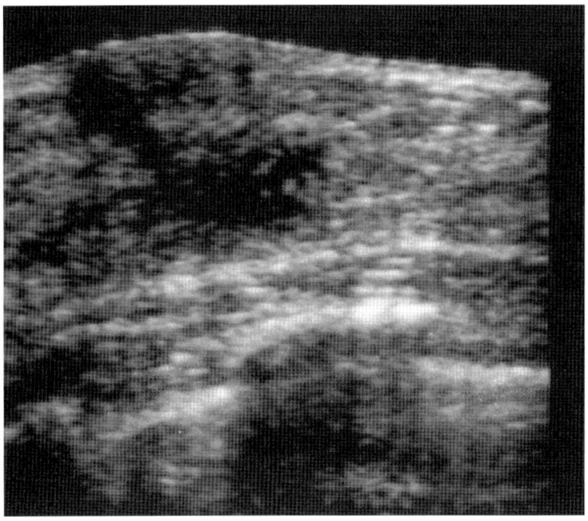

Fig. 12.**9 a** Abscess formation with skin fistula.

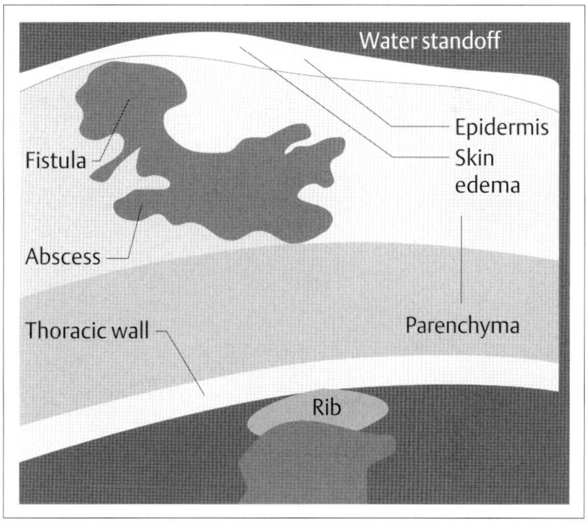

Fig. 12.**9 b** Line drawing.

Carcinoma

Basic Facts

- Most breast cancers are diagnosed after menopause, but 20–30% of patients are premenopausal.
- Clinical findings vary and are unreliable; palpation does not allow early diagnosis.
- In 20–40% of cases multiple tumors arise in different regions of the breast (multifocal or multicentric lesions).
- Primary screening mammography will detect up to 20% of cancers while still in the preinvasive stage.
- Microcalcifications are the leading sign in some of the carcinomas.
- Tumor spread frequently reaches beyond the area of calcification.
- Mammographic diagnosis of tumor spread and of multifocal/multicentric lesions is inaccurate.

Problem cases:

- About 2% of carcinomas have a smooth margin and are easily mistaken for benign tumors. This applies in particular to medullary, mucinous, and tubular carcinomas, but also to solid, invasive ductal carcinomas.
- Diffusely infiltrating, lobular invasive, and comedo carcinomas will occasionally display higher echogenicity and thus are more difficult to recognize. Only careful assessment of the glandular structure may reveal the architectural abnormalities. For the final assessment of a sonogram without abnormal findings, all other available information must always be taken into account as well.
- Carcinomas may easily be overlooked in the presence of other, more obvious changes.
- Sonography can detect only those in-situ carcinomas that have resulted in ductal dilatation. If the mammogram shows polymorphic clustered calcifications, further investigations are mandatory even if ultrasound proves normal.
- Advanced lymph node metastases are hypoechoic. In early stages, cortical or hilar asymmetry may be evident. Micrometastases usually cannot be delineated.

Sonographic Criteria for Assessment (Figs. 12.**10**, 12.**11**)

- Shape (irregular).
- Long tumor axis (vertical).
- Margin (indistinct).
- Boundary (echogenic halo).
- Echo pattern (hypoechoic).
- Sound transmission (shadowing).
- Elasticity (not compressible).
- Mobility (moderately mobile).
- Surrounding tissue (architectural distortion).
- Lymph node metastasis (hypoechoic, loss of hilar structure).

Note: Taking all findings into account including mammography, in preoperative planning one has to decide if the palpatory finding is sufficient or whether mammographic or US-guided preoperative wire localization is required. If multifocal cancer is suspected (Fig. 12.**12**), the diagnostician must be contacted on how to confirm this either preoperatively or during surgery. Excision of lesions delineated exclusively on sonography must be marked on a sonogram of the resected specimen so that the pathologist can identify the individual lesions during pathological workup.

Consequences for Surgical Treatment

Diagnosis	Characteristic Findings	Management
Suspicious	Suspicious mammogram	Surgery
Suspicious	Normal mammogram	Surgery; in case of doubt, preoperative confirmation by FNAB or core biopsy
Ambivalent		In case of doubt, diagnostic confirmation by FNAB or core biopsy
Benign(?)	Benign mammogram	Diagnostic confirmation by minimally invasive means, since scar formation after open biopsy may result in diagnostic problems during follow-up

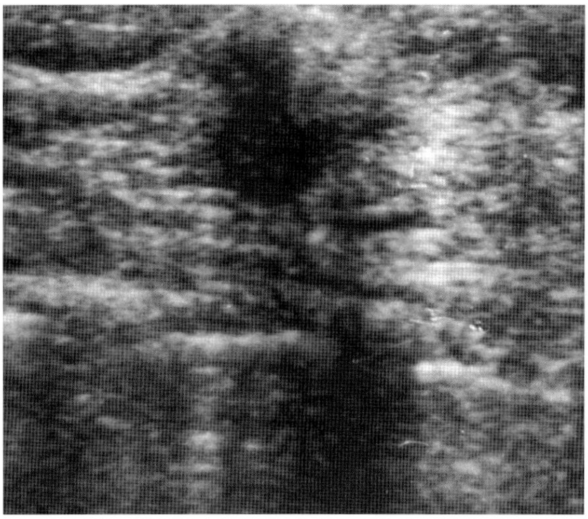

Fig. 12.**10 a** Varied sonomorphology in invasive ductal carcinoma of the breast. Irregular hypoechoic tumor with indistinct border and posterior shadowing.

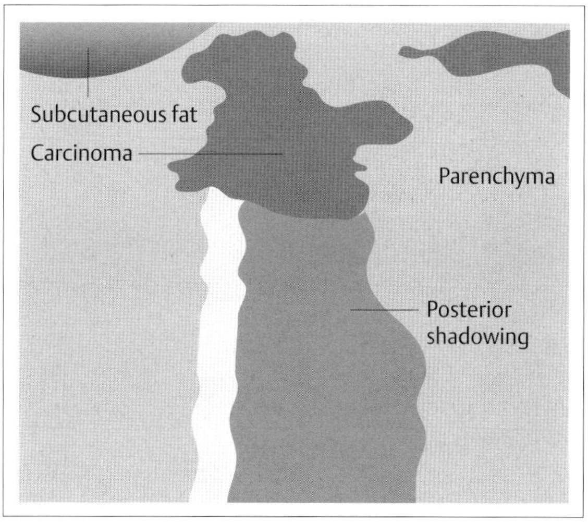

Fig. 12.**10 b** Line drawing.

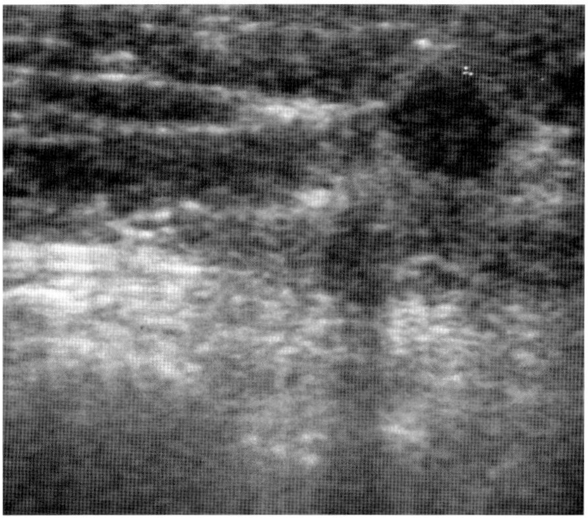

Fig. 12.**11 a** Varied sonomorphology in invasive ductal carcinoma of the breast. Irregular hypoechoic tumor with sharp border and good sound transmission.

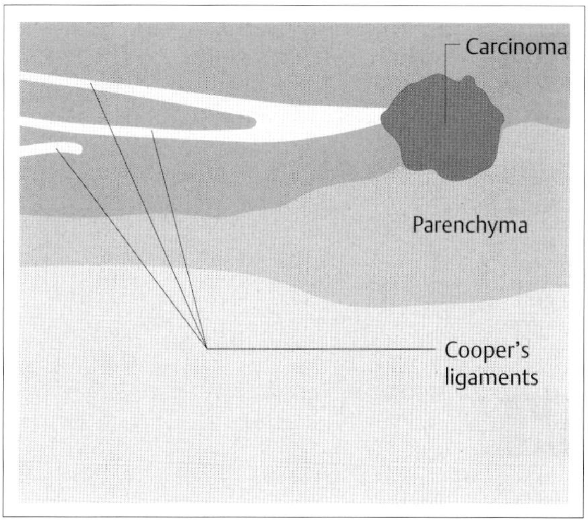

Fig. 12.**11 b** Line drawing.

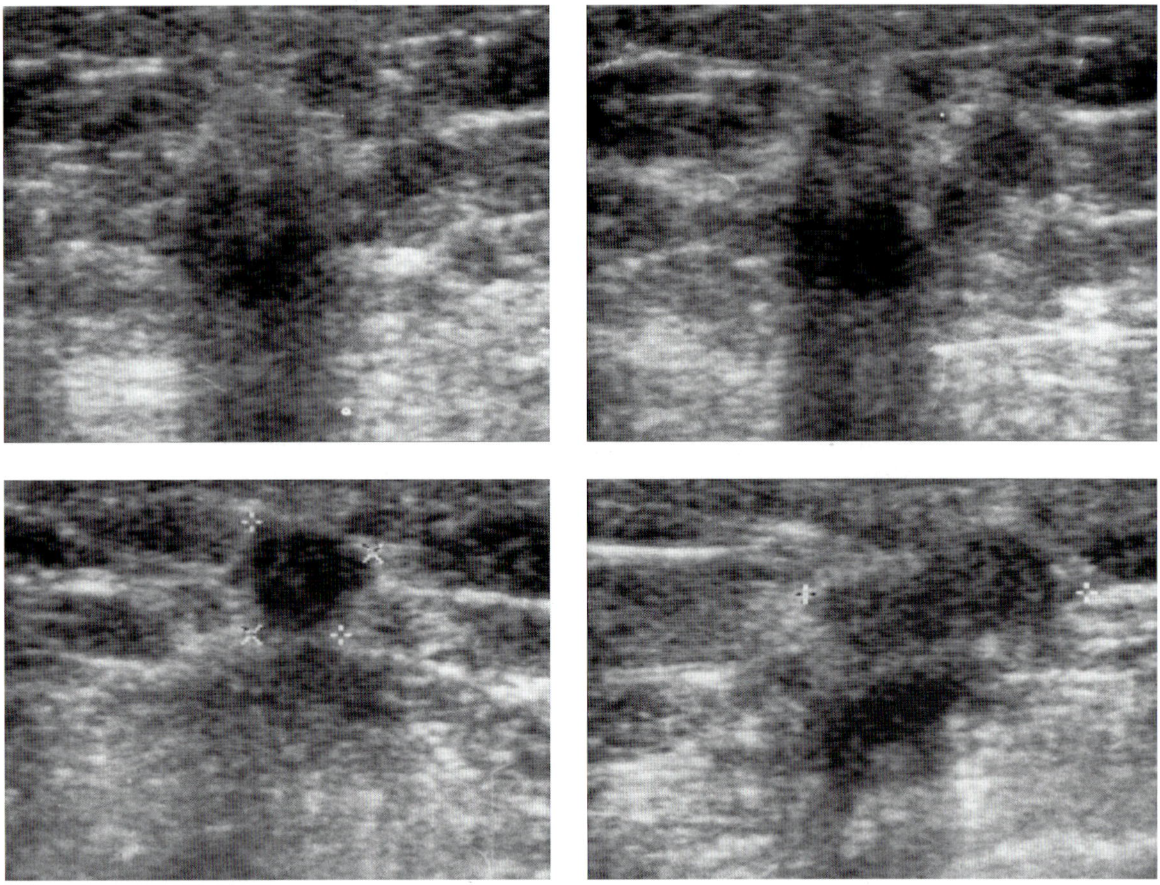

Fig. 12.**12 a** Multiple views of a breast with multifocal, partly ductal and partly lobular invasive carcinoma.

Interventional Techniques

Procedures

- Fine-needle aspiration.
- Core biopsy.
- US-guided minimally invasive tumor resection (vacuum-assisted biopsy).
- Preoperative wire localization of nonpalpable tumors.
- Sonography of the specimen to confirm complete excision.

Indications for Interventional Procedures

- Cysts that are painful or suspicious of proliferation.
- Smoothly defined solid tumors, confirmation of their benign nature.
- Preoperative confirmation of malignancy of suspicious lesions, in order to optimize surgical strategy when frozen section is not a useful option.
- Confirmation of suspected multifocality in order to plan surgical strategy.
- US-guided minimally invasive resection in probably benign lesions if avoidance of troublesome scar formation is important.

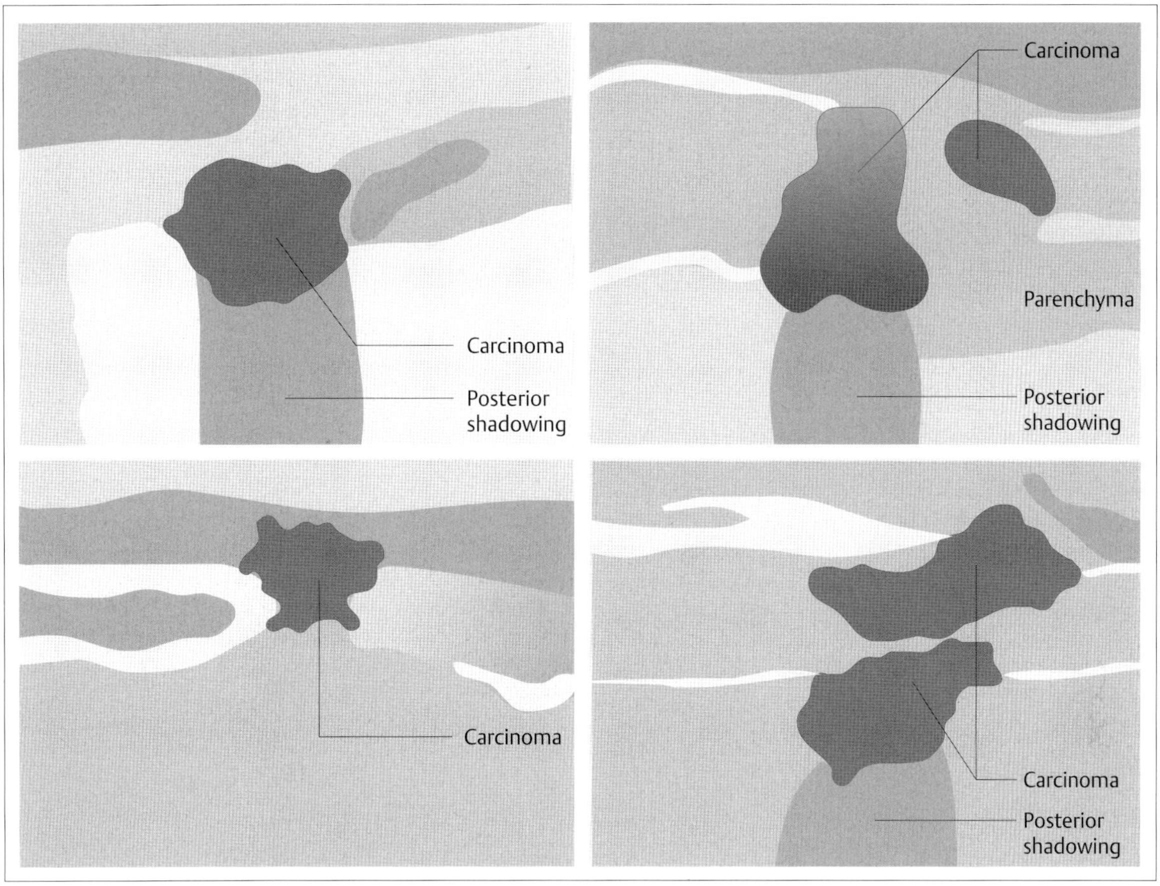

Fig. 12.**12 b** Line drawings corresponding to the images in Fig. 12.**12 a**.

Needle Aspiration and Biopsy in Practice (Figs. 12.**13**, 12.**14**)

- Needle direction within the imaging plane and along the ultrasound field.
- Needle direction paralleling the thoracic wall in order to avoid deep injuries and for optimum delineation of the needle (beam angle of inclination orthogonal to the needle).
- Always work under real-time visual control.
- During FNA of tumors the needle should be fanned within the tumor while constantly aspirating.
- For core biopsies, high-speed biopsy systems should be employed.
- In core biopsies, the needle tip is introduced into the tumor prior to firing the system, so that the tumor cannot move out of range during the procedure.

Final Remarks

Sonography may be of significant help in preoperative planning. In addition, it optimizes diagnostic workup in young women with dense breasts as well as in inflammatory and postirradiation changes that do not lend themselves to accurate mammographic assessment. This is complemented by the option of interventional procedures in diagnosis and treatment. Nevertheless, it should be noted that the breast is subject to numerous physiological variants and pathological changes. The performance of this modality depends on the experience of the operator and the quality of the equipment. This brief chapter can only offer basic insights into this field. For a more detailed understanding of the diagnostic workup of the breast, the reader is referred to the appropriate textbooks.

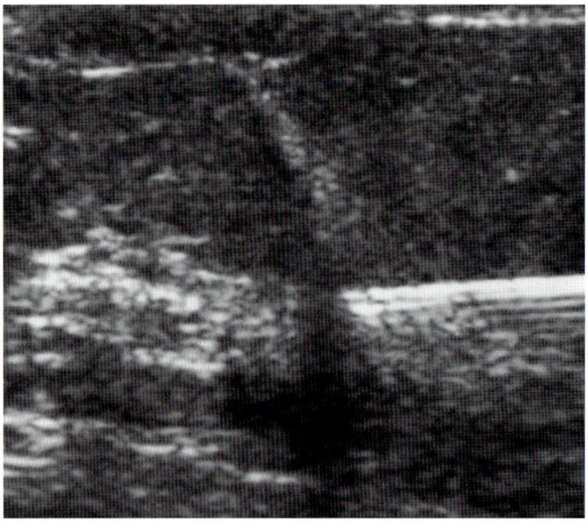

Fig. 12.**13 a** Ultrasound guided fine-needle aspiration. Optimum direction of the needle–within the imaging plane and paralleling the thoracic wall.

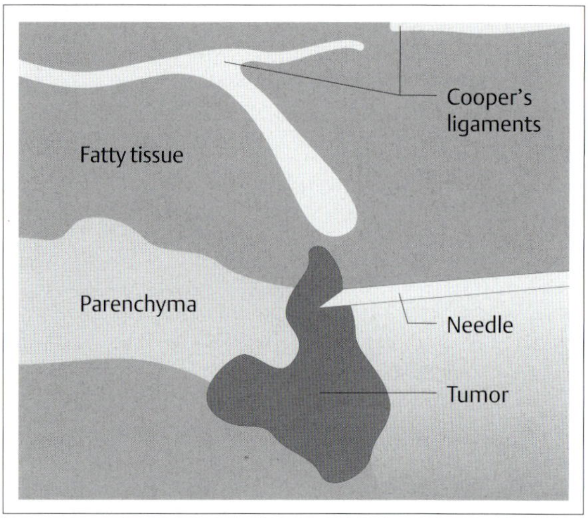

Fig. 12.**13 b** Line drawing.

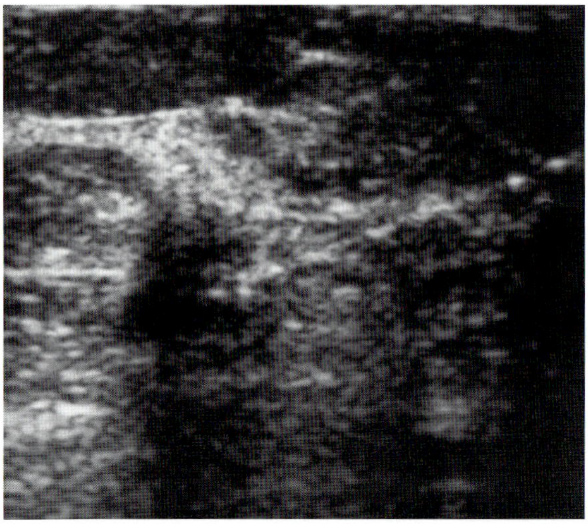

Fig. 12.**14 a** Poor needle direction: the needle enters the breast adjacent to the probe and must be angled downward rather steeply. This results in poor visualization of the needle.

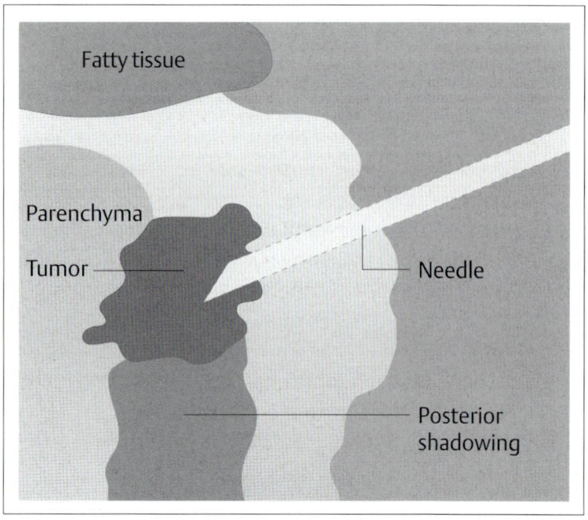

Fig. 12.**14 b** Line drawing.

Bibliography

American College of Radiology (ACR). ACR BI-RADS®-Ultrasound. In: ACR Breast Imaging Reporting and Data System, Breast Imaging Atlas. Reston, VA: American College of Radiology; 2003.

Gordon PB, Goldenberg SL. Malignant breast masses detected only by ultrasound: a retrospective review. Cancer. 1995; 76: 626–30.

Kolb TM, Lichy J, Newhouse JH. Comparison of the performance of screening mammography, physical examination, and breast US and evaluation factors that influence them: an analysis of 27 825 patient evaluations. Radiology. 2002; 225: 165–75.

Leucht D, Madjar H. Atlas Mammasonographie. 2nd ed. Stuttgart: Georg Thieme Verlag; 1995.

Madjar H. The Practice of Breast Ultrasound. New York: Thieme; 2000.

Madjar H, Rickard M, Jellins J, Otto R. IBUS guidelines for the ultrasonic examination of the breast. Eur J Ultrasound. 1999; 9: 99–102.

Madjar H, Teubner J, Hackelöer BJ. Breast Imaging Update. Basel: Karger; 1994.

Merritt CRB. Future directions in breast ultrasonography. Sem Breast Dis. 1999; 2(1): 89–96.

Porrath S. A Multimodality Approach to Breast Imaging. Rockwell, MD: Aspen Publishers; 1986.

Sohn Ch, Blohmer JU. Mammasonographie. Stuttgart: Georg Thieme Verlag; 1996.

Stavros AT. Breast Ultrasound. Philadelphia: Lippincott Williams and Wilkins; 2004.

Stavros AT, Thickman D, Rapp CL, et al. Solid breast nodules: use of sonography to distinguish between benign and malignant nodules. Radiology. 1995; 196: 123–34.

Teboul M, Halliwell M. Atlas of Ultrasound and Ductal Echography of the Breast. Oxford: Blackwell Science; 1995.

Tohno E, Cosgrove DO, Sloane JP. Ultrasound Diagnosis of Breast Disease. London: Churchill Livingstone; 1994.

13 Sonography of the Musculoskeletal System

K. Mahlfeld, G. Pap, H. R. Merk

Introduction

Together with the ever-expanding skills of sonographers, rapid advances in technology, resulting in high-performance ultrasound units, have made sonography an increasingly important imaging modality in the diagnosis of musculoskeletal disease. Following history-taking and physical examination, sonography of joints, bones, and adjacent soft tissues should be an integral part of today's basic work-up and should precede any other imaging modalities in the diagnostic algorithm.

Sonography is an easy-to-use, noninvasive, cost-effective modality resulting in a quick differential diagnosis of diseases and injuries of muscles and bones, and also permitting objective follow-up of treatment. Its diagnostic power depends on the experience of the sonographer as much as on correct interpretation of the ultrasound findings as part of the overall clinical picture.

Sonography of Muscles and Tendons

Sonography in Muscular Injuries

Basic Facts

- Sonographic assessment of normal skeletal muscles and any pathology is easily possible due to their rather superficial anatomy.
- As always, image in two planes; however, there are no standard views as in arthrosonography.
- Examination should routinely include a dynamic assessment: minor pathologies might otherwise remain undetected.
- For most myosonographic questions, the 7.5 MHz linear transducer is superior to a 5 MHz probe; however, the latter is indispensable for delineation of deeper structures and lesions, e.g., within the thigh muscles.
- Healthy muscle is of intermediate echogenicity, but its fibers cannot be visualized individually.
- Comprising numerous fibers, the fasciculi are almost anechoic; while on longitudinal views their perimysium is delineated as a thin line, on cross-sections they appear as dots.
- On longitudinal views, the fascial septa (epimysium) may give the muscle a striated or fibrillar appearance.
- Muscle septa are few in early childhood, increasing to the adult number at about age 5 years.
- Echogenicity of muscles depends primarily on the angle of insonation; in case of nonorthogonal insonation this will result in echogenicity changes lacking any morphological correlation.
- This phenomenon of echo reversal and echo migration is physiologically inherent to some muscles because of the course of their fibers (e.g., infraspinatus, brachial, and triceps brachii muscles).
- Distribution of hypoechoic and hyperechoic areas varies from muscle to muscle as well as between people; it also depends on age and physical fitness.
- *Additional workup:* plain radiography in soft-tissue mode, MRI, angiography, biopsy.

Sonographic Criteria of Assessment

- Fresh **muscular contusions** ("bruises") can only be demonstrated if they are sufficiently large. The concomitant intramuscular edema results in hypoechoic structural changes; sometimes there is intramuscular hemorrhage with indistinct delineation of the septa.
- **Muscle strain** (distraction injury grade 1) is characterized by partial hyperextension of the fibers without a break in continuity. Local swelling results in circumscribed volume increase of up to 50% of the cross-sectional area of the muscle. In severe strains there may be anechoic hematoma, while minor strains may present as normal sonographic findings.
- **Partial muscle tears** (distraction injury grade 2) correspond to a more severe injury of the fiber, breaks in the septa, and intercalated hematoma. Ruptured muscle stumps possibly floating in the hematoma (bell-clapper sign) are echogenic. Dehiscence increases on isometric contraction, frequently accompanied by local muscle spasms. Injuries affecting the muscle over a length of > 1 cm are reliably demonstrated on sonography.

- **Complete muscle tears** (distraction injury grade 3) with total loss of continuity are characterized by extensive accompanying hematoma with posterior enhancement, bell-clapper sign, and fascial injury. Ruptured ends are likely to retract. Permanent sequelae in the form of persistent loss of parallel septa and calcifications in the scar may remain after healing (Figs. 13.**1**, 13.**2**).
- Tumors are usually hypoechoic; reliable differentiation between benign and malignant processes is impossible, as is tissue typing. Precise US-guided biopsy of tumors in these areas is possible.
- Acute **compartment syndrome** is diagnosed primarily on clinical findings. The sonographic findings include increase in echogenicity and volume of the muscle while intramuscular septa remain intact.
- **Myopathies** are essentially characterized by changes in the normal echotexture of the muscle; transverse views yield more relevant information than longitudinal sections. Fascial planes lose their distinct delineation. Generalized neuromuscular disease results in increased muscular echogenicity.
- Congenital abnormalities, such as **aplasia/hypoplasia**, are sonographically well demonstrated by contralateral reference. Accessory muscles appear as soft-tissue masses with the characteristic echotexture of muscles.
- **Muscle hernias** are well visualized as protrusions through fascial gaps, differing from other soft-tissue tumors by their isomuscular echotexture.

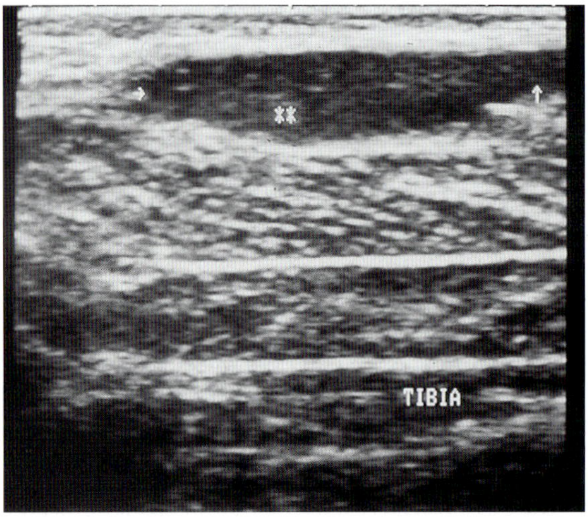

Fig. 13.**1 a** Longitudinal view of the posterior lower leg: Hypoechoic mass at the medial head of the gastrocnemius muscle, with the sonogram suspicious for a partial muscle tear.

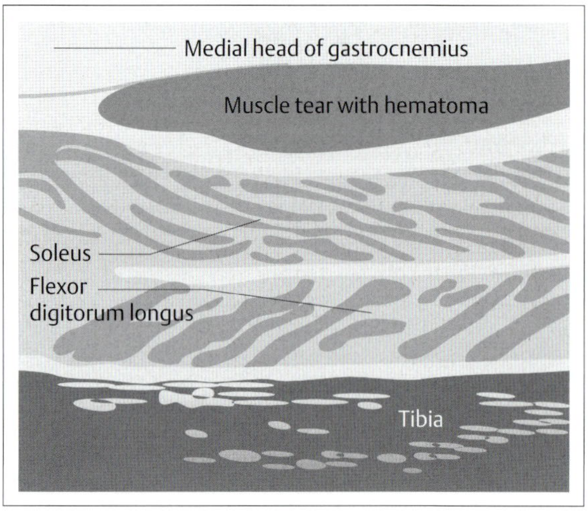

Fig. 13.**1 b** Line drawing.

Consequences for Surgical Treatment

Diagnosis	Characteristic Findings	Management
Contusion	Hypoechoic change in echotexture	Conservative
Strain	Circumscribed increase in volume, anechoic areas	Conservative
Tear	Large anechoic area, bell-clapper sign	Conservative
Compartment syndrome	Increase in volume and echogenicity	Emergency fasciotomy
Myopathy	Increased echogenicity	Conservative

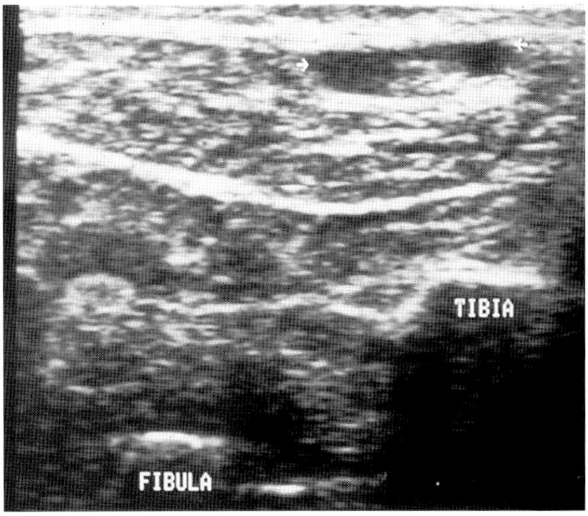

Fig. 13.**2a** Transverse view through the lower leg: This hypoechoic mass within the medial head of the gastrocnemius muscle is seen posterior to the tibia (same patient as in Fig. 13.**1**).

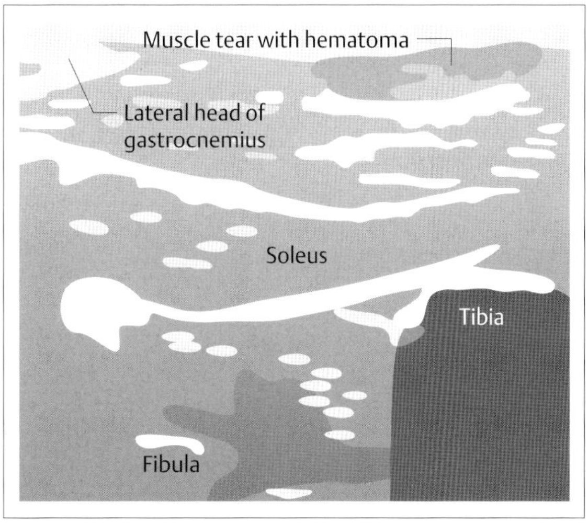

Fig. 13.**2b** Line drawing.

Disorders and Injuries of the Tendons

Examination of the tendons in the upper extremity is discussed in more detail later in this chapter, while the following paragraphs deal primarily with the large tendons of the leg.

Basic Facts

- Ultrasound is the modality of choice in the differential diagnosis of disorders and injuries of the large tendons of the lower limb.
- It follows the patient's history and physical examination.
- Tendons are imaged with a 5 or 7.5 MHz linear probe; because of the sometimes difficult coupling, the use of a standoff pad is recommended.
- Initial static evaluation should be followed by a dynamic examination of the tensed tendon as this allows assessment of its contractility and mobilization.
- Evaluate tendons in two orthogonal planes (longitudinal and transverse views) and check the contralateral tendon for reference.
- Most common pathological findings: rupture, bursitis, tendonitis, peritendonitis.
- Rupture of the Achilles tendon is a rather common injury, while rupture of the quadriceps and patellar tendons occurs less frequently.
- In longitudinal scans, tendons are easily recognized as an echogenic band with homogeneous border and characteristic fibrillar echotexture, being rather hyperechoic to the surrounding muscles and only slightly hyperechoic to the adjacent fatty tissues.
- In dynamic examinations, the hyperechoic border of the tendon (peritendineum) is well demarcated from the surrounding tissue.
- The ultrasound beam must be strictly perpendicular to the tendon's axis, since the slightest obliquity causes scattering of the beam resulting in an artifactual hypoechogenicity.
- On transverse views, tendons assume an oval shape and produce spotlike echoes; their area of insertion into the bone appears hypoechoic and should not be mistaken for an effusion.
- For reference measurements, see Table 13.**1**.
- *Additional workup:* plain radiographs, MRI.

Table 13.**1** Reference measurements for tendons

Tendon	Thickness (mm)	Width (mm)
Quadriceps	4–8	30–50
Patellar	3–6	15–25
Achilles	4–9	8–16

Sonographic Criteria of Assessment

- The change in sonomorphology diagnostic of a **tendon tear** (Figs. 13.**3**,13.**4**) is a break in its continuity. Since they may retract and contract, the torn tendon fragments appear hyperechoic and thicker. Clear sonographic signs of acute tendon tear include discontinuity; zonal defect filled with hypoechoic hemorrhagic fluid; echogenic margins of the fragments; and length of gap increasing on dynamic examination. In older tears, the zonal defect becomes hyperechoic as the hematoma undergoes organization.
- In **peritendonitis of the Achilles tendon**, the peritendinous tissue becomes hypoechoic, the tendon echo becomes splayed, and its sagittal diameter may double. In chronic cases, calcifications with posterior shadowing may develop around and within the tendon. **Acute tendonitis** manifests with edematous swelling of the tendon, at least initially, which in the chronic phase may involve the peritendineum and result in increasing echogenicity and heterogeneity.
- In **bursitis** (inflammation of, e.g., the calcaneal and retrocalcaneal bursa) (Figs. 13.**5**, 13.**6**), sonograms can demonstrate the normally sonolucent walls of the bursa now separated by hypoechoic fluid. The bursa will then be visualized in typical location as an ellipsoid hypoechoic structure. In the chronic stage there is progressive echogenic wall thickening.
- In **jumper's knee** (patellar enthesopathy/enthesitis or patellar tendonitis/tendinosis; inflammation of the insertion of the patellar tendon into the patella) (Fig. 13.**7**), the sonographic changes depend on the age of the lesion. If the history is brief, the sagittal diameter of the tendon at its insertion is only slightly wider than the contralateral reference; over time, the entire tendon may become thickened. In the chronic stage, hyperechoic intratendinous changes with posterior shadowing point to focal calcification (Table 13.**2**).

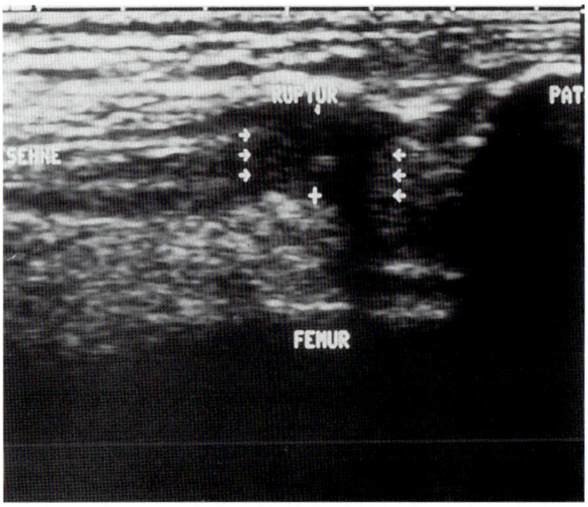

Fig. 13.**3a** Longitudinal suprapatellar view of the left knee in a 76-year-old patient. Rupture of the quadriceps tendon.

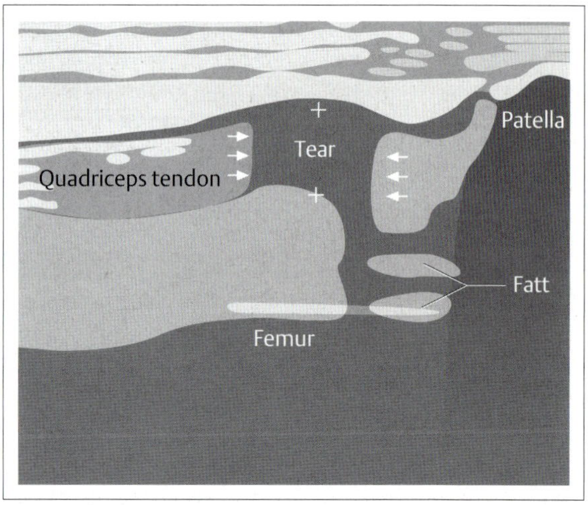

Fig. 13.**3b** Line drawing.

Table 13.**2** Sonographic classification of jumper's knee

Tendon Morphology	Stage
Thickening of the apical patellar insertion, with difference of 2 mm on contralateral comparison	1
Thickening of the apical patellar insertion, with difference of > 2 mm on contralateral comparison	2
Thickening of the tendon over its entire course	3
Thickening of the tendon with focal calcification	4
Partial tear	5
Complete tear	6

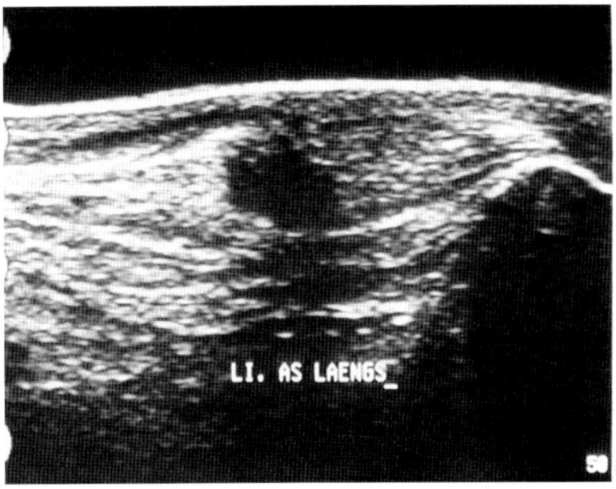

Fig. 13.**4 a** Longitudinal view of the left Achilles tendon. Hyperechoic fragment margins and hypoechoic defect in a torn Achilles tendon.

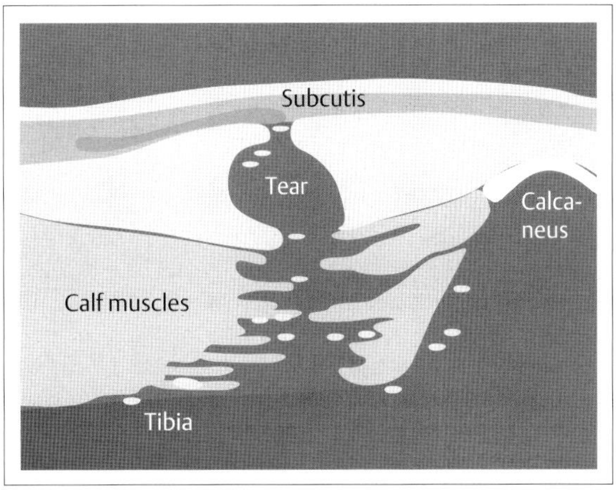

Fig. 13.**4 b** Line drawing.

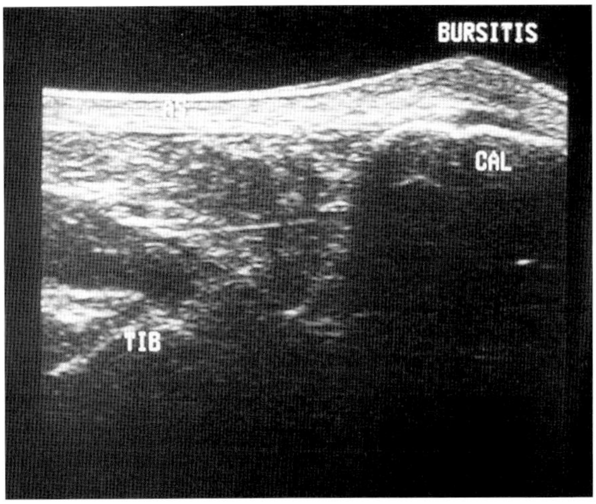

Fig. 13.**5 a** Longitudinal view of the right Achilles tendon. Suspected subcutaneous bursitis on sonography with hyperechoic changes immediately posterior to the calcaneus.

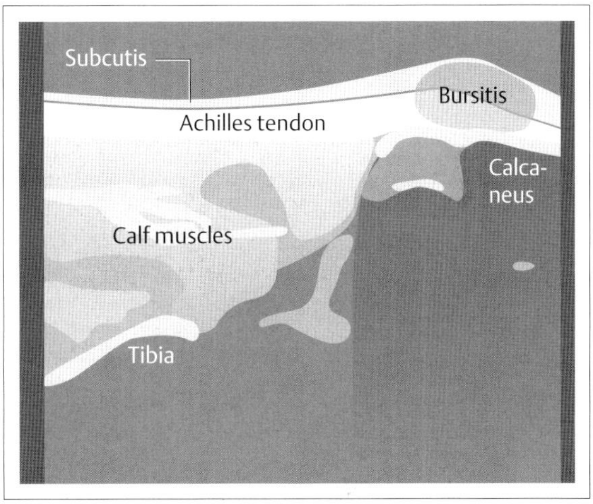

Fig. 13.**5 b** Line drawing.

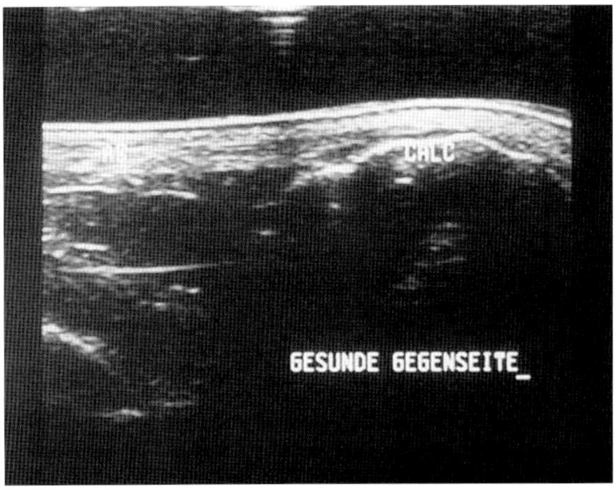

Fig. 13.**6 a** Longitudinal view of the right Achilles tendon. Healthy contralateral reference of the patient in Fig. 13.**5** with characteristic fibrillar echotexture of the Achilles tendon.

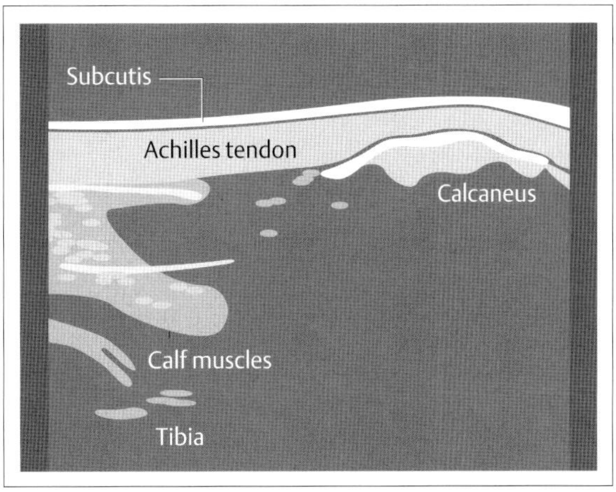

Fig. 13.**6 b** Line drawing.

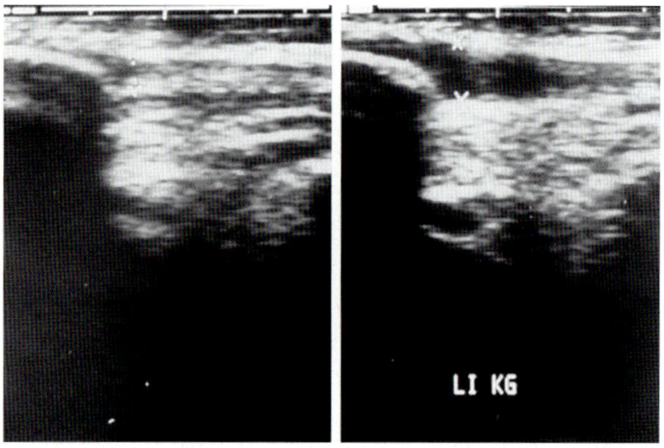

Fig. 13.7 a Longitudinal infrapatellar view of both knees. Normal finding (right knee) on the left, while the sonogram of the left knee, on the right, demonstrates a splayed patellar insertion of the tendon–jumper's knee stage II.

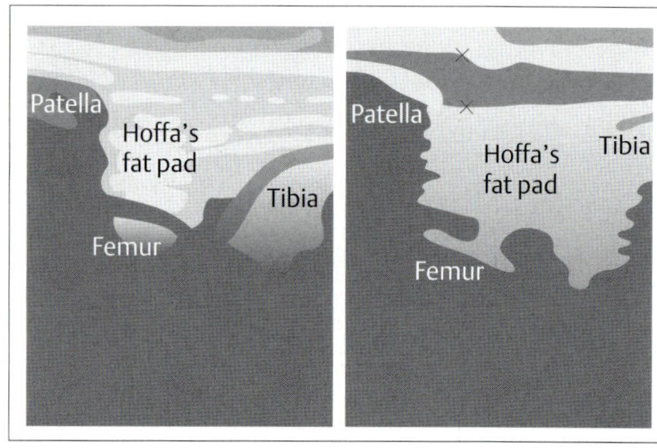

Fig. 13.7 b Line drawing.

Consequences for Surgical Treatment

Diagnosis	Characteristic Findings	Management
Jumper's knee	Hypoechoic splaying of the tendinous insertion into the patella	Conservative
Achilles peritendonitis	Hypoechoic halo around thickened tendon	Conservative; in chronic cases surgical tenolysis
Bursitis	Hypoechoic mass (fluid) at location of bursa	Conservative; bursectomy in chronic cases
Tendon tear	Hypoechoic discontinuity with hyperechoic margins of the torn fragments	Surgical repair

Arthrosonography

Humeroscapular and Acromioclavicular Joint

Basic Facts

- The shoulder is particularly amenable to sonographic evaluation because of its extensive soft tissue coat in which numerous pathologies may be found.
- Scanning planes must be adapted to the different locations of the various joint disorders.
- The central landmark is the head of the humerus.
- Sonography of the shoulder relies on 5 or 7.5 MHz linear transducers; tendon examinations (biceps, supraspinatus, and infraspinatus tendons) are enhanced by dynamic evaluation.
- Always document findings in two planes, ideally with contralateral reference.
- Relevant guidelines recommend that shoulder sonography be performed in three standard views, with two orthogonal scans in each view:
  - Anterior (transverse plus longitudinal scan)
  - Lateral (transverse plus longitudinal scan)
  - Posterior (transverse plus longitudinal scan)
- Though not mandatory, a consistent uniform examination proceeding from anterior to lateral and finally posteriorly is recommended.
- For anterior scans the slightly pronated arm should dangle freely, while for examinations of the lateral planes the arm is positioned as in Apply's scratch test, and for assessment of the posterior planes the arm is adducted completely with the lower arm resting on the abdomen.
- Pathologies of the long biceps tendon are imaged in the anterior plane (longitudinal plus transverse views). Isometric contraction of the biceps brachii muscle with

forearm in pronation and supination permits dynamic sonographic assessment.

- Rotator cuff and subacromial pathologies are best investigated in the standard lateral planes. Crossing the hands behind the back with the palms facing posteriorly results in maximum pronation and improves exposure of the supraspinatus tendon. Dynamic examination primarily involves rotation of the upper arm.
- The acromioclavicular joint is visualized by aligning the transducer along the longitudinal axis of the clavicle and placing it directly onto the palpable joint. If acromioclavicular joint injury is suspected, a coracoclavicular view should be obtained, with the probe placed orthogonal to the coracoid process and visualizing the inferior border of the clavicle. Use of a standoff device is recommended.
- *Additional workup:* plain radiographs, MRI, arthro-CT, possibly arthroscopy.

Sonographic Criteria of Assessment

- Sonographic signs of **supraspinatus tendon tears** vary depending on the extent (total/partial) and acuteness (acute traumatic/degenerative) of the tear. Generally, in longitudinal and transverse scans there are definite and ambivalent signs exhibiting the same characteristics. Definite signs: defect; narrowing; contour inversion (from convex to concave); abrupt change in caliber; step-off; hypoechoic area with echogenic fragment margins (particularly in acute tears). Ambivalent signs: hyperechoic, hypoechoic, or mixed changes; discontinuity of the bursal outline; impaired mobilization of the tendon on dynamic examination (Fig. 13.**8**).
- Subacromial bursitis is characterized by widening of the capillary gap between the bursal walls to > 2 mm, possibly with wall thickening (callosity, contralateral comparison).
- In **rotator cuff calcification** (calcific tendonitis) echogenic focal calcification with posterior shadowing is common; during resorption there may also be echogenic foci without posterior shadowing (Fig. 13.**9**).
- In *transverse views*, **tendonitis of the long biceps tendon** is characterized by enlarged halo, convex retinaculum, and transverse diameter of > 10 mm. In *longitudinal views*, there is a hypoechoic halo along the tendon. Tendonitis of the long biceps tendon may also be indicative of a SLAP tear (Fig. 13.**10**).
- In *transverse views*, an acute **tear of the long biceps tendon** is visualized as hypoechoic hemorrhagic ballooning of the retinaculum, while it cannot be displayed in old tears (ambivalent sign) or rupture of the retinaculum. In *longitudinal views*, an acute tear is displayed as a hypoechoic (hemorrhage) zonal defect with hyperechoic margins of the torn fragments, while it cannot be delineated in old ruptures.
- In *transverse views*, incomplete and complete **dislocation of the long biceps tendon** from the bicipital groove can be triggered by forced supination of the lower arm against resistance.
- Arthritis of the **acromioclavicular joint** is characterized by ballooning of the joint capsule (contralateral comparison) with posterior enhancement and possibly pressure lesions/erosions in the articular surfaces.
- The sonographic picture in **acromioclavicular joint separations** is characterized by joint space widening (contralateral comparison), distinct prominence of the clavicle over the acromion (contralateral comparison), and frequently by joint effusion, depending on the extent of the injury. In Tossy type I injuries, there will always be concomitant effusion and thus ballooning of the joint capsule, while clavicular prominence and joint space widening cannot be demonstrated (Fig. 13.**11**). Tossy type II is characterized by joint space widening and a hypoechoic effusion with only mild clavicular prominence over the acromion. On contralateral comparison, there is normally only slight widening of the coracoclavicular gap (Fig. 13.**12**). In Tossy type III injuries, sonography demonstrates hypoechoic effusion with joint space widening. Clavicular displacement is quite marked, with a severely widened coracoclavicular gap. There may be a hypoechoic rim (hematoma) around the coracoclavicular ligament.

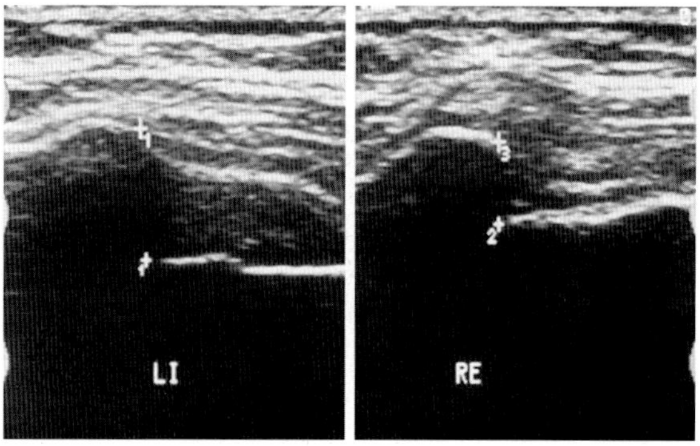

Fig. 13.**8 a** Lateral longitudinal view of the shoulder. In the **left image**, normal sonographic findings with a 10.6 mm gap between the head of the humerus and the acromion; in the **right image**, this gap has narrowed to 6.6 mm, and the subacromial bursa abuts the humeral head while the supraspinatus muscle is not delineated. These findings are consistent with a complete tear of the right supraspinatus tendon.

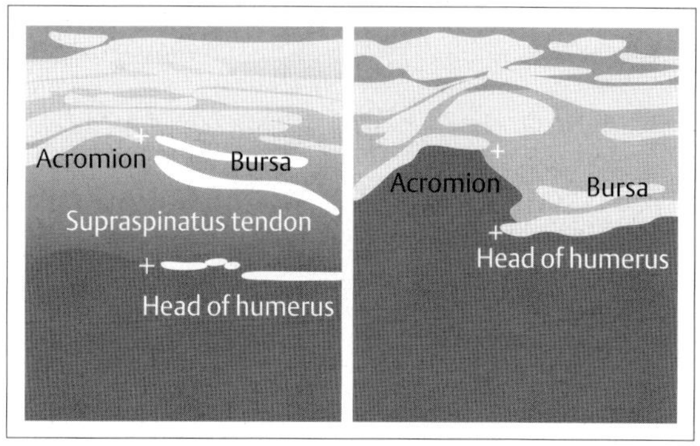

Fig. 13.**8 b** Line drawing.

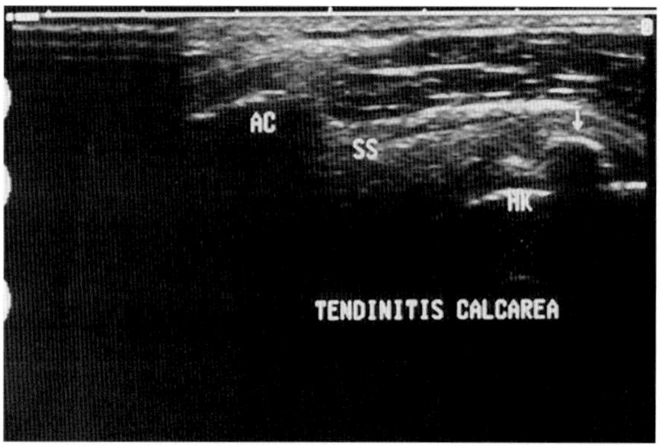

Fig. 13.**9 a** Lateral longitudinal view of the shoulder. Echogenic mass within the supraspinatus muscle (SS) with posterior shadowing at the humeral head (HK); calcific tendonitis of the supraspinatus muscle.

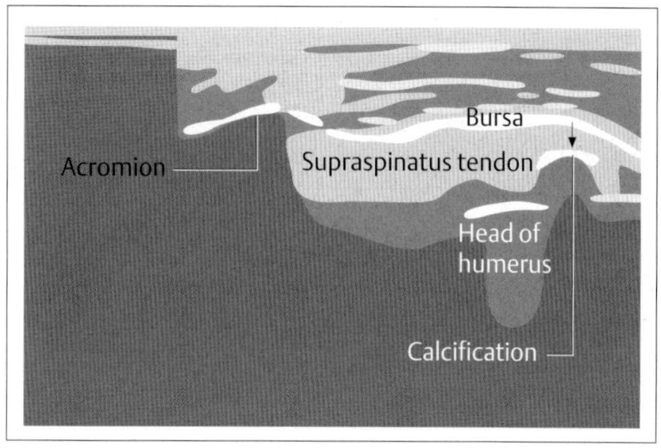

Fig. 13.**9 b** Line drawing.

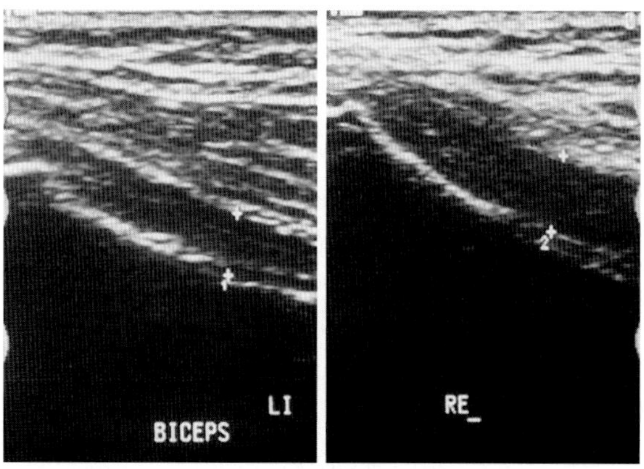

Fig. 13.**10 a** Anterior longitudinal view. On the **left**, normal view of the long biceps tendon; on the **right**, it is encased by a large echogenic mass, the sonomorphological correlate of tendonitis.

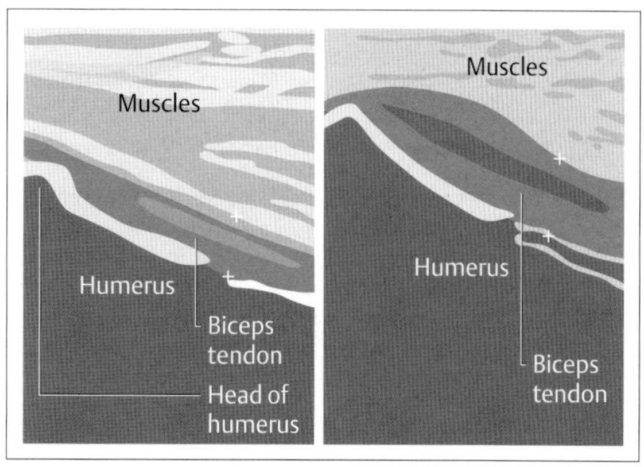

Fig. 13.**10 b** Line drawing.

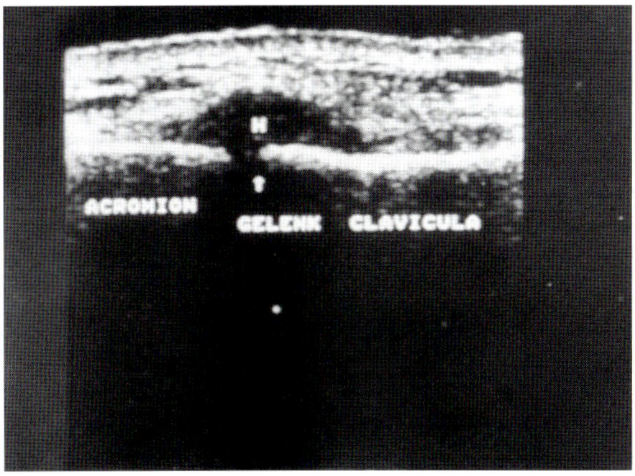

Fig. 13.**11 a** Longitudinal view of the acromioclavicular joint. Ballooning of the capsule by an echogenic mass; sonographically, this is highly suspicious for a Tossy type I injury.

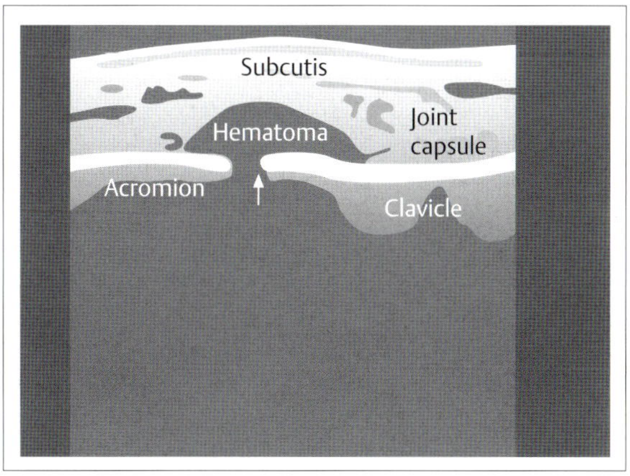

Fig. 13.**11 b** Line drawing.

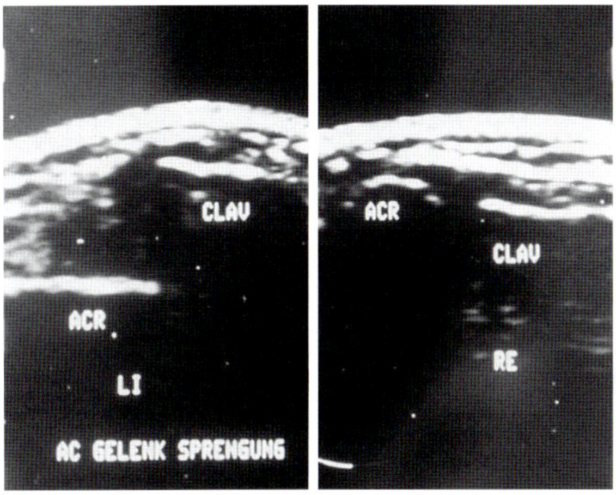

Fig. 13.**12 a** Longitudinal view of the acromioclavicular joint. The **left image** demonstrates the left acromioclavicular joint of a 42-year-old patient with a clavicle (CLAV) distinctly prominent above the acromion (ACR) and a hypoechoic joint effusion; these sonographic findings are consistent with a Tossy type III injury. **Right image:** The intact contralateral right side of the same patient is depicted.

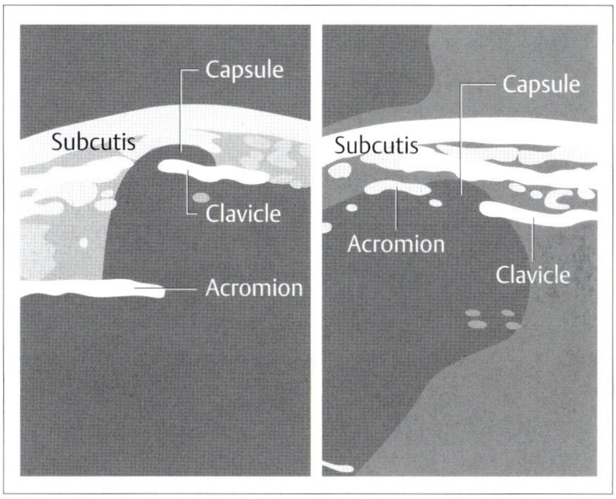

Fig. 13.**12 b** Line drawings.

Consequences for Surgical Treatment

Diagnosis	Characteristic Findings	Management
Bicipital tendonitis	Hypoechoic halo around the tendon	Conservative
Biceps tendon tear	Hypoechoic ballooning of the retinaculum	Conservative in proximal tears, surgical in distal ruptures
Supraspinatus tendon tears	Defect; narrowing; contour inversion (from convex to concave); abrupt change in caliber; step-off; hypoechoic area with echogenic fragment margins	Conservative, possibly arthroscopy plus tendon repair
Subacromial bursitis	Widening of the gap between the bursal wall > 2 mm	Conservative; arthroscopic bursectomy in chronic cases
Calcific tendonitis	Echogenic mass with posterior shadowing	Conservative; arthroscopic resection in chronic cases
Acromioclavicular joint separation	Joint space widening, step-off, hypoechoic intra-articular mass (hematoma)	Conservative; in Tossy type III injuries possibly surgical repair

Sternoclavicular Joint and Sternum

Basic Facts

- Swelling and physical signs related to the sternoclavicular joint are rare symptoms and disorders.
- Possible causes are traumatic or chronic dislocation as well as inflammatory, degenerative, and neoplastic processes.
- As a rule, clinical diagnosis of a fresh traumatic separation of the sternoclavicular joint is easy if the history is known; otherwise, swellings in the sternoclavicular joint region are difficult to assess.
- Radiological demonstration of a sternal fracture may often be ambivalent. Fissures and fractures with minor displacement are particularly easy to miss on plain radiographs.
- Use a 7.5 MHz linear transducer with standoff pad.
- Landmarks in sonographic assessment of the sternoclavicular joint are the clavicle and manubrium.
- Measurements include the width of the joint space and the distance between the clavicle and the manubrium of the sternum.
- Assessment includes any intra-articular effusion, ballooning of the joint capsule, intra-articular calcifications, and changes in the cortical texture of the clavicle and manubrium.
- Sternal assessment must be performed in longitudinal and transverse views.
- With the transducer applied anteriorly in the longitudinal plane, a strong cortical echo will be seen.
- At the transition between manubrium and corpus of the sternum there will be a small physiological defect of the otherwise contiguous cortical outline: the fibrous sternal synchondrosis.
- *Additional workup:* plain radiographs, MRI, CT.

Sonographic Criteria of Assessment

- An overview of pathologies affecting the sternoclavicular joint is presented in Table 13.**3**.
- Depending on the degree of **separation**, joint space widening and prominence can be demonstrated in all fresh injuries. The capsule lacks any changes in echogenicity with posterior shadowing akin to calcifications. The bone echo, too, appears to be homogeneous. Contrary to fresh injuries, in long-standing separations there will only be clavicular prominence without intra-articular hematoma. Recurrent separation can be clearly differentiated from injuries by dynamic assessment, where clavicular prominence can be triggered depending on the position of the arm; the result should be documented (Figs. 13.**13**, 13.**14**). Degenerative pseudo-separation is due to ballooning of the sternal end of the clavicle. In this case, sonography will depict not only the prominent end of the clavicle but also hyperechoic echoes within the capsule-ligamentous structures, signifying small calcifications. The osseous echo of the sternal end of the clavicle is heterogeneous, while articular effusions are atypical.
- Sonographic signs of **arthritis** are marked sternoclavicular joint effusions, ballooning of the joint capsule, and soft-tissue inflammation. The osseous echo is heterogeneous with defects in the cortical outline.
- Sonographic signs of **sternal fracture** include:
  - Break in the cortical echo.
  - Hypoechoic anterior area signifying a concomitant hematoma.
  - In dislocated fractures the cortical echo will demonstrate step-off.
  - On careful pressure application with the probe, the fracture gap will demonstrate a springy resistance (Fig. 13.**15**).

Table 13.**3** Sonographic findings in the sternoclavicular joint

Diagnosis	Joint Space Widening	Step-off	Intra-articular Fluid Collection	Calcified Joint Capsule	Bone Echo
Fresh traumatic separation	+	+	+	–	Homogeneous
Chronic traumatic separation	+	+	–	–	Homogeneous
Recurrent separation	+	+	–	–	Homogeneous
Degenerative separation	(+)	+	–	+	Heterogeneous
Benign tumor	–	–	–	–	Homogeneous
Malignancy	(+)	–	–	–	Heterogeneous
Bacterial arthritis	–	–	+	–	Heterogeneous

+ = present; – = absent; (+) = possibly present

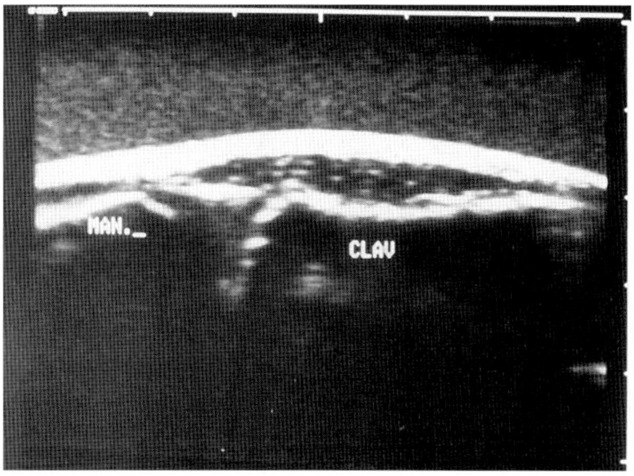

Fig. 13.**13 a** Longitudinal view of the right sternoclavicular joint of a 15-year-old girl. The clavicle and manubrium of the sternum are aligned.

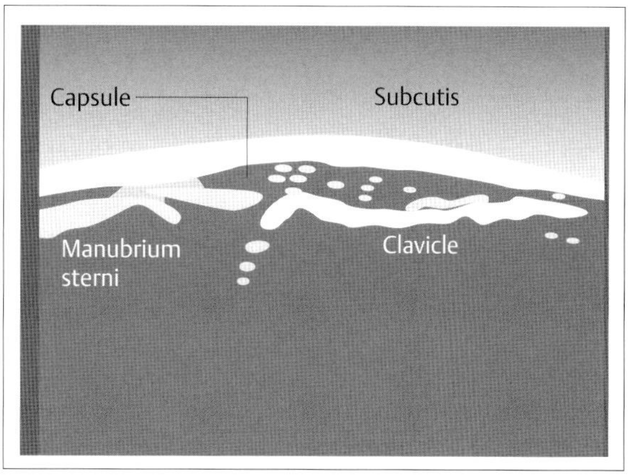

Fig. 13.**13 b** Line drawing.

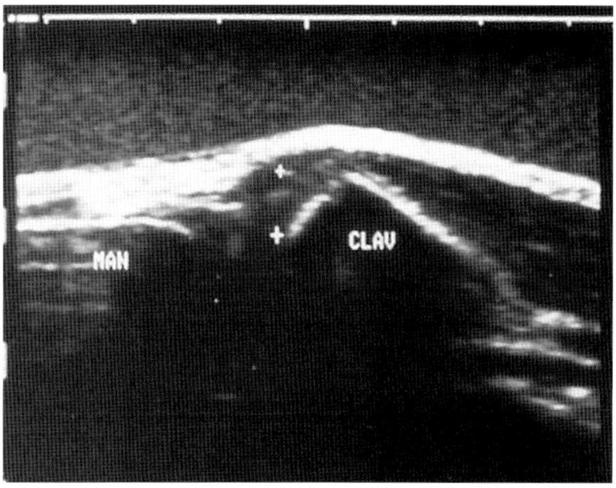

Fig. 13.**14 a** Longitudinal view of the right sternoclavicular joint in the same patient as in Fig. 13.**13**. On external rotation the clavicle is prominent by 7 mm anterior to the manubrium; chronic sternoclavicular joint separation.

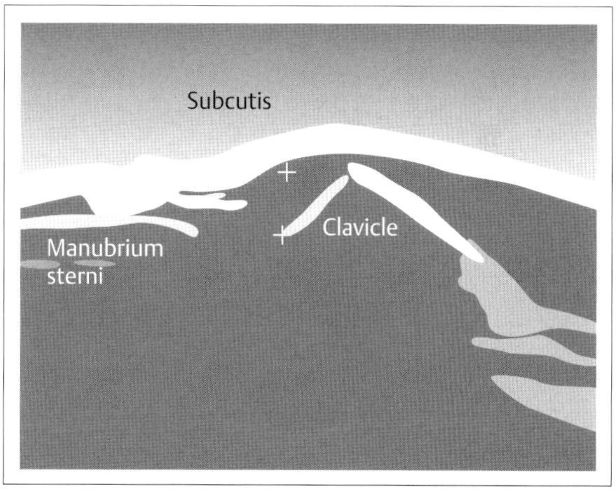

Fig. 13.**14 b** Line drawing.

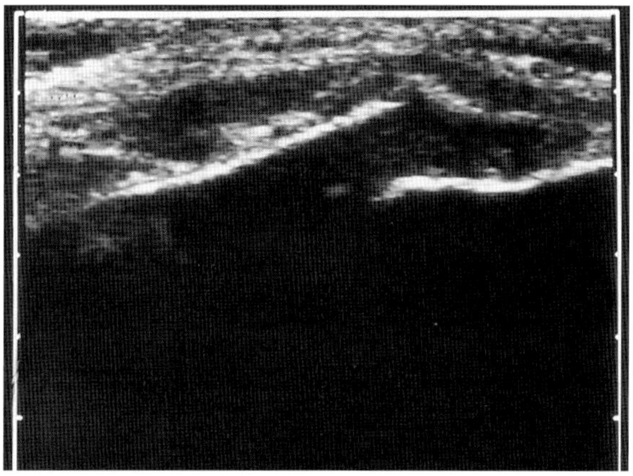

Fig. 13.**15 a** Longitudinal anterior view of the sternum. Distinct defect in the cortical echo, anterior fragment dislocated cephalad, hypoechoic mass cephalad of the posterior cortical echo. Fracture of the sternum in a 30-year-old man.

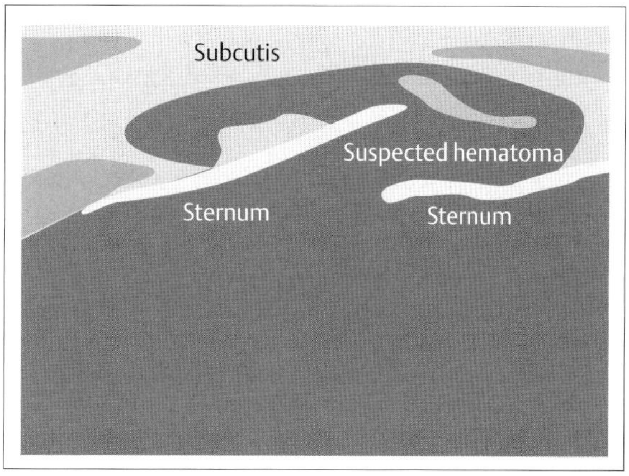

Fig. 13.**15 b** Line drawing.

Consequences for Surgical Treatment

Diagnosis	Characteristic Findings	Management
Sternoclavicular joint separation	Joint space widening, step-off, effusion	Conservative; open reduction and fixation rarely required
Arthritis	Effusion, possibly soft-tissue inflammation	Conservative; surgical excision rarely required
Sternal fracture	Break in cortical outline with anterior hypoechoic area signifying hematoma	Conservative

Elbow

Basic Facts

- The elbow joint can be examined with a 5 MHz as well as a 7.5 MHz transducer. Better coupling is achieved through a standoff device but this is not mandatory.
- For sonography the elbow joint should rest on a folded or rolled towel to render full extension of the arm more comfortable.
- The DEGUM guidelines recommend five standard views:
  - Three anterior planes (humeroradial and humero-ulnar longitudinal as well as anterior transverse view) with the elbow extended.
  - Both posterior planes (longitudinal and transverse view) with the elbow flexed at about 90°.
- The main indication for sonography of the elbow is confirmation or elimination of suspected elbow joint effusion.
- *Additional workup:* plain radiographs, MRI, possibly arthroscopy.

Sonographic Criteria of Assessment

- Depending on the condition, **effusion** (e.g., in cubital arthritis) may be demonstrated in one or more of the three cubital compartments. The larger the fluid collection, the more pronounced the ballooning of the joint capsule. Contralateral reference is mandatory in order to measure the true increase in the gap between capsule and cortex (Fig. 13.**16**).
- Depending on the kind of effusion, in **olecranon bursitis** a hypo-/hyperechoic mass can be delineated posterior to the olecranon. Serous effusion (hypoechoic bursal contents) results in posterior enhancement and increased change in impedance from the bone beneath.
- In **Panner disease** there may be a defect in the cortical contour with a small step in the bone and ballooning of the overlying joint capsule signifying effusion.

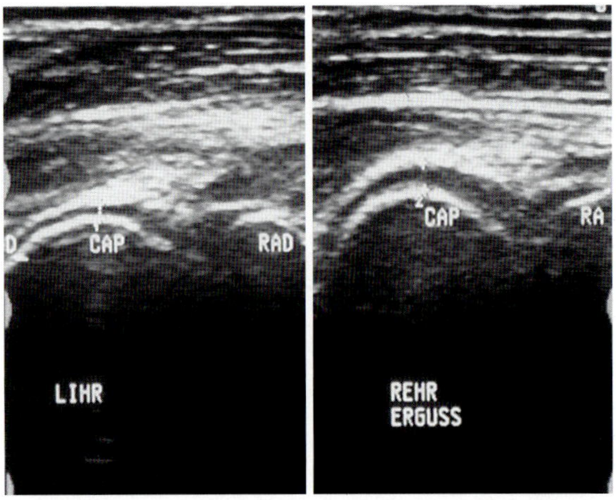

Fig. 13.**16a** Longitudinal humeroradial view. The sonogram on the left depicts a normal left humeroradial joint (LIHR), while the sonogram on the right demonstrates the capsule ballooning off the capitulum (CAP) as well as intra-articular effusion (erguss) in the right humeroradial joint. RAD, radius; CAP, capitulum.

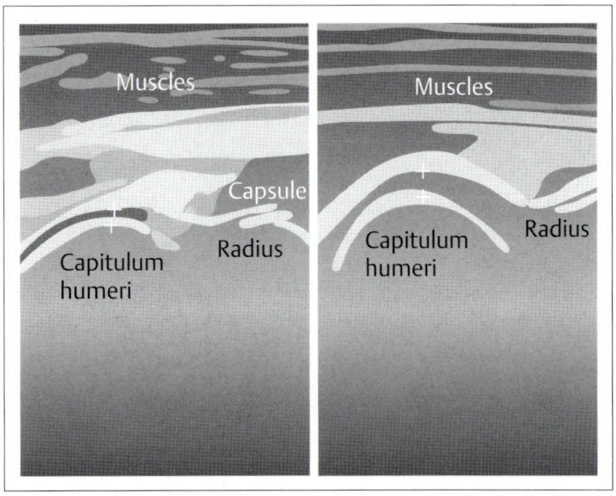

Fig. 13.**16b** Line drawing.

Consequences for Surgical Treatment

Diagnosis	Characteristic Findings	Management
Effusion	Ballooning of the capsule	Conservative, possibly arthrocentesis
Olecranon bursitis	Hypo-/hyperechoic mass posterior to the olecranon	Conservative, bursectomy rarely required
Panner disease	Break in cortical contour with ballooning of capsule above it signifying effusion	Conservative, possibly arthroscopic drilling and removal of loose bodies

Joints of the Hand

Basic Facts

- Joints of the hand are examined with a linear 7.5 MHz transducer.
- Standoff device and contralateral reference are mandatory.
- Dynamic examinations are recommended, particularly when delineating changes in the palmar tendons.
- Digital and metacarpal joints are assessed from a posterior and palmar view, each in the longitudinal and transverse plane, while at the wrist an additional radio-ulnar view is required.
- Common findings easily visualized on sonography include ganglion (demonstration of size and location) and effusion (usually in the distal radio-ulnar joint), although for these only semiquantitative diagnosis is possible.
- *Additional workup:* plain radiographs, MRI.

Sonographic Criteria of Assessment

- **Effusion** is demonstrated as an anechoic or hypoechoic mass between lower arm and the carpals.
- **Tenosynovitis** results in an anechoic or hypoechoic halo around the tendon (corresponding with the synovia).
- **Ganglia** are fluid-filled (i.e., hypoechoic) masses with smooth borders.
- **Foreign bodies** usually are characterized by a bright hyperechoic echo with complete posterior shadowing, surrounded by hypoechoic tissue (inflammatory reaction).

Consequences for Surgical Treatment

Diagnosis	Characteristic Findings	Management
Effusion	Anechoic/hypoechoic intra-articular mass	Conservative, possibly arthrocentesis
Tenosynovitis	Anechoic/hypoechoic halo around the tendon	Conservative, possibly synovectomy
Ganglia	Anechoic/hypoechoic mass with smooth borders	Resection
Foreign body	Bright hyperechoic echo with posterior shadowing	Surgical removal

Adolescent and Adult Hip

Basic Facts

- Due to the joint's deep anatomy and surrounding coat of soft tissues, palpation reveals only very little diagnostic information.
- Particularly when joint effusion is suspected, sonography of the adolescent and adult hip has a high degree of sensitivity and specificity and thus should be the initial imaging modality of choice, following history-taking and physical examination.
- Prime indication for hip sonography in children/adolescents and adults is suspected effusion and diagnostic workup of any disorder with concomitant effusion (Perthes disease, slipped capital femoral epiphysis), since almost all disorders of the juvenile hip demonstrate hip joint effusion, at least initially.
- Examine with the patient supine, employing a 5 MHz linear transducer and usually imaging the joint in two planes.
- In the anterior longitudinal view, the probe parallels the femoral neck and is applied at right angles to the inguinal canal. Owing to femoral antetorsion and anterior flattening of the acetabulum, sonography can visualize a rather large section of the hip joint.
- Transverse views through the hip joint are at right angles to the longitudinal plane.
- In special cases (e.g., Perthes disease) a coronal plane will offer a third view; to this end, the probe is applied in the longitudinal direction, its inferior end resting on the greater trochanter.
- Landmarks in sonography of the adult hip are the contour of the femoral head, femoral neck, and joint capsule.

Sonographic Criteria of Assessment

- In **hip joint effusion** the joint capsule displays anterior ballooning off the femoral neck, the capsule no longer paralleling the femur. Effusions appear as hypoechoic masses. The distance between joint capsule and femoral neck is measured. Differences ≥ 2.5 mm between affected and contralateral side are pathognomonic for effusion. In transient synovitis of the hip there are usually only slight differences between both joints (rarely > 5 mm), while in septic arthritis the difference may jump to 8–12 mm. In chronic cases, the capsule will be breached and the abscess can be traced into the soft tissues (Fig. 13.**17**).
- All acute cases of **slipped capital femoral epiphysis** are characterized by effusion, prominence of the epiphysis over the metaphysis, and distinct widening of the growth plate on contralateral reference. In chronic and subacute forms, effusion often may be rather small, occasionally even missing, while the usually semispherical contour of the epiphysis appears flattened. The amount of prominence of epiphysis over metaphysic yields an indirect measure of the angle of slippage (1 mm gap size corresponds to an angle of slippage of about 7°) on radiographs (frog lateral projection) (Fig. 13.**18**).
- The typical course in **Perthes disease** passes through different stages, each with its characteristic sonographic features:
  - *Initial stage:* Effusion always present, in some cases mild flattening of the femoral head, jumbled cortical echotexture, and widening of the epiphyseal plate.
  - *Condensation stage:* Effusion always present. Additionally, the size of the femoral head is diminished and the cortical structure beginning to show defects, widening of the growth plate. Subchondral fracture lines are seen (doubled epiphyseal contour), and possibly metaphyseal changes.
  - *Fragmentation stage:* Effusion in 80–90% of cases, definite breaks in the cortical outline, heterogeneous epiphyseal plate possibly with anterolateral displacement. Predominance of the hyperechoic (old sclerotic) bone undergoing resorption.
  - *Regenerative stage:* Effusion is rare and the newly forming hypoechoic bone predominates. Otherwise, the changes resemble those of the fragmentation stage.
  - *Terminal stage:* Effusion is rare and the cortical outline is continuous once more As sequelae after healing, the epiphysis may display anterior and/or lateral displacement signifying coxa magna, or it may recover an entirely normal shape in case of complete reconstitution (Fig. 13.**19**).
- **Fractures of the femoral neck** always result in breaks of the cortical outline, as well as intra-articular effusion (hematoma).
- Depending on the type of **hip arthroplasty** implanted, an echogenic stepped echo (neck of the femoral component) is demonstrated in the course of the femoral neck. After two months at the earliest, a neocapsule can be distinguished from the surrounding tissue. Septic infections may balloon this pseudocapsule so that it assumes a convex shape. With tissue necrosis in prolonged courses, the capsule may be breached, with inflammatory exudate spreading into the surrounding muscles. Loosening of the implant is usually also accompanied by effusion.

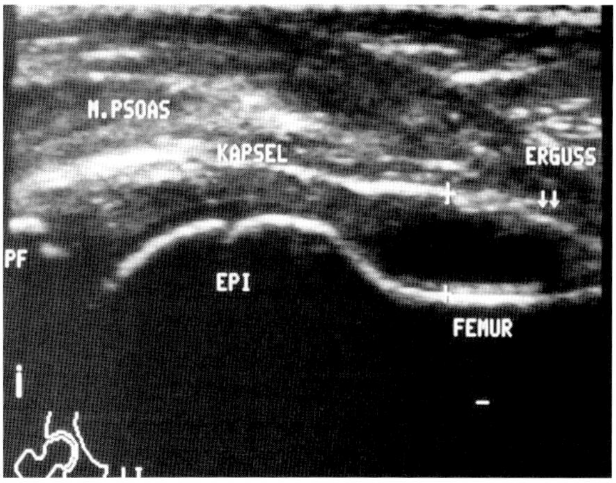

Fig. 13.**17 a** Anterior longitudinal view of the hip in a 12-year-old boy. Ballooning of the joint capsule (KAPSEL) of the femur by a hypoechoic effusion (ERGUSS), the sonomorphology being suspicious for coxitis.

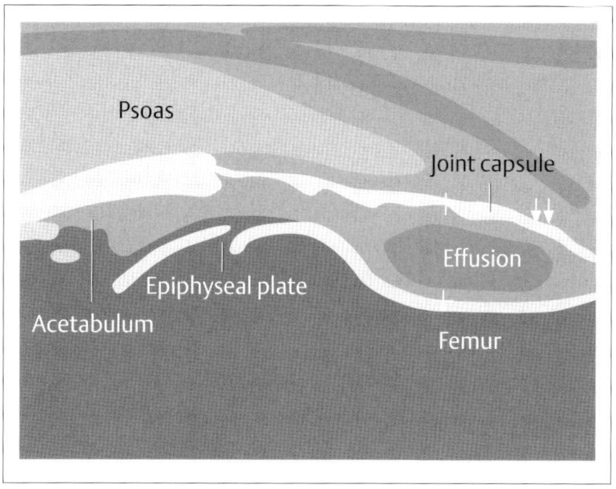

Fig. 13.**17 b** Line drawing.

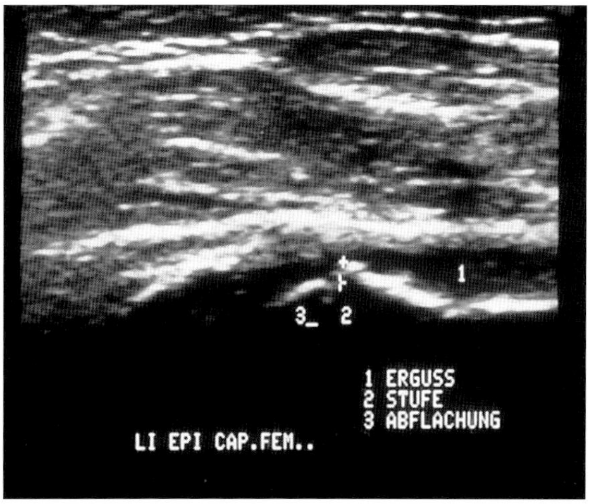

Fig. 13.**18 a** Anterior longitudinal view of the left hip in a 13-year-old boy. There is a 3.1 mm step between metaphysis and epiphysis and marked ballooning of the joint capsule signifying intra-articular effusion. Sonographic confirmation of slipped left capital femoral epiphysis. 1, Effusion; 2, step; 3, flattening.

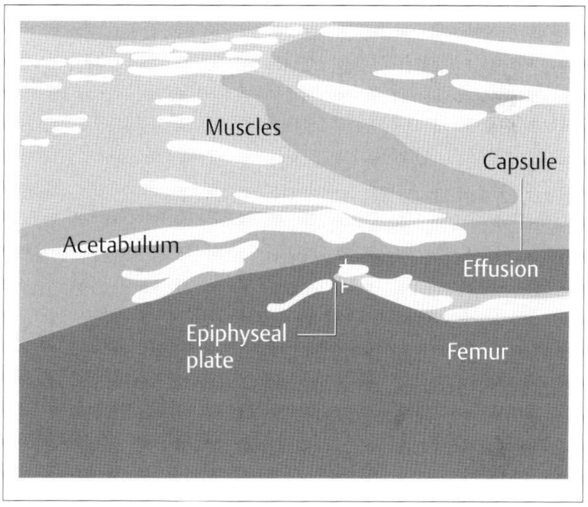

Fig. 13.**18 b** Line drawing.

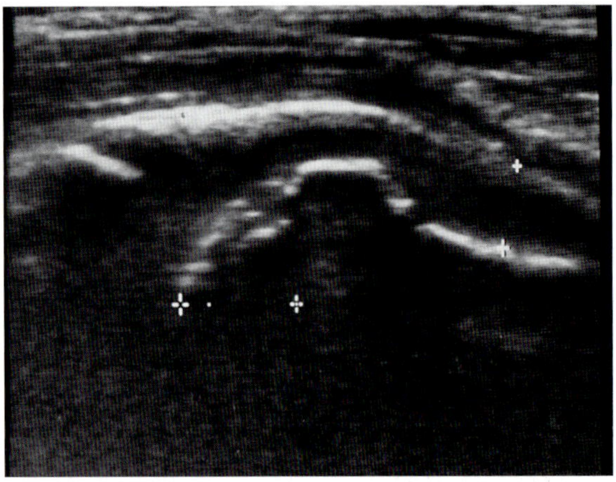

Fig. 13.**19 a** Anterior longitudinal view of the right hip in an 8-year-old boy. Ephyseal fragmentation and diminution, joint capsule ballooning signifying intra-articular effusion. Sonographic confirmation of Perthes disease in the fragmentation stage.

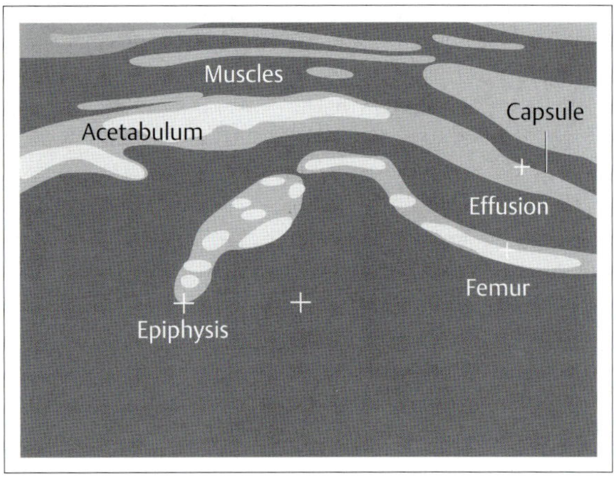

Fig. 13.**19 b** Line drawing.

Consequences for Surgical Treatment

Diagnosis	Characteristic Findings	Management
Hip joint effusion	Ballooning of the capsule, hypoechoic mass around the femoral neck, contralateral difference > 2.5 mm	Conservative, possibly arthrocentesis; synovectomy in bacterial effusion
Perthes disease	Sonographic characteristics depending on stage (see above)	Conservative with off-loading braces, or surgery (corrective osteotomy)
Slipped capital femoral epiphysis	Effusion, epiphyseal step-off, widened epiphyseal plate	Kirschner wire fixation; Imhäuser osteotomy in angles of slippage > 50 °
Fracture of the femoral neck	Broken cortical outline, intra-articular effusion	Reduction and fixation, hip arthroplasty

Knee

Basic Facts

- Sonographic examination of the knee with 5 or 7.5 MHz linear transducers (sector scanner for meniscal sonography) employing anterior, lateral, and posterior views according to the recommendations of the Working Committee on the Musculoskeletal System of DGOT.
  - *Anterior views* (suprapatellar and infrapatellar longitudinal scan, suprapatellar transverse scan).
  - *Lateral views* (lateral and medial longitudinal scan).
  - *Posterior views* (medial, intercondylar, and lateral longitudinal scan, transverse scan through the popliteal fossa).
- Patient supine for anterior and lateral views.
- Patient prone for posterior views.
- Depending on the clinical picture, the examination encompasses additional views, femur and tibia always being the landmarks.
- Bursitis counts among the most common pathologies assessed by sonography, predominantly seen deep to the gastrocnemius muscle in conjunction with Baker's cyst. Prepatellar bursitis is frequently accompanied by prepatellar effusion. Extra-articular bursitis is rather rare
- Delineation of the menisci is another common application of knee sonography. Its segments (anterior and posterior cornu, intermediate section) are examined in longitudinal scans, separately as well as in continuity.

- For examination of the anterior horns, as for the intermediate sections, a supine position is best (knee flexed at about 90°), while the posterior horns are more favorably assessed in the prone patient with mild knee flexion of about 30°.
- Both linear and sector scanners may be used, but the latter are clearly superior.
- *Additional workup:* plain radiographs, MRI, arthroscopy.

Table 13.**4** Types of bursitis with corresponding sonomorphology

Type of Bursitis	Sonomorphology
Serous	Increased hypoechoic echotexture
Suppurative	Increased hyperechoic echotexture
Chronic	Increased echogenicity of the bursal wall
Calcifying	Hyperechoic lamella with posterior shadowing
Rheumatoid	Villous internal texture

Sonographic Criteria of Assessment

- The most common **synovial herniations** are popliteal (Baker's) cysts in the typical dorsomedial location between the heads of the gastrocnemius muscle. Anechoic cysts will display posterior enhancement. Septations (polycystic form) are easily visualized. As part of chronic polyarthritis, increased echogenicity due to exudate rich in fibrin (Figs. 13.**20**, 13.**21**).
- Because of the interlinked bursae, knee joint **effusion** first appears as an anechoic suprapatellar mass. The scanning plane of choice is the suprapatellar longitudinal view. Distinct lifting of the patella can also be demonstrated. Dynamic examination is recommended and fluctuation should be documented. Hemarthrosis or empyema must be suspected in hyperechogenicity.
- **Synovitis** increases synovial consistency and can first be demonstrated in the suprapatellar recess. The structure is thickened and hyperechoic (synovial edema). Its thickness can best be measured on transverse views. It may reach 1 cm in chronic proliferative synovitis, e.g., in the context of chronic polyarthritis.
- Depending on the bursal contents, there are several types of **bursitis** (Fig. 13.**22**) with different features on sonography (Table 13.**4**).
- **Loose bodies** visible only in the suprapatellar recess or within the joint space, appearing as hyperechoic round structures with posterior shadowing.
- In **Osgood–Schlatter disease**, the osseous contour of the tibial tuberosity loses its usual smooth border. The echo of the bone becomes discontinuous and somewhat fluffy. The insertion of the patellar tendon into the tuberosity is splayed and heterogeneous. The cartilaginous anlage of the pretibial apophysis is thickened, sometimes being twice the size of the contralateral side. Infrapatellar bursitis is present in 50% of cases (Figs. 13.**23**, 13.**24**).
- **Fresh ligamentous tears** are typically accompanied by hematoma and instability of the joint, often displaying the break in the hyperechoic ligament. Documentation of collateral ligament tears is of greater relevance than those of the cruciate ligaments. For stress loading of the knee, the help of an assistant is useful.
- For the easily visualized quadriceps tendon tears, see the earlier section Disorders and Injuries of the Tendons, p. 273.
- **Meniscal tears** stand out distinctly in the homogeneous grayish meniscal triangle by their hyperechoic echotexture. A bright double line with a hypoechoic gap in between indicates a cleft with high diagnostic reliability; if the fragments are separated, there may instead be a single echo line without interwoven hypoechoic gap.
  - The margins in **fresh meniscal tears** are bright and sharply defined sonographically; the echotexture (single or double line echo) must be reproducible across several views.
  - **Chronic meniscal tears** with degenerative changes in the surrounding tissues lose their clear-cut outline but must also be reproducible across several views. Frequently, a meniscal ganglion in the posterior horn will be visualized as a hypoechoic cystic mass.
  - **Meniscal degeneration** will also be hyperechoic, but in contrast to the sharp outline of fresh tears it usually gives rise to a cloudy image. When examined in several views, it cannot be expected to appear at the same position in the sonogram but will change its position with each new scanning plane. Differential diagnosis has to include loose bodies, which also appear as hyperechoic masses but stay outside the meniscal triangle.

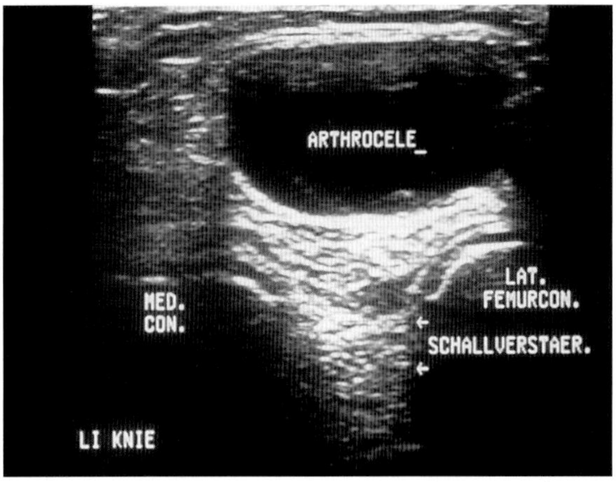

Fig. 13.**20 a** Posterior transverse view through the popliteal fossa. Hypoechoic roundish mass in the popliteal fossa with posterior enhancement (arrows); sonographically suspicious for synovial herniation.

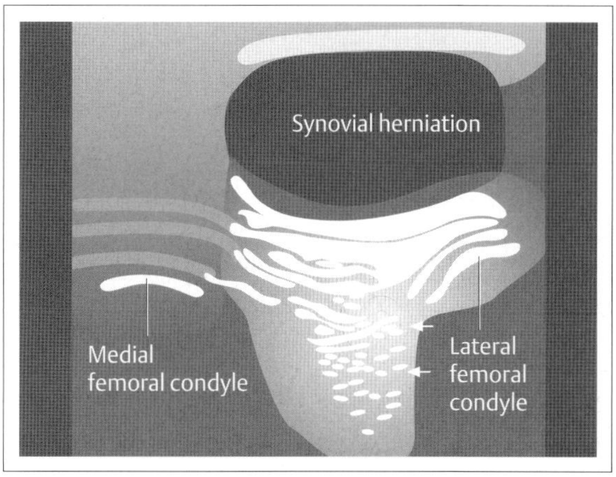

Fig. 13.**20 b** Line drawing.

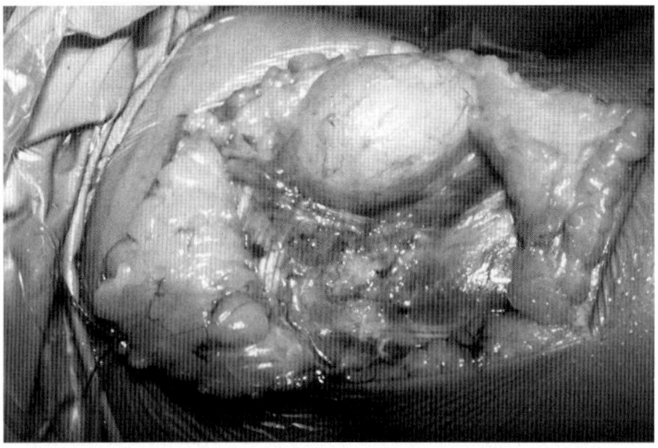

Fig. 13.**21** Same patient as in Fig. 13.**20**. Intraoperative finding of synovial herniation into the popliteal fossa.

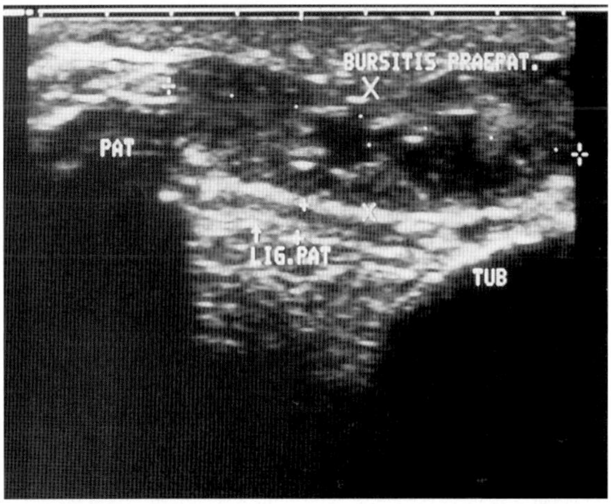

Fig. 13.**22 a** Longitudinal infrapatellar view in a 50-year-old female patient: 5 × 63 × 18 mm encapsulated mass anterior to and displacing the patellar ligament (LIG. PAT); this finding is consistent with prepatellar bursitis.

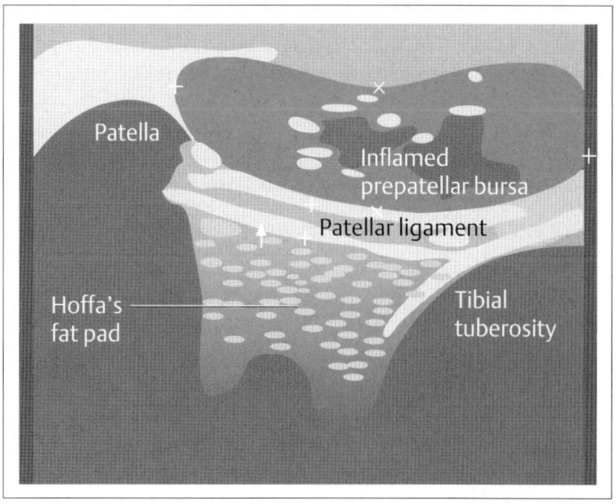

Fig. 13.**22 b** Line drawing.

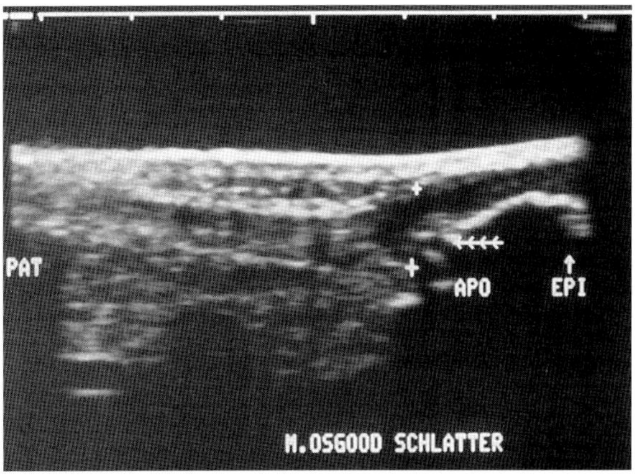

Fig. 13.**23 a** Longitudinal infrapatellar view in a 14-year-old girl. At the insertion of the patellar tendon into the tibial tuberosity the apophysis (APO) is fragmented and the tendon is splayed; sonographic features suspicious for Osgood–Schlatter disease.

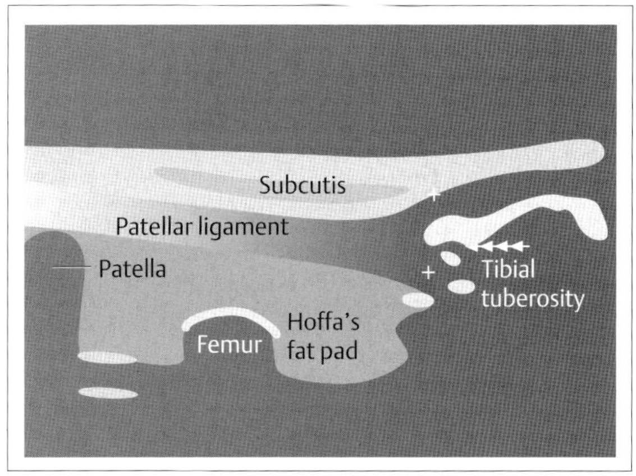

Fig. 13.**23 b** Line drawing.

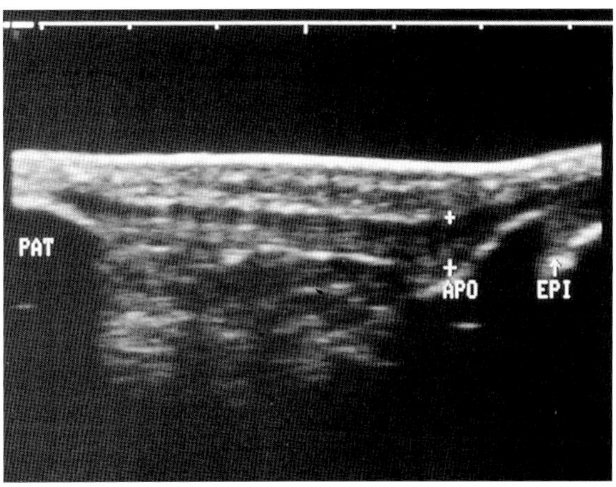

Fig. 13.**24 a** Longitudinal infrapatellar view of the left knee: Normal contralateral joint of the same girl as in Fig. 13.**23**.

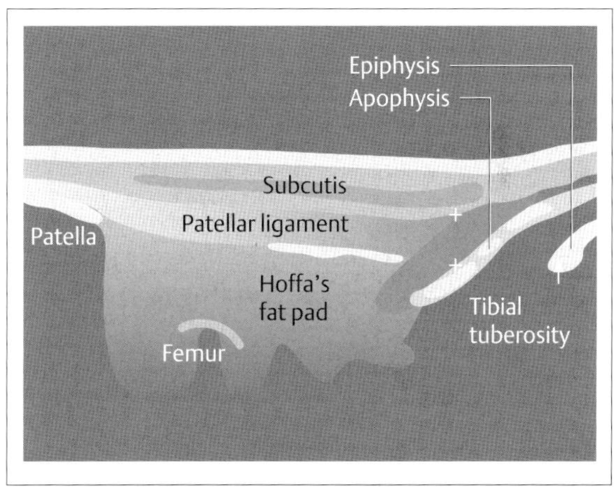

Fig. 13.**24 b** Line drawing.

Consequences for Surgical Treatment

Diagnosis	**Characteristic Findings**	**Management**
Synovial herniation	Anechoic, well-defined mass with posterior enhancement	Repair of any underlying internal knee damage and resection
Knee joint effusion	Anechoic suprapatellar mass	Arthrocentesis, diagnostic workup
Synovitis	Hyperechoic thickening (1 mm) of the synovium	Conservative or synovectomy
Prepatellar bursitis	Depending on the type of bursitis (Table 13.**4**), demonstration of a hypo-/hyperechoic bursa which normally is sonolucent	Conservative, possibly bursectomy
Osgood–Schlatter disease	Thickening of the patellar ligament (caudad) and apophysis with fluffy cortical echotexture	Conservative
Meniscal tear	Hyperechoic echo within the homogeneous meniscal triangle	Arthroscopy, suture repair of the meniscus or partial resection

Ankle

Basic Facts

- The primary purpose of sonography of the ankle is to gain additional information complementary to other modalities.
- Diagnostic workup of ligament injuries is the prime indication.
- 7.5 MHz linear transducer with standoff device is recommended.
- The DEGUM guidelines recommend five standard views:
  - *Two anterior views* (transverse plus longitudinal scan).
  - *One lateral view* (diagonal scan).
  - *Two posterior views* (transverse plus longitudinal scan).

Sonographic Criteria of Assessment

- **Joint effusion** is characterized by the capsule ballooning off the bones and is most easily demonstrated in both anterior views. Contralateral reference is mandatory.
- **Tenosynovitis** results in an anechoic or hypoechoic halo around the tendon (corresponding with the synovia).
- **Hematomas** are recognized as hypoechoic fluid collections in the adjacent soft tissue whose echogenicity gradually increases with organization.
- **Loose bodies** are identified by their bright echogenicity, usually accompanied by total posterior shadowing.
- Fresh **tears of the talofibular ligament** may be suggested by the presence of a localized hematoma. Ankle stress radiographs (using appropriate devices) will demonstrate an increased distance between both bony landmarks.

Consequences for Surgical Treatment

Diagnosis	Characteristic Findings	Management
Joint effusion	Ballooning of the capsule	Conservative, diagnostic workup
Tenosynovitis	Anechoic/hypoechoic halo around the tendon	Conservative
Talofibular ligament tear	Hematoma around the ligament	Conservative, surgery rarely required

Sonography in Particular Disorders of the Musculoskeletal System

Inflammatory Diseases

Basic Facts

- Diagnostic workup of inflammatory diseases of the musculoskeletal system relies primarily on history, physical examination, and laboratory parameters.
- As an imaging modality, sonography complements this basic assessment in an appropriate and economic fashion.
- In inflammatory disorders of the musculoskeletal system, the various organs/organ systems are examined sonographically according to the guidelines already described in the related sections.
- Use of 5 or 7.5 MHz linear transducers is recommended and the findings are documented in two orthogonal planes.
- Because of the major impact of inflammatory disease of the musculoskeletal system, the essential pathologies are briefly summed up below.
- *Additional workup:* plain radiographs, MRI, scintigraphy.

Sonographic Criteria of Assessment

- In **osteomyelitis** the affected bone segment displays a heterogeneous echotexture, typically with cortical defects and subperiostal abscess formation (fusiform hypoechoic ballooning beyond the cortical outline with elevated periostal echo). These changes may be accompanied by soft tissue involvement.
- In septic **arthritis** there is ballooning of the joint capsule, as is true in all intra-articular effusions. Thickening of the capsule, synovial villi, and hypoechoic or even relatively hyperechoic intra-articular fluid collections provide further evidence of inflammation. Sonography may demonstrate osseous defects (pressure lesion, erosion).
- **Soft tissue abscesses** may arise as an isolated process as part of osteomyelitis or spondylitis. On the sonogram, they appear as an ovoid hypoechoic intramuscular mass displacing the septa. The early stage is characterized by diffuse infiltration, while the late stages display smooth delineation with increased hyperechoic internal echotexture. Focal calcifications may be present in some cases.
- **Rheumatoid arthritis** causes changes similar to those described above for septic arthritis. Differences include more pronounced changes of the synovial membrane, with marked synovial villi formation and additional bursitis (hypo-/hyperechoic fluid collections within the bursae).

Consequences for Surgical Treatment

Diagnosis	Characteristic Findings	Management
Osteomyelitis	Irregular bone texture deep to fusiform hypoechoic ballooning signifying subperiostal abscess formation	Surgical debridement and irrigation-suction drainage
Arthritis	Joint capsule ballooning, intra-articular hypo-/hyperechoic fluid collection	Arthrocentesis, diagnostic workup
Soft-tissue abscess	Ovoid hypoechoic intramuscular mass displacing the septa	Incision and drainage
Rheumatoid arthritis	Synovial thickening with bursal villi	Conservative, surgery depending on type and extent of finding

Soft-Tissue and Bone Tumors

Basic Facts

- Despite there being numerous alternatives for visualizing and assessing bone and soft-tissue tumors with ultrasound, reliable differentiation between benign and malignant tumors has remained impossible with the technology available to date. Thus, in sonography of bone and soft-tissue tumors accurate description of the sonograms is of paramount importance. According to Graf (1988) this should always include the following details: consistency (solid, cystic) of the process; internal texture (homogenous, heterogeneous, possibly calcification); delineation from the surrounding tissue (smooth, irregular, tuberous, displacing, invasive, etc.); three-dimensional size (in metric measurements, if possible); and topographic relations.
- Because of the total reflection of ultrasound by bone, neoplastic osseous lesions can be visualized and evaluated only if the tumor has altered the outline of the bone or if cortical defects are present.
- Soft-tissue tumors are best visualized if their echotexture is either particularly hypoechoic or hyperechoic.
- Cysts (e.g., Baker's cysts) and hyaline cartilage structures (e.g., the chondrous parts of cartilaginous exostoses) are particularly hypoechoic, the former usually being well defined by their capsule.
- Heterotopic ossifications (e.g., rotator cuff calcification and myositis ossificans) are especially hyperechoic and by their posterior shadowing are easily delineated from the surrounding soft tissues.
- If the tumor is ill defined against the surrounding tissues and its relation to anatomical structures proves difficult, dynamic examination may help in directly visualizing soft-tissue structures by their movement.
- In bone tumors cortical defects result in discontinuity of the bone contour and thus are indicative. Apart from the visible break in the sonographic echo, such gaps may provide access to deeper sites and may thus provide insight into intraosseous parts of the tumor.
- Particularly in metaphyseal and epiphyseal areas, appraisal of such changes can be difficult because quite often the bone surface displays an irregular shape. Cortical defects visible on sonography may occur in benign as well as malignant tumors; they are, however, overwhelmingly more common in malignant lesions.
- *Additional workup:* plain radiographs, CT, MRI, histology (diagnostic resection/biopsy).

Sonographic Criteria of Assessment

- The majority of **soft-tissue tumors** are hypoechoic (Tables 13.**5**, 13.**6**). Inferences about a tumor visualized on sonography may be drawn from its (characteristic) location and the patient's history rather than its echotexture (Tables 13.**1**, 13.**2**). If tumor impedance does not differ from that of the surrounding soft tissues (e.g., as in subcutaneous lipoma), a surrounding capsule (if present) may permit delineation. Since such a capsule is infrequent in invasive tumors, e.g., at the margin of metastases, exact outlining has proved rather difficult (Figs. 13.**25**, 13.**26**).
- Apart from their typical cortical discontinuity, in most cases **bone tumors** (Tables 13.**5**, 13.**6**) display a heterogeneous echotexture. Most often, sonography demonstrates anechoic, hypoechoic, and hyperechoic areas. In bone tumors, posterior shadowing frequently signals calcification. Sonography can be of great assistance in visualizing any para-osseous parts of bone tumors. The question of the extent to which an indistinct interface between tumor and neighboring anatomical structures harbors tumor spread or simply edema may remain unanswered. Apart from the criteria for sonographic assessment of bone tumors described above, the behavior of the periosteum in the transition zone between normal and altered bone segments also plays an important role. For example, periosteal elevation with subperiosteal calcifications, corresponding to the Codman triangles seen on plain radiographs (Fig. 13.**27**), is sometimes seen in osteosarcoma and Ewing sarcoma.
- Owing to the extremely low echogenicity of hyaline cartilage, **osteochondromas** permit excellent assessment of the cartilaginous cap of an exostosis and its exact size. As the cartilaginous parts of exostoses are barely, if at all, visible on radiographs, ultrasonography is considered the modality of choice in these cases.

Table 13.**5** Sonographic characteristics of benign tumors (modified from Reimers, 2005)

Tumor	Echogenicity	Note
Hemangioma	Solid part of medium echogenicity with hypo-/hyperechoic parts, homogeneously hypo-/hyperechoic	Possibly multilocular; possibly hyperechoic phleboliths; change in shape on contraction; increase in size after physical acitivity
Lipoma	Hypoechoic with hyperechoic structures (pointlike or arc-shaped)	Encapsulated and therefore easily delineated; typical subcutaneous location facilitates diagnosis
Angiomyolipoma	Hypoechoic or hyperechoic	
Fibrous histiocytoma	Hypoechoic	
Fibroma	Homogeneously hypoechoic	Include in differential diagnosis if encountered close to strong fascia
Myxoma	Hypoechoic	Posterior enhancement, sometimes cystic internal structures in the millimeter range
Desmoid	Hypoechoic	Possibly complete ultrasound reflection at the surface of the tumor
Arteriovenous malformation	Hyperechoic	Localized muscular hypertrophy
Osteochondroma	Anechoic structure on top of the bone	Often massive focal elevation of the bone surface; shadowing posterior to the spurlike base; well defined from the surrounding tissue

Table 13.**6** Sonographic characteristics of malignant tumors (modified from Reimers, 2005)

Tumor	Echogenicity	Note
Liposarcoma	Mostly hyperechoic	Possibly difficult delineation from the surrounding muscles due to similar echogenicity
Other sarcomas	Hypoechoic	Well-defined
Malignant fibrous histiocytoma	Hypoechoic and hyperechoic areas	Heterogeneous texture, ill-defined transition zones
Lymphoma	Hypoechoic or mixed echogenicity	Sometimes well-defined
Osteosarcoma	Hyperechoic with alternating hypoechoic and anechoic areas	Only visible in case of cortical defects; often multiple adjacent ill-defined cortical defects; periostal calcification at the margins (Codman's triangle)
Chondrosarcoma	Hypoechoic with large-sized hyperechoic internal echoes	Visualization possible only in case of cortical defects; highly irregular echotexture; extraosseous parts smoothly delimited from the surrounding tissue; shadowing posterior to the focal ossifications
Metastases	Hypoechoic or heterogeneous	

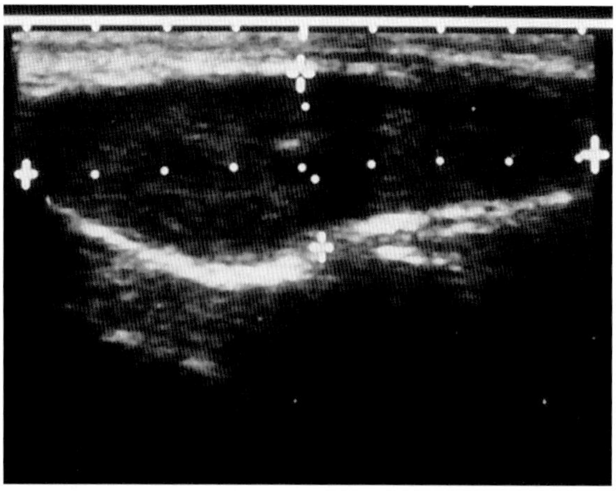

Fig. 13.**25 a** Longitudinal plantar view at the metatarsal level. Encapsulated echogenic mass measuring 82 × 24 mm; sonographic features consistent with soft-tissue tumor.

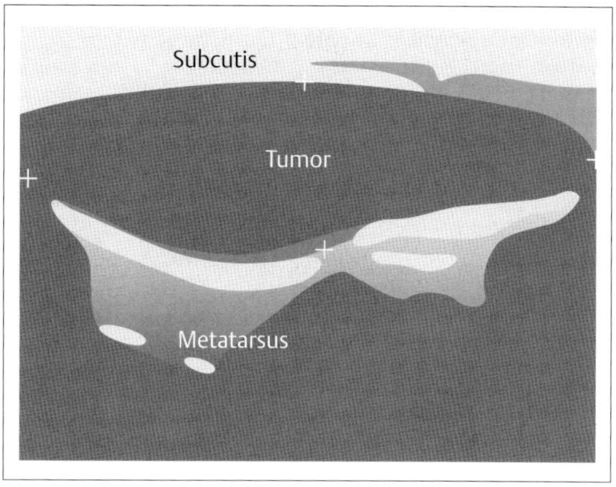

Fig. 13.**25 b** Line drawing.

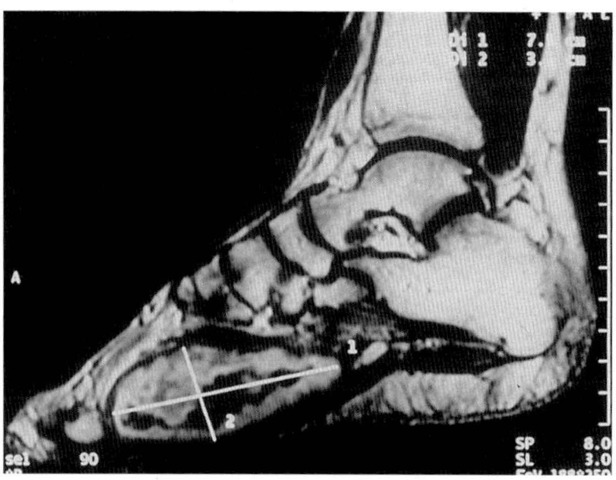

Fig. 13.**26** Same patient as in Fig. 13.**25**. MRI confirmed the sonographic finding of tumor, which on histopathology was identified as benign schwannoma.

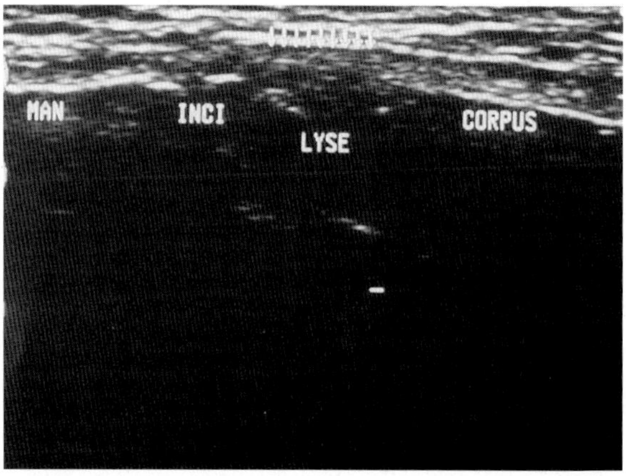

Fig. 13.**27 a** Anterior longitudinal view of the sternum in a 33-year-old patient. Caudal of the sternal synchondrosis the cephalic part of the sternal body displays a lytic lesion; histopathology identified the tumor as plasmocytoma. INCI, angle; LYSE, lysis.

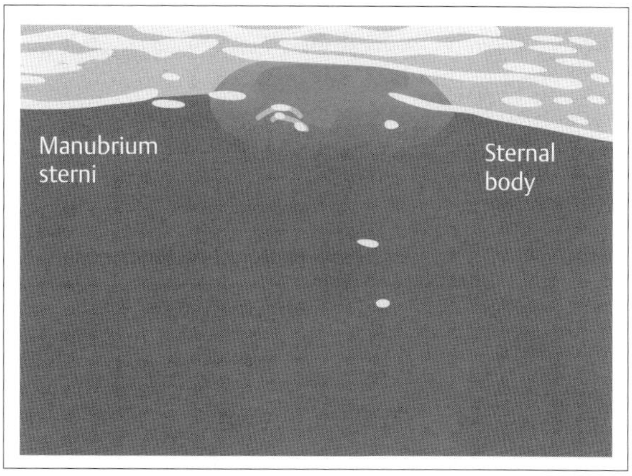

Fig. 13.**27 b** Line drawing.

Consequences for Surgical Treatment

Diagnosis	Characteristic Findings	Management
Soft-tissue tumor	Most often hypoechoic (for differentiation see Tables 13.**5**, 13.**6**)	Biopsy; histopathology will decide on further necessity of treatment
Bone tumor	Cortical discontinuity, echogenic heterogenicity (for differentiation see Tables 13.**5**, 13.**6**)	Biopsy; histopathology will decide on further necessity of treatment
Osteochondroma	Anechoic structure on top of the bone	Resection in case of clinical complaints

Bibliography

Azzoni R, Cabitza P, Parrini M. Sonographic evaluation of subacromial space. Ultrasonics. 2004; 42: 683–7.

Beekman R, Visser LH. High-resolution sonography of the peripheral nervous system–a review of the literature. Eur J Neurol. 2004; 1: 5–14.

Benson LS, Donaldson JS, Carroll NC. Use of ultrasound in management of posterior sternoclavicular dislocation. J Ultrasound Med. 1991; 10: 115–8.

Bialik R. Sonography and diagnosis in painful hips. Int Orthop. 1991; 15: 155–9.

Casser HR, Sohn Ch, Kiekenbeck A. Current evaluation of sonography of the meniscus. Results of a comparative study of sonographic and arthroscopic findings. Arch Orthop Trauma Surg. 1990; 109: 150–4.

Finlay K, Ferri M, Friedman L. Ultrasound of the elbow. Skeletal Radiol. 2004; 33: 63–79.

Fornage BD. Musculoskeletal Ultrasound. New York: Churchill Livingstone; 1995.

Freyschmidt J, Ostertag H, Jundt G. Ultrasonographie. In: Freyschmidt J, Ostertag H, Jundt G, eds. Knochentumoren. Klinik, Radiologie, Pathologie. Berlin, Heidelberg: Springer; 1998: 37–8.

Graf R, Schuler P. Sonographie bei Weichteiltumoren. Orthopäde. 1988; 17: 128–133.

Gruber G, Konermann W, Müller-Miny H, Gruber GM. Standardized ultrasound study of the knee joint. Ultraschall Med. 1997; 18: 52–61.

Hoffmann V. Ultraschalldiagnostik in Pädiatrie und Kinderchirurgie. Stuttgart: Thieme; 1996.

Heyde CE, Mahlfeld K, Stahel PF, Kayser R. Ultrasonography as a reliable diagnostic tool in old quadriceps tendon ruptures: a prospective multicenter study. Knee Surg Sports Traumatol Arthrosc. 2005; 13: 564–8.

Jacobson JA, Lancaster S, Prasad A, van Holsbeeck MT, Craig JG, Kolowich P. Full-thickness and partial-thickness supraspinatus tendon tears: value of US signs in diagnosis. Radiology. 2004; 230: 234–42.

Kayser R, Hampf S, Pankow M, Seeber E, Heyde CE. Validity of ultrasound examinations of disorders of the shoulder joint. Ultraschall Med, 2005; 26: 291–8.

Kayser R, Mahlfeld K, Heyde CE. Partial rupture of the proximal Achilles tendon: a differential diagnostic problem in ultrasound imaging. Br J Sports Med. 2005; 39: 838–42.

Kayser R, Mahlfeld K, Heyde C, Graßhoff H. Ultrasonographic imaging of fractures of the clavicle in newborn infants. J Bone Joint Surg [Br]. 2003; 85B: 115–6.

Kayser R, Mahlfeld K, Scheller W, Müller J, Schmidt W, Heyde CE. The ultrasound examination of the distal biceps tendon–an anatomical and clinical study. Eur J Ultrasound. 2005; 26: 17–23.

Konermann W, Gruber G. Septic coxitis in childhood. Differential ultrasound diagnoses. Orthopade. 1997; 26: 830–7.

Konermann W, Gruber G. Standard ultrasound sections of the upper extremity–shoulder and elbow joint. Ultraschall Med. 1998; 19: 130–8.

Mahlfeld A, Franke J, Mahlfeld K. Ultrasound diagnosis of sternum fractures. Zentralbl Chir. 2001; 126: 62–4.

Mahlfeld A, Merk H, Franke J, Kayser R, Mahlfeld K. Diagnostic ultrasonography of the sternoclavicular joint. Ultraschall Med. 1999; 20: 74–7.

Mahlfeld K, Franke J, Awiszus F. Postcontraction changes of muscle architecture in human quadriceps muscle. Muscle Nerve. 2004; 29: 597–600.

Mahlfeld K, Franke J Graßhoff H Bilateral and simultaneous quadriceps tendon rupture in secondary hyperparathyroidism. A case report. Zentralbl Chir. 1999; 124: 1045–48.

Mahlfeld K, Franke J, Schaeper O, Graßhoff H. Bilateral and simultaneous rupture of the quadriceps tendon–a diagnostic problem? Ultraschall Med. 2000; 21: 226–8.

Mahlfeld K, Graßhoff H, Jentsch-Ulrich K, Röcken C, Franke J. Visualization of a solitary myeloma of the sternum by ultrasonography. Zentralbl Chir. 2004; 129: 63–6.

Mahlfeld K, Kayser R, Franke J. Ultrasonographic visualization of a Baker-cyst as cause of a peroneal nerve palsy in a patient with rheumatoid arthritis. Unfallchirurg. 2004; 107: 429–32.

Mahlfeld K, Kayser R, Franke J, Merk H. Ultrasonography of the Osgood-Schlatter disease. Ultraschall Med. 2001; 22: 182–5.

Mahlfeld K, Kayser R, Mahlfeld A, Graßhoff H, Franke J. Value of ultrasound in diagnosis of bursopathies in the area of the Achilles tendon. Ultraschall Med. 2001; 22: 87–90.

Mahlfeld K, Kayser R, Mahlfeld A, Merk H. Ultrasound findings of the patellar tendon and its insertion sites. Ultraschall Med. 1997; 18: 249–53.

Mahlfeld K, Mahlfeld A, Kayser R, Franke J, Merk H. Ultrasonography as a diagnostic tool in cases of quadriceps tendon rupture. Ultraschall Med. 1999; 20: 22–5.

Matter HP, Gruber G, Konermann W, Gruber GM, Litzelbauer HD. Standardized ultrasound examination of the ankle joint. Clarification of ultrasound standard image sections by corresponding MRI sections. Ultraschall Med. 1998; 19: 34–9.

Merk H, Wissel H, Merkel M. Ultrasound follow-up after surgically managed Achilles tendon ruptures. Ultraschall Med. 1997; 18: 254–7.

Pollock RC, Bankes MJ, Emery RJ. Diagnosis of retrosternal dislocation of the clavicle with ultrasound. Injury. 1996; 27: 670–1.

Reimers CD, Gaulrapp H. Muskel- und Sehnensonographie. Köln: Deutscher Ärzteverlag; 2005.

Roberts D, Miller TT, Erlanger SM. Sonographic appearance of primary synovial chondromatosis of the knee. J Ultrasound Med. 2004; 23: 707–9.

Schmidt WA, Schmidt H, Schicke B, Gromnica-Ihle E. Standard reference values for musculoskeletal ultrasonography. Ann Rheum Dis. 2004; 63: 988–94.

Sofka CM, Adler RS. Sonography of cubital bursitis. AJR Am J Roentgenol. 2004; 183: 51–3.

Sugimoto K. Ultrasonographic evaluation of the Bankart lesion. J Shoulder Elbow Surg. 2004; 13: 286–90.

Stürmer I, Merk H, Witt HJ. Ultraschalldiagnostik bei Arthritiden und Osteomyelitiden. Ultraschalldiagnostik 91. Berlin, Heidelberg: Springer; 1992: 249–53.

Teefey SA, Rubin DA, Middleton WD, Hildebolt CF, Leibold RA, Yamaguchi K. Detection and quantification of rotator cuff tears. Comparison of ultrasonographic, magnetic resonance imaging, and arthroscopic findings in seventy-one consecutive cases. J Bone Joint Surg Am. 2004; 86-A: 708–16.

Weishaupt D, Berbig R, Prim J, Brühlmann W. Ultrasound findings after shoulder dislocation. Ultraschall Med. 1997; 18: 129–34.

Zehetgruber H, Lang T, Wurnig C. Distinction between supraspinatus, infraspinatus and subscapularis tendon tears with ultrasound in 332 surgically confirmed cases. Ultrasound Med Biol. 2002; 28: 711–7.

14 Sonography of the Abdominal Wall

W. Grechenig, J. Mayr, W. Pichler

Indications for Sonography

In abdominal sonography, the abdominal wall acts as acoustic window to the underlying organs. Extensive scarring (after repeated laparotomies) or excessive subcutaneous fat (obesity, abdominal pannus) may hinder the sonographic view into the abdominal cavity. Cutaneous emphysema (in case of accompanying chest trauma) may even render the examination altogether impossible.

Conscientious sonographic evaluation of the abdominal wall is an integral part of the diagnostic workup in blunt abdominal trauma as well as in the acute abdomen. Sonography immediately follows the physical examination and is best performed by the same examiner.

In hematomas, tumors, hernias, penetrating foreign bodies, and abscesses of the abdominal wall, as well as in postoperative wound surveillance, sonography is the initial imaging modality of choice and can help verify a clinical diagnosis. Under ideal circumstances it may yield significant additional information regarding extent, size, and localization of pathological lesions of the abdominal wall.

Specific Technique and Diagnostic Evaluation

- Patient in standard (supine) position.
- High frequency linear transducers of at least 5–7.5 MHz are recommended.
- Longitudinal, transverse, and oblique views following the course of the abdominal wall muscles.
- Differentiated delineation of the individual muscles, fascias, and vessels according to their anatomy.
- Isometric contraction permits further functional assessment of the paired muscles of the abdominal wall.
- Wounds in the abdominal wall can be examined with the probe covered by a sterile disposable glove, using alcohol or sterile ultrasound jelly as the coupling medium. Alternatively, the wound may be covered with a sterile sonolucent OpSite drape.
- Always start the examination with a 5 MHz transducer, surveying the rectus abdominis muscles in longitudinal and transverse views (the larger area covered facilitates anatomical relation and orientation); specific questions may be addressed subsequently with higher-frequency probes (smaller sector).
- The anterior abdominal wall comprises the paramedian rectus abdominis muscles running in a longitudinal direction and, laterally, three layers of obliquely oriented muscle. As these muscles are layered and run obliquely to each other, the ultrasound beam may not always be orthogonal to all muscle segments displayed on the monitor. However, for assessment of muscular and fascial echogenicity it is mandatory that the axis of insonation be orthogonal to the structures examined (otherwise artifactual misinterpretation is possible).

Abdominal Wall Trauma–Rectus Sheath Hematoma

Basic Facts

- The most common causes are posttraumatic hemorrhage or spontaneous bleeding under anticoagulant therapy.
- Rare causes are coagulopathy, perforation of a subcutaneous vascular prosthesis, and fractures.
- Rectus sheath hemorrhage is frequently misdiagnosed as acute abdomen.
- Most of the fluid is limited to the muscular segment between adjacent tendinous intersections.
- Hematoma cannot spread into the pelvis and retroperitoneum as there are no infraumbilical tendinous intersections.
- Since the advent of blunt handlebars, mandatory wearing of seatbelts, and child safety/booster seats, abdominal wall injury in children has become rather infrequent.
- In children, lap-belt trauma of the abdominal wall (straplike transverse ecchymosis, most often at the umbilical level) may signify a lap-belt complex (intestinal and lumbar spine injury with or without paraplegia).
- Abdominal wall hematoma should undergo clinical and sonographic follow-up until complete resolution, as development of a posttraumatic abdominal wall hernia and its differentiation from a muscle tear may initially be rendered difficult by hematoma-induced swelling of the abdominal wall.

- Blunt abdominal wall trauma must be monitored clinically and calls for sonographic assessment of the abdominal cavity and retroperitoneum as well as laboratory workup.

Table 14.**1** Muscular trauma–sonographic findings

Bruise (inter-/intramuscular hematoma)
Compact hematoma or diffuse bleeding
No splaying of the fibers on dynamic examination
Muscle fibers displaced by the more hypoechoic hematomas
Diffuse hemorrhage may also result in increased echogenicity
Strain–muscle tear
Thin discontinuous longitudinal echoes
On contraction the muscle fibers become splayed
On palpation with probe, a possible noticeable dent that can be expanded
Floating muscle fibers (bell-clapper sign)
Complete muscle tear
Fluid collection within the fascial sleeve lacking any muscle texture
Further retraction of the muscle stumps on isometric contraction

Sonographic Criteria of Assessment

- **Intramuscular abdominal wall hematoma** results in circumscribed thickening of the abdominal muscles, which assume a heterogeneous echotexture with hyperechoic as well as hypoechoic areas and display discontinuous echoes of the longitudinal muscle fibers (Figs. 14.**1** and 14.**2**).
- **Fluid collection in the rectus sheath** can be identified with certainty by eliciting fluctuation on active muscle contraction or external compression (by probe or fingers).
- For classification of muscular injury, see Table 14.**1** and Fig. 14.**3**.
- Major **bleeding into the lower abdomen** and rupture of the symphysis is quite often accompanied by extensive prevesical hematoma, complicating differential diagnosis. In most cases both sides are affected, thus making contralateral reference impossible.
- *Later course:* frequently a mixed sonographic picture (Fig. 14.**4**); later, liquefaction with subsequent abdominal wall seroma or absorption with scarring and possibly secondary calcifications.
- *Differential diagnosis of hypoechoic areas:* hemorrhage, edema, artifact (nonorthogonal insonation of the muscles).
- *Lap-belt complex:* usually free sonolucent fluid within the abdominal cavity (primarily in the pouch of Douglas) and signs of retroperitoneal hematoma (widening of the retroperitoneal space with ill-defined hypoechoic or hyperechoic areas).

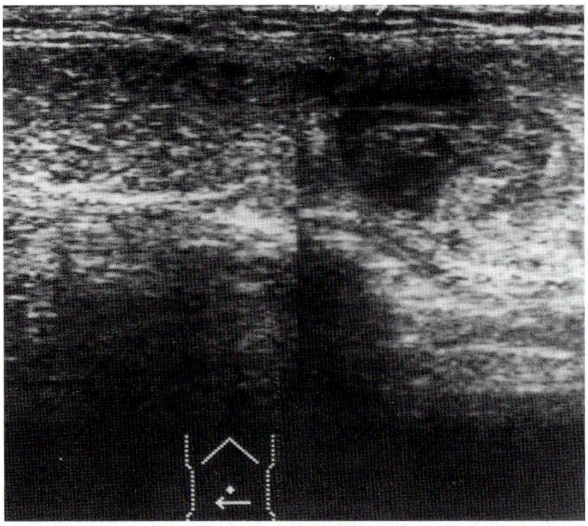

Fig. 14.**1 a** Transverse view of the lower abdomen. Rectus sheath hematoma (right image) with normal contralateral reference (left image).

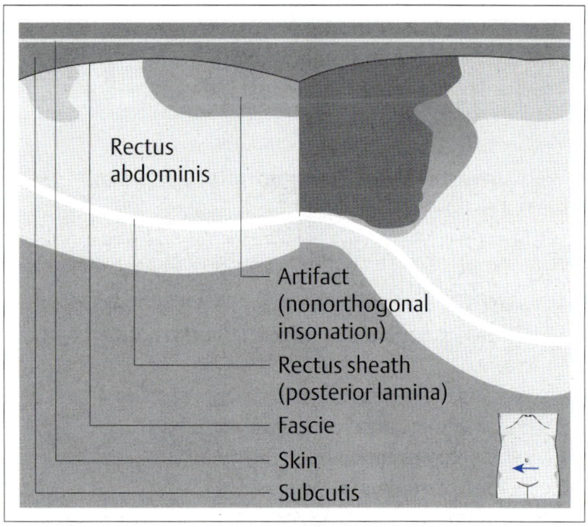

Fig. 14.**1 b** Line drawing.

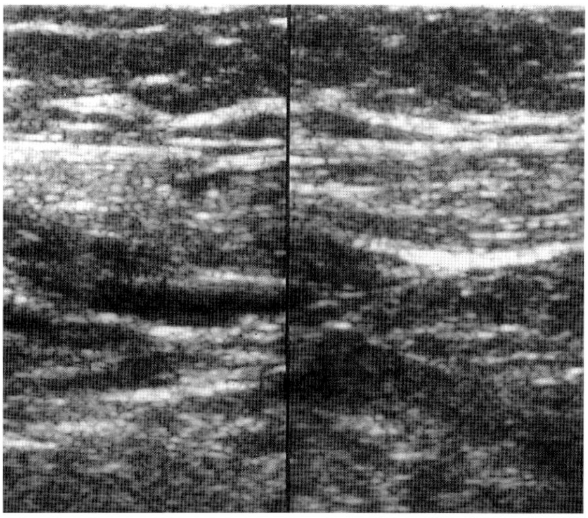

Fig. 14.**2a** Longitudinal view of the lower abdomen. Rectus sheath hematoma (**left image**) with normal contralateral reference (**right image**).

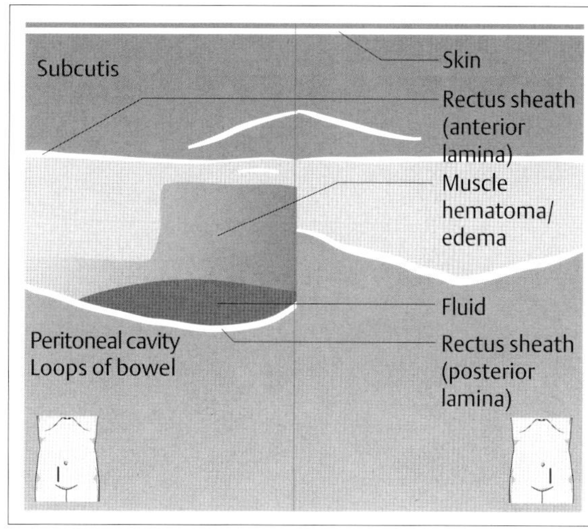

Fig. 14.**2b** Line drawing.

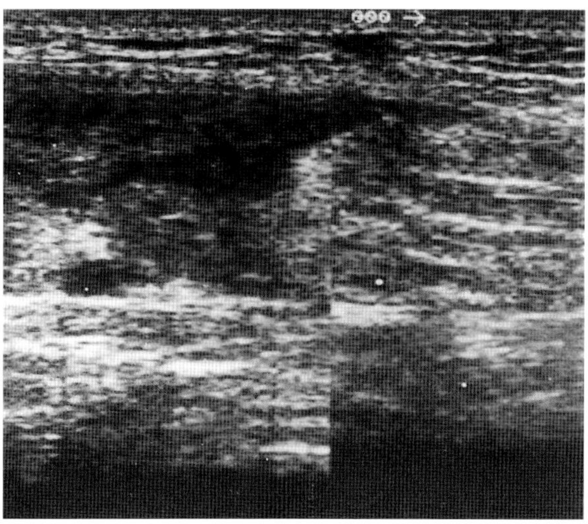

Fig. 14.**3a** Longitudinal view of the lower abdomen. Extensive rectus sheath hematoma with torn left rectus abdominis muscle.

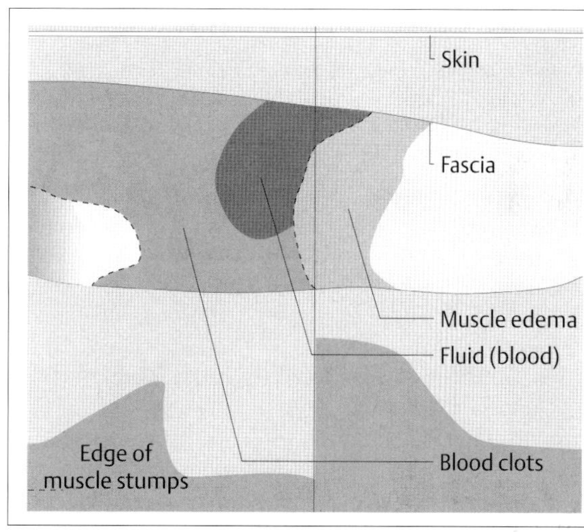

Fig. 14.**3b** Line drawing.

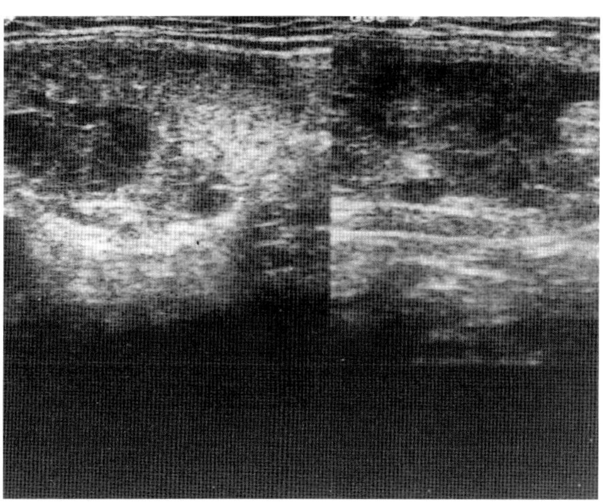

Fig. 14.**4a** Rectus sheath hematoma treated conservatively–three weeks post trauma (transverse view on the left, longitudinal view on the right).

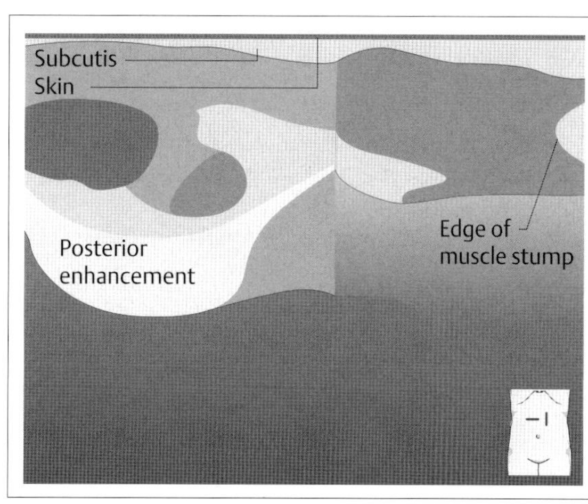

Fig. 14.**4b** Line drawing.

Consequences for Surgical Treatment

Diagnosis	Characteristic Findings	Management
Intramuscular abdominal wall hematoma/muscle tear	Heterogeneous echogenicity with ballooning of the muscle and discontinuous muscle fibers	Serial follow-up, laboratory parameter checks; in case of concomitant blunt abdominal trauma, possibly more extensive workup
Complete muscle tear with severe swelling and pain	Complete break in muscular continuity, marked hemorrhage (hypoechoic–anechoic), massive clot formation (hyperechoic, possibly heterogeneous echotexture)	Surgical evacuation and drainage; possibly repair of muscle and refixation to the symphysis
Myolysis and seroma formation in the later course	Hypoechoic to anechoic fluid collection	Possibly US-guided aspiration and drainage (seromas frequently recur, calling for repeated aspiration)
Traumatic abdominal wall hernia	Intestinal wall (gas echoes, hyperechoic areas [omentum, fatty tissue]) in the hernial orifice	In case of narrow orifice, urgent surgical repair, otherwise postponed until after absorption of hematoma
Lap-belt complex (neurological deficits, acute abdomen possible)	Free intraperitoneal fluid and/or retroperitoneal hematoma	Internal fixation of unstable lumbar fractures. In hollow viscus perforation or acute abdomen, laparotomy. Free intra- or retroperitoneal fluid with intact renal perfusion or in acute abdomen, watchful waiting

Postoperative Fluid Collections, Abdominal Wall Abscess

Basic Facts

- In a palpable mass, sonography can reliably differentiate between solid parts and fluid.
- Fluid assessed by US-guided aspiration (differentiation of blood, seroma, and pus).
- Even if clinical appraisal is impaired (e.g., by obesity), fluid can almost always be localized sonographically.
- During the first few postoperative weeks, artifacts (e.g., due to sutures) may hinder sonographic evaluation of the abdominal wall.
- Fresh surgical incisions are examined through a sonolucent sterile drape (e.g., OpSite), employing alcohol as coupling medium.
- For the most common causes of abdominal wall abscesses, see Table 14.**2**.

Sonographic Criteria of Assessment

- **Postoperative fluid collections** are anechoic or hypoechoic
- Fluctuation can be elicited by pressure with the probe or fingers, the latter permitting assessment of consistency.
- **Abscess:** Anechoic or hypoechoic mass, possibly with floating echoes ("snowstorm"), irregular hyperechoic mural contour, in case of gas internal echoes with posterior shadowing or reverberation, possibly hypoechoic margin due to edema and invasion; point of maximum tenderness can be located with the probe (Fig. 14.**5**).
- **Cellular debris, tissue necrosis, and pus** sediment in fluid result in increased echogenicity, and become turbulent on compression.
- For *planned aspiration,* sonography can identify the optimum point of needle entry (anechoic area–fluid).
- For *planned drainage* or incision, sonography can spot the most dependent part of the fluid collection.

Table 14.2 Abdominal wall abscess–causes

Infected wound	Acute pancreatitis
Status post surgery	Leukemia, chemotherapy, AIDS
Status post injection, diabetes	Infected subcutaneous vascular prosthesis
Insect bite	Infection secondary to abdominal wall hematoma
Foreign body	After transcutaneous insertion of leads or drains
Sutures	

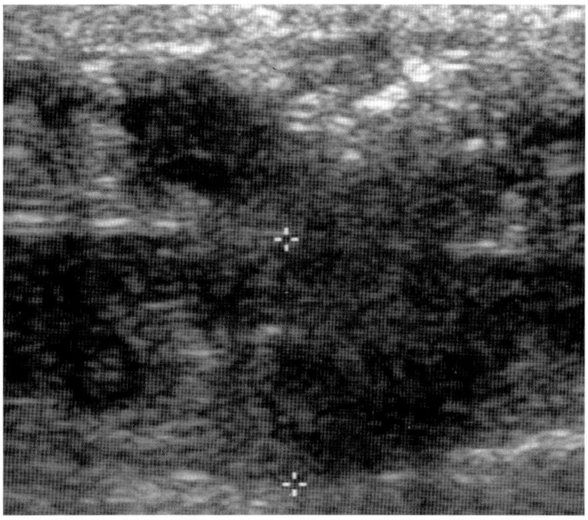

Fig. 14.5 a Subcutaneous abscess (hypoechoic, irregular outline). Longitudinal view of the lower abdomen, with strong echoes and reverberation due to gas collection. The abdominal muscles deep to it are inflamed, thickened, and edematous (between the calipers).

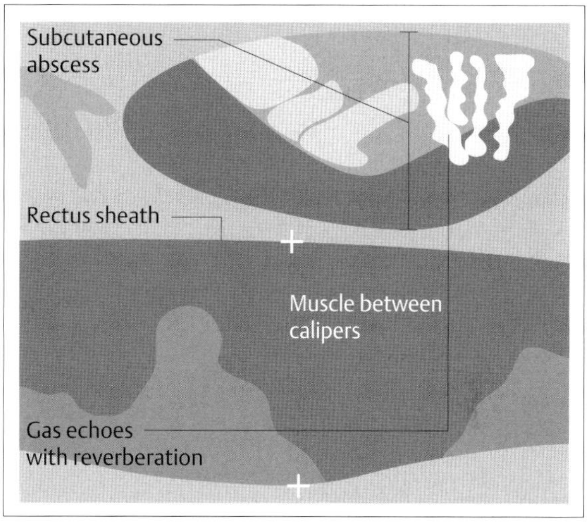

Fig. 14.5 b Line drawing.

Consequences for Surgical Treatment

Diagnosis	Characteristic Findings	Management
Asymptomatic localized postoperative fluid collection	Well-defined hypoechoic areas	Observation, aspiration, MCS
Localized postoperative fluid collection with clinical signs of inflammation	Hypoechoic areas with sedimentation	Cloudy fluid on aspiration, positive culture; surgical evacuation and drainage, antibiotics
Abdominal wall abscess	Anechoic or hypoechoic mass, internal echoes, localized tenderness, irregular wall contour	Surgical evacuation and drainage

Abdominal Wall Hernias

Basic Facts

- Hernias are protrusions of the parietal peritoneum through a preformed or secondary orifice.
- The parts of a hernia most important to the surgeon include:
  - Hernial orifice
  - Hernial sac
  - Hernial contents
  - Hernial layers
- Strangulation is the most dangerous complication of hernia. Congestion (small orifice, relatively voluminous sac) or strangulation will compromise the vascularity of the protruded viscus.
- Most important sites of herniation: inguinal (indirect hernia in 99% of children and adolescents), femoral, epigastric, spigelian, lumbar, umbilical, incisional.
- In posttraumatic hernias of the abdominal wall, sonography can help in assessing the urgency of operation (the smaller the orifice the more urgent the operation) as well as in delineating the extent of the hematoma.
- Small hernias may better be demonstrated on active straining and contralateral comparison.

Sonographic Criteria of Assessment

- Localization of the **defect in abdominal wall continuity** (Fig. 14.**6**) is facilitated by exact anatomical mapping of the various layers of the abdominal wall and peritoneum (Figs. 14.**7** and 14.**8**); frequently, the characteristic structures of the intestinal wall with central gas reflexes and some free fluid between them can be demonstrated at the level of the hernia (Figs. 14.**9** and 14.**10**).
- Peristalsis may be evident.
- By tilting the probe, the **loops of bowel** can be traced from the hernial sac through the neck and into the abdominal cavity.
- **Omentum** appears as an immobile hyperechoic (Fig. 14.**11**) or hypoechoic (edema) structure.
- In **strangulation** and aperistalsis, mural edema and lack of gas echoes may render reliable differentiation between bowel and omentum difficult.
- Sonography can document **successful taxis** in reducible hernia.
- Sonographic identification of the femoral vessels can help in preoperative differentiation between **direct** and **indirect** hernia. On straining, the hernial sac will protrude medially (direct) or laterally (indirect) to the vessels.

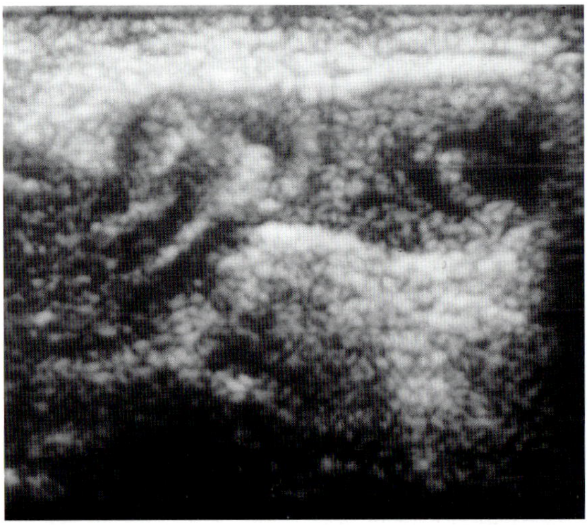

Fig. 14.**6a** Longitudinal view of the inguinal canal in inguinal hernia.

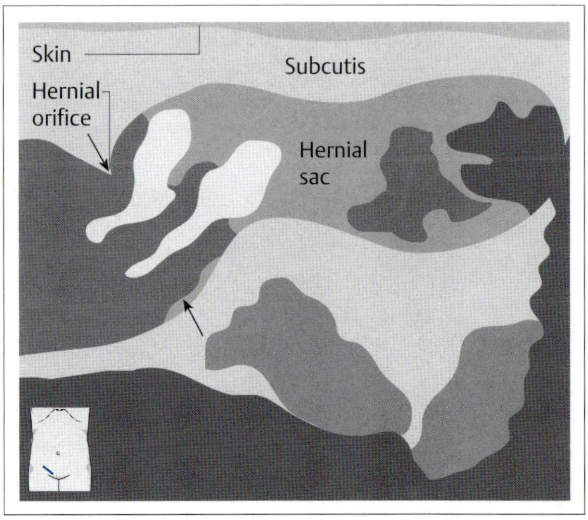

Fig. 14.**6b** Line drawing.

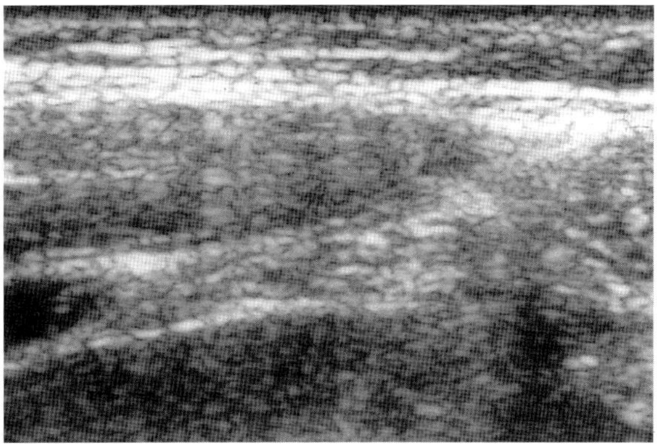

Fig. 14.**7** and 14.**8** An 8-year old boy with traumatic hernia of the left lower abdominal wall after handlebar injury.

Fig. 14.**7 a** Normal abdominal wall on comparison.

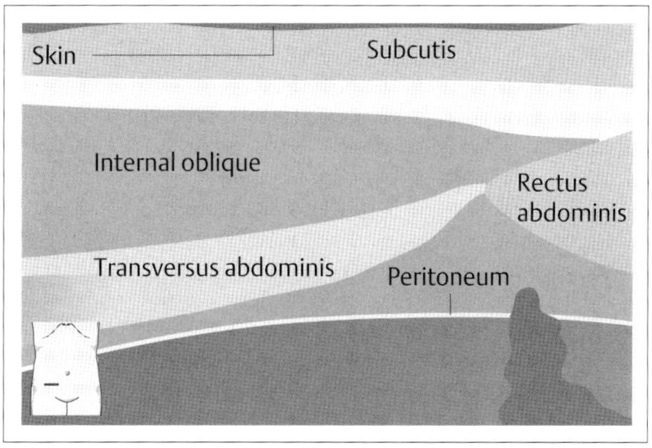

Fig. 14.**7 b** Line drawing.

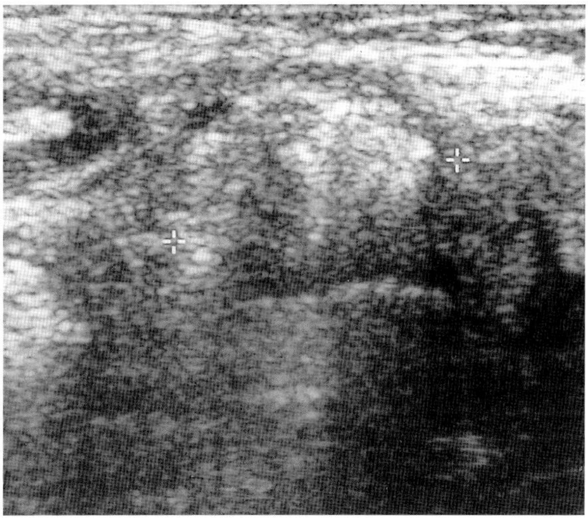

Fig. 14.**8 a** Transverse view of the hernia.

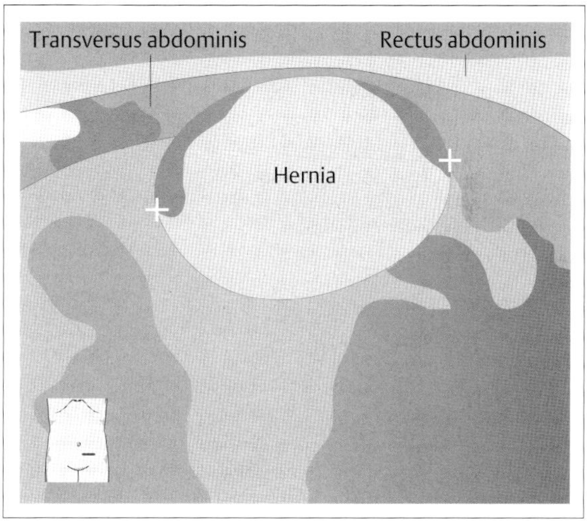

Fig. 14.**8 b** Line drawing.

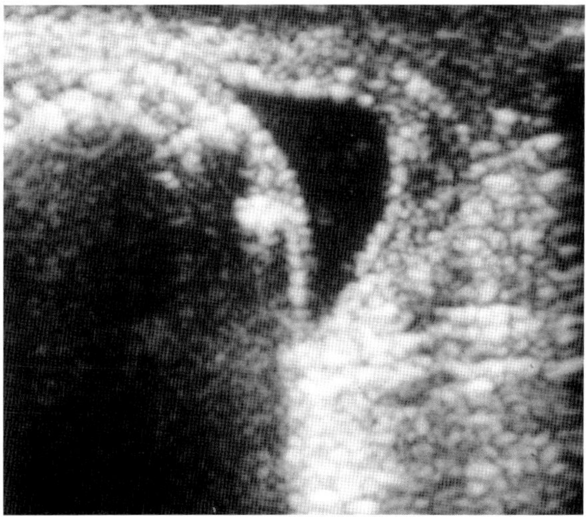

Fig. 14.**9 a** Right inguinal hernia.

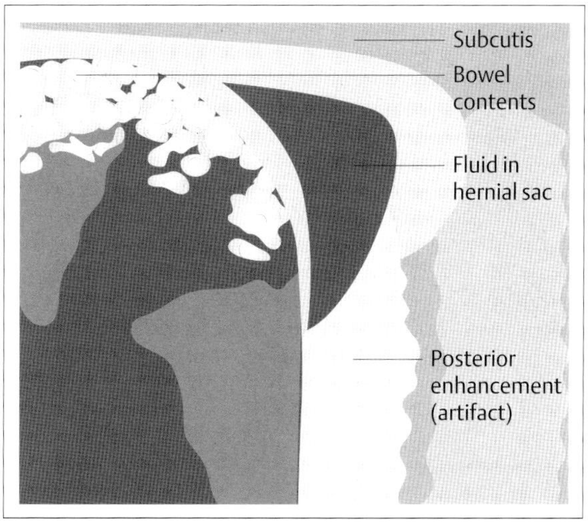

Fig. 14.**9 b** Line drawing.

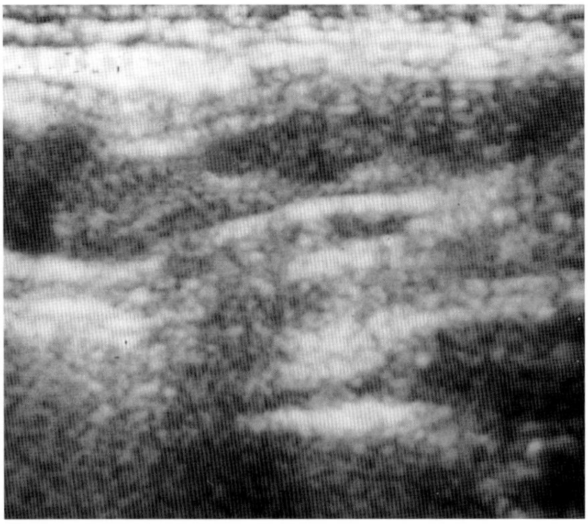

Fig. 14.**10 a** Longitudinal view of the inguinal canal. Large inguinal hernia containing bowel in the sac.

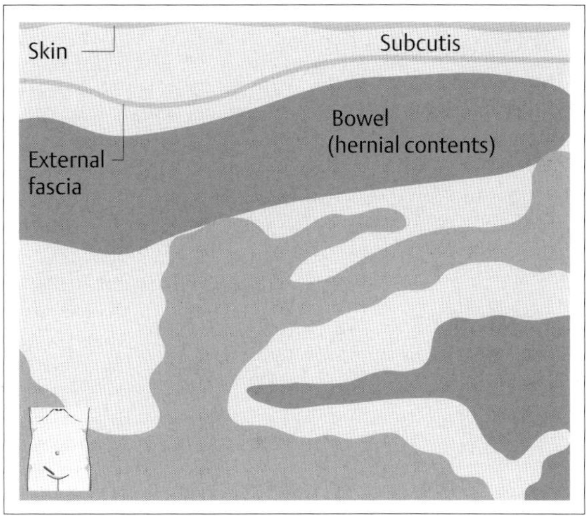

Fig. 14.**10 b** Line drawing.

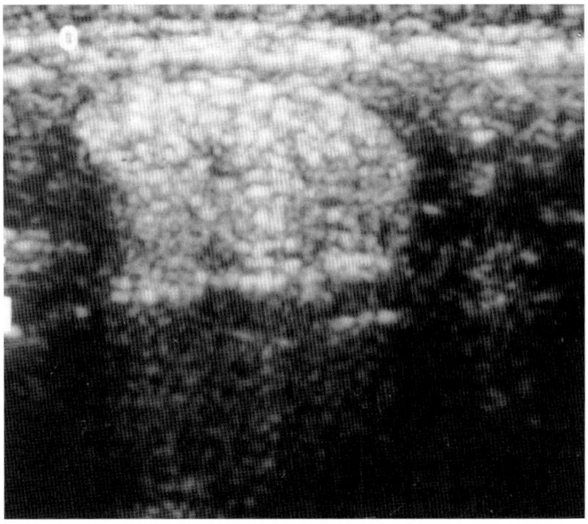

Fig. 14.**11 a** Transverse view of the inguinal canal in strangulated inguinal hernia.

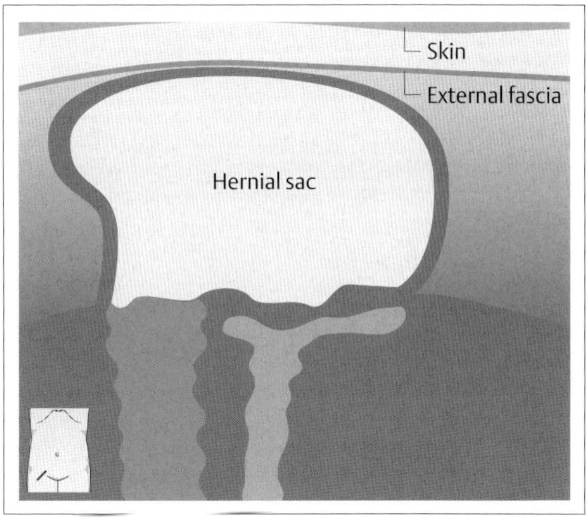

Fig. 14.**11 b** Line drawing.

Consequences for Surgical Treatment

Diagnosis	Characteristic Findings	Management
Strangulated hernia	Abdominal wall defect, hernial sac ± definite sign of bowel contents	Early surgery
Hernia without strangulation	Enlargement of hernial sac on straining, sonographic assessment of neck diameter, possibly demonstration of bowel contents	Surgery depending on general condition and complaints; elective surgery preferred in order to prevent strangulation–if low risk operation is possible

Soft-Tissue Tumors

Basic Facts

- In most cases benign (lipoma, fibroma, atheroma), suture granuloma.
- Most often subcutaneous localization.
- Frequently visible swelling or palpable nodule.
- Tumor demonstrated on longitudinal, transverse, and oblique views.
- If ambivalent further workup, possibly with resection if mandated.

Sonographic Criteria of Assessment

- Size and shape of benign tumors can be determined exactly by sonography; hypoechoic/hyperechoic echogenicity, heterogeneous echotexture is common (Fig. 14.**12**).
- **Foreign body granulomas** frequently display a bright central echo with posterior echo phenomena (shadowing, reverberation, comet-tail) and hypoechoic rim (edema, invasion).

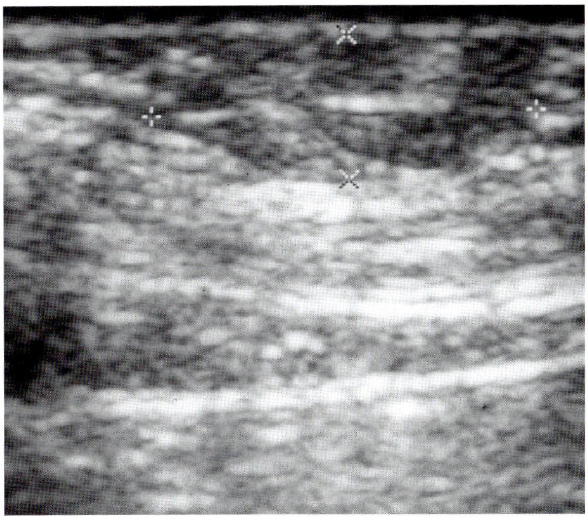

Fig. 14.**12 a** Longitudinal view of the right lower abdomen. Subcutaneous fibroma (between the calipers) of heterogeneous hyperechoic echotexture, compressing the abdominal wall and muscles deep to it.

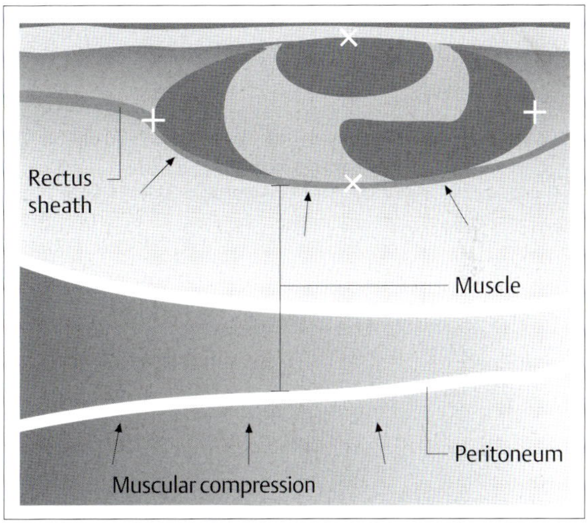

Fig. 14.**12 b** Line drawing.

Table 14.**3** Possible causes of hypoechoic areas in the post-laparotomy abdominal wall

Localized subcutaneous or intramuscular edema or hematoma
Localized seroma as inflammatory reaction to sutures being absorbed
Dehiscence of individual segments of the abdominal wall
Artifacts due to nonorthogonal insonation of the abdominal wall segment after wound closure

Consequences for Surgical Treatment

Diagnosis	Characteristic Findings	Management
Small soft-tissue tumor	Hypo-/hyperechoic, often heterogeneous, well-defined margin	Sonographic differentiation of benignity/malignancy is impossible; exact localization (epifascial/subfascial) is helpful regarding surgery under local or general anesthesia
Soft-tissue tumor of uncertain benignity	Hypo-/hyperechoic, heterogeneous, possibly ill-defined plus invasion	Further workup and resection according to oncological standards

Bibliography

Benson M. Rectus sheath hematomas: ultrasonographic diagnosis. AJR Am J Roentgenol. 1982; 128: 283–5.

Beyer D, Mödder U. Diagnostik des Akuten Abdomens mit bildgebenden Verfahren. Heidelberg: Springer; 1985.

Bonnaire F, Berwarth H, Paul C, Muller B, Kumer H. Einsatz der Sonographie zur Akut- und Verlaufsdiagnostik in der septischen Unfallchirurgie. Unfallchirurgie. 1994; 97: 164–70.

Furtschegger A, Lungenschmid D. Einfluß der Sonographie auf das therapeutische Vorgehen bei posttraumatischen, postoperativen und entzündlichen Weichteilläsionen. Radiologe. 1990; 30: 337–42.

Grechenig W, Clement H, Bahadori K, Freigassner M, Grechenig M. Sonographie und Pathologie der Bauchdecke. Ultraschall Klinik und Praxis. 1997; 11: 60–7.

Kaftori JK, Rosenberger A, Pollack S, Fish JW. Rectus sheath hematomas: ultrasonographic diagnosis. AJR Am J Roentgenol. 1977; 128: 283–5.

Weber K, Mahlfeld A, Otto W. Stellenwert der Ultraschalluntersuchung bei Verletzung der Symphyse. Unfallchirurgie. 1996; 22: 36–8.

15 Sonography of Peripheral Arteries and Veins

R. Mantke, Th. Bürger, M. Pross

Color Flow Doppler Imaging of the Peripheral Vascular System

R. Mantke, Th. Bürger

Sonography is part of the standard diagnostic workup in most vascular pathologies.

Its essential benefits are that it is noninvasive and may be repeated at short intervals and with no risk. In addition to assessment of vascular morphology, color-flow Doppler imaging (CFDI) permits functional appraisal of the circulatory system. Due to the gain in information yielded by this modality, Doppler imaging has become an integral component of higher specialist training in vascular as well as in GI tract surgery. Every physician should have basic knowledge of the opportunities and limitations of this technique.

Basic Facts

- **Continuous Wave (CW) Doppler Mode**
  - Uses two transducers that transmit and receive ultrasound continuously.
  - No depth discrimination, all moving echo sources (e.g., erythrocytes) inducing frequency shifts contribute to the Doppler signal (if vessels are in line they become superimposed).
  - Precise measurement even of very high velocities (in kHz).
- **Pulsed Wave (PW) Doppler Mode**
  - Pulsed wave Doppler imaging uses the same crystal to send and receive.
  - Using pulses of sound permits use of the time interval between the transmission of a pulse and the return of its echo as a means of determining the depth from which the Doppler shift arises; before the next pulse is emitted, the echo of the previous one must have been received.
  - The deeper the region to be examined, the longer the transmission–reception cycle and the lower the pulse repetition frequency (PRF, the number of pulses per time); the fraction of time spent transmitting sound is referred to as the *duty factor*.
  - The sample volume defines the spatial dimensions of the area from which signals are collected and in PW mode the area of the sample volume can be modified.
  - The benefit of precise depth discrimination of the sample volume in PW mode is paid for by an upper limit of the correctly measured maximum velocity; in symmetric positive and negative scaling this corresponds to one-half the pulse repetition frequency (Nyquist limit = PRF/2).
  - If the baseline is downshifted (demonstration of only one flow direction) the range of velocities measured correctly will be doubled. Example: For a PRF of 6000 Hz the Nyquist limit is ± 3000 Hz, i.e., frequency shifts/velocities of up to 3 kHz will be recorded correctly, while higher velocities will result in aliasing.
- **Aliasing**
  - Velocities higher than the Nyquist limit defined by the selected sample depth and PRF are cut off and reappear in opposite flow direction.
  - Aliasing is encountered in PW as well as CFDI; once the maximum recordable velocity has been passed, the color will turn into the brightest shade of the opposite flow direction (e.g., from red-orange to turquoise-blue).
- **CFDI** (Color Flow Doppler Imaging)
  - Flow information is displayed two-dimensionally.
  - By convention, flow toward the transducer is encoded in red and flow away from it in blue color; the higher the velocity the brighter the shade.
  - With the addition of yellow, high velocities in the red range appear orange while in the blue range a transition toward turquoise is observed.
- **Power Doppler**
  - In power mode Doppler imaging, a color map displays the integrated power of the Doppler signal instead of its mean frequency shift.
  - One color suffices as the image does not provide any information related to flow direction or velocity.
  - Power mode is particularly well suited for imaging of small vessels with slow flow.
- **Spectral Waveform**
  - In contrast to the analogue Doppler waveform, the spectral waveform encompasses all flow information.
  - The envelope of the spectrum represents the maximum frequencies present at any given point in time, and the width of the spectrum at any point indicates the range of frequencies present; the amplitude of each frequency component is displayed in gray scale.
  - Maximum and mean Doppler shift can be displayed, and if the Doppler angle is known flow velocity can be estimated.

Table 15.**1** Characteristics of the major veins in the lower limb

Vein	Characteristics	US Access
Common iliac vein	Results from the union of the external and internal iliac veins and terminates in the inferior vena cava; often masked by bowel and difficult to visualize	+ (other probe 3.5 MHz)
External iliac vein	Begins behind the inguinal ligament and ascends along the brim of the lesser pelvis to end in front of the sacroiliac joint where it is joined on its medial aspect by the internal iliac vein to form the common iliac vein	++ (other probe 3.5 MHz)
Common femoral vein	Results from the union of the profunda femoris and femoral vein and ends at the level of the inguinal ligament shortly after receiving the longer saphenous vein on its medial aspect	+++
Femoral vein	Begins as the continuation of the popliteal vein, and after it has received the profunda femoris vein it becomes the 'common' femoral vein; paired in 20–30% of cases; a thick coat of soft tissue severely restricts visualization in the adductor canal	++
Deep vein of thigh; profunda femoris vein	Drains 2/3 of the posterior thigh muscles; joins the 'superficial' femoral vein about 8–10 cm inferior to the inguinal ligament (caudad to the arterial bifurcation) to form the femoral vein; in 30–40% of cases it communicates directly with the popliteal vein	++
Popliteal vein	Results from the union of the anterior and posterior tibial veins with the fibular veins; paired in 30% of cases; on entrance into the adductor canal it becomes the 'superficial' femoral vein	+++
Anterior tibial veins	Drain the anterior compartment of the lower leg and course on the interosseous membrane	+++
Posterior tibial veins	Run deep from the medial malleolus to the soleus; in the proximal third of the lower leg they are more difficult to demonstrate as they course deep to the medial head of the gastrocnemius	++
Fibular veins	Course posterior and medial to the fibula, deep to the soleus, gastrocnemius, and flexor hallucis longus	+
Soleus veins	Drain the soleus and are tributaries either to the fibular veins or to the posterior tibial veins	++
Gastrocnemius veins	Drain the gastrocnemius and join the popliteal vein	++
Perforating veins	Link the superficial with the deep veins. Major groups are: – Cockett (superior to the medial malleolus) – Boyd (medial aspect inferior to the knee) – Hunter (medial aspect, lower thigh) – Dodd (medial aspect, mid-thigh)	+++
Long saphenous vein	Courses subcutaneously from anterior to the medial malleolus, draining the medial aspect of the leg and joining the femoral vein just below the inguinal canal	+++
Short saphenous vein	Runs subcutaneously, draining the lateral aspect of the calf and joining the popliteal vein	+++
Femoropopliteal vein	Recurrent course, originating in the deep flexors of the thigh and joining the popliteal vein	+++

- **Contrast Harmonic Imaging**
  - For better imaging of blood flow (enhanced echo) encapsulated bubbles of gas (e.g., ultrasound contrast agent Levovist) are administered intravenously.
  - In contrast harmonic imaging mode, the system normally transmits at one frequency, but is tuned to preferentially receive echoes at double this frequency, where the echoes from the bubbles lie (this enhances flow detection).

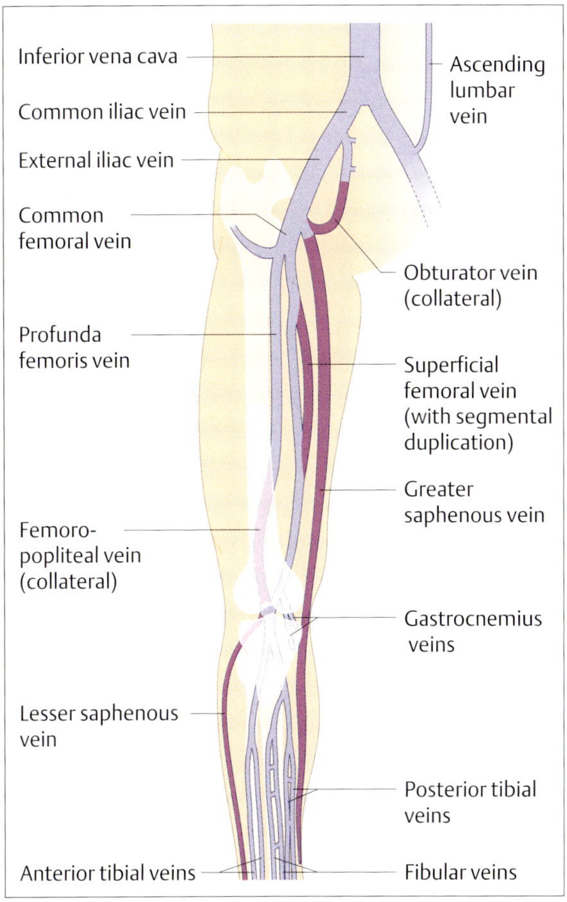

Fig. 15.**1** Major veins of the lower limb; potential collateral vessels in thrombosis are marked in purple.

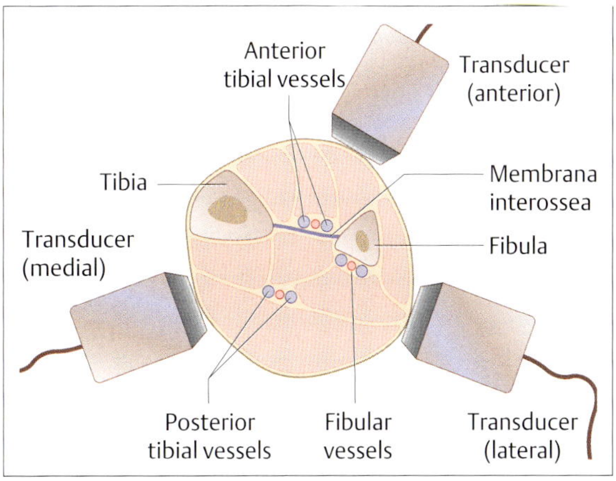

Fig. 15.**2** Topography and suitable probe positions for the vessels of the lower leg; transverse view through the left lower leg from caudad.

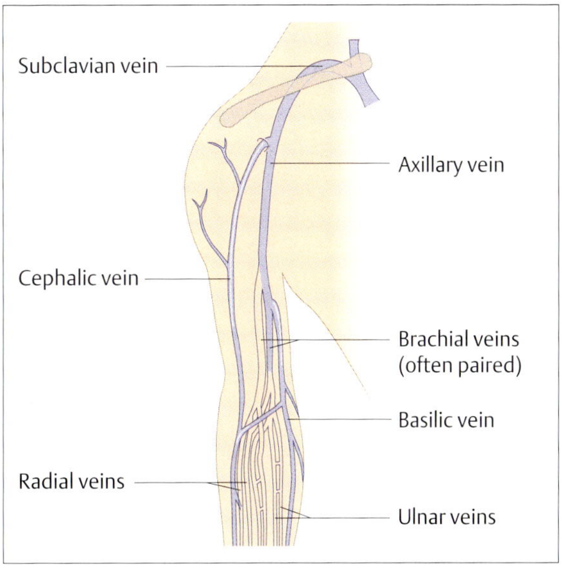

Fig. 15.**3** Anatomy of the major veins in the upper limb.

Peripheral Veins

Basic Facts

- Blood from the lower limb is drained via a deep and a superficial venous system.
- In the lower leg, the deep veins are almost always paired (posterior tibial veins, anterior tibial veins, fibular veins [also termed peroneal veins]).
- Fibular veins are the most difficult to assess with CFDI because of their location dorsomedial to the fibula.
- The popliteal vein originates at the union of the posterior tibial, anterior tibial, and fibular veins (Figs. 15.**1**, 15.**2**).
- Veins from the soleus are tributaries either to the fibular veins or posterior tibial veins.
- Veins from the gastrocnemius often join the popliteal vein directly
- Table 15.**1** gives a general overview of the major veins of the lower limb.
- All deep and superficial veins of the upper extremity drain via the axillary vein (Fig. 15.**3**).
- The axillary vein is formed by the union of the brachial and basilic veins.
- The subclavian vein is the continuation of the axillary vein, extending from the first rib to its union with the internal jugular vein; the distal part of the subclavian vein is examined with the probe inferior to the clavicle, while its medial segment is scanned via a supraclavicular window.
- Due to its location behind the clavicle, the subclavian vein is not amenable to compression testing.
- The axillary vein is visualized from the axilla with the arm abducted to 70–90°.
- Upper limb veins are followed from the forearm up to the medial third of the clavicle.

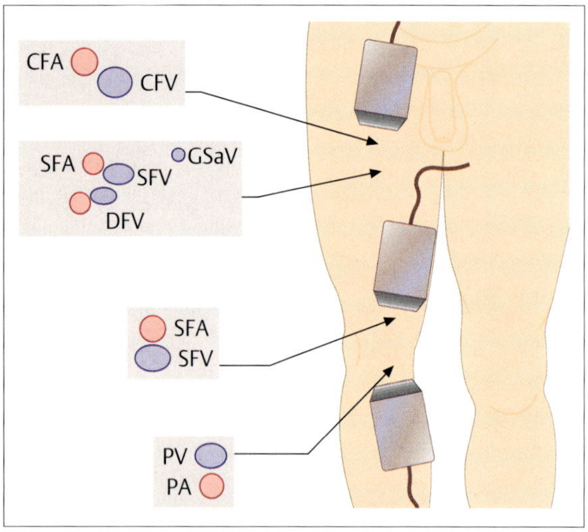

Fig. 15.**4** Topographic relations of arteries and veins at thigh and knee; transverse view in typical diagnostic workup in thrombosis.

CFA/CFV	common femoral artery/common femoral vein
DFA/DFV	deep femoral artery/deep femoral vein
SFA/SFV	superficial femoral artery/superficial femoral vein
PA/PV	popliteal artery/popliteal vein
GSaV	greater saphenous vein

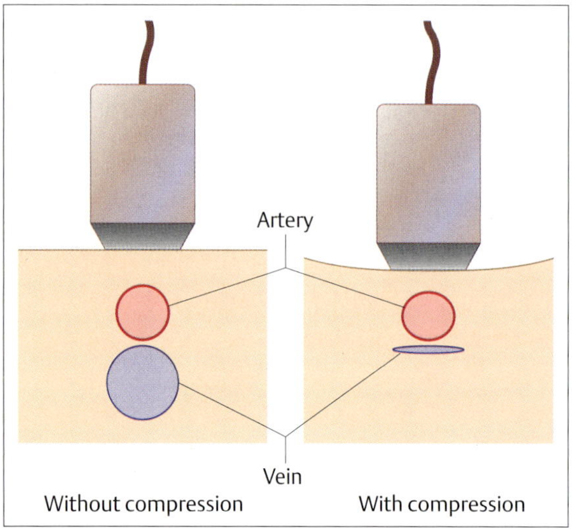

Fig. 15.**5** Complete compressibility in a normal vein; transverse view ruling out thrombosis.

Table 15.**2** Valsalva maneuver

Patient	Effect
Normal breathing	Blood flow with variations on respiration
Deep inspiration with pressing the abdomen outward (increases intra-abdominal pressure)	Brief flow reversal followed by no flow, if the valves are competent
Normal breathing resumed	Marked centripetal flow on expiration

- For assessment of the leg veins, the upper body of the supine patient should be level (good access to the inguinal region and unimpeded venous return to the heart).
- The legs should be straight and in mild external rotation.
- Examination starts at the groin at the distal external iliac/proximal femoral vein and progresses caudad (Fig. 15.**4**).
- The veins of the calf and popliteal vein are best assessed in prone position with mild knee flexion of 10–20°; alternatively in lateral decubitus or with the leg elevated.
- Linear transducers with a frequency of 5–7.5 MHz are recommended.
- Comprehensive examination of the veins of the lower extremities, including those of the lower leg, may be expected to take around 10 minutes per limb.
- Usually, in the large deep veins of the lower extremity, most markedly in the femoral vein, the continuous antegrade blood flow characteristically varies with respiration (inspiration increases the abdominal pressure and thus slows down the venous flow, while on expiration the flow quickly returns to baseline). This phenomenon is not regularly observed in the popliteal and posterior tibial veins, and it does not occur at all in the anterior tibial and fibular veins.
- Blood flow can be accelerated by compression of the calf and by dorsiflexion or plantar flexion of the ankle; prompt flow augmentation provides evidence of a patent venous system caudad of the recording site.
- Distal compression is indispensable for identification of the lower leg veins; since the arteries of the lower leg usually are easy to identify, these serve as landmarks.
- While B-mode imaging may suffice to rule out thrombosis of the femoral and popliteal veins, evaluation of the lower leg veins requires CFDI.
- Bilateral examination is always indicated, in order not to miss a silent thrombosis in the other leg and for comparison of the anatomical structures of both limbs.
- The greater saphenous vein can always be delineated, while a normal lesser saphenous vein is not always identified due to its more variable course.
- Patency of the iliac vein may also be tested indirectly: in examination of the distal external iliac vein, during the Valsalva maneuver there is a period of no flow, followed by venous dilatation and abrupt increase in forward venous flow with quick return to baseline; in case of symmetric findings this indirectly proves patency of the iliac vein.
- Beside variation with respiration and the characteristic spectral profile of venous flow during the Valsalva maneuver (Table 15.**2**), compressibility of the vein is an essential diagnostic criterion in ruling out thrombosis (Fig. 15.**5**).

Venous Thrombosis

Basic Facts

- Without prophylactic heparin, the risk of deep venous thrombosis (DVT) averages 10–30% in general surgery, reaching 54% in hip surgery (Lippert, 1998).
- In Germany, the incidence of DVT is 160 per 100 000 individuals.
- Incidence of pulmonary embolism is 60 per 100 000 individuals.
- More than 80% of pulmonary embolisms are caused by DVT.
- Isolated thrombosis of the lower leg induces pulmonary emboli in only 15–26% of cases, but iliofemoral thrombosis in 56–85%; however, only 0.1–5% of pulmonary embolisms are fatal (depending on the risk group; Polak, 1992).
- Thrombus location plays a decisive role in the clinical picture (Fig. 15.**6**).
- Thrombi usually originate in the venous sinusoids of the calf muscles or at the cusps of the popliteal and femoral veins behind which the flow is rather slow (Fig. 15.**7**).
- Venous thrombosis proceeds through several stages, starting with a small nonobstructive thrombus, e.g., at a valve; in only about 20% of cases will it extend proximally, finally occluding the lumen of the vein. Painful swelling of the leg may be part of the clinical symptoms.
- 3–7 days after formation, the thrombus is firmly attached to the venous wall.
- Fresh echogenic thrombus initially consists of erythrocytes and platelets, followed by fibrin scaffolding a few hours later.
- After a few days, hemolysis and partial fibrin degradation follow, making the thrombus become heterogeneous on sonography.
- Thrombosed venous segments either slowly reopen by intrinsic thrombolysis or remain permanently occluded (in up to 30%).
- Partial recanalization results in an irregular venous wall, the valves becoming fibrotic and nonfunctional.
- In diagnostic workup of thrombosis the following four diagnostic criteria are relevant:
  - Direct visualization of a thrombus
  - Distension of the venous lumen in case of fresh thrombosis
  - Loss of complete compressibility of the normal vein
  - Changes in the blood flow

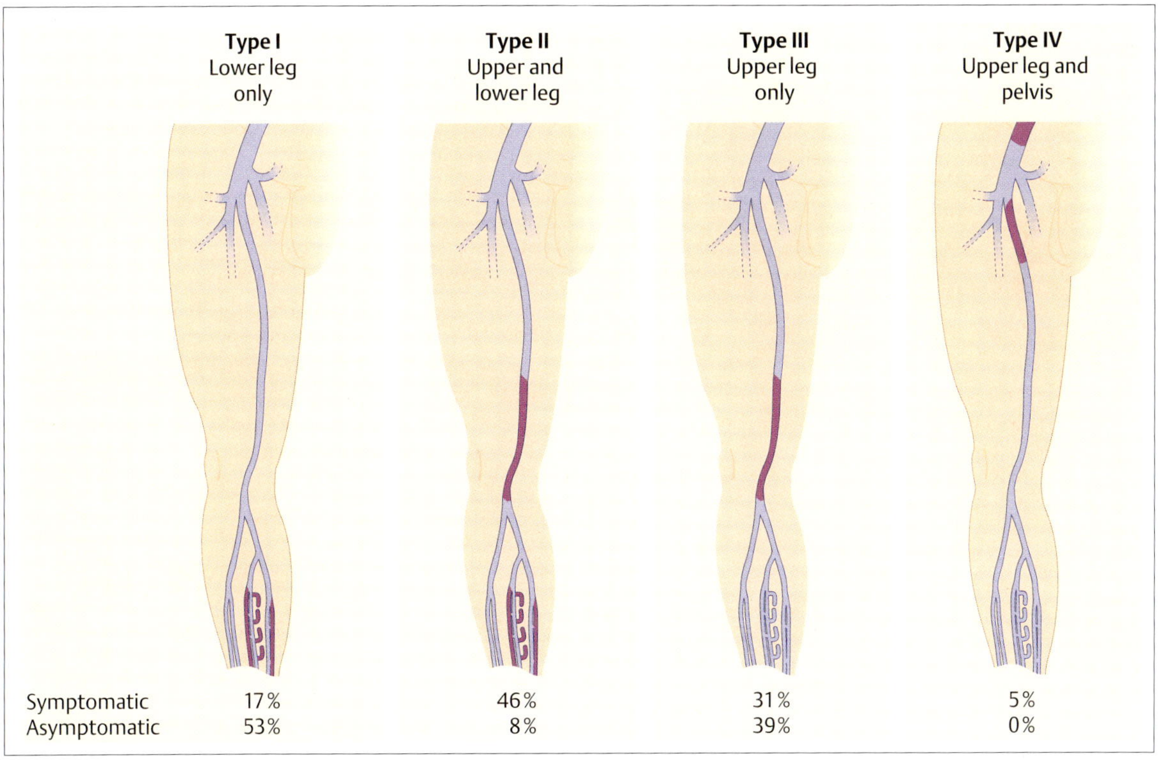

Fig. 15.**6** Sites and symptoms in DVT (phlebothrombosis) (modified from Polak, 1992). Out of all primarily symptomatic patients, 46% present with DVT type II, while 53% of all asymptomatic DVTs are restricted to the lower leg (type I).

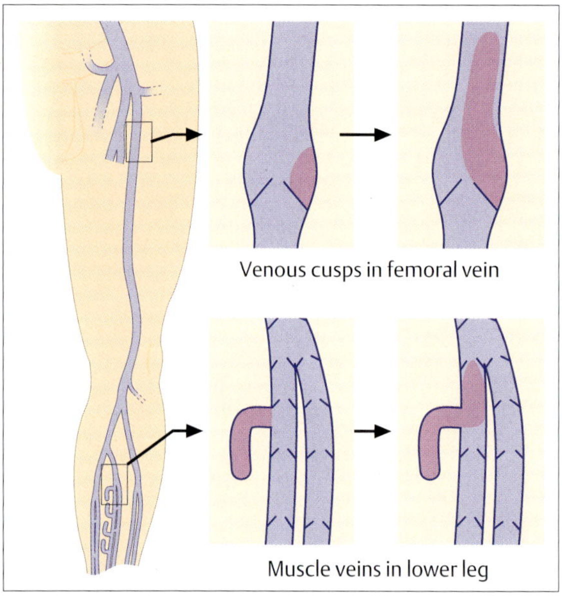

Fig. 15.7 Sites prone to thrombus formation.

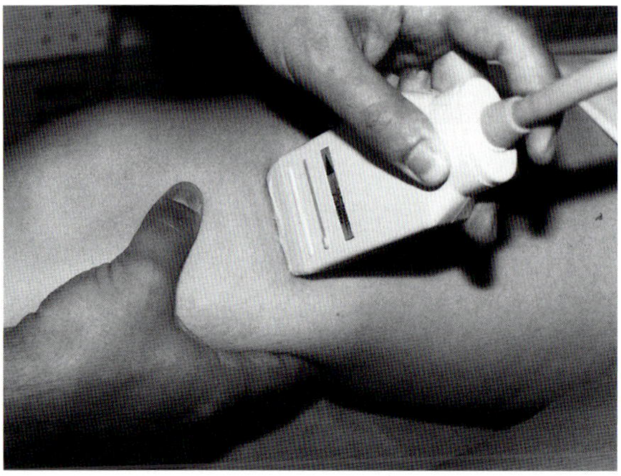

Fig. 15.8 Elevation of the soft tissues of the posteromedial thigh will improve the view into the adductor canal.

- Sonographic determination of thrombus age is difficult as thrombus formation is an asynchronous process, and the individual thrombi may undergo quite different stages of their development. Fibrinolysis, always paralleling coagulation, may partially dissolve a thrombus, contributing further to the sonographic heterogeneity and giving rise to the strong interindividual variations observed.
- The deeper the veins and the more obese the patient, the less reliable sonographic determination of thrombus age becomes (due to artifacts, absorption, scattering).
- Based on our own experience, one reliable parameter for estimating the age of the last thrombus triggering the symptoms is the time of onset of symptoms.
- Thrombus echogenicity also is decisively determined by the frequency of the probe employed (it appears less echogenic the lower the frequency).
- Thus, a homogeneous thrombus of low or high echogenicity is more indicative of recent-onset thrombosis (1–3 days), while heterogeneous thrombi with hypoechoic areas (fibrinolysis induced) are more characteristic of older thrombosis.
- Thrombus age may also be estimated based on the diameter of the thrombosed vein (Wolf and Fobbe, 1993).
- Fresh thrombosis results in significant distension of the vein, and sonographic comparison with the corresponding artery permits exact assessment.
- Fobbe et al. (1991) have suggested an index based on the ratio of the largest diameter of the thrombosed vein (under compression) to the largest diameter of the corresponding artery; an index value of 2 and higher would indicate thrombosis probably no older than 10 days.
- In the later stages, the vein shrinks due to retraction of the fibrin scaffolding and therefore this ratio diminishes.
- On the whole, sonographic determination of thrombus age must be treated with caution.
- In practical terms, the simplest but at the same time most important criterion confirming thrombosis is the inability to obliterate a thrombosed vein on probe compression.
- Compression testing is always carried out in the transverse view (where the vein cannot slip out of the viewing sector) and pressure is applied in such a fashion that it will not significantly deform the accompanying artery.
- The probe is then shifted caudad in steps of 1–2 cm under repeated compression testing.
- Thromboses within the popliteal and femoral veins can reliably be ruled out with this test.
- Potential sources of error in probe compression testing include infrapopliteal thrombi, thrombi in the adductor canal, postphlebitic syndrome, incomplete thrombosis, and venous duplication.
- Probe compression testing is ill-suited for assessment of the profunda femoris and iliac veins.
- So far, no clinically relevant thrombus dislocation due to probe compression has been observed in the approximately 2000 patients examined by us to date.
- Assessment of the adductor canal is facilitated by manually elevating the soft tissues from posterior (Fig. 15.**8**).
- Potential sources of error lie in longitudinal examination of the veins and in compression testing (Fig. 15.**9**).
- Thrombosis also changes the characteristics of venous flow.
- Venous flow is assessed by duplex sonography/CFDI.
- Loss of flow variation with respiration in the major veins of the leg may be due to thrombosis or external venous obliteration proximal to the recording site (also: low blood volume, pressure increase in the right heart, and even unfavorable patient position–contralateral reference is mandatory!).

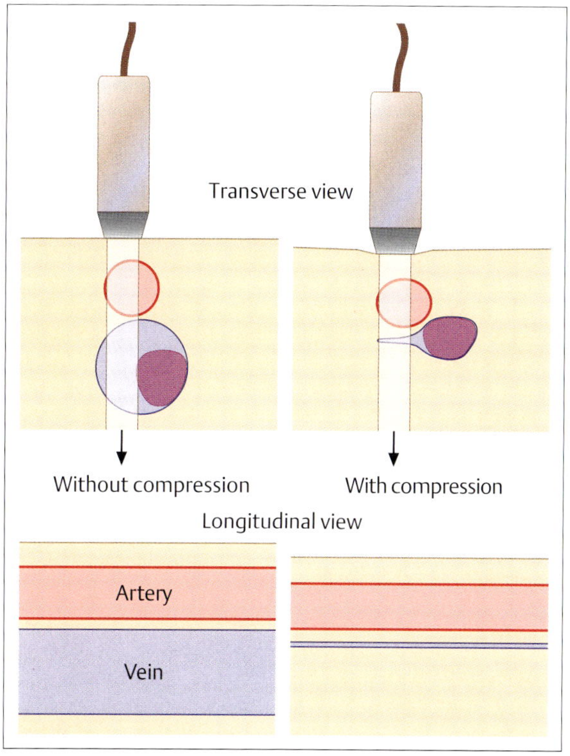

Fig. 15.**9** Potential sources of error in the longitudinal evaluation of veins suspected for thrombosis.

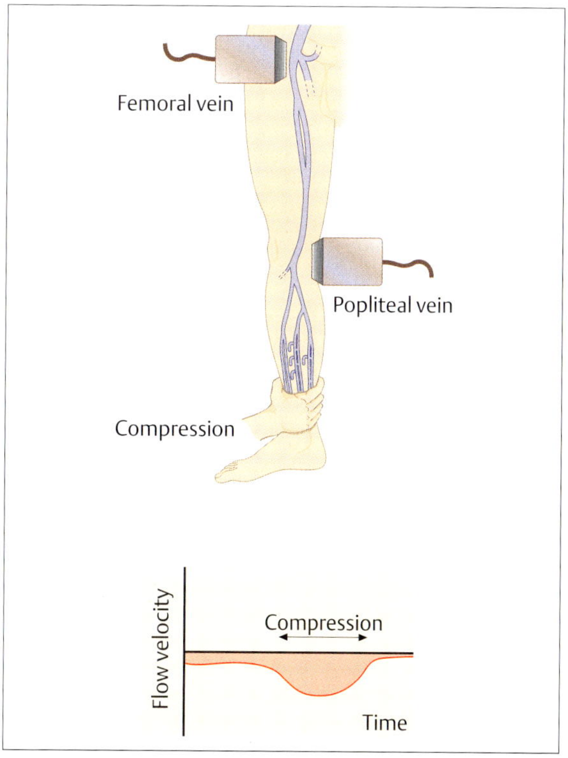

Fig. 15.**10** Normal findings on venous compression above the ankle.

- Patency of the iliac vein may also be tested indirectly: in examination of the distal external iliac vein, during the Valsalva maneuver there is a period of no flow, followed by venous dilatation and abrupt increase in forward venous flow with rapid return to baseline. If this is the case and there is no difference on contralateral comparison, patency of the iliac vein may be assumed indirectly.
- Finally, prompt increase in proximal blood flow on external compression of the lower leg ("augmentation test") confirms normal patency of the veins caudal to the recording site and to some extent proximally to this site as well (Figs. 15.**10,** 15.**11**).
- Incomplete venous thrombosis or thrombosis with extensive collaterals may yield a false-negative result for this external compression test.
- Caudal compression is indispensable for identification of the calf veins; the arteries of the lower leg can serve as rough landmarks as they are easily identified on CFDI in the supine patient.
- Compression triggers an immediate increase in blood flow, which is reflected by equally prompt color shifts on CFDI.
- Table 15.**3** compares the sensitivity and specificity of CFDI with that of phlebography (gold standard in 10 studies).

Sonographic Criteria of Assessment

- Compared with blood, fresh thrombus appears as a homogeneous hyperechoic intraluminal structure; on compression, vein diameter remains unchanged at about twice the size of the accompanying artery; in complete thrombosis no blood flow can be demonstrated (Figs. 15.**12**–15.**15**).
- If the vein cannot be obliterated on probe compression, this is a definite sign of thrombosis (Fig. 15.**16**).
- In incomplete venous obliteration, partial compressibility and a flow signal on CFDI are seen (Figs. 15.**17**, 15.**18**).
- In case of a floating thrombus, the vein is only partially compressible, and during the Valsalva maneuver the diameter of the vein will increase significantly, with the thrombus seeming to float within the lumen.
- Normal CFDI finding in a lower leg vein (Fig. 15.**19**).

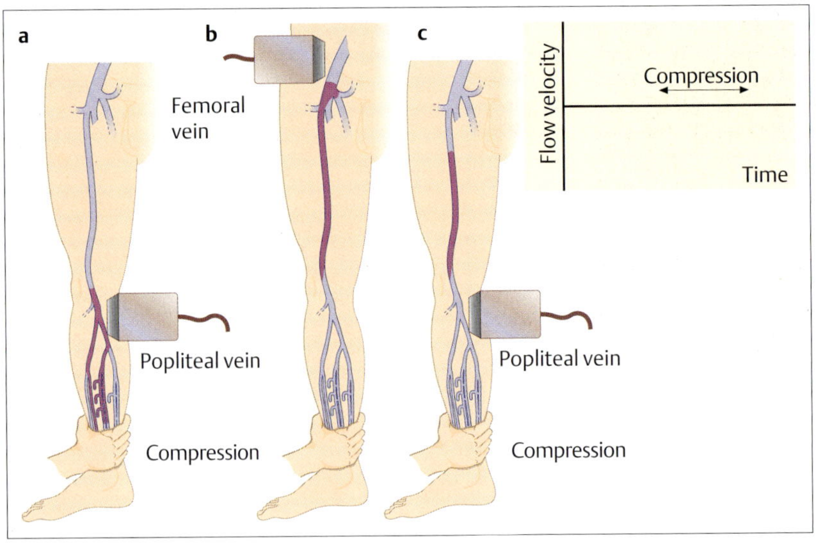

Fig. 15.**11** On compression of the lower leg in patients with thrombosis, flow velocity will not increase at the level of the thrombus (**a**), proximally to it (**b**), or caudad to the thrombus (**c**).

Table 15.**3** Sensitivity and specificity of CFDI

Modality	Sensitivity	Specificity
CFDI proximal veins	90–100%	91.7–100%
CFDI calf	67–87.5%	93–100%

- Indications for CFDI:
  - Clinical suspicion of thrombosis or pulmonary embolism
  - Standard modality in the diagnostic workup of suspected thrombosis (taking into account site-related accuracy, which is lower below the knee; possibly combined with strain gauge plethysmography)
- Indications for phlebography:
  - Definite clinical suspicion of thrombosis despite negative duplex analysis
  - Baseline status before fibrinolysis or thrombectomy
  - Legal issues
- In principle, the arm veins can be assessed for thrombosis in much the same way as the lower extremity veins.
- In the arm, too, lack of compressibility (basilic, cephalic, brachial, axillary, and jugular veins) is the most important criterion of thrombosis and, at the same time, the easiest to demonstrate.
- Only the lateral third of the clavicle can be obliterated by probe compression, while assessment of the central and medial third must be based on the echogenicity of the vascular lumen and the flow parameters (lack of venous flow variation with respiration in case of complete central obstruction, and no flow at the thrombus).
- The central and medial thirds of the subclavian vein may be difficult to evaluate, and frequently it is impossible to definitely rule out thrombosis in this area.
- Examination of the jugular vein starts at the carotid bifurcation and follows the vessel caudad; it can be evaluated quite well throughout its entire course.
- Pathogenesis of upper extremity thrombosis:
  - Central venous catheter or pacemaker lead
  - Intravenous administration of (in particular cytotoxic) drugs
  - Fractures of the clavicle or ribs
  - Status post axillary lymph node dissection
  - Thoracic inlet syndrome
  - Malignancy
  - Cardiac failure
  - Mediastinal tumor
- *Additional workup:*
  - Phlebography, strain gauge plethysmography, (scintigraphy, MRI), D-dimers.
  - Confirmation of etiology, coagulation workup, malignoma?

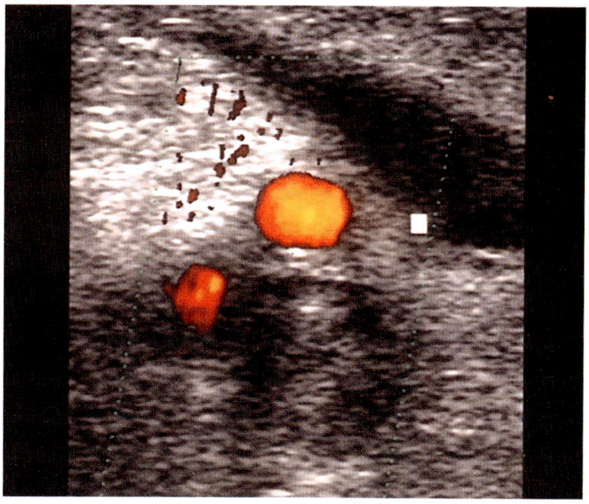

Fig. 15.**12 a** Complete thrombosis of the femoral vein, clinically 3 days old; dilated hyperechoic lumen of the vein, which remains noncompressible. Status post liver transplantation with a bio-pump introduced via the femoral vein; transverse view.

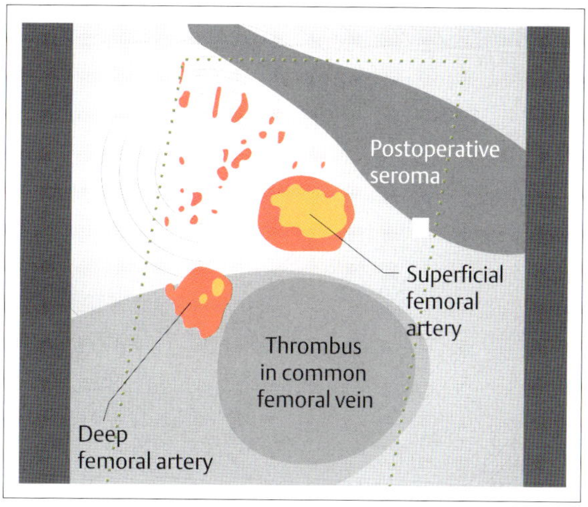

Fig. 15.**12 b** Line drawing.

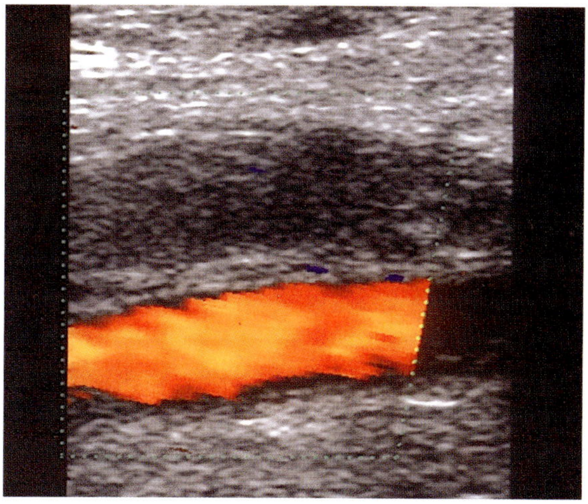

Fig. 15.**13 a** Complete thrombosis of the popliteal vein, clinically 3 days old; longitudinal view of the markedly dilated vein. The lumen is obliterated by rather homogeneous hyperechoic material.

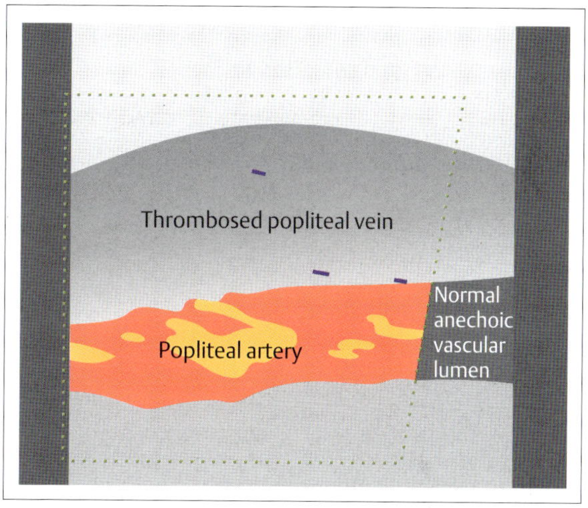

Fig. 15.**13 b** Line drawing.

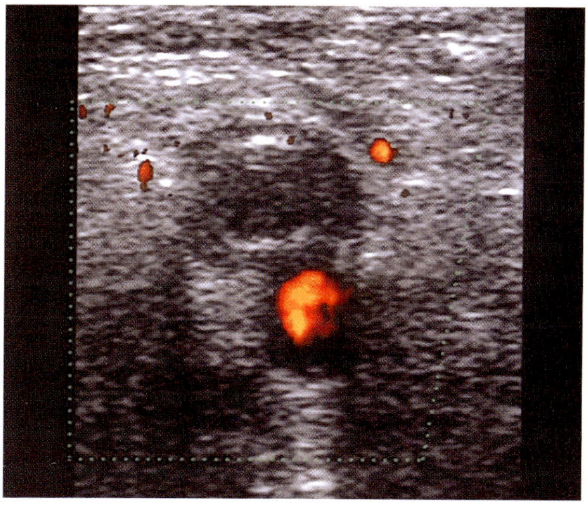

Fig. 15.**14 a** Same patient as in Fig. 15.**13,** but now on transverse view. Compression of the vein is impossible; no flow detected in the popliteal vein, which is rather distended.

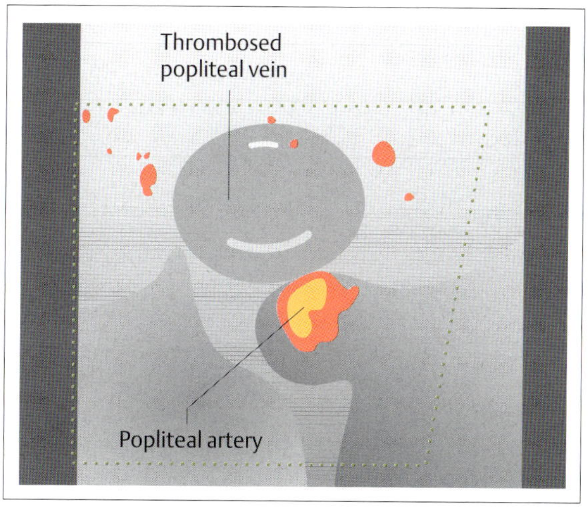

Fig. 15.**14 b** Line drawing.

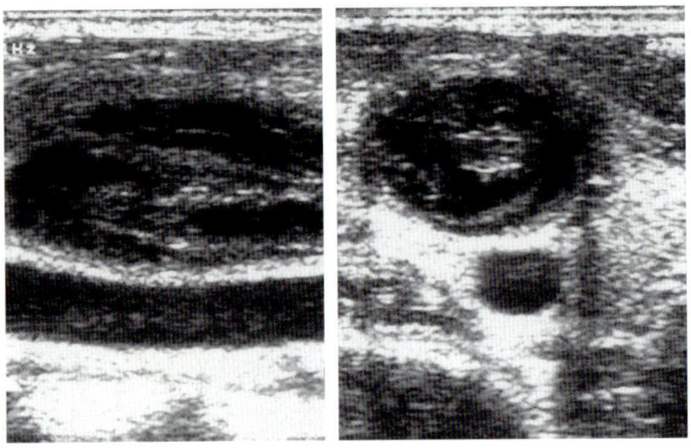

Fig. 15.**15 a** Longitudinal and transverse views of a left internal jugular vein completely occluded by an older heterogeneous thrombus due to central venous catheterization.

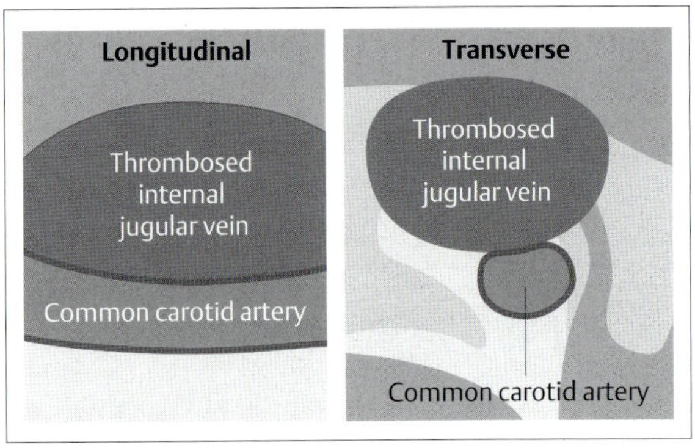

Fig. 15.**15 b** Line drawing.

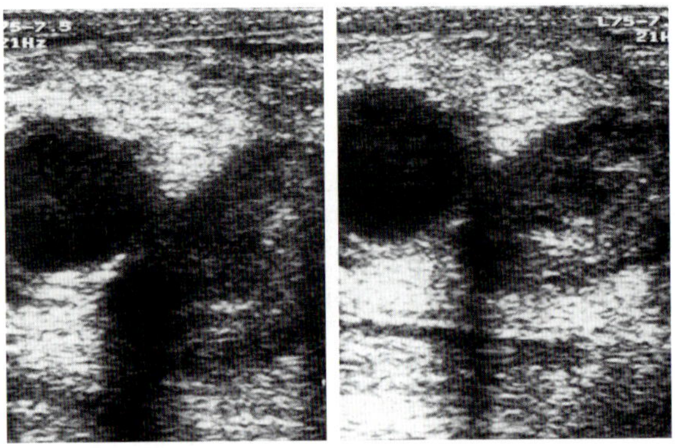

Fig. 15.**16 a** Side-by-side comparison of the transverse views through a thrombosed common femoral vein, with and without probe compression; the lumen cannot be obliterated on probe compression and is occluded by heterogeneous material.

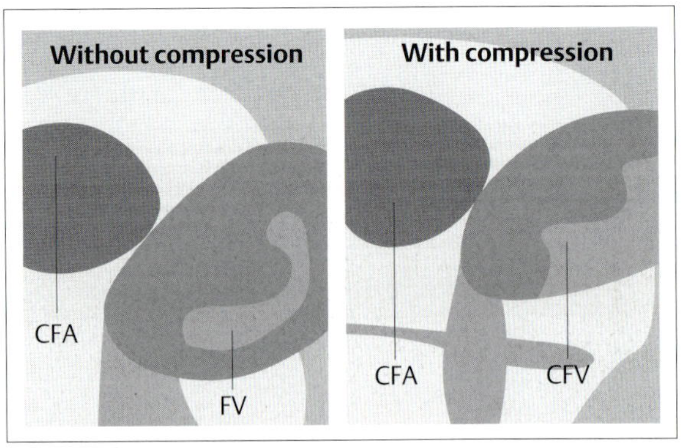

Fig. 15.**16 b** Line drawing.

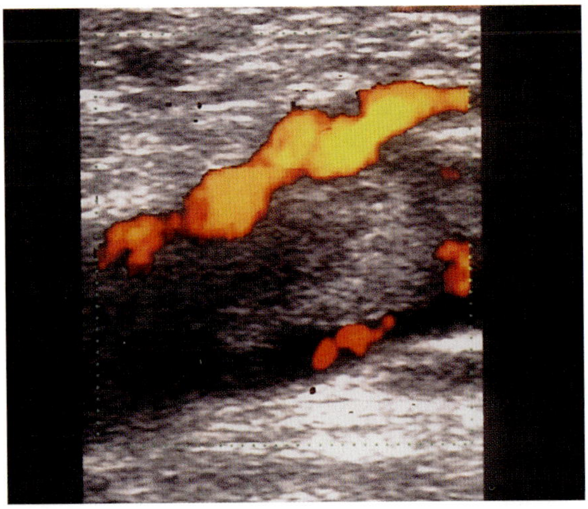

Fig. 15.**17 a** Power Doppler image (transverse view) of a partially thrombosed common femoral vein with (clinically) 7-day old thrombus, around which blood flow can be demonstrated on CFDI.

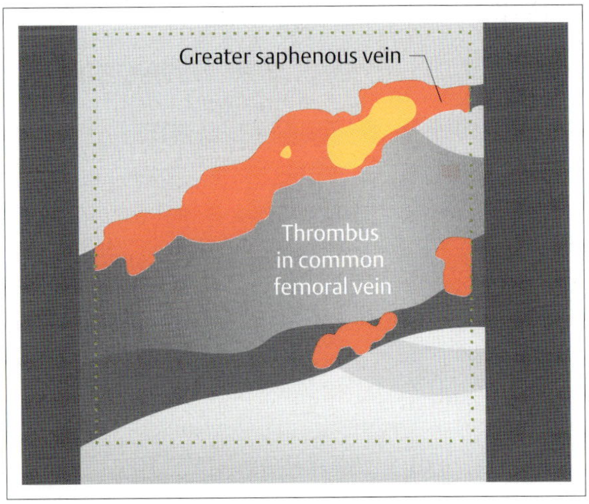

Fig. 15.**17 b** Line drawing.

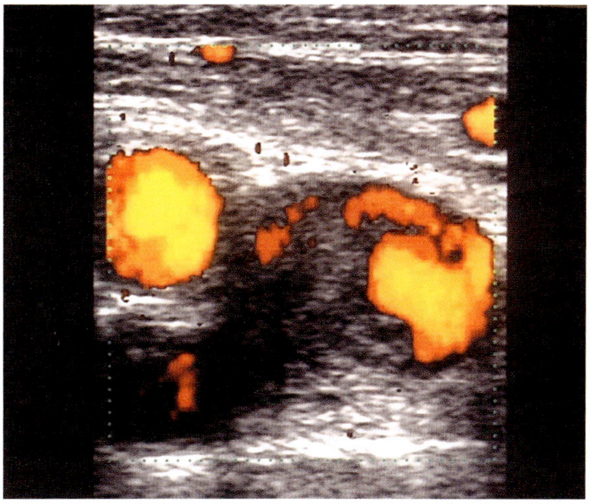

Fig. 15.**18 a** Same patient as in Fig. 15.**17**, but now in transverse view at the level of the femoral bifurcation; Power Doppler imaging clearly identifies the thrombosed and perfused parts of the lumen.

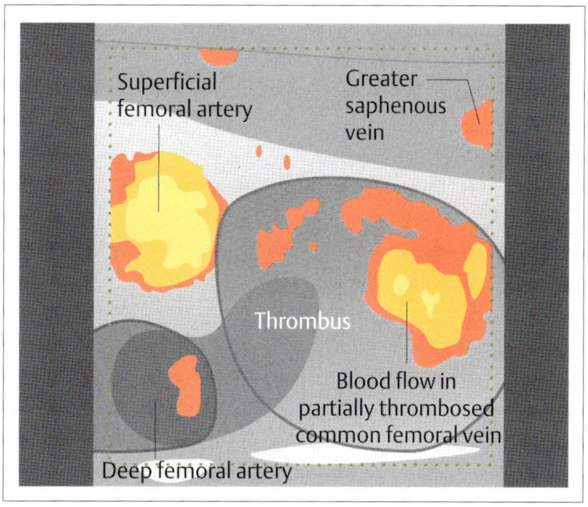

Fig. 15.**18 b** Line drawing.

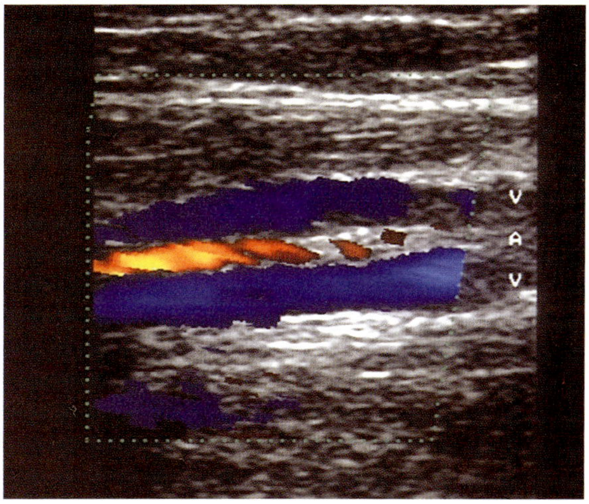

Fig. 15.**19 a** Longitudinal view of the paired normal posterior tibial veins; marked blood flow on CFDI after compression at the ankle, easy identification of the landmark artery.

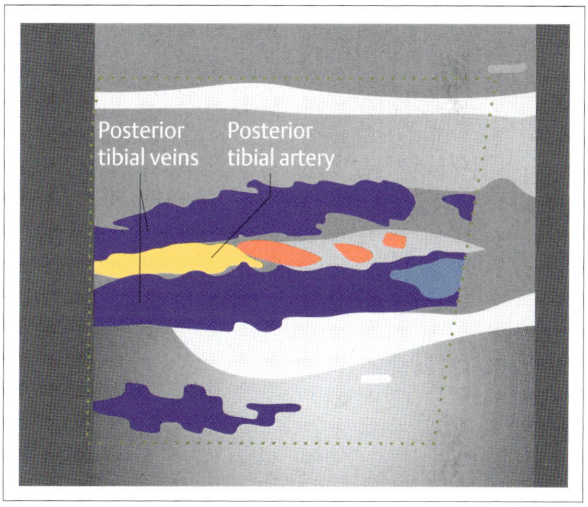

Fig. 15.**19 b** Line drawing.

Consequences for Surgical Treatment

Diagnosis	Characteristic Findings	Management
Acute DVT of the leg	Total thrombosis of lower limb (all levels), duration of symptoms < 7 days **Clinical presentation:** Painful calf Sensation of heaviness Unilateral swelling {100,0,0,101}osis Tachycardia, fever, restlessness	Bed rest, short-stretch compression bandages, lower limb elevation, full intravenous heparinization with overlapping switch to coumarin for 6–12 months DVT is also treated more and more with approved LMWH Possibly fibrinolysis, coagulation workup
Acute DVT of the leg	Development of phlegmasia coerulea dolens	Venous thrombectomy Full heparinization Fibrinolysis in selected cases
Acute DVT of the leg	Restricted to calf (possibly involving popliteal vein)	LMWH (approval!), elastic compression, ambulation, repeat CFDI follow-up, subsequent anticoagulation with coumarin for 6–9 months, outpatient treatment possible; or hospitalization with therapeutic full heparinization, leg compression with short-stretch bandages, lower limb elevation, followed by anticoagulation with coumarin for 6–9 months
Arm DVT	Involving brachial, axillary, or subclavian vein (approx. 2% of all extremity thromboses), superficial collaterals frequently prominent	Arm elevation, compression bandage, anticoagulation (heparin including LMWH, followed by coumarin for 3 months) Fibrinolysis or thrombectomy (phlegmasia) in selected cases, possibly surgery of underlying cause (thoracic inlet syndrome)
Superficial venous thrombosis	In the arm or leg, thrombophlebitis of varicose veins, posttraumatic or after i.v. infusions	Compression, ambulation, analgesics, NSAIDs (e.g., ASA), cooling; if extensive treat with LMWH as outpatient; stab incision rarely needed; for ascending and floating thrombi at the saphenofemoral junction, resection of the saphenofemoral junction

Chronic Venous Insufficiency

- Combination of changes affecting veins and skin (in permanent venous hypertension).
- Stages:
  - Edema tendency, corona phlebectatica paraplantaris (a flare of fine spider webs at the ankle)
  - Hyperpigmentation and hyperkeratosis, scleroderma
  - Leg ulcer
- Causes:
  - Postphlebitic syndrome in status post DVT with secondary varicose veins.
  - Primary varicose veins.

Postphlebitic Syndrome (PPS)

Basic Facts

- Venous insufficiency (inability of normal valvular closure and thus direct transmission of the hydrostatic pressure of the standing column of fluid in the venous system to the distal leg) of the deep leg veins may result from venous valvular damage following DVT (Fig. 15.**20**).
- Due to thrombosis secondary to CVI (chronic venous insufficiency), PPS may develop with the clinical signs and symptoms outlined below.
- About 5% of the German population suffer from PPS.
- Depending on the severity and site of the thrombosis, 10–50% of cases will progress to PPS (Kappert, 1989).
- Evidence of CVI has been found in as many as 75% of patients 5–6 years after extensive DVT of the popliteal and femoral veins (Polak, 1992).

- PPS symptoms (latency 1–20 years):
  - Swelling, sensation of heaviness
  - Dull tearing leg pain
  - Dystrophic skin changes (induration, atrophy, pigmentation)
  - Leg ulcer
- Even if a thrombosed vein becomes fully recanalized, there is endothelial damage stimulating proliferation and sclerosis of the venous wall ("neointima" formation).
- Solitary veins with high flow velocities (e.g., femoral vein) will become recanalized faster than paired veins of which only one is thrombosed (e.g., paired superficial femoral vein or the veins of the lower leg).
- Incompetence of the valves in the deep veins will increase the hydrostatic pressure; this will lead to reflux into the superficial venous system via the perforating veins, resulting in dilatation and development of secondary varicose veins.
- Secondary varicose veins may also result from volume overload (acting as collateral vessel) when deep leg veins are permanently occluded.
- *Additional workup:* phlebography, strain-gauge plethysmography, LRR, phlebodynamometry.

Sonographic Criteria of Assessment

- A narrow flow channel with homogeneous thrombus well visible in the venous lumen signifies **incomplete recanalization**, in which case the vein is only partially compressible (Fig. 15.**21**).
- **Venous incompetence** as part of PPS is characterized by marked **backflow** during the Valsalva maneuver (Figs. 15.**22**, 15.**23**).
- Reflux in a major vein (femoral or popliteal vein) during the Valsalva maneuver or on release after compression of the leg caudad to the recording site: < 0.5 s normal, 0.5–1 s borderline, > 1 s definitely pathological = **venous insufficiency**.
- Owing to *retraction* and organization, permanently occluded veins may be difficult or almost impossible to identify, which is not true for their collaterals (if needed, examination with the patient standing and with distal compression).
- Particularly in the popliteal vein, *valvular function* can also be *tested* by compression upstream and downstream of the recording site.

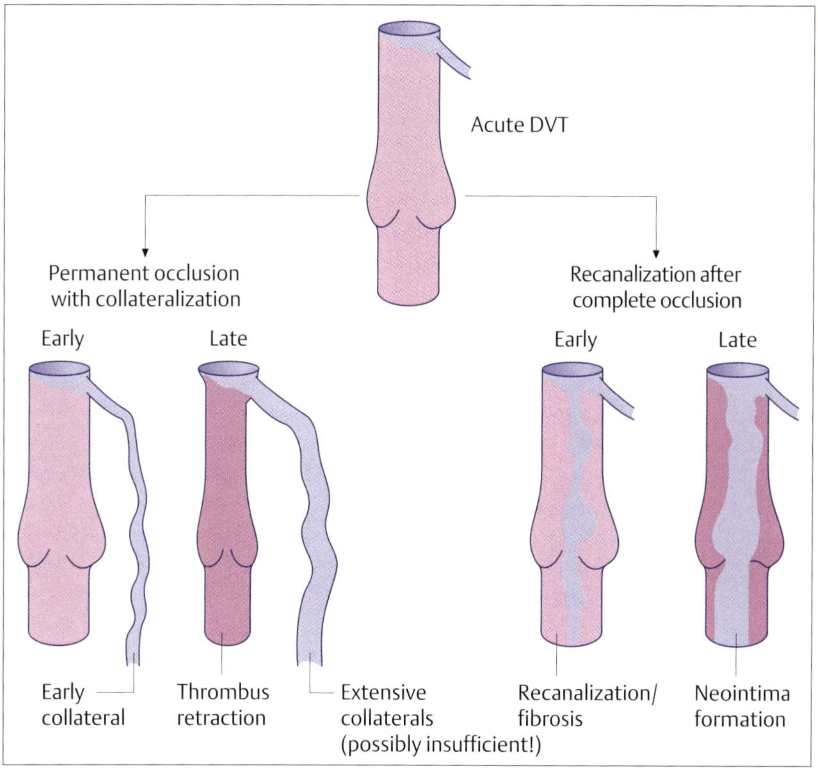

Fig. 15.**20** Possible course of total DVT in the lower extremity.

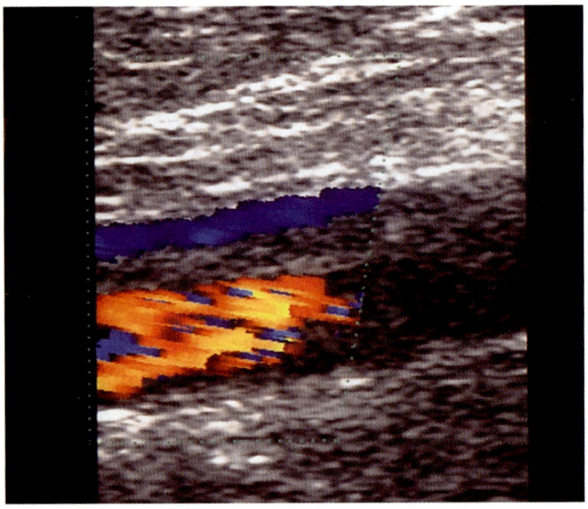

Fig. 15.**21 a** Longitudinal view of the popliteal vein 16 years after DVT. Only about one-third of the vein has become recanalized, while the remainder is filled with a homogeneous hyperechoic thrombus.

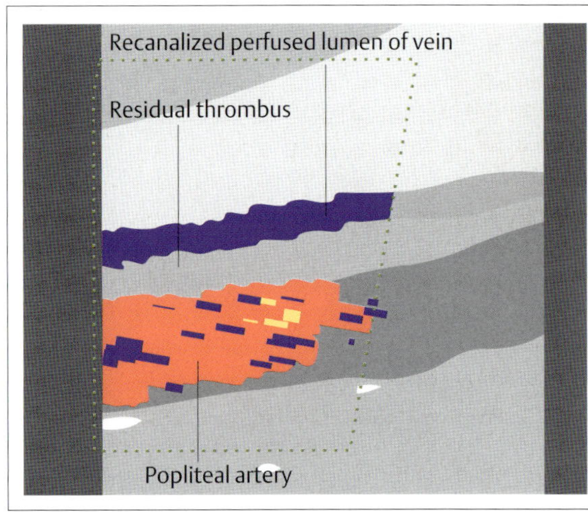

Fig. 15.**21 b** Line drawing.

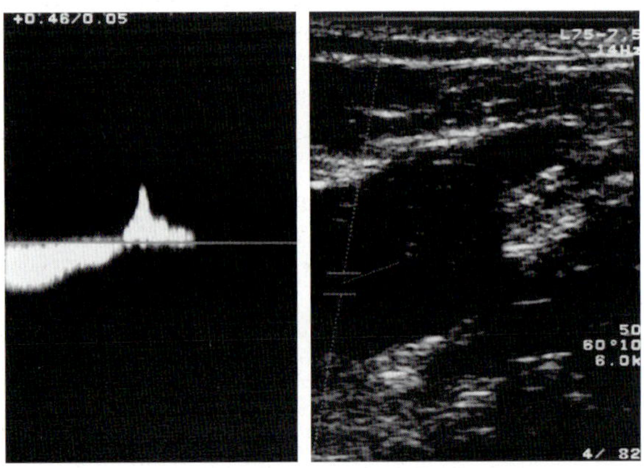

Fig. 15.**22 a** Longitudinal view of the femoral vein in a healthy man. Flow variations with respiration, regular valvular competence during the Valsalva maneuver with a reflux of < 1 s.

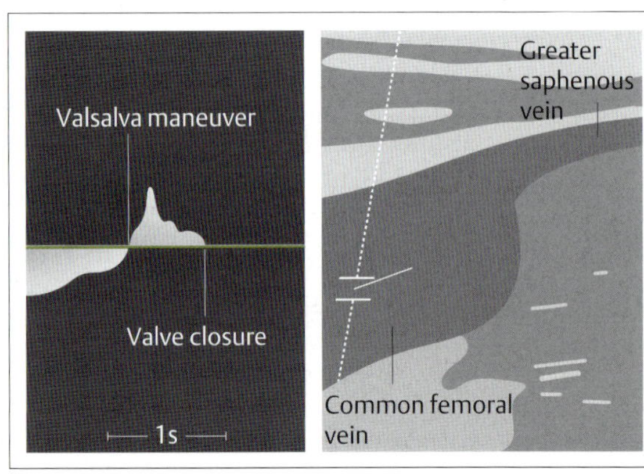

Fig. 15.**22 b** Line drawing.

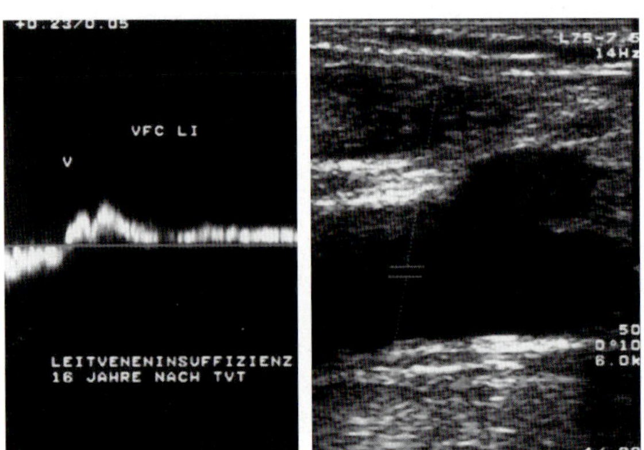

Fig. 15.**23 a** Marked reflux (> 1 s) in the femoral vein during the Valsalva maneuver in a patient with postphlebitic syndrome (CVI stage II) 16 years after total DVT. Longitudinal view, duplex study.

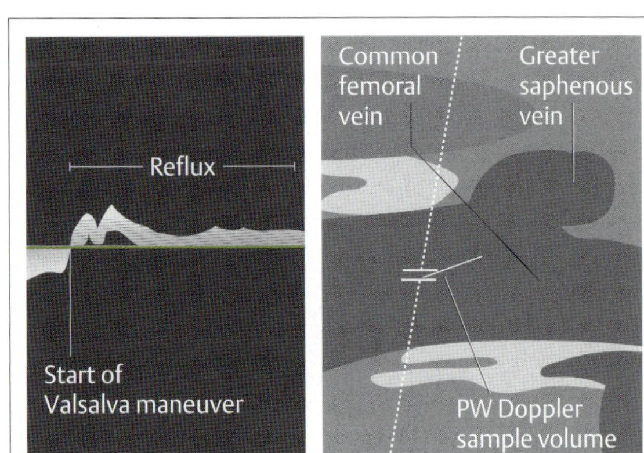

Fig. 15.**23 b** Line drawing.

Consequences for Surgical Treatment

Diagnosis	Characteristic Findings	Management
Venous insufficiency post DVT	Femoral and popliteal veins; symptoms corresponding to CVI stage I–II	Supportive compression hose or thigh-high compression stockings grade II
Venous insufficiency post DVT	Femoral and popliteal veins; symptoms corresponding to CVI stage III	Supportive compression hose or thigh-high compression stockings grade II Special ulcer treatment Possibly division of perforating veins Possibly reconstructive valve surgery (direct repair or transfer)
Venous insufficiency post DVT	Restricted to the calf, more proximal valves competent	Knee-high compression stockings grade II
Deep venous insufficiency in primary varicose veins	Due to volume overload of the deep veins, no signs of thrombosis	Varicose vein surgery Thigh-high compression stockings grade II

■ Varicose Veins in the Lower Extremity

Basic Facts

- Degenerative venous disorders (risk factors: genetic disposition, obesity, pregnancy) with atrophy of the muscles in the venous wall, increase in collagen, and fibrosis, resulting in loss of the elastic qualities of the venous walls with subsequent dilatation.
- Hyperextension of the cusps degrades valvular competence and results in a standing column of blood in the lower extremity veins; via the perforating veins, this volume overload also damages the deep veins with development of secondary CVI of the deep venous system.
- Age of clinical onset of primary varicose veins is usually the 2nd to 3rd decades of life.
- Manifestations: spider veins (telangiectasias), reticular veins, varicosities, incompetent perforating veins, saphenous varicose veins (greater and lesser saphenous vein).
- Any examination of the superficial veins should be preceded by evaluation of the deep venous system, in order to rule out deep CVI and past, possibly silent, DVT with persistent secondary changes in the deep venous system.
- Clinical examination of the standing patient prior to duplex sonography provides a basic overview of the varicose veins.
- Valvular competence is checked with the Valsalva maneuver, which should not yield any reflux in either saphenous vein (reflux 0.5 s = normal, > 1 s = definitely pathological), and with distal compression (transient flow augmentation without subsequent reflux in either saphenous vein).
- The saphenofemoral and saphenopopliteal junctions and their valvular competence may also be examined in the supine patient.
- However, the upright position (weight supported by the contralateral leg) better reflects physiological conditions and is therefore preferred
- Greater and lesser saphenous vein are scanned caudad in longitudinal views, beginning at their junction with the deep veins; reflux is ruled out with the Valsalva maneuver as well as by distal and possibly proximal compression of the limb.
- Evaluation of the entire course is of major importance, as there may be reflux from the deep venous system via incompetent perforatoring veins, despite a competent valve at the saphenofemoral junction, (Table 15.**4**).

Table 15.**4** Suggested examination sequence for the sonographic assessment of varicose veins

Vessel assessed	Issue
1. Distal external iliac vein, femoral vein, popliteal vein, anterior and posterior tibial veins	Looking for sequelae of past DVT and possible deep CVI
2. Greater saphenous vein	Competent saphenofemoral junction? Course of greater saphenous vein – extent of insufficiency, incompetent perforating veins
3. Lesser saphenous vein	Competent saphenopoliteal junction? Venous insufficiency along the course
4. Perforating veins	Venous insufficiency at the typical sites

- Due to their superficial course, examination of varicose veins is delicate since even mild pressure with the probe will make them collapse.
- Varicose veins are a clinical diagnosis, and CFDI/duplex sonography is employed in the assessment of the deep venous system, in localization of the most proximal and distal sites of venous insufficiency, and for identification of incompetent perforators, thereby serving to assure stage-adapted varicose vein surgery.
- Phlebography as the gold standard in diagnostic workup of varicose veins has mostly been replaced by CFDI.
- CFDI is also suitable for evaluation of recurrent varicose veins (in up to 27% of patients by 10 years after saphenous vein stripping; Mantke et al., 1993).
- *Additional workup:* phlebography, strain-gauge plethysmography, LRR, phlebodynamometry.

Sonographic Criteria of Assessment

- **Reflux** < 1 s in the Valsalva maneuver, if there is **valvular competence** at the saphenofemoral junction (Fig. 15.**24**).
- CFDI of the saphenofemoral junction with flow variation on respiration, **normal finding** (Fig. 15.**25**).
- In **junctional valvular incompetence**, the greater saphenous vein will demonstrate reflux during the Valsalva maneuver (Fig. 15.**26**).
- **Varicose veins** appear distended and demonstrate reflux after distal compression.
- Testing for **venous insufficiency** by distal compression (Fig. 15.**27**).
- Stump of greater saphenous vein too long; improperly performed varicose vein surgery (Fig. 15.**28**).

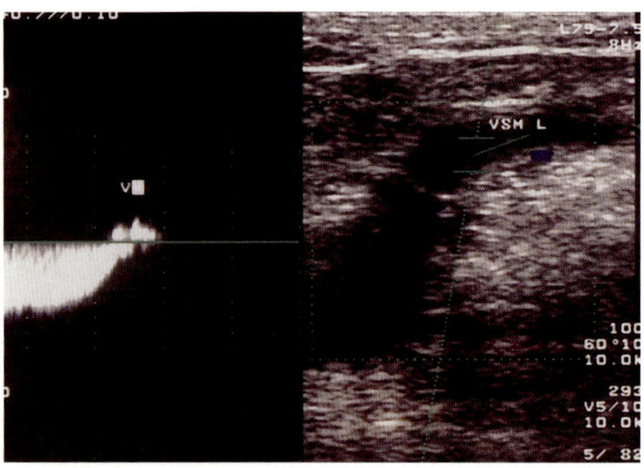

Fig. 15.**24 a** Longitudinal view of the greater saphenous vein and saphenofemoral junction with valvular competence and only minimal reflux on Valsalva maneuver (significantly less than 1 second).

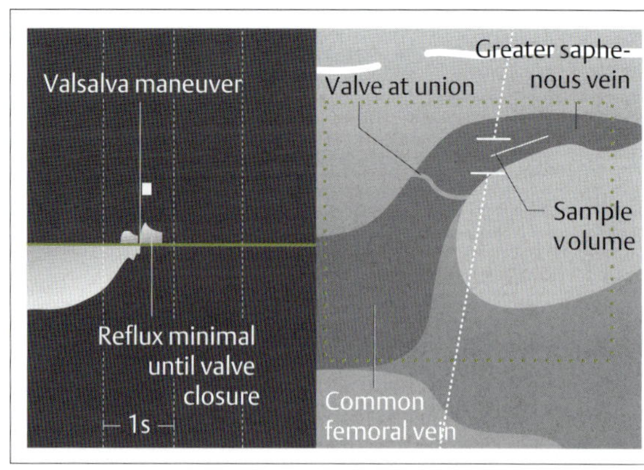

Fig. 15.**24 b** Line drawing.

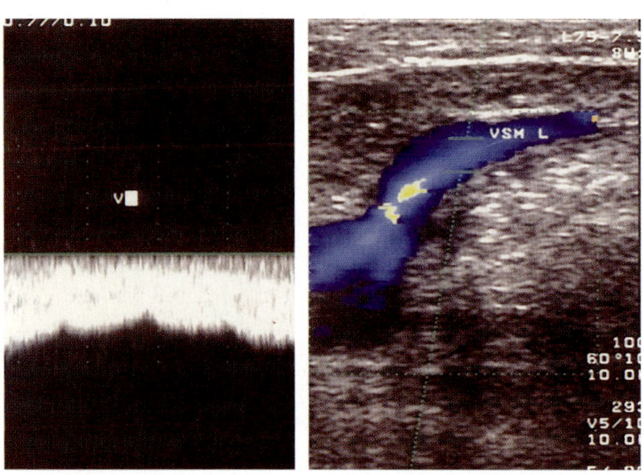

Fig. 15.**25 a** CFDI of the saphenofemoral junction with flow variation on respiration; longitudinal view. Normal finding.

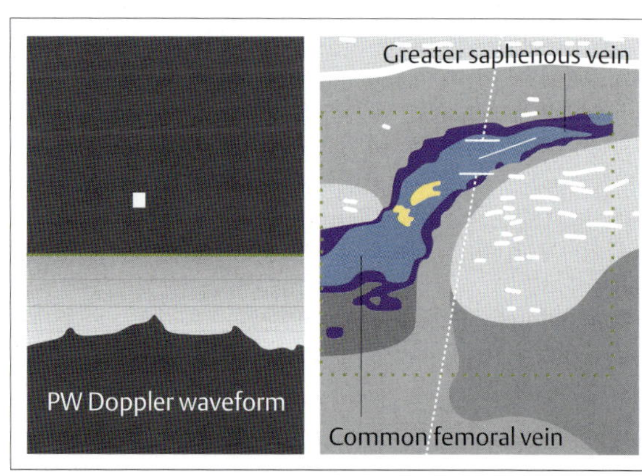

Fig. 15.**25 b** Line drawing.

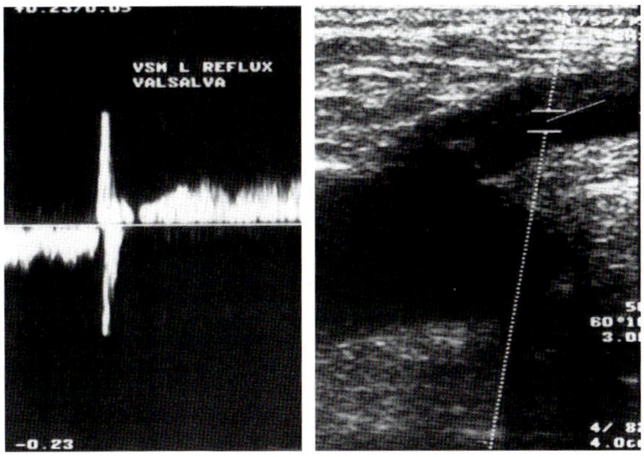

Fig. 15.**26 a** Incompetent valve at the saphenofemoral junction with reflux in the greater saphenous vein during the Valsalva maneuver.

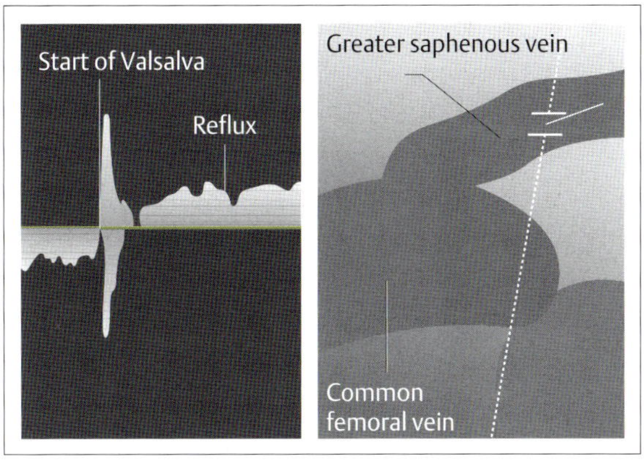

Fig. 15.**26 b** Line drawing.

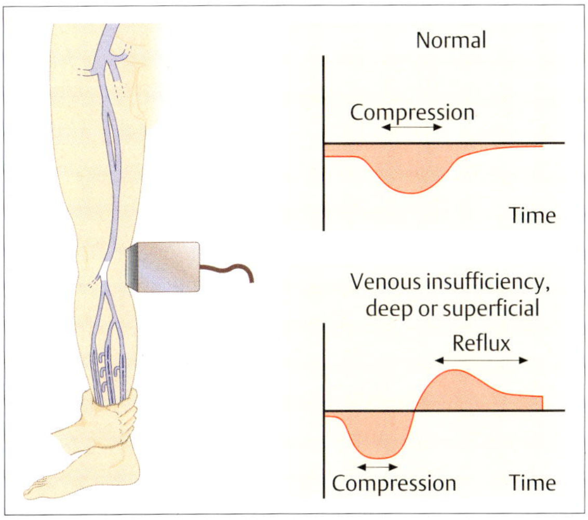

Fig. 15.**27** Blood flow in a leg vein on distal compression with competent (upper diagram) versus incompetent valves (lower diagram).

Consequences for Surgical Treatment

Diagnosis	Characteristic Findings	Management
Spider veins	No insufficiency at the saphenofemoral junction, no deep CVI, no DVT	Sclerotherapy Possibly bipolar cautery or laser therapy
Reticular veins	No insufficiency at the saphenofemoral junction, no deep CVI, no DVT	Possibly sclerotherapy
Varicosities	No insufficiency at the saphenofemoral junction, no deep CVI, no DVT	Compression stockings grade II, sclerotherapy or stab avulsion
Greater saphenous vein insufficiency	No DVT	Isolated insufficiency of saphenofemoral junction = dissection Insufficiency of saphenofemoral junction plus greater saphenous vein = dissection of junction + stripping of insufficient segments Compression stockings grade II
Lesser saphenous vein insufficiency	No DVT	1. Dissection of saphenofemoral junction + stripping of insufficient segments 2. Compression stockings grade II
Incompetent perforating veins	No DVT Competent saphenofemoral junction	1. Dissection of incompetent perforating veins 2. Compression stockings grade II

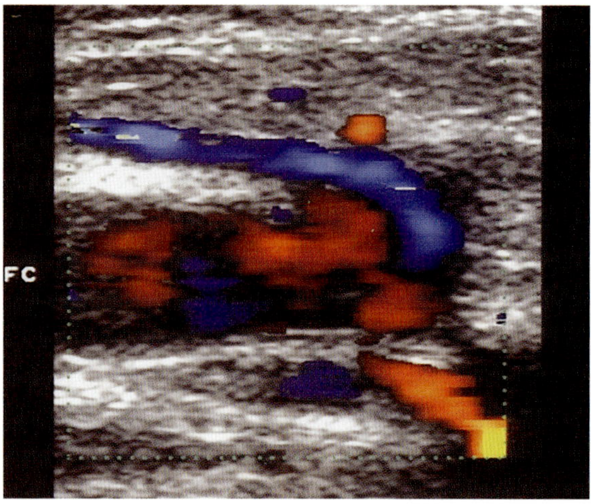

Fig. 15.**28 a** Stump of the greater saphenous vein is too long, resulting in recurrent varicose veins at the saphenofemoral junction three years after varicose vein surgery. Longitudinal view.

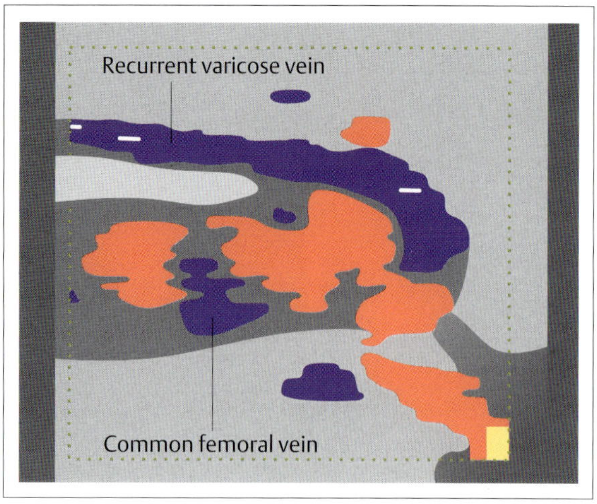

Fig. 15.**28 b** Line drawing.

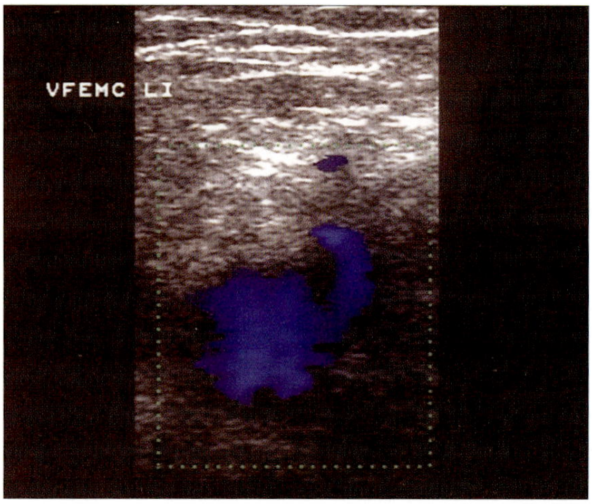

Fig. 15.**28 c** Same patient as in Fig. 15.**28 a**. Transverse view.

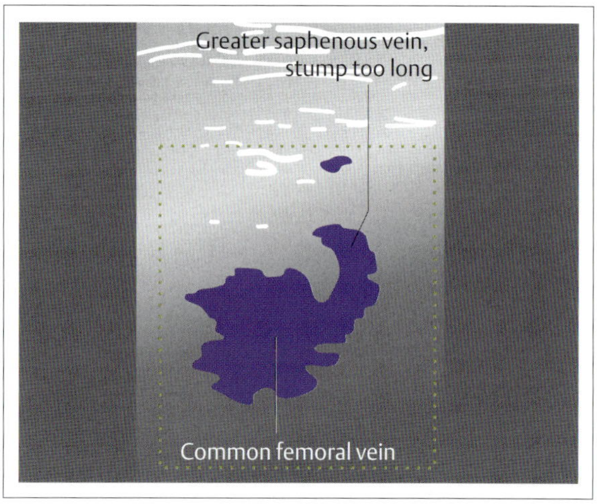

Fig. 15.**28 d** Line drawing.

Peripheral Arterial System–Basics

- Indications for CFDI in the arterial system:
  - Hemodynamically significant stenoses and occlusions
  - True and false aneurysms
  - Hematomas
  - AV fistulas
  - Monitoring of autologous and synthetic grafts
- Examination of pelvic and lower limb arteries starts with the patient supine.
- Iliac arteries can be fully visualized in only 40–50% of patients and should be assessed with a 3.5 MHz probe.
- The distal part of the external iliac artery and the other arteries in the lower extremity are scanned with 5–7.5 MHz probes
- For primary orientation on location and course, transverse views have proven most suitable; however, PW Doppler analysis requires longitudinal delineation of the vessels.
- Progressing in a caudal direction, each arterial segment is conscientiously imaged with CFDI; any region with turbulent flow or velocity changes on CFDI is further assessed with PW Doppler imaging; for each of the common femoral, femoral, and popliteal arteries Doppler analysis should be documented.
- Collateral vessels bypassing occlusive arterial lesions will impair any CFDI appraisal.
- The popliteal artery examined with the patient supine and the leg slightly flexed at the knee and in external rotation, as well as in the prone position (in the authors' experience, the latter more suitable).
- About 6–7 cm below the knee, the popliteal artery bifurcates into the anterior tibial artery, which perforates the interosseous membrane to reach the frontal aspect of

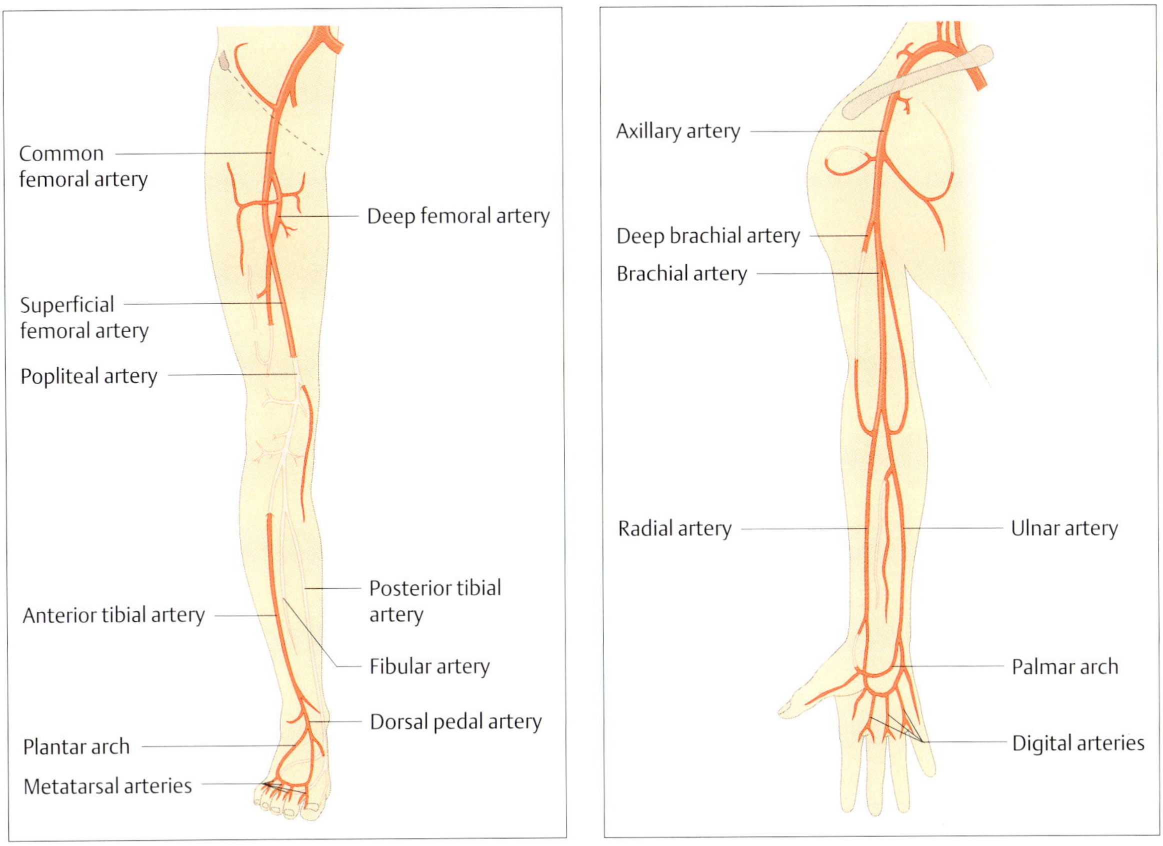

Fig. 15.**29** Arterial anatomy of the limbs: anterior aspect, depicting the posterior vessels as lighter lines.

the lower leg, and its direct continuation proper, the posterofibular trunk (comprising the fibular and the posterior tibial arteries) (Fig. 15.**29**).

- The posterior tibial artery is best viewed medially, and the anterior tibial artery from anterior; both vessels can easily be traced down to the level of the ankle.
- Since the fibular artery courses deep to the muscles, at times it may be hard to delineate.
- Limb arteries characteristically display a triphasic flow profile (rapid systolic rise, drop and slight reflux, followed by another, this time-low amplitude, forward flow during diastole).
- Magnitude of backward blood flow decreases in the arteries below the knee.
- Deviations from this ideal triphasic Doppler waveform may be encountered even in individuals with a normal arterial system (Fig. 15.**30**).
- The third phase (mid- to end-diastolic forward flow) depends on the elasticity of the vessel wall and may disappear in advanced age.
- Doppler waveform amplitude does differ significantly on contralateral comparison.
- At rest, the end-diastolic level of the Doppler waveform is zero (= no arterial flow).

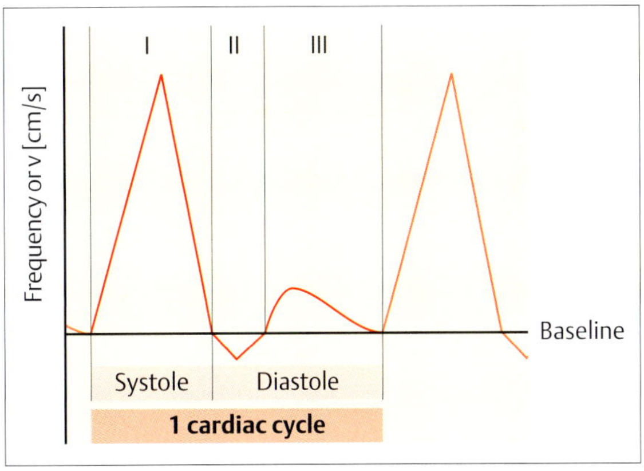

Fig. 15.**30** Diagram of an ideal Doppler waveform of an extremity artery.

- Under physiological conditions, the following changes are seen in the Doppler waveform on exercising and in the subsequent recovery period (Table 15.**5**):
  - Increased peak systolic velocity (PSV).
  - Early diastolic backward flow is lifted just above the zero baseline but keeps its emphasis.
  - Increased end-diastolic flow velocity (EDV).

Table 15.5 Parameters influencing the arterial Doppler waveform (modified from Kopp and Ludwig, 1999)

Parameter	Decrease	Increase
Peak systolic frequency (peak velocity)	The steeper the angle of insonation, the smaller the amplitude	Vascular spasms and within/behind stenoses
	Venous superposition	Hyperthyroidism
Systolic signal width	–	In stenoses of > 70% or in occlusions upstream of the recording site
Early diastolic backward flow	In decreased peripheral vascular resistance, proximal stenosis	–
End-diastolic frequency (flow velocity)	–	By decreased outflow resistance
Bandwidth of frequency spectrum	–	Impaired laminar blood flow at stenoses, branches, kinks, or dilatations

Pseudoaneurysms, Aneurysms, and Arteriovenous Fistulas

Basic Facts

- Pseudoaneurysms can develop after trauma, surgical procedures, and, most frequently, after cardiac catheterization, angiography, or direct arterial pressure monitoring.
- Since the femoral artery is preferred for puncture, it represents the predominant site of pseudoaneurysms (incidence 0.5–1%).
- Pseudoaneurysms are in direct contact with the puncture site and demonstrate direct communication with the arterial lumen (Fig. 15.**31**).
- Arterial punctures superior to the inguinal ligament are at higher risk of complications, including development of pseudoaneurysms, than those of the femoral artery. Insufficient compression, obesity, and anticoagulation medication also increase the risk of pseudoaneurysm formation.
- Clinically, simple para-arterial hematomas may be mistaken for pseudoaneurysms because of transmitted pulsations.
- True aneurysms primarily develop in patients > 60 years because of the decreased strength of the arterial wall (due to atherosclerosis [> 90%], inflammation, or genetic disposition) (Fig. 15.**31**).
- In the limbs, popliteal and femoral artery aneurysms are most common, being bilateral in 35–50% of cases, and combined with abdominal aortic aneurysms (AAAs) in 20–35% of patients.
- CFDI has become the gold standard as diagnostic modality of this region, since it has proved more sensitive than angiography where sessile thrombi often mimic a normal lumen.
- Popliteal artery aneurysms may remain asymptomatic for a long time; apart from rare rupture with acute hemorrhage, their main danger is progressive arterial thromboembolism of the lower leg.
- Arterial diameter increase of at least 50% definitely confirms the diagnosis of an aneurysm; in the popliteal artery, the complication rate increases significantly with diameters > 2 cm.
- Arteriovenous (AV) fistulas are identified clinically by vibrations of the venous walls (thrill), which are palpable and can be heard on auscultation.
- Principal cause of AV fistulas are femoral artery punctures (incidence about 0.5%) and congenital malformations (e.g., Klippel–Trenaunay syndrome).
- AV fistula is a rather rare complication of trauma and surgery.
- Transverse CFDI views are well suited for confirmation and documentation of the fistula.
- *Additional workup:* DSA, angio-CT, angio-MRI.

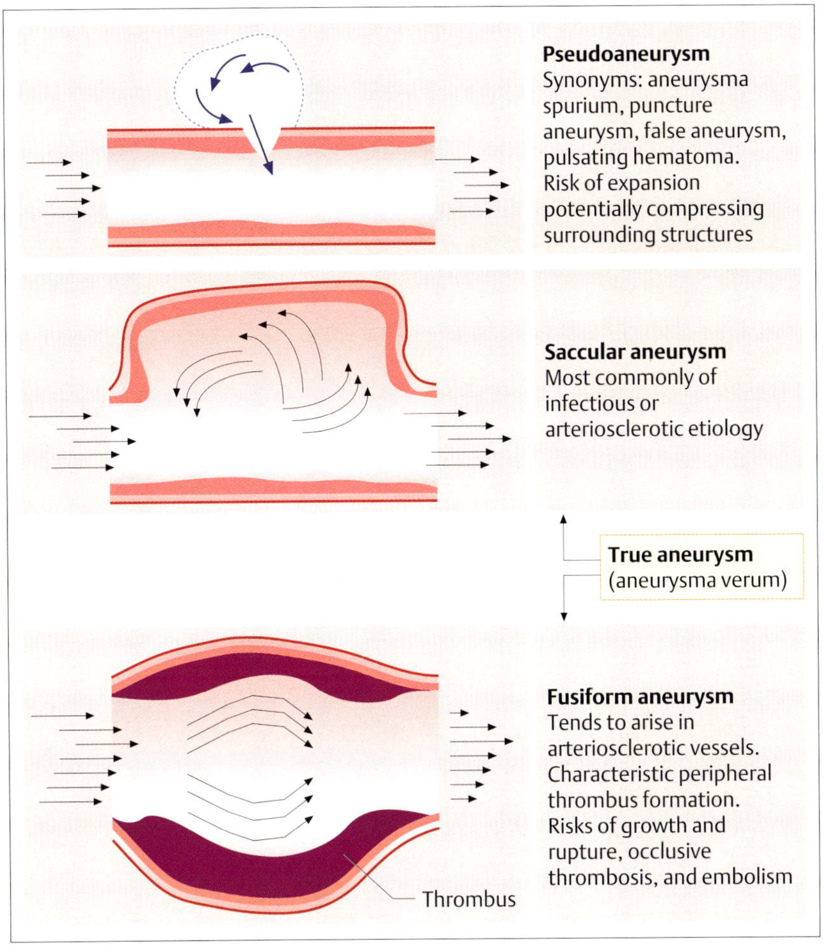

Fig. 15.**31** Schematic illustration of the most common arterial aneurysms.

Sonographic Criteria of Assessment

- **Pseudoaneurysms** appear as hypoechoic para-arterial masses with hyperechoic outline (hematoma).
- With CFDI, pulsatile turbulent blood flow is demonstrated within the pseudoaneurysm on systolic inflow and diastolic outflow (Fig. 15.**32**).
- CFDI can delineate the communication between the arterial lumen and the pseudoaneurysm (Fig. 15.**33**).
- **Thrombosed pseudoaneurysms** appear as heterogeneous hypoechoic/hyperechoic masses (Fig. 15.**34**).
- **True aneurysms** are fusiform or saccular dilatations of the artery, often demonstrating moderately hyperechoic intraluminal thrombi; frequently, the perfused lumen is significantly smaller than the outside diameter of the aneurysm.
- In **AV fistulas,** there is a permanent high-velocity flow signal in the vein (contralateral reference), which in larger fistulas will not disappear during the Valsalva maneuver. Typically, on Doppler spectral analysis, the frequency range broadens, the anechoic window vanishes, and there is no flow variation with respiration (Fig. 15.**35**).

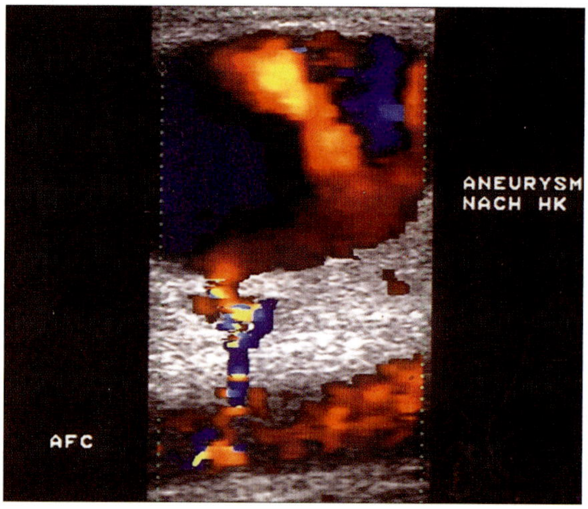

Fig. 15.**32 a** Pseudoaneurysm of the femoral artery four days after cardiac catheterization, with characteristic turbulent blood flow.

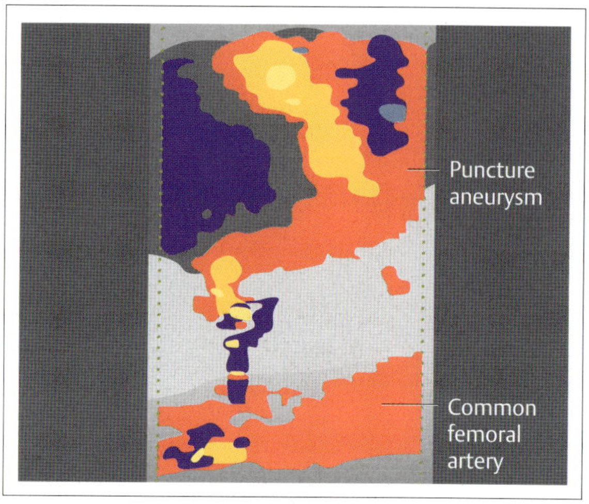

Fig. 15.**32 b** Line drawing.

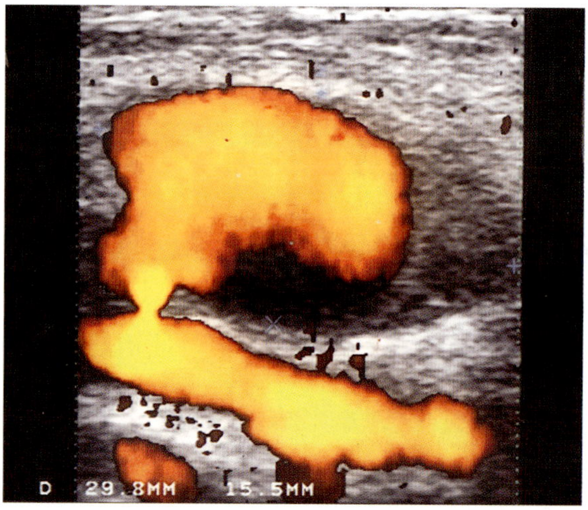

Fig. 15.**33 a** Pseudoaneurysm of the femoral artery with partial thrombosis after cardiac catheterization, with demonstration of the communication on power Doppler imaging.

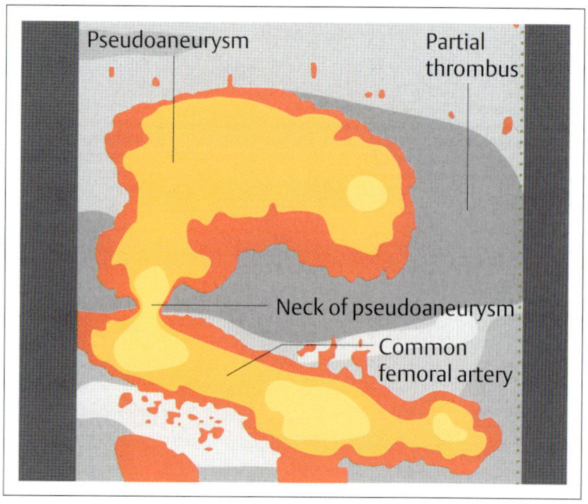

Fig. 15.**33 b** Line drawing.

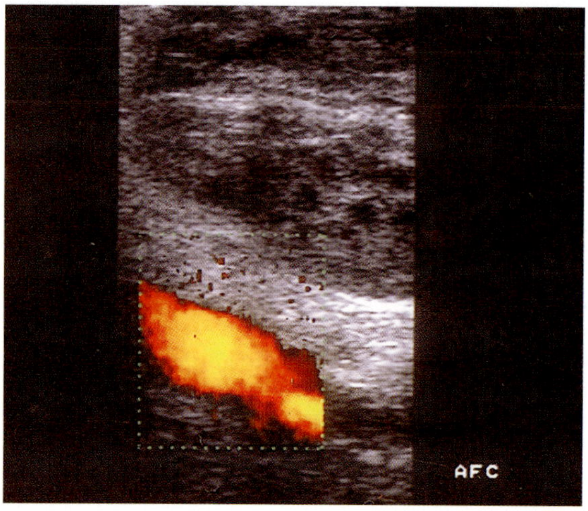

Fig. 15.**34 a** Pseudoaneurysm of the femoral artery with spontaneous thrombosis after two months; same patient as in Fig. 15.**33**; power Doppler imaging.

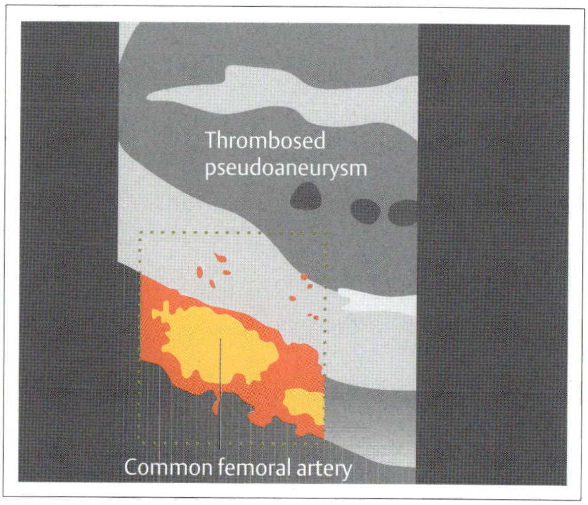

Fig. 15.**34 b** Line drawing.

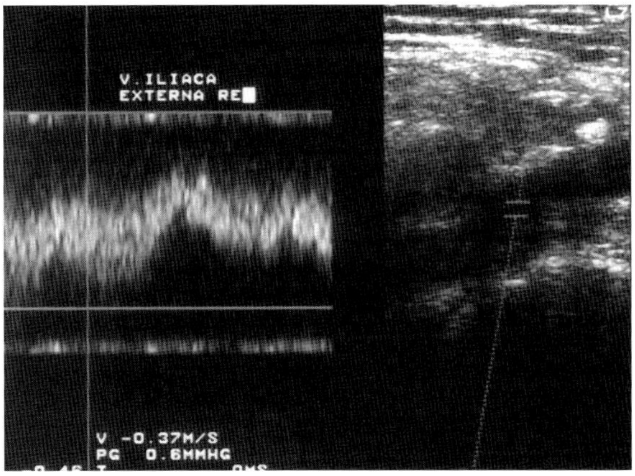

Fig. 15.**35 a** Delineation of the right external iliac vein with Doppler imaging of an iatrogenic AV fistula at the level of the inguinal ligament. Permanent high blood flow, not influenced by the Valsalva maneuver.

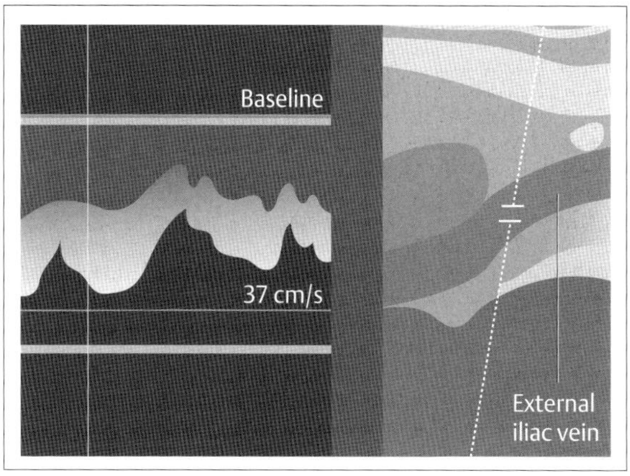

Fig. 15.**35 b** Line drawing.

Consequences for Surgical Treatment

Diagnosis	Characteristic Findings	Management
Pseudoaneurysm	Stable size, no sign of displacement	Expectant; usually spontaneous thrombosis within 3 months US-guided compression of the neck of the pseudo-aneurysm to induce thrombosis (arterial flow should not be impaired; 10–60 min per session, depending on size)
Pseudoaneurysm	Progressive increase in size, extending into the iliac region, with signs of compression or ischemia or persisting for more than 3 months	Surgical repair (direct suture or patch angioplasty)
Popliteal aneurysm	Asymptomatic, diameter < 2 cm (no peripheral embolism)	Follow-up, possibly platelet inhibitors
Popliteal aneurysm	Symptomatic or significant increase in size, > 2 cm, suspected rupture	Ligation of aneurysm and its tributaries and graft interposition
AV fistula	Shortly after intervention, no venous flow on Valsalva maneuver, no clinical symptoms	Close follow-up with CFDI
AV fistula	Significant flow (even during Valsalva maneuver), symptomatic, persisting for > 4 weeks	Surgery with reconstruction of the arterial and venous wall Radiological intervention if possible

Peripheral Arterial Occlusive Disease (PAOD)

Basic Facts

- In western industrialized countries, symptomatic PAOD affects 5–10% of the population over 70 years.
- About 2.5% of the population between 40 and 64 years show signs of PAOD (Kappert, 1989).
- CFDI is particularly well suited for assessment of the aortoiliac and femoropopliteal segments in PAOD of the lower extremities.
- Fontaine's classification of claudication is listed in Table 15.**6**.
- Both legs are affected in 70% of patients.
- Around 50% of all occlusions of lower limb arteries are located within the femoropopliteal segment.
- CW Doppler examination with a pen probe, including measurement of the ankle-brachial index (ABI) or of segmental arterial pressure, is used in screening for hemodynamically significant stenoses of the aortoiliac and femoropopliteal arteries; however, it cannot accurately quantify either severity or extent of PAOD.
- ABI (ankle brachial index) = RR systolic at the ankle/RR systolic at the arm
  - ABI > 1: normal
  - ABI < 1: suggests PAOD
  - ABI < 0.5: probably multilevel disease, critical ischemia
- Critical ischemia: persistent or recurring rest pain with or without necrosis of the foot or toes, typically associated with a systolic pedal artery pressure < 50 mmHg (except in diabetic subjects).
- In PAOD occluded, stenotic, and normal segments may be found in the same limb and even in the same vessel.
- Because of their length, complete CFDI of the lower limb arteries is rather time-consuming, but still does not give the surgeon comprehensive insight into possible vascular reconstruction.
- Decisions on invasive therapy still hinge primarily on the clinical presentation plus angiography (DSA or angio-MRI); the latter permits more precise delineation of the pelvic vessels upstream (run-in) and the arterial segments downstream (run-off), of the extent of the occlusions, and of any collateralization.
- CFDI detects femoropopliteal stenoses of > 50% and occlusions with a sensitivity and specificity of about 90% each (Ranke et al., 1992; Whelan et al., 1992) Table 15.**7** may be used as rough guideline.
- In principle, the arteries of the lower leg may also be examined by CFDI for stenoses and occlusions; however, as this is extremely time-consuming without providing clinically relevant information, this step is largely omitted in our institution.
- Peak systolic velocity decreases the further caudally the artery is assessed (femoral artery 1.1 m/s, superficial femoral artery 0.9 m/s, popliteal artery 0.7 m/s, arteries below the knee 0.4–0.5 m/s).

Table 15.**6** Fontaine's classification of PAOD

Stage	Symptoms
I	Asymptomatic
II a	Intermittent claudication, walking distance > 200 m
II b	Intermittent claudication, walking distance < 200 m
III	Rest pain, trophic changes
IV	Gangrene

Table 15.**7** Normal flow velocities in the major arteries of the leg and their increase in stenosis

Artery	Normal Peak Systolic Velocity	Stenosis if Peak Systolic Velocity Higher than
Femoral artery	< 110 cm/s	200 cm/s
Popliteal artery	< 70 cm/s	150 cm/s

- Assessment of the iliac arteries is frequently limited by bowel gas between probe and vessel.
- Diagnostic criteria for the much less common arteriosclerotic occlusive disease in the arteries of the upper extremity are the same as those in the leg.
- Hemodynamic significance and reduced cross-section of the perfused lumen can be estimated by the ratio of the peak systolic velocity in the stenosis to that 2–4 cm further upstream.
  - Maximum systolic velocity in the stenosis/maximum systolic velocity 2–4 cm upstream > 3 means Stenosis > 75%
- *Additional workup:* DSA (gold standard), ABI, plethysmography, angio-MRI.

Sonographic Criteria of Assessment

- Absence of coloring on duplex B-mode images and of PW Doppler signals provides evidence of **vascular occlusion** (high Doppler gain and low velocity scale [PRF ↑] in order to detect low velocities as well); segments upstream and downstream of the occlusion plus the corresponding veins should also be imaged; possibly echogenic intraluminal material (Figs. 15.**36**, 15.**37**).
- **Stenoses of more than 50%** of the luminal cross-section are hemodynamically significant; they demonstrate a significant increase of the peak systolic velocity at the site of maximum stenosis as well as immediately downstream; CFDI facilitates detection at these areas because of the color changes (possibly also by aliasing).

- Compared with the corresponding normal peripheral arterial segment, a **stenosis of 50%** almost doubles the peak systolic velocity while a stenosis of 75% increases it by 370% (Ranke et al., 1992) (Fig. 15.**38**).
- Peak systolic velocities of more than 200 cm/s correspond to a proximal femoral artery stenosis of 50% and a stenosis of about 75% in the popliteal region (Polak, 1998).
- **Stenoses of less than 50%** demonstrate broadening of the Doppler spectrum.
- Decreased peak systolic velocities with persisting monophasic forward flow indicate an **occlusion/stenosis** upstream of the recording site (Fig. 15.**39**).
- **Calcifications** in the arterial wall with their characteristic posterior shadowing are part of PAOD and may significantly restrict sonographic assessment of morphology and function.
- **Popliteal artery entrapment** results from a developmental defect in which the popliteal artery passes medial to and beneath the medial head of the gastrocnemius muscle or a slip of that muscle, with consequent compression of the artery; in case of stenosis on dorsal or plantar flexion, the Doppler waveform will change (peak systolic velocity at least doubled).

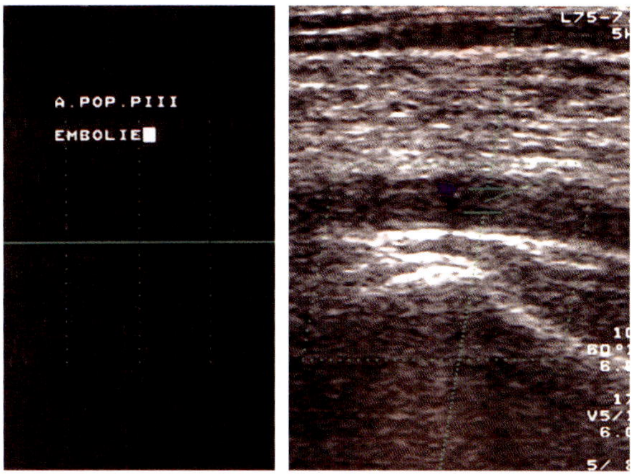

Fig. 15.**36 a** Longitudinal view of acute total occlusion in segment III of the popliteal artery; no flow on CFDI and PW Doppler sonography.

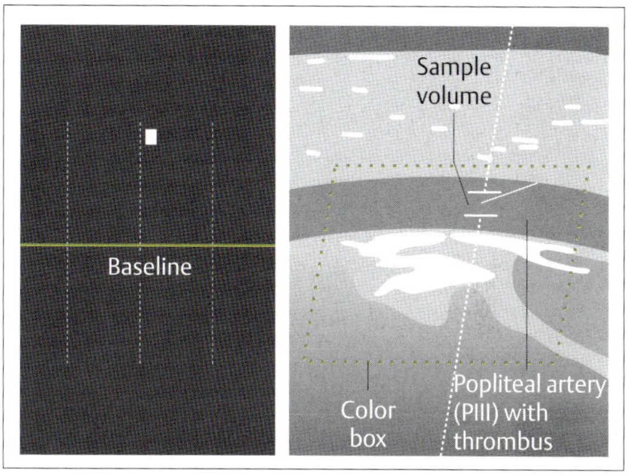

Fig. 15.**36 b** Line drawing.

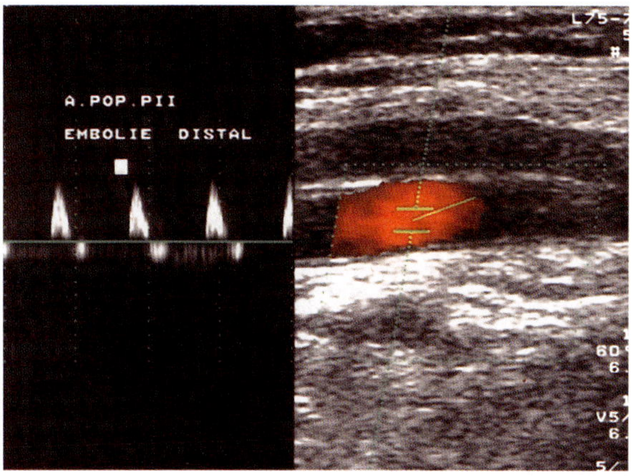

Fig. 15.**37 a** Same patient as in Fig. 15.**36**. Only systolic flow and slight reflux in segments I–III of the popliteal artery; the occlusion downstream forestalls any antegrade diastolic flow.

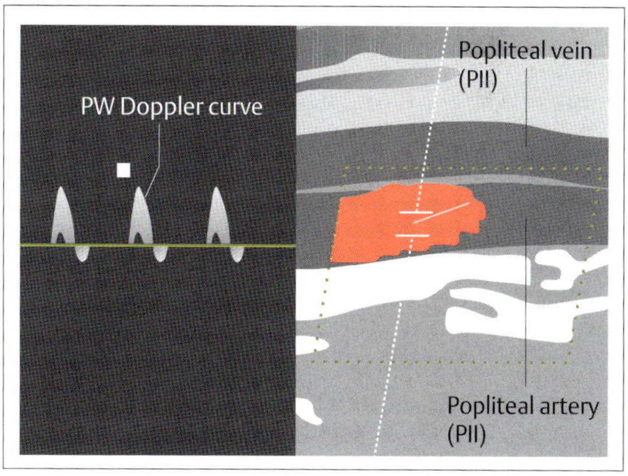

Fig. 15.**37 b** Line drawing.

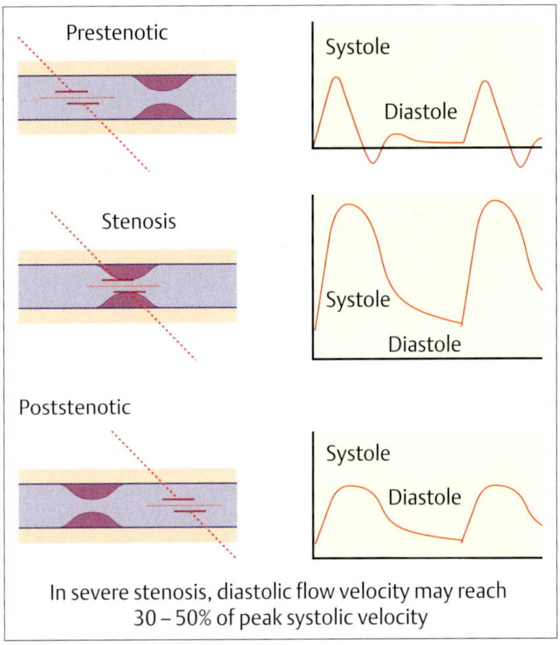

Fig. 15.**38** Characteristic Doppler waveform of a stenosis.

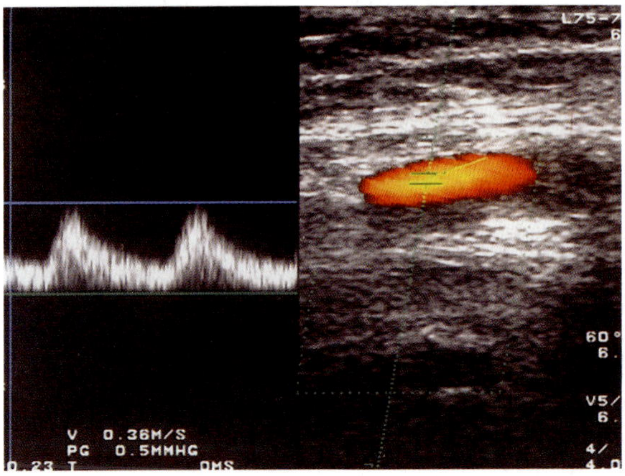

Fig. 15.**39 a** Femoral artery with only monophasic flow in a patient with PAOD and proximal stenosis.

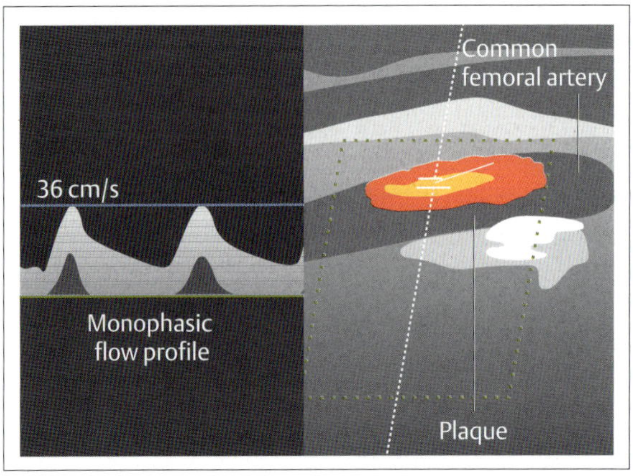

Fig. 15.**39 b** Line drawing.

Consequences for Surgical Treatment

Diagnosis	Characteristic Findings	Management
Femoropopliteal PAOD	Stage I	None, possibly platelet inhibitor
Femoropopliteal PAOD	Stage II a	Walking regime, pentoxifylline, platelet inhibitor; vascular reconstruction in selected cases only in nonresponders
Femoropopliteal PAOD	Stages II b, III, and IV	PTA, stent grafting, vascular arterial surgery, bypass surgery Thrombendarterectomy plus patch angioplasty primarily at the origin of the profunda femoris artery

CFDI and Reconstructive Vascular Surgery for PAOD

Basic Facts

- Options include open and semi-closed thrombendarterectomy, autogenous vein bypass or prosthetic graft, and more recently endovascular stent grafting.
- In the early postoperative phase, air bubbles or hematomas not yet absorbed may impair sonographic delineation of the reconstructed vessel.
- Hematomas and pseudoaneurysms after bypass surgery may also be demonstrated rather easily by CFDI.
- CFDI reliably identifies stenosis and graft thrombosis.
- Stenosis after prosthetic bypass grafting is primarily of the anastomotic type, i.e., fibrotic intimal hyperplasia of the native artery (manifestation about two years postoperatively).
- Diameter of a vein bypass may vary significantly, and in the reversed vein graft the diameter of the proximal segment is smaller than that of its distal end.
- Flow characteristics of a well-functioning bypass with both good run-in and run-off may correspond to those of a normal artery in this same segment, although the early diastolic reflux is often missing or minute.
- Vein graft thrombosis within the first 30 days (early graft failure) usually results from technical errors (poorly fashioned anastomosis, vascular trauma due to clamping, insufficient run-in or run-off).
- In the later course, fibrotic intimal hyperplasia at the no longer functional cusps and at the anastomoses may give rise to stenosis and thrombosis.
- Stenosis of more than 70% of the lumen in infrainguinal vein grafts is likely to result in graft thrombosis within 3–6 months (Idu et al., 1993).
- Regular follow-up by CFDI and early intervention can significantly increase graft lifetime.
- Patients scheduled for vein graft with a history of thrombosis, varicose vein surgery, or vein harvesting should undergo preoperative CFDI of the veins in order to assess their complete vascular status.
- Veins with a diameter > 2–3 mm are usually suitable for arterial replacement.
- *Additional workup:* DSA, angio-MRI, ABI, CW Doppler.

Sonographic Criteria of Assessment

- **Stenosis** is signaled by an increase in peak systolic velocity within the narrowed lumen and immediately distal to the stenosis where aliasing takes place. Doubling of the peak systolic velocity is tantamount to a stenosis of about 75% (Fig. 15.**40**).
- Due to the various techniques of fashioning anastomoses, quite often an increase of up to 50% in peak systolic velocity can be observed at the distal anastomosis.
- Peak systolic velocities of < 45 cm/s in a normal graft (diameter 3 mm) suggest **impaired blood flow**, the cause of which may be insufficient run-in or run-off, or problems within the graft itself: Follow-up is mandatory in such cases!
- Absence of coloring on duplex B-mode images and of PW Doppler signals provides evidence of **vascular occlusion** (high Doppler gain and low velocity scale [PRF ↑] in order to detect low velocities as well).
- **Prosthetic PTFE grafts** are characterized by a hyperechoic double line, while Dacron produces a saw-tooth-like image (Fig. 15.**41**).

Consequences for Surgical Treatment

Diagnosis	Characteristic Findings	Management
Status post infrainguinal reconstruction	Always good blood flow in routine follow-ups	No interventional measures
Status post infrainguinal reconstruction	ABI declined by > 0.15 **and** peak systolic velocity < 45 cm/s (with or without clinical symptoms) Possibly local peak systolic velocity > 200 cm/s	Surgical repair of stenosis. If revascularization is contraindicated, anticoagulation with vitamin K antagonist
Status post infrainguinal reconstruction	Acute graft thrombosis	DSA for objective demonstration of vascular situation Surgical repair or possibly interventional catheterization
Status post infrainguinal reconstruction	Chronic graft failure/thrombosis	Surgery (new graft) depending on clinical situation and technical feasibility

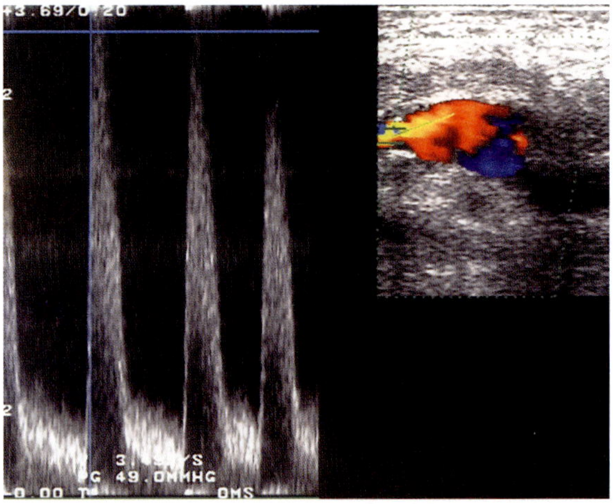

Fig. 15.**40 a** Longitudinal CFDI of a femoral artery stenosis in PAOD, with peak systolic velocity = 349 cm/s: aliasing, and monophasic flow. Status post thrombendarterectomy.

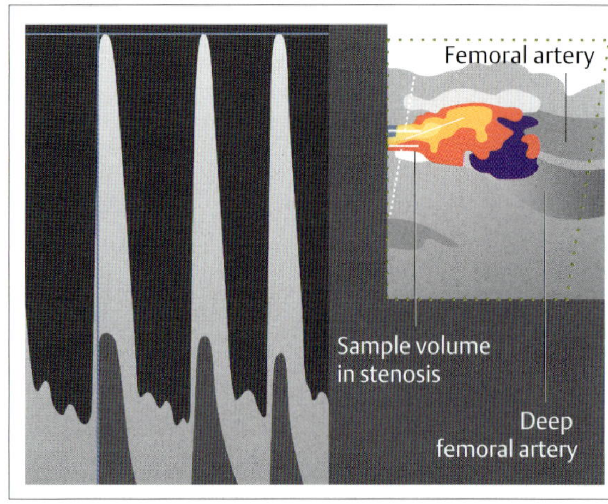

Fig. 15.**40 b** Line drawing.

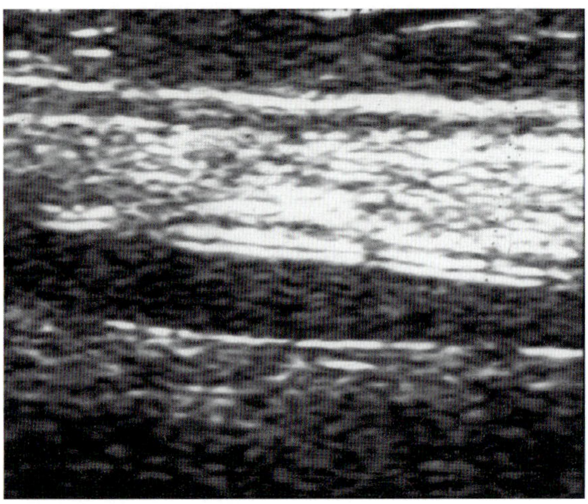

Fig. 15.**41 a** Longitudinal view of a thrombosed PTFE graft, five days after occlusion: no flow on CFDI, and presence of homogeneous hyperechoic intraluminal thrombus.

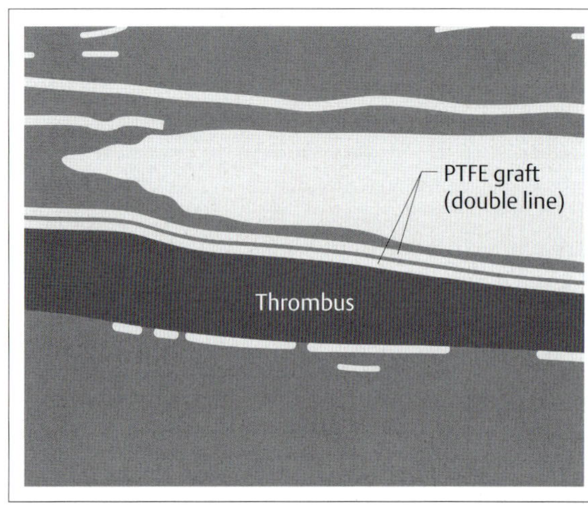

Fig. 15.**41 b** Line drawing.

CFDI of the Supra-aortic Vessels

Basic Facts

Carotid Artery

- Figure 15.**42** outlines the normal anatomy of the supra-aortic vessels.
- Carotid bifurcation is roughly at the level of upper edge of the thyroid cartilage (in a short neck even higher).
- Patient position is variable
- We favor the following: Patient supine, investigator sitting beyond the head of the patient, whose neck is mildly hyperextended and slightly turned to the contralateral side (Fig. 15.**43**).
- Examination comprises three equally important phases:
  - B-mode imaging
  - Doppler imaging with spectral analysis
  - CFDI
- CFDI facilitates localization of hemodynamically significant stenoses and helps to resolve discrepancies between B-mode and Doppler imaging.
- Small linear 5–10 MHz probes are employed.
- First the common, internal, and external carotid artery are imaged in a longitudinal view and duplex scans (flow signals corrected for Doppler angle) obtained in order to document normal blood flow; CCA, ECA, and ICA are also scanned in the transverse plane; pathological findings are documented in longitudinal and transverse views.

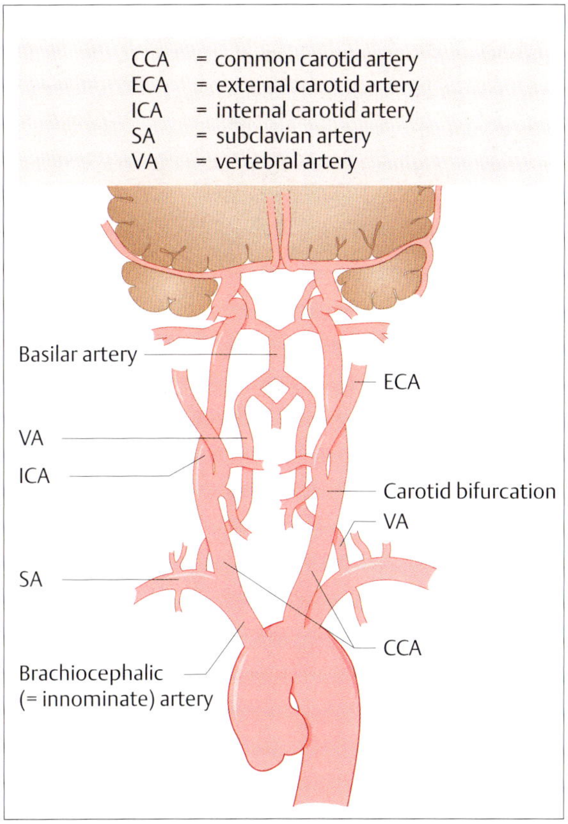

Fig. 15.**42** Normal anatomy of the supra-aortic vessels.

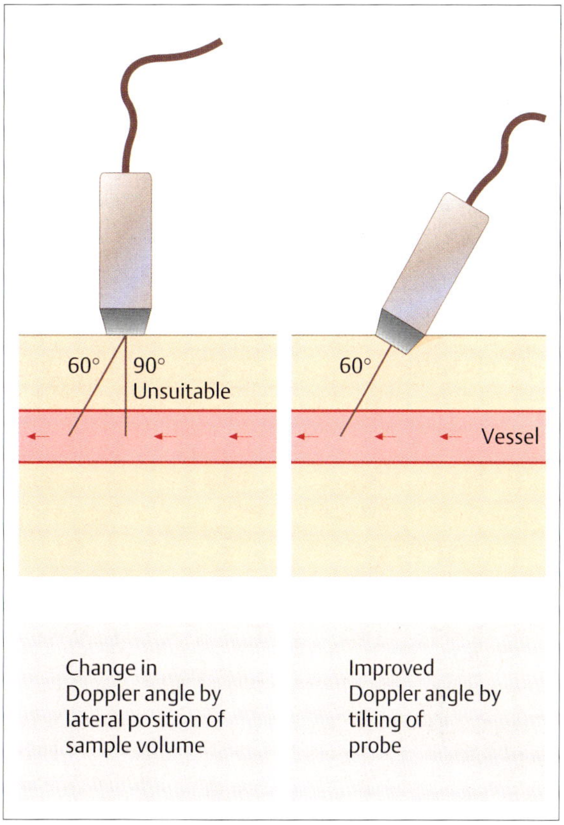

Fig. 15.**44** Optimum Doppler angle.

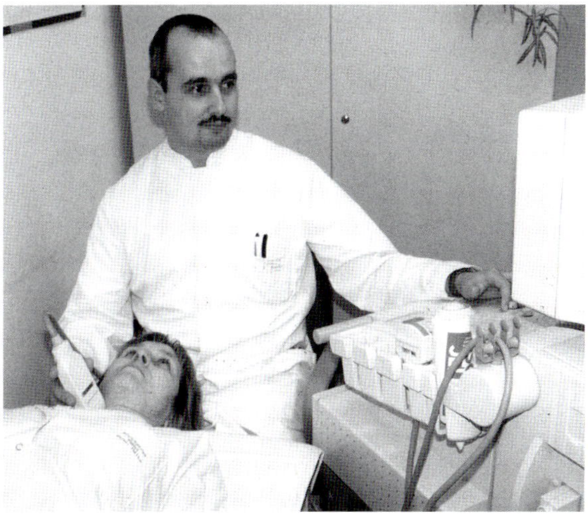

Fig. 15.**43** Suggested patient and investigator positions for CFDI of the carotid artery bed.

- Longitudinal assessment of the carotid artery involves anteroposterior as well as lateroposterior insonation.
- If the anatomy remains ambivalent (meandering vessel, kinking, extreme posterior shadowing), the artery should first be scanned in transverse views in order to identify its approximate course.
- Bilateral blood pressure measurement is an integral part of any supra-aortic vascular assessment (subclavian stenosis).
- Between the ages of 45 and 65 years, luminal narrowing by < 50% is observed in 25–30%, and highly stenotic lesions in 5% of the normal population.
- Principal site of arteriosclerotic changes is the carotid bifurcation (extending into the ICA for up to 2 cm).
- Plaques and stenoses in the CCA are found in no more than 2% of patients referred for carotid assessment.
- Around 60% of all TIAs, PRINDs, and strokes are caused by lesions in the CCA or ICA.
- Diffuse intimal thickening in the CCA or at the carotid bifurcation is considered a sign of generalized arteriosclerosis, and only rarely is it due to inflammation or Takayasu's disease.
- Recurrent carotid stenoses secondary to fibrotic intimal hyperplasia may develop in 5–10% of patients within

Table 15.**8** Sonographic assessment of the carotid artery

B-mode Imaging	Spectral Doppler Imaging	CFDI
– Transverse and longitudinal view from cephalad of clavicle to mandible – On the right, by tilting the probe the origin of the CCA behind the clavicle can frequently be visualized (left origin is lower) – Delineation of plaques (location, extent, size of residual lumen, plaque morphology) – Size of residual lumen relative to normal lumen is difficult to assess due to posterior shadowing – Longitudinal view of carotid bifurcation from anterolaterally and posterolaterally for reliable identification even of small plaques	– If CFDI is not available, the entire carotid trunk should be Doppler imaged (wide sample volume) – Document flow profiles of CCA, ECA, ICA, and vertebral artery (narrow sample volume) – In luminal stenosis, perform Doppler analysis within as well as immediately upstream and downstream of presumed maximum stenosis (adjust correction of Doppler angle so that it parallels main flow) – Setting of Doppler angle correction affects the Doppler angle, which is needed for converting Doppler frequency into velocity – Doppler shift is maximum if Doppler angle of insonation is 0°; in practice, angles of 30–60° are acceptable; angles > 60° should not be included in the measurement, and for a theoretical angle of 90° the Doppler shift will be zero (Fig. 15.**44**) – Vertebral artery followed from origin and between the transverse processes up to the base of the skull (note direction of flow)	– CFDI permits comprehensive overview of vascular and velocity abnormalities of the carotid artery bed (longitudinal and transverse views) – Sites with turbulence (color change) and high velocities (brighter color or aliasing) – Once sites of abnormal velocities have been identified, precise measurement is performed by spectral analysis – B-mode imaging often overlooks hypoechoic plaques, which can be identified by corresponding color-sparing – CFDI can delineate even a minute residual lumen and thus rule out occlusion

one year of carotid catheterization or thrombendarterectomy.
- Overview: Table 15.**8**.
- Indications for carotid Doppler imaging:
  • Symptomatic carotid stenosis suspected (stroke or TIA)
  • Bruit over cervical vessels
  • Follow-up after carotid surgery
  • Follow-up of known arteriosclerosis in the carotid vascular bed
  • Prior to major surgery, particularly cardiovascular procedures
  • Controversial: Screening in patients with known arteriosclerosis or risk factors
- The NASCET (North American Symptomatic Carotid Endarterectomy Trial) and ECST (European Carotid Surgery Trial) documented significantly better results with carotid endarterectomy than with medical therapy alone in symptomatic stenoses ≥70% (Rothwell and Warlow, 2003).
- Rothwell and Warlow in 1999 suggested taking into account further risk factors: additional TIAs, irregular plaques, short history, female sex, coexisting PAOD, and arterial hypertension.
- One essential aspect in establishing the indication for carotid surgery is the estimated degree of stenosis; various classification systems are in use and still under discussion.
- Since angiography is no longer part of routine workup in patients with carotid stenosis, modalities based on Doppler and duplex imaging have been developed, using peak systolic velocity and end-diastolic or minimal diastolic velocity as criteria for estimating the degree of stenosis.
- Compared with angiography, accuracy is at 90–95%.
- Numerous classifications for US-based estimation of carotid stenosis have been proposed (Abu Rahma et al., 1998; Bluth et al., 1988; Carroll, 1991; Neale et al., 1994; Neuerburg-Heusler and Hennerici, 1999; Taylor and Strandness, 1987; Withers et al., 1990; Zwiebel, 1992) (Tables 15.**9**–15.**13**).
- A PSV > 270 m/s correlates with a stenosis > 70% (sensitivity 96%, specificity 86%); an EDV > 110 m/s also correlates with a stenosis > 70% (sensitivity 91%, specificity 93%). Combining both criteria results in a sensitivity of 96% and a specificity of 93% (Neale et al., 1994).

Table 15.**9** Neale's classification of carotid artery stenosis (Neale et al., 1994)

Severity	Stenosis (%)	PSV (cm/s)	EDV (cm/s)
Moderate	50–59	120–130	20–40
Severe	60–79	131–250	40–100
Critical	80–99	> 250	> 100

Table 15.**10** Abu Rahma's classification of carotid artery stenosis (Abu Rahma et al., 1998)

Severity	Stenosis (%)	PSV (cm/s)	EDV (cm/s)	Sensitivity (%)	Specificity (%)
Mild	30–49	> 120	–	93	67
Moderate	50–59	> 140	–	92	95
Moderate	60–69	> 150	> 65	82	97
Severe	70–99	> 150	> 90	85	95

Table 15.**11** Strandness's classification of carotid stenosis (Strandness, 1990)

Stenosis (%)	Criteria
1–15	No effect
16–49	Spectral broadening
50–79	PSV > 125 cm/s, EDV < 140 cm/s
80–99	PSV > 125 cm/s, EDV > 140 cm/s

Table 15.**12** Carroll's classification of carotid stenosis (Carroll, 1989)

Stenosis (%)	PSV (cm/s)	EDV (cm/s)
0–40	> 25, < 110	< 40
41–59	> 120	< 40
60–79	> 130	> 40
80–99	> 250	> 80–135

Table 15.**13** Classification of carotid stenosis according to Neuerburg-Heusler and Hennerici (1999)

Degree of Stenosis	Stenosis (%)	PSV (cm/s)	EDV (cm/s)
Nonstenosing plaques	< 40	< 120	< 40
Minor	40–60	> 120	< 40
Moderate	60–70	> 120	> 40
Severe	70–90	> 240	> 135
Subtotal	> 90	Varied	Varied

- Angiography provides a two-dimensional image of the perfused stenotic lumen; because of the differences in plaque surface, the exact cross-sectional area of a stenosis cannot be determined precisely (Fig. 15.**45**).
- Peak systolic velocity, though, represents a reproducible parameter that correlates well with the degree of stenosis.
- This chapter will not discuss the published alternatives for estimating the severity of a stenosis based on indices.
- Due to plaque irregularity, limited spatial resolution, and frequent presence of calcifications with concomitant posterior shadowing, direct sonographic assessment of a stenosis on transverse views (ratio of residual lumen to actual lumen of artery) has proved impractical.
- Angiography offers the essential advantage of simultaneous demonstration of cerebral perfusion (revealing any "tandem" stenoses downstream); accordingly, if the indication for surgery relies on carotid CFDI, the latter should always be complemented with transcranial Doppler sonography.
- Any plaque narrows the luminal cross-section; however, hemodynamic significance (measurable increase in flow velocity on Doppler imaging) only results in stenoses ≥ 40–50%. A plaque is defined as a lesion *without* hemodynamically significant stenosis.
- Characteristic features of plaques and their behavior are listed in Table 15.**14**.
- Possible plaque development is outlined in Fig. 15.**46**.
- Table 15.**15** lists the sonographic criteria for differentiation between ECA and ICA.
- In elderly patients and those with chronic hypertension, the carotid arteries sometimes become tortuous and elongated.
- In a short neck, the carotid bifurcation (flow divider) may be situated so far cephalad that it cannot be visualized at all or not appropriately with the CFDI probe.
- Even if there is reduced diastolic flow velocity in all supra-aortic vessels (symmetrical), it more likely reflects low cardiac output than manifestation of a high-grade stenosis downstream.
- In arrhythmia, PSV and EDV should be determined during a regular cardiac cycle.
- Constant diastolic reflux is a sign of aortic valve insufficiency.
- Causes of symmetrical high blood flow velocities in the absence of carotid stenosis include arterial hypertension, systemic AV fistulas, and intracardiac shunts.
- Subtotal stenoses are characterized by low residual flow; usually, definite detection is only possible by CFDI.
- Small systolic "blips" may correspond to pulsations transmitted via thrombi/plaques.
- In imaging of the supra-aortic vessels, the Doppler angle should also be between 30° and 60°.
- Within the stenosis, the cursor for Doppler angle correction should not parallel the arterial wall but rather the direction of flow in the stenosis.

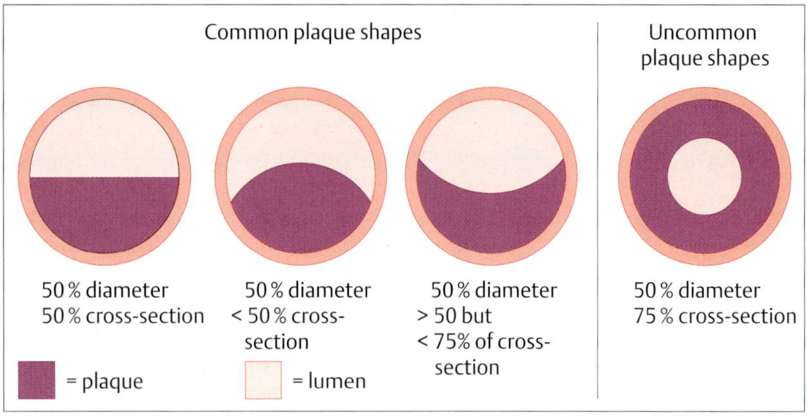

Fig. 15.**45** Correlation between plaque surface condition, diameter of the stenosis, and reduction in cross-sectional area of the lumen (= actual degree of stenosis) (modified from Stavros et al., 1994).

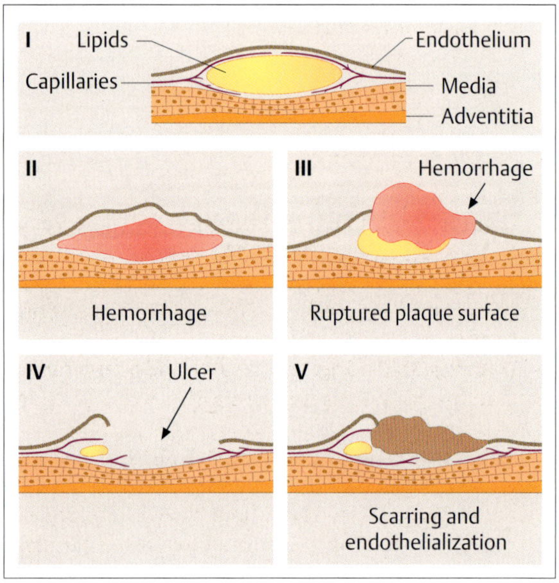

Fig. 15.**46** Possible plaque formation and development.

Table 15.**14** Sonographic characteristics of plaques and their behavior

Plaque	Heterogeneous Plaques	Homogeneous Plaques
Characteristics	Comprise hemorrhagic areas	May comprise calcifications
Sonogram	Heterogeneous, low-level echoes, with hypoechoic and anechoic areas	Homogeneous, hyperechoic to blood
Behavior	Increased risk of thromboembolism	Lower risk of embolism

Table 15.**15** Sonographic criteria for differentiating internal from external carotid artery

Criterion	ICA	ECA
Course	Posterior to spine (in about 95 % of cases)	Anterior in the direction of the face
Branches	None	Yes
Transmission of finger tapping on temporal artery	No	Yes
Doppler waveform	Low vascular resistance (large end-diastolic flow)	Large vascular resistance (low end-diastolic flow)

- Depending on the US unit, the color-flow Doppler signal will overwrite the arterial wall and thus is not useful in determining the residual lumen.
- Spectral broadening need not imply the presence of a stenosis but depends to a large extent on the location of the sample volume, its size, blood flow velocity, and the course of the vessel (branching, curves).
- Turbulence and other changes in the blood flow may be observed not only in pathological vascular lesions, but also at branchings, curves, and widened vascular diameter (e.g., partial flow reversal in the carotid bulb).
- Carotid body tumor: rare disorder; semimalignant tumor of the chemoreceptors at the carotid bifurcation (paraganglioma); clinically, possibly palpable tumor, bradycardia, syncope, and occasionally fistula bruit on auscultation, highly vascularized with AV shunts.
- Carotid dissection: detachment of the intima from the media resulting in a false as well as true lumen; possibly traumatic but also spontaneous in Marfan syndrome, collagen disease, fibromuscular dysplasia, or hypertension with possible concomitant neurological deficit.
- Carotid artery aneurysms are rare and usually traumatic or sequelae of an inflammatory vascular lesion.

- Kinking and coiling, mainly of the ICA, may be congenital or signify advanced arteriosclerosis; neurological symptoms are possible.
- Transcranial PW Doppler recording may provide intraoperative monitoring of cerebral blood flow during carotid endarterectomy and can help decide on the necessity of temporary shunting.
- Intracranial microembolism, e.g., during shunt insertion, may be responsible for late neurological deficits (Ackerstaff et al., 1995).
- Table 15.**16** gives an overview of the clinical stages of carotid artery stenosis.

Subclavian Artery

- Subclavian steal syndrome is caused by stenosis (or occlusion) of the proximal subclavian artery with subsequent retrograde filling of the subclavian artery via the vertebral artery, which demonstrates permanent or temporary flow reversal.
- On arm exercise, subclavian steal syndrome may result in vertebrobasilar insufficiency.
- In total subclavian steal syndrome, there is permanent retrograde blood flow in the vertebral artery; in the subtotal type, retrograde flow can only be demonstrated on arm exercise.
- Provocation testing for subtotal subclavian steal syndrome: At the ipsilateral arm, the blood pressure cuff is inflated to above systolic RR and kept at that pressure for 1–2 minutes; on subsequent release, vasodilation in the hypoxic arterial bed triggers hyperemia and compensation is by flow reversal in the vertebral artery. (Caveat: The vertebral artery is always accompanied by a vein.)
- Proximal stenosis of the subclavian artery may cause arm claudication, concomitant vertigo, or RR differences of > 20 mmHg on contralateral comparison (stenosis becomes symptomatic if > 70%).
- In total subclavian steal syndrome, the danger of cerebral embolism during PTA of the subclavian artery stenosis is less than in the subtotal type or in forward flow.

Table 15.**16** Clinical stages of carotid artery stenosis

Stage I	Asymptomatic carotid stenosis (Stroke frequency at 5%, under conservative medical management at 2% per year, ACAS study 1995)
Stage II	Symptomatic carotid stenosis with temporary clinical deficits (TIA, PRIND) (spontaneous stroke rate at 15% per year; NASCET study)
Stage III	Manifest stroke with increasing or resolving neurological symptoms
Stage IV	Past stroke with residual symptoms

Vertebral Artery

- Stenoses or occlusions are usually are located at or close to the origin.
- Typical symptoms of vertebrobasilar ischemia are drop attacks, dysarthria, dysphagia, nystagmus, and ataxia.
- Bilateral RR measurement mandatory: subclavian steal syndrome?
- The most common pathological changes in the vertebral artery are steal syndrome, hypoplasia, agenesis, arterial occlusions and stenoses at branch-offs.
- Vertebral arteries can be followed with CFDI from their origin throughout almost their entire course; only at the level of the atlas will a pen probe gain better access than the larger CFDI transducer.
- *Additional workup* in the examination of all supra-aortic vessels: transcranial Doppler imaging, angiography, CT, MRI, angio-MRI, SPECT.

Sonographic Criteria of Assessment

Carotid Artery Bed

- **Normal Doppler spectral waveforms** of CCA, ICA, and ECA are presented in Figs. 15.**47** and 15.**48**.
- There is flow separation in the **carotid bulb** because dilatation of the artery interrupts the laminar flow pattern.
- Tapping with the finger on the temporal artery results in retrograde undulations in the ECA, thus helping to identify the vessel (Fig. 15.**49**).
- Stenosis of 60–70% (moderate) is characterized by marked plaque formation, spectral broadening, distorted Doppler waveform, and typical increase of peak systolic and end-diastolic flow velocities (Figs. 15.**50**, 15.**51**).
- In stenoses of 70–90% with little calcification, the residual lumen can be outlined on CFDI or power Doppler imaging (Fig. 15.**52**).
- In critical stenoses (lumen reduced by > 90%), there may be no recordable flow in the ICA, and the PSV may remain normal due to distortion of the Doppler waveform; diastolic flow in the CCA falls (increased resistance), while it rises in the ECA (resistance falls–collateral flow), and therefore the systolic–diastolic difference is lowered.
- ICA occlusion: no visible or measurable flow on Doppler analysis, possibly visible thrombus and small systolic spikes correlating with pulsations transmitted onto the thrombus, externalization of the CCA (little or no diastolic flow) and internalization of the ECA (Figs. 15.**53**, 15.**54**).
- In carotid dissection, there is antegrade blood flow in the true lumen (frequently compressed) and oscillating turbulent flow in the false lumen (anterior to the intima); within the lumen of the artery a membrane

pulsating synchronously with the cardiac cycle can be demonstrated.

- Carotid body tumor is a highly vascularized tumor of low to high echogenicity splaying the carotid bifurcation (Fig. 15.**55**).
- Intimal thickening (> 0.6 mm) signals early arteriosclerosis (Fig. 15.**56**).
- Following carotid thrombendarterectomy, laminar flow in the ICA is frequently lost. Recurrent stenosis is characterized by the same velocity criteria as in primary stenosis; frequently it is characterized by diffuse fibrotic intimal hyperplasia, and almost exclusively occurs in the first postoperative year.
- Kinking and coiling are best visualized on CFDI, and stenosis is ruled out according to the criteria above by measuring PSV and EDV (Fig. 15.**57**).

Subclavian and Vertebral Arteries

- Distal to the lesion in subclavian artery stenosis, the Doppler waveform changes from triphasic to monophasic; in the stenosis itself (often not accessible to the ultrasound beam), a typical stenotic signal with increased flow velocity is seen.
- On contralateral reference, increased blood flow in Doppler imaging of the vertebral artery may signal high-grade carotid stenosis or hypoplasia of the contralateral vertebral artery, while flow reversal is characteristic of subclavian steal syndrome (Fig. 15.**58**).
- Normal vertebral artery with its accompanying vein between the transverse processes of the cervical vertebrae (Fig. 15.**59**).
- Visualization of the vertebral artery without blood flow is pathognomonic of occlusion (distal refilling possible via collaterals).
- Decreased amplitude of the Doppler signal in the vertebral artery (contralateral reference) may be caused by a more distal stenosis (Fig. 15.**60**).
- Hypoplasia of the vertebral artery is characterized by a marked difference in diameter on contralateral reference, measuring < 2 mm on the affected side, and is associated with a low amplitude flow signal.
- In stenoses > 75%, the PSV increases by > 250% (>180 cm/s).

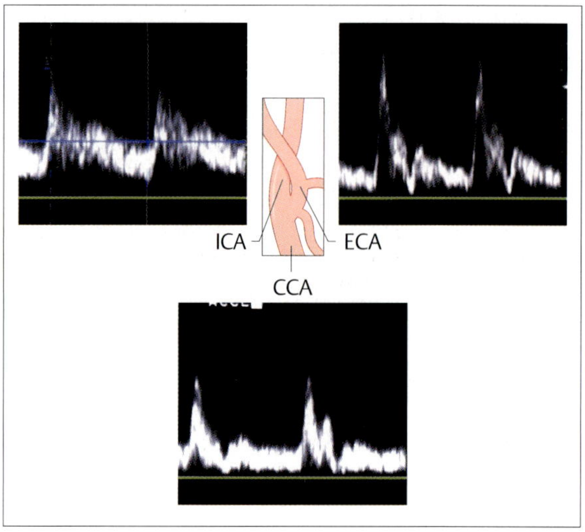

Fig. 15.**47** Normal Doppler spectral waveforms in the carotid region.

Vessel	Characteristic features of the Doppler curve
ICA	Low outflow resistance results in monophasic antegrade flow, which is relatively high also in the diastole. The waveform is gentle. PSV = 0.6–1 m/s.
ECA	Flow is usually also antegrade throughout but, owing to higher peripheral resistance, the diastolic flow is significantly lower. A sharp waveform results with a steep rise to a high but narrow systolic peak, and not quite so rapid a fall to a brief early diastolic notch, followed by continuous low diastolic flow.
CCA	Corresponding to a combination of the flow characteristics of ICA and ECA, the waveform is sharper than that of the ICA and diastolic flow is higher than in the ECA.

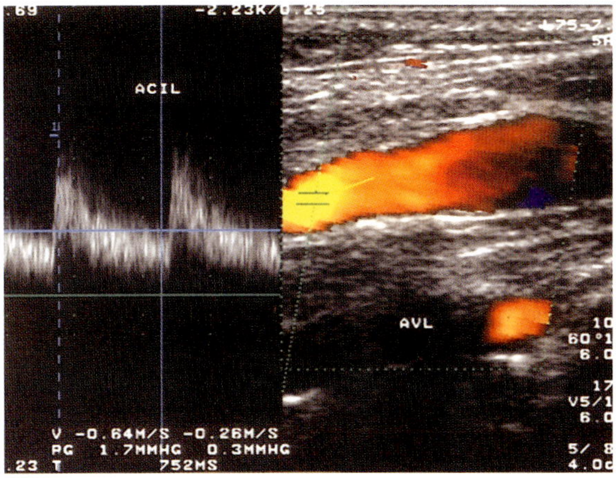

Fig. 15.**48 a** Longitudinal view of normal ICA on CFDI: spectral Doppler waveform with free systolic window; PSV 64 cm/s, EDV 26 cm/s; ipsilateral vertebral artery also displayed in color window.

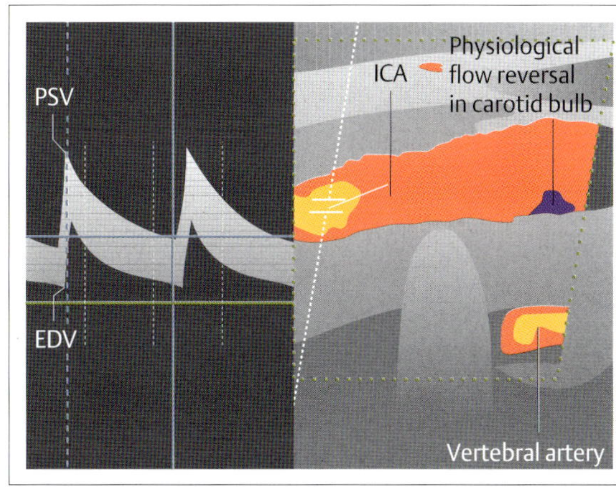

Fig. 15.**48 b** Line drawing.

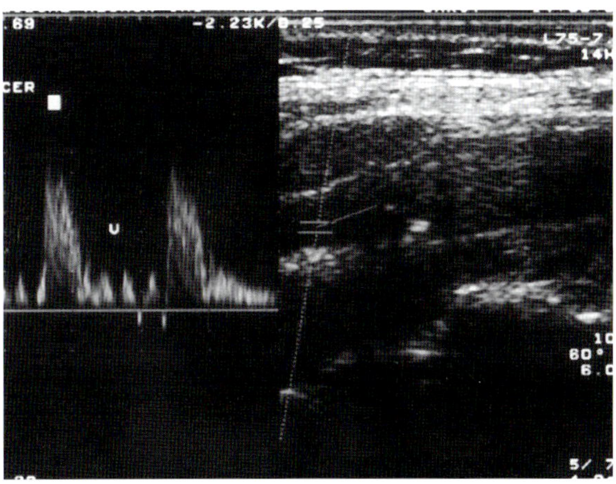

Fig. 15.**49 a** Longitudinal view of the ECA with retrograde transmission of the undulations originating in the temporal artery, permitting reliable identification of the ECA; sharply defined Doppler waveform and low diastolic flow.

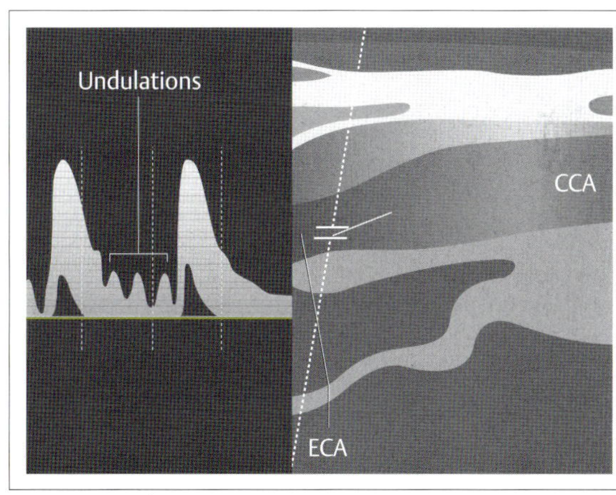

Fig. 15.**49 b** Line drawing.

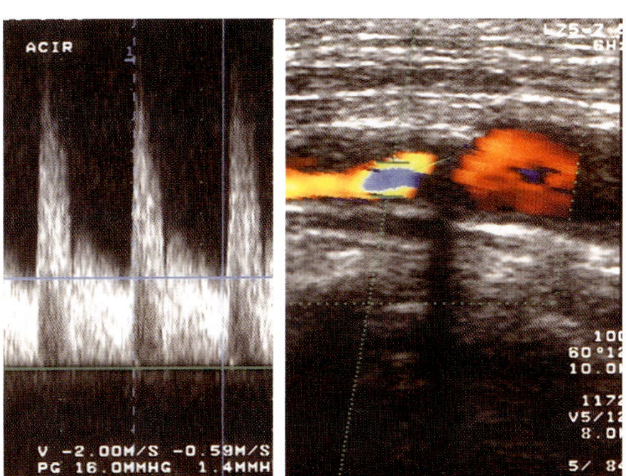

Fig. 15.**50 a** Longitudinal view of ICA with moderate stenosis on CFDI: loss of free systolic window beneath the Doppler waveform; PSV 200 cm/s, EDV 59 cm/s; clear-cut luminal stenosis in the ICA, aliasing on CFDI, posterior shadowing.

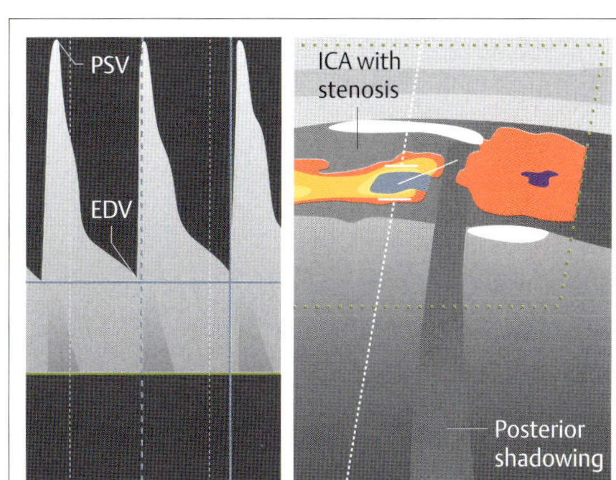

Fig. 15.**50 b** Line drawing.

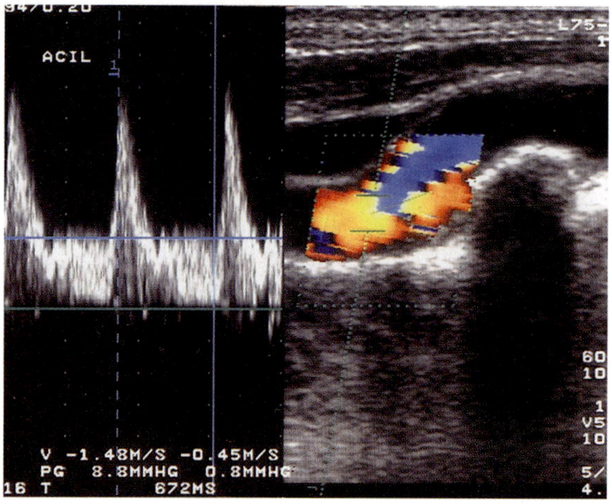

Fig. 15.**51 a** Longitudinal view of the ICA in moderate stenosis with marked posterior shadowing: PSV 148 cm/s, EDV 45 cm/s; spectral broadening.

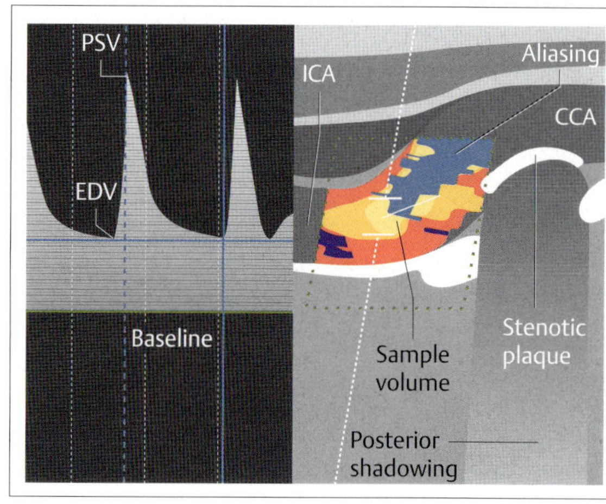

Fig. 15.**51 b** Line drawing.

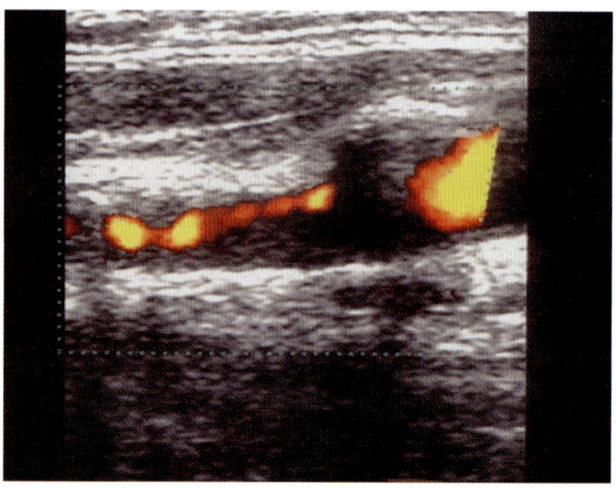

Fig. 15.**52 a** Longitudinal view of the ICA in severe stenosis (70–90 %) with delineation of the residual lumen on power Doppler imaging, incomplete posterior shadowing, and clinical symptoms.

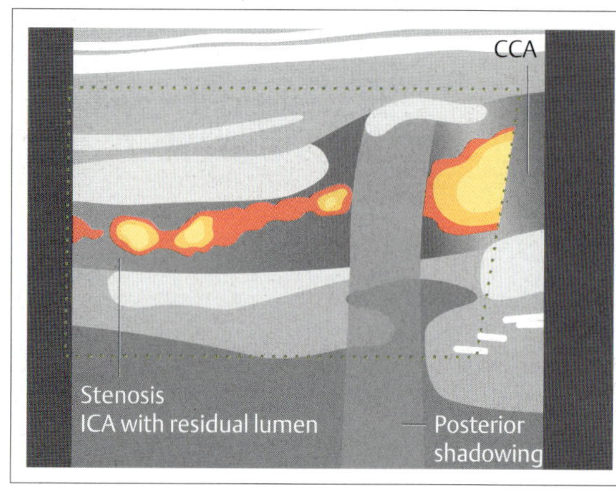

Fig. 15.**52 b** Line drawing.

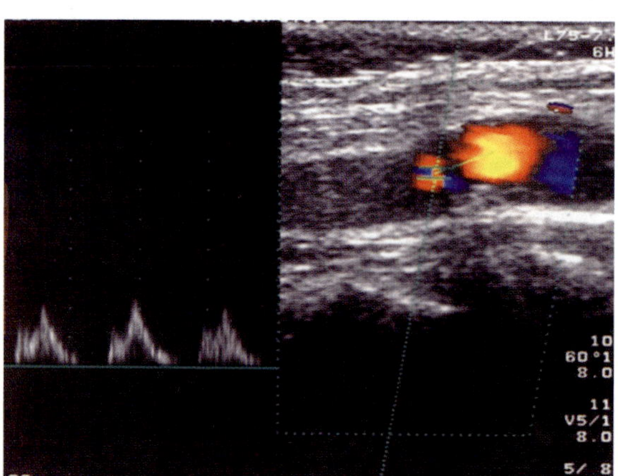

Fig. 15.**53 a** Longitudinal view of a 4-week old symptomatic occlusion of the ICA with definite intraluminal thrombus and minimal palpable transmitted pulsations.

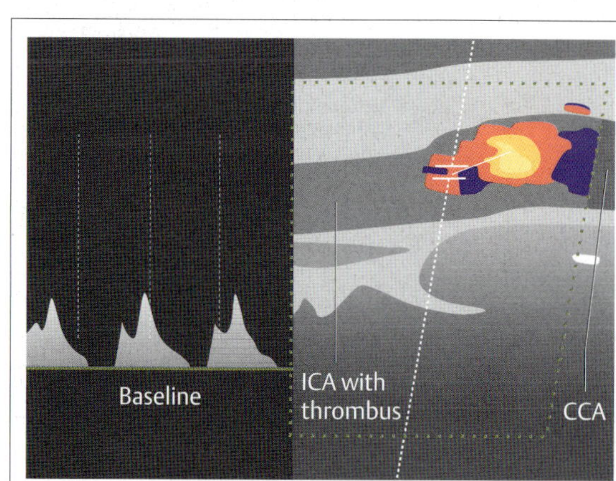

Fig. 15.**53 b** Line drawing.

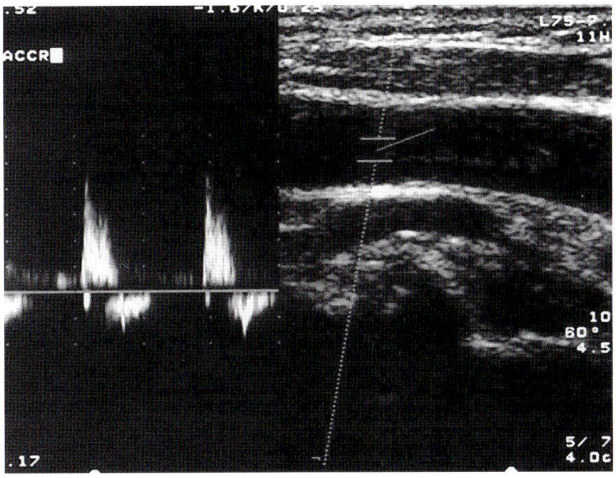

Fig. 15.**54 a** Longitudinal view of the CCA in case of occluded ICA with externalization of the CCA, reduced diastolic flow, and partial reflux.

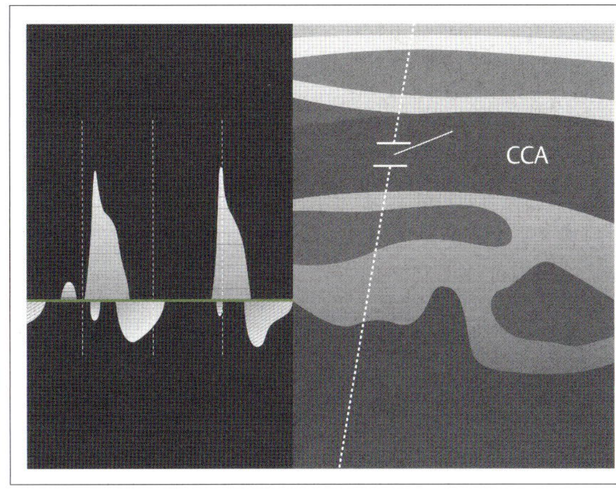

Fig. 15.**54 b** Line drawing.

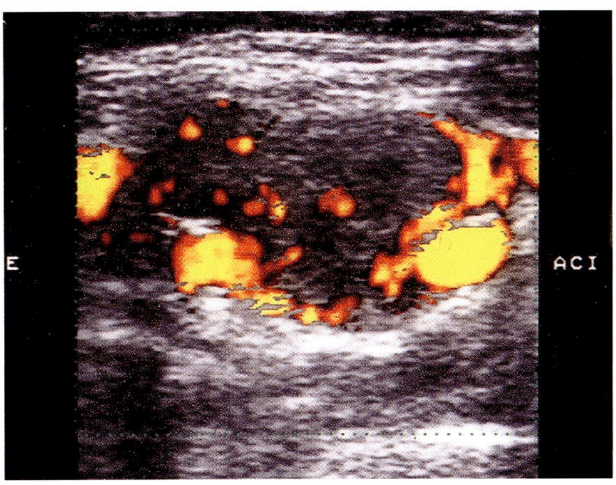

Fig. 15.**55 a** Transverse view of the carotid bifurcation with hypoechoic carotid body tumor splaying the ECA and CCA, well vascularized on power Doppler imaging.

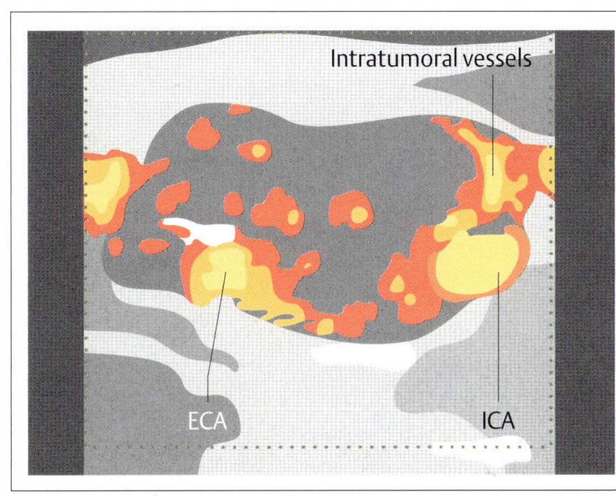

Fig. 15.**55 b** Line drawing.

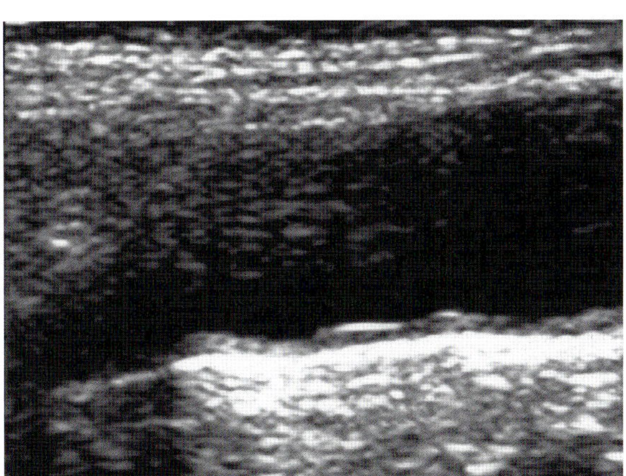

Fig. 15.**56 a** Longitudinal B-mode view of the CCA with marked intimal thickening at the posterior arterial wall.

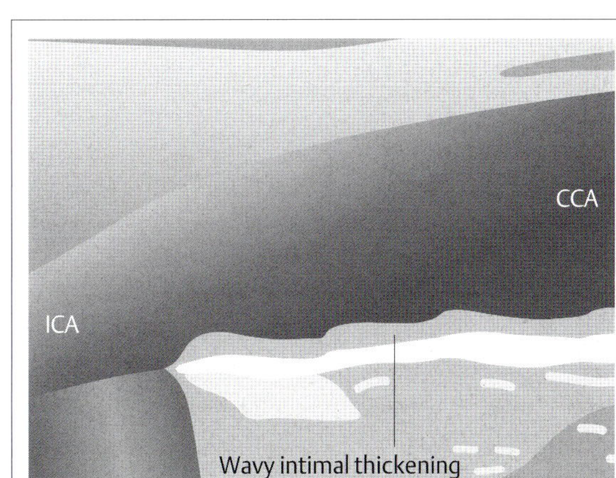

Fig. 15.**56 b** Line drawing.

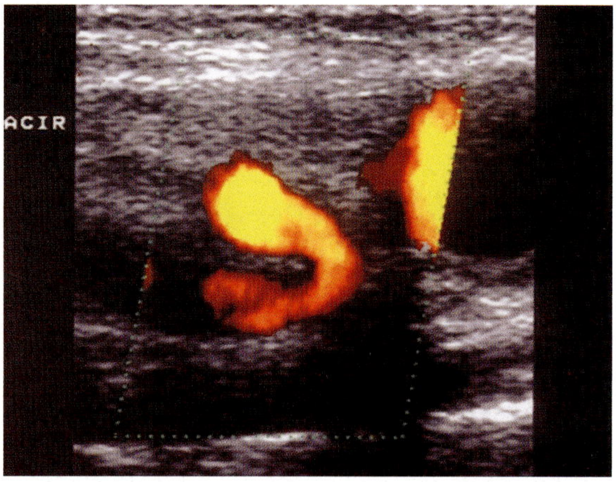

Fig. 15.**57 a** On power Doppler imaging, coiling of the ICA with demonstration of hemodynamically moderate degree of stenosis and lack of neurological symptoms; dilated carotid bifurcation.

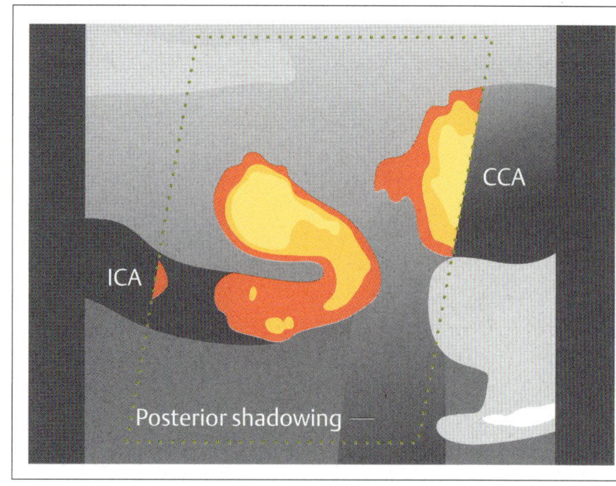

Fig. 15.**57 b** Line drawing.

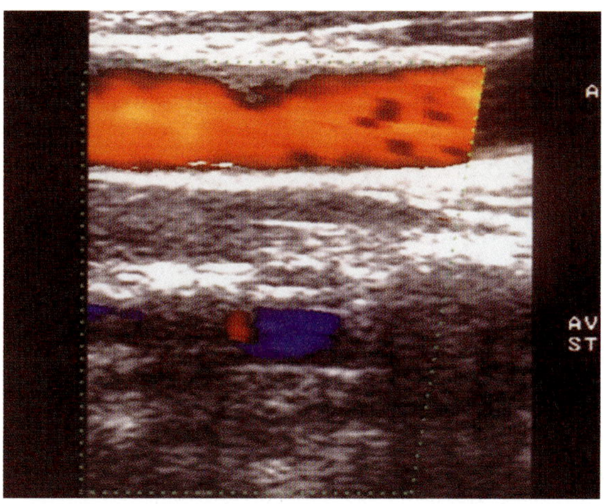

Fig. 15.**58 a** Longitudinal view of the CCA and vertebral artery with permanent retrograde flow in the vertebral artery; total subclavian steal syndrome in subclavian artery stenosis, Caveat: The vertebral artery is easily mistaken for the parallel vertebral vein.

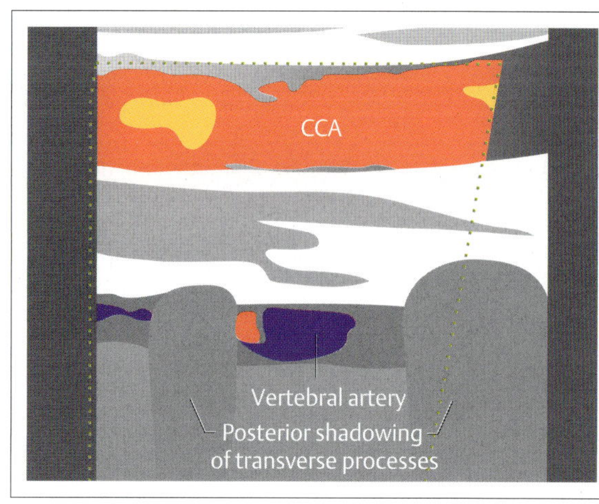

Fig. 15.**58 b** Line drawing.

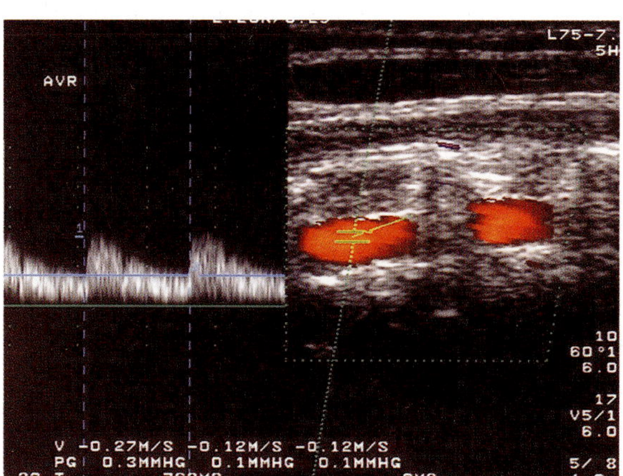

Fig. 15.**59 a** Longitudinal view of the normal vertebral artery, CFDI between the transverse processes of the cervical spine: PSV 27 cm/s, EDV 12 cm/s, with free systolic window.

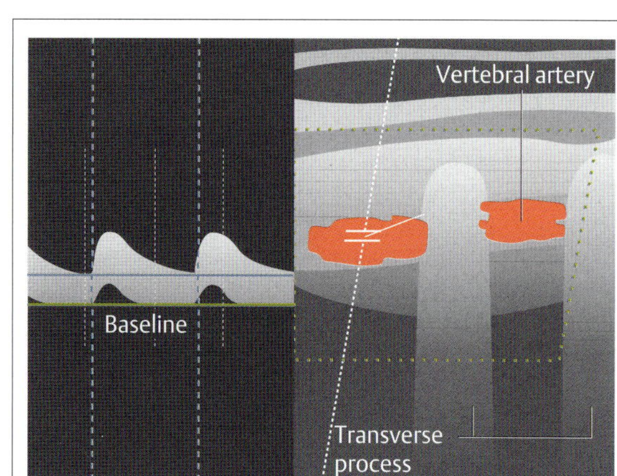

Fig. 15.**59 b** Line drawing.

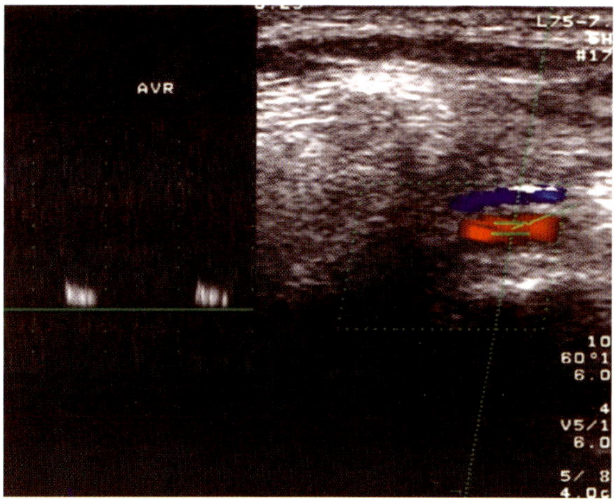

Fig. 15.**60 a** Longitudinal view of the vertebral artery and vein; on contralateral reference, spectral Doppler analysis demonstrates a marked decrease in amplitude and loss of the diastolic phase, suggesting downstream stenosis or occlusion.

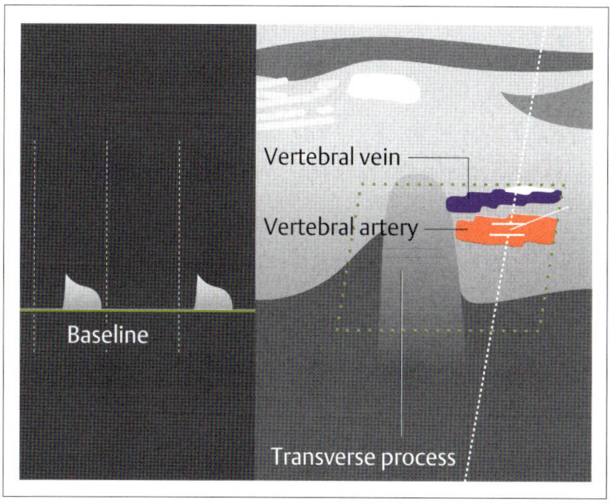

Fig. 15.**60 b** Line drawing.

Consequences for Surgical Treatment

Diagnosis	Characteristic Findings	Management
Plaque	No hemodynamically relevant stenosis, asymptomatic or symptomatic	Nonsurgical, medical therapy
Plaque	Recurrent; symptomatic despite medical therapy, ulceration	Reconstructive vascular surgery
ICA stenosis	Grade II and stenosis > 70%	TEA, possibly with patch angioplasty or eversion endarterectomy
ICA stenosis	Grade I, stenosis > 70% (asymptomatic)	Slight benefit for surgery in stenosis (> 70%); spontaneous stroke rate under medical treatment 2% per year, after surgery 1% per year (ACAS study). Surgery only indicated if life expectancy of patient is > 5 years
ICA stenosis	Grade III, if no loss of consciousness, acute onset (4–6 hours), carotid artery occlusion, normal CCT	Emergency surgery possible Neurological symptoms may resolve in up to 50% of patients, but mortality of up to 9% is rather high; thrombectomy + TEA and possibly patch angioplasty
ICA stenosis	Grade IV almost complete resolution of symptoms	Surgical repair of stenosis about 2–6 weeks after the event In ICA occlusion, a low-key approach to surgery, possibly extra-intracranial graft (individual decision)
Subclavian artery stenosis	Symptomatic, steal syndrome, arm claudication	PTA Extrathoracic bypass grafting or transposition
Carotid body tumor	Well-vascularized tumor at the carotid bifurcation, confirmed by CFDI and angiography	Resection of complete tumor

Consequences for Surgical Treatment *(continuation)*

Diagnosis	Characteristic Findings	Management
Carotid dissection	Asymptomatic, no floating intima or thrombi	Watchful waiting, anticoagulation, reattachment of dissecting membrane to obliterate the false lumen
Carotid dissection	Symptomatic plus neurological deficit, floating intimal fragments	Reattachment, possibly resection of dissecting membrane or resection of the dissected arterial segment with graft interposition
Kinking or coiling	Asymptomatic, no sign of stenosis	Conservative, follow-up
Kinking or coiling	Symptomatic or sign of hemodynamically significant stenosis	Excision
Vertebral artery occlusive disease	Bilateral occlusion or stenosis, marked symptoms, nonvascular causes ruled out (ENT, cardiology, neurology)	Central: Local TEA or transposition into CCA Peripheral: Carotidovertebral C1 graft (restricted indication)

Intravascular Sonography (IVUS)

M. Pross, Th. Bürger

Continuing technical progress with refinement and miniaturization of instrumentation has made possible percutaneous as well as transluminal and intravascular ultrasound (IVUS) examinations. Employing thin catheter systems and guide wires, these specialized probes are positioned into central or peripheral vessel segments. This permits direct assessment of vascular lumen and wall, and of neighboring anatomical structures. IVUS in particular may be able to close the gap in diagnostic workup for suspected mural involvement. However, the main areas are diagnostic workup and treatment follow-up of arterial lesions, particularly in (coronary) catheterization.

Sonographic Criteria of Assessment

- The most important parameter is delineation of the wall layering. The normal vessel wall comprises the inner hyperechoic intima, the hypoechoic media in the middle, and the hyperechoic adventitia on the outside (Fig. 15.**61**); loss of this triple layering may indicate tumor invasion (Fig. 15.**62**).
- Assessment of elasticity of the arterial wall during the pulse wave.

Basic Facts

- The patient is supine.
- Vascular access is usually gained in the groin, with placement of a 6–8 Fr introducer sheath in Seldinger technique and subsequent advancement of a guide wire into the target area.
- The IVUS probe is introduced over the wire and brought into the desired position under fluoroscopic control.
- Usually, IVUS will only be performed in specialized centers and in conjunction with vascular contrast studies, since it is a technically demanding and expensive investigation.
- In tumor patients, IVUS is indicated only if contrast-enhanced CT and angiography or vena cavography are ambivalent regarding possible tumor invasion (e.g., of the vena cava, aorta, or portal vein).
- IVUS provides information on arteriosclerotic lesions of the arterial wall
- IVUS allows follow-up in interventional catheterization.

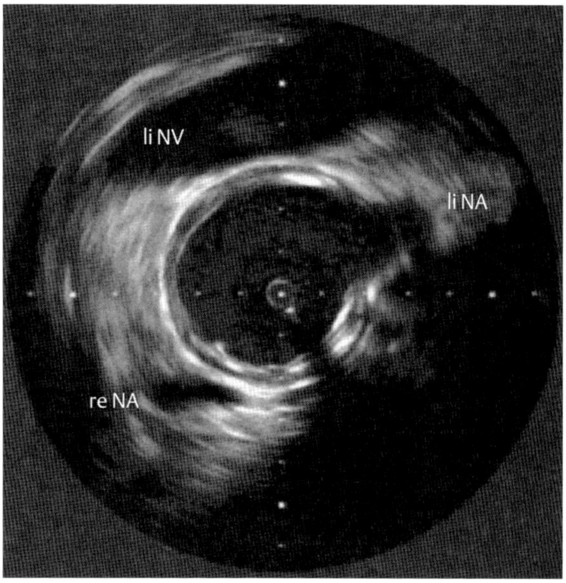

Fig. 15.**61 a** Normal make-up of the aortic wall. The ultrasound catheter is visible at the center of the vessel. The layers of the aortic wall are concentric to the catheter: hyperechoic intima on the inside, hypoechoic media in the middle, and hyperechoic adventitia on the outside.

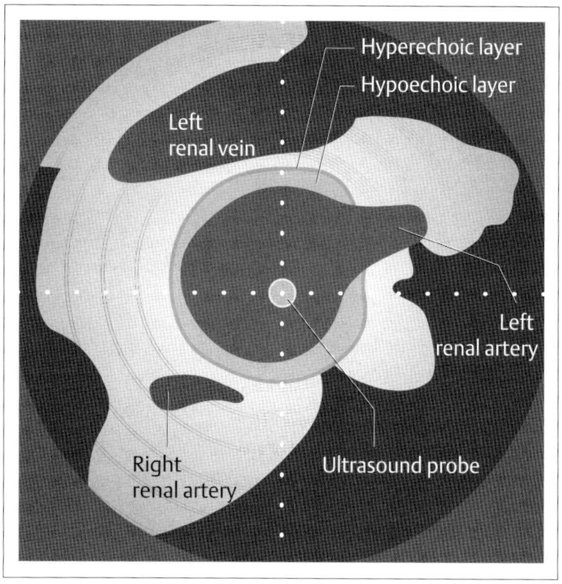

Fig. 15.**61 b** Line drawing.

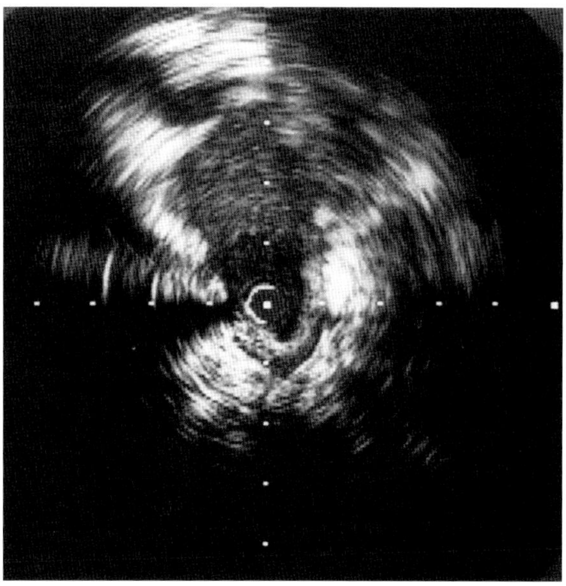

Fig. 15.**62 a** Intravascular view demonstrates loss of wall layering in the vena cava. The wall is no longer mobile due to tumor invasion.

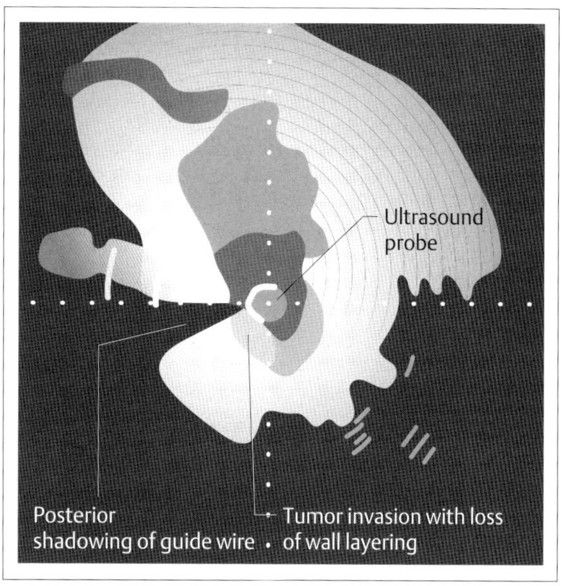

Fig. 15.**62 b** Line drawing.

Consequences for Surgical Treatment

Vessel Wall	Characteristic Findings	Consequences for Treatment
No tumor invasion of vessel wall	Demonstration of characteristic wall layering	Resection of tumor desirable
Tumor invasion of vessel	Wall layering interrupted, the tumor breaching the lumen	Resection of tumor only if this includes resection of vessel and graft interposition
Determining degree of arteriosclerosis and stenosis	Bright hyperechoic outline = calcified plaques; cross-sectional view of lumen possible	Influences treatment options
Catheterization follow-up	Segment open, dissection membrane	Success/failure/broadening of treatment

Bibliography

Armstrong PA, Bandyk DF, Wilson JS, Shames ML, Johnson BL, Back MR. Optimizing infrainguinal arm vein bypass patency with duplex ultrasound surveillance and endovascular therapy. J Vasc Surg. 2004; 40: 724–30; discussion: 730–1.

Calligaro KD, Doerr KJ, McAfee-Bennett S, Mueller K, Dougherty MJ. Critical pathways can improve results with carotid endarterectomy. Semin Vasc Surg. 2004; 17: 253–6.

Devalia K, Riches J, Hands L, Handa A. Preoperative duplex on admission prevents unnecessary carotid surgery. Eur J Vasc Endovasc Surg 2004; 28: 634–5.

Fils V, Miksic K, Tetizkovie E. Outcome of stenosis of the internal carotid artery after contralateral endarterectomy. Wien Klin Wochenschr. 2004; 116 (Suppl 2): 44–50.

Fobbe F, Ruhnke-Trautmann M, v. Gemmeren D, Hartman CA, Kania U, Wolf KJ. Altersbestimmung venöser Thromben im Ultraschall. Fortschr Röntgenstr. 1991; 155: 344–8.

Hannesson PH, Stridbeck H, Lundstedt C, Dawiskiba S, Andren-Sandberg A, Ihse I. Intravascular ultrasound for evaluation of portal venous involvement in pancreatic cancer. Eur Radiol. 1997; 7: 21–5.

Idu MM, Blankenstein JD, de Gier P, Truyen E, Buth J. Impact of a color-flow duplex surveillance program on infrainguinal vein graft patency: a five-year experience. J Vasc Surg. 1993; 17: 42–52.

Kaneko T, Nakao A, Funahashi H, et al. Intracaval ultrasonography in the diagnosis of tumours involvement of the vena cava. Br J Surg. 1995; 82: 1655–9.

Kaneko T, Nakao A, Inove S, et al. Intraportal endovascular ultrasonography in the diagnosis of portal vein invasion by pancreatobiliary carcinoma. Ann Surg. 1995; 222: 711–8.

Kappert A. Lehrbuch und Atlas der Angiologie. 12th ed. Bern, Stuttgart, Toronto: Hans Huber; 1989.

Kopp H, Ludwig M. Checkliste Doppler- und Duplexsonographie. Stuttgart: Thieme; 1999.

Lippert H. Praxis der Chirurgie. Stuttgart: Thieme; 1998.

Mantke R, Lindner F. Rezidivvarikose nach Babcock-Operation–10 Jahre postoperativ. Phlebologie. 1993, 22: 156–8.

McGahan P, Goldberg BB. Diagnostic ultrasound: a logical approach. Philadelphia: Lippincott-Raven; 1998.

Neuerburg-Heusler, Hennerici M. Gefäßdiagnostik mit Ultraschall. Stuttgart: Thieme; 1999.

Nguyen LL, Conte MS, Menard MT, Gravereaux EC, Chew DK, Donaldson MC, Whittemore AD, Belkin M. Infrainguinal vein bypass graft revision: factors affecting long-term outcome. J Vasc Surg. 2004; 40: 916–23.

North American Symptomatic Carotid Endarterectomy Trial (NASCET) Steering Committee. North American symptomatic carotid endarterectomy trial: methods, patient characteristics, and progress. Stroke. 1991; 22: 711.

North American Symptomatic Carotid Endarterectomy Trial Collaborators. Beneficial effect of carotid endarterectomy in symptomatic patients with high grade carotid stenosis. N Engl J Med. 1991; 325: 4–15.

Passman MA, Moneta GL, Nehler MR, et al. Do normal early color-flow duplex surveillance examination results of infrainguinal vein grafts preclude the need for late graft revision? J Vasc Surg. 1995; 22: 476–81.

Polak JF. Peripheral arterial disease. Evaluation with color flow and duplex sonography. Radiol Clin North Am. 1995; 33: 71–90.

Polak JF. Peripheral vascular sonography. Baltimore: Williams & Wilkins; 1992.

Ranke C, Creutzing A, Alexander K. Duplex scanning of the peripheral arteries: correlation of the peak velocity ratio with angiographic diameter reduction. Ultrasound Med Biol. 1992; 18: 433–40.

Rothwell PM, et al. Prediction of benefit from carotid endarterectomy in individual patients: a risk-modelling study. Lancet. 1999; 353: 2105–10.

Westerband A, Mills JL, Kistler S, Berman SS, Hunter GC, Marek JM. Prospective validation of threshold criteria for intervention in infrainguinal vein grafts undergoing duplex surveillance. Ann Vasc Surg. 1997; 11: 44–8.

Whelan JF, Barry MH, Moir JD. Color flow Doppler ultrasonography: comparison with peripheral arteriography for the investigation of peripheral vascular disease. J Clin Ultrasound. 1992; 20: 369–74.

Wolf KJ, Fobbe F. Farbkodierte Duplexsonographie. Stuttgart: Thieme; 1993.

Yock PG, Fitzgerald PJ. Intravascular ultrasound: state of the art and future directions. Am J Cardiol. 1998; 81: 27–32.

16 Sonography of the Kidney, Liver, and Pancreas Transplant

H. Lang, R. Lück, A. Weimann, A. Weimann

Kidney Transplantation

Basic Facts

- In 2005, 2712 kidneys were transplanted in Germany, of which 522 were from living-related donors (Deutsche Stiftung Organtransplantation [German Foundation of Organ Transplantation: www.dso.de]).
- **Surgical technique:** The donor organ is implanted into the iliac fossa, except for very small recipients for whom retroperitoneal transplantation (usually on the right) is carried out; in selected cases also within the peritoneal cavity.
- Most commonly, vascular supply is created from an end-to-side anastomosis of the donor artery and vein to the external iliac artery and vein, respectively (Fig. 16.**1**).
- Exception: Very small recipients → abdominal aorta and inferior vena cava.
- The donor ureter is implanted into the urinary bladder, except that if the donor ureter is ischemic or too short the recipient ureter may be used as conduit into bladder; this is also a possible option in case of postoperative necrosis of the donor ureter.
- Recommended **sonographic views**: sagittal and transverse scans through the transplant, in practice along the skin incision (scar) and orthogonal to it → renal transplant with vessels easily delineated even in obesity. The view of the ureter is mostly obstructed by bowel gas. Assessment of lesser pelvis → perigraft masses, changes in urinary bladder, psoas hemorrhage.
- **Recommendation:** immediate postoperative sonography, including Duplex analysis, for baseline documentation → sonographic follow-up every 3–4 days even if the transplant functions well.
- CFDI permits easy differentiation between vessels and fluid collections.
- Based on peak systolic and end-diastolic flow velocities (PSV and EDV), the resistance index (RI) is calculated as: RI = (PSV – EDV)/PSV → diagnostic value in suspected rejection is controversial (biopsy mandatory). Additional information through use of microbubbles for contrast enhancement.
- *Additional workup:* renal scintigraphy if sonographic assessment is not sufficient (extreme obesity, extensive healing by second intention) or equivocal → assessment of perfusion and function, detection of urine leak; biopsy (always US guided) → rejection; DSA → arterial stenosis.

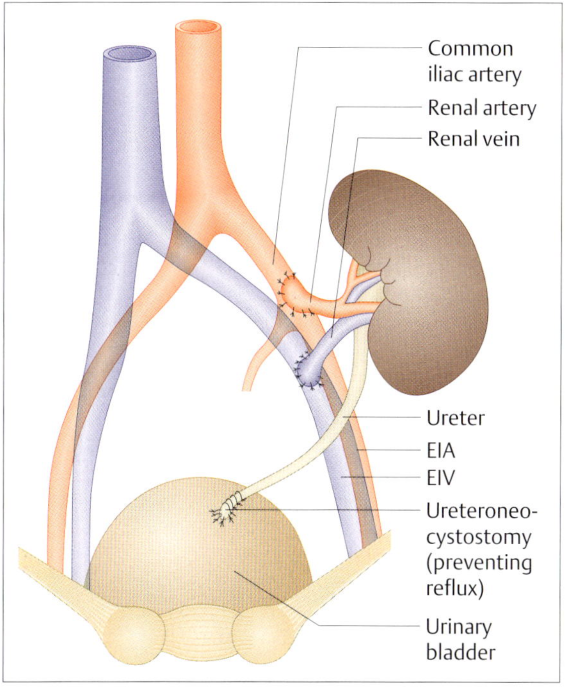

Fig. 16.**1** Kidney transplantation: typical anastomoses. EIA = external iliac artery; EIV = external iliac vein.

Sonographic Criteria of Assessment

- **Hypertrophy** and mild to moderate pelvocaliectasis as in hydronephrosis grades I and II is common (caused by denervation of the pelvocaliceal system; initially often increased diuresis in a well-functioning transplant)
- Evaluation of **shape** (regular), **echotexture** (homogeneous), **pelvocaliceal system**, arterial and venous **perfusion** (follow arterial flow into interlobar arteries). Assessment of surrounding tissue: localized fluid collection (hematoma, urinoma, seroma, lymphocele), free fluid, evaluation of urinary bladder (Figs. 16.**2**–16.**6**).
- **Caveat:** Arterial oscillation = flow reversal during diastole in impaired venous run-off → e.g., kinking or thrombosis of the renal graft vein (Fig. 16.**7**).
- High RI > 0.85, particularly if increasing over time, signals change flow profile due to parenchymal changes, e.g., in rejection.
- In old transplants, **cortical** hyperechogenicity may indicate chronic rejection → no increase in RI.

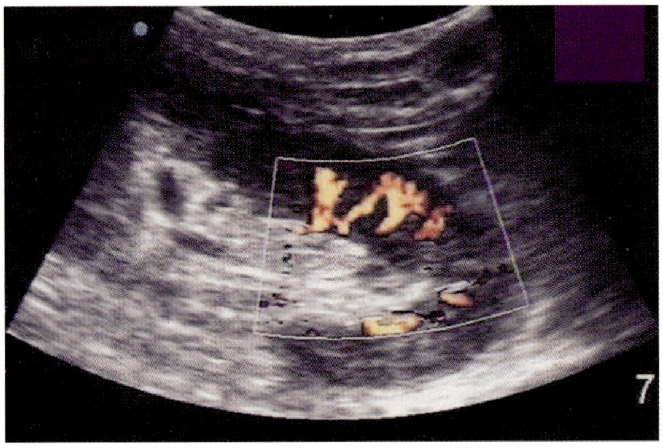

Fig. 16.**2a** Normal transplant parenchyma with confirmed perfusion on power Doppler imaging.

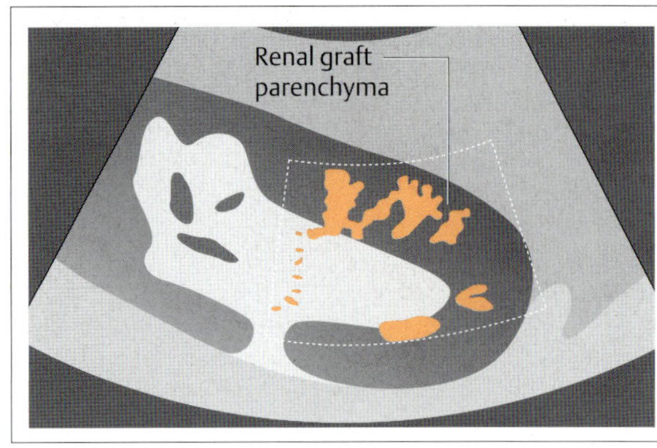

Fig. 16.**2b** Line drawing.

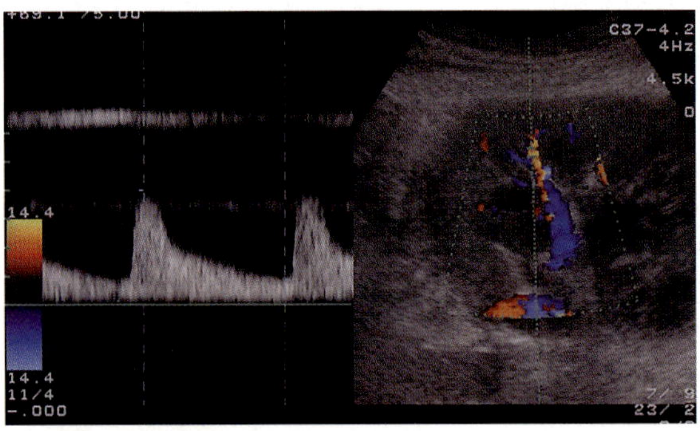

Fig. 16.**3a** Kidney transplant in right iliac fossa; homogeneous parenchyma with interlobar artery and Doppler waveform–normal finding: V_{max} 40 cm/s; V_{min} 9 cm/s, and RI = 0.78.

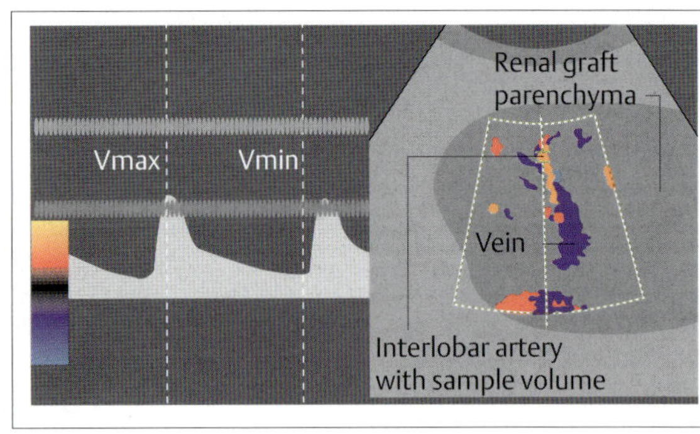

Fig. 16.**3b** Line drawing.

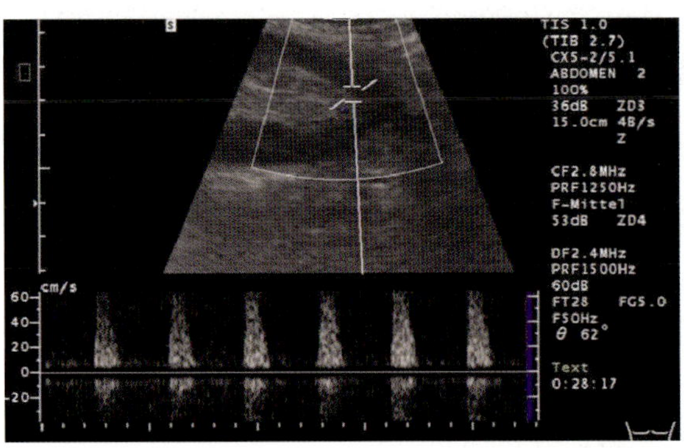

Fig. 16.**4a** Kidney transplant with RI rising to around 1.0 over time, signaling parenchymal damage. DD: rejection, calcineurin inhibitor (CNI) toxicity.

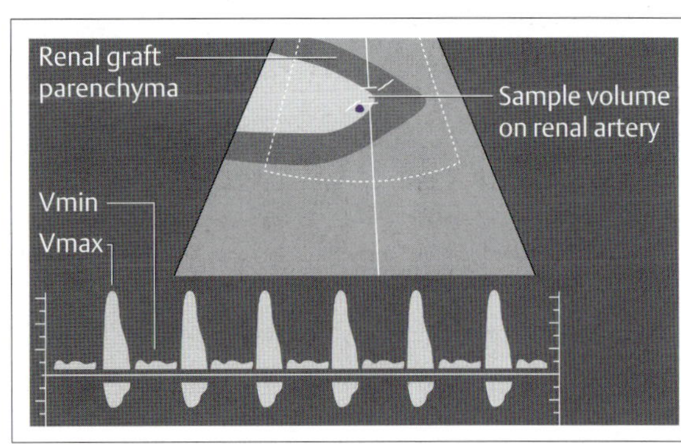

Fig. 16.**4b** Line drawing.

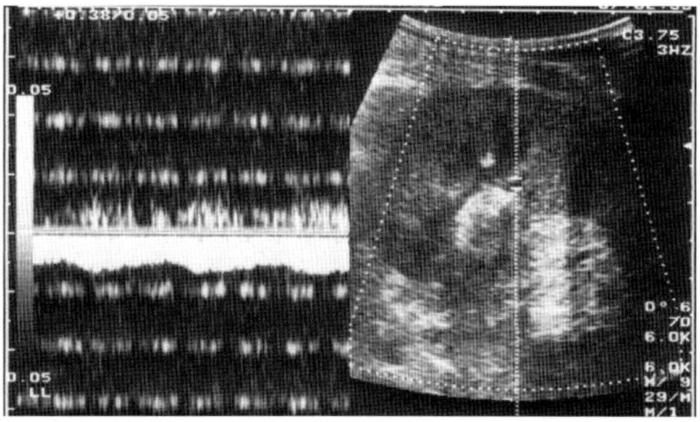

Fig. 16.5 a Normal monophasic venous signal of a renal transplant, with no variation on respiration.

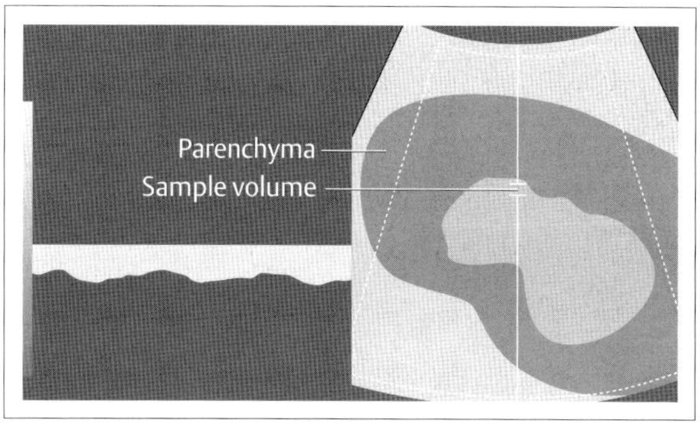

Fig. 16.5 b Line drawing.

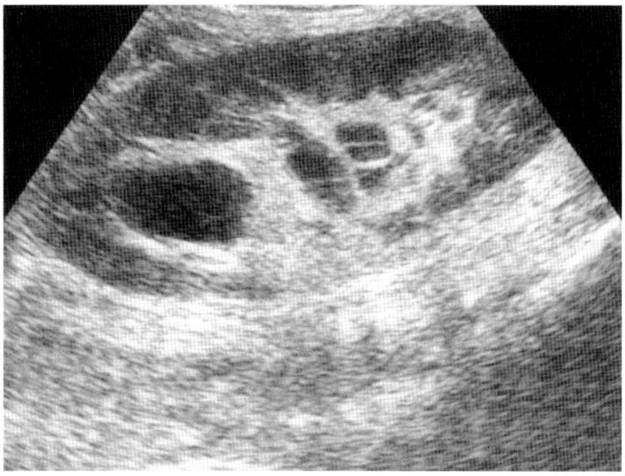

Fig. 16.6 a Dilated renal pelvis with suspected stenosis of the ureteroneocystostomy.

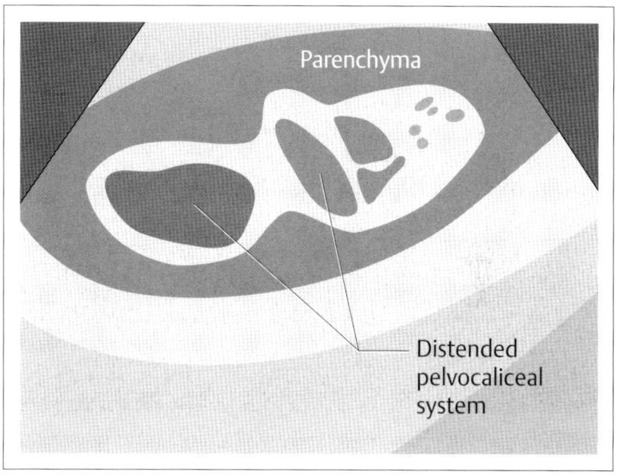

Fig. 16.6 b Line drawing.

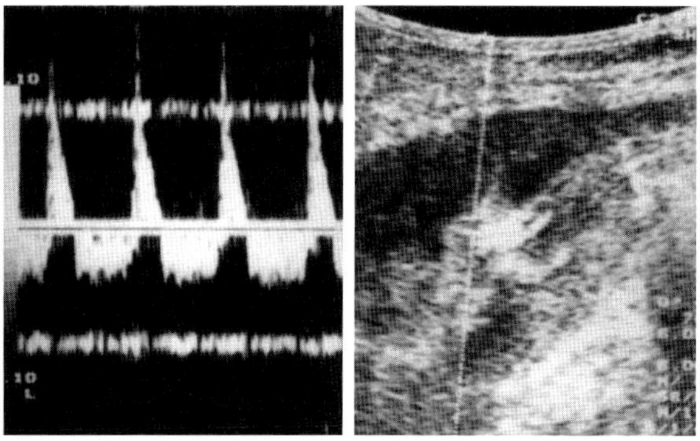

Fig. 16.7 a Arterial oscillation (diastolic flow reversal) in occlusive renal vein thrombosis of the transplant.

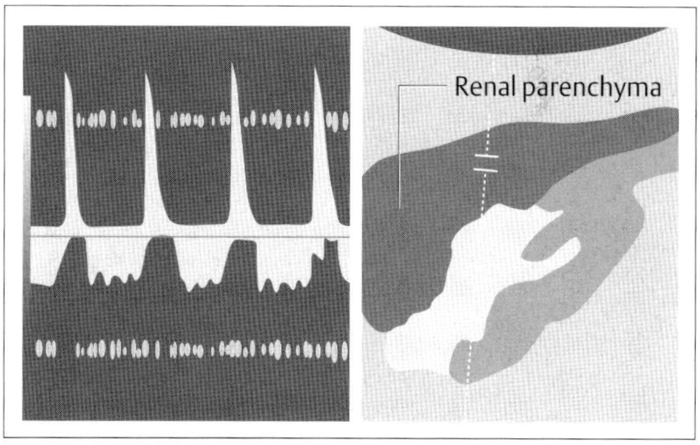

Fig. 16.7 b Line drawing.

Consequences for Surgical Treatment

Diagnosis	Characteristic Findings	Management
Early postoperative phase		
Difficult vascular anastomoses	Immediately post-Tx oscillating arterial flow or no arterial signal	Immediate reoperation
No urine output	Vessels OK, bladder full, hyperechoic structure–suggestive of bladder tamponade	Check urine catheter, bladder irrigation
No urine output	Vessels OK, bladder empty	Suggestive of initially nonfunctional graft; watchful waiting
No urine output	Oscillating arterial flow	Impaired venous run-off–possible thrombosis of graft vein, immediate reoperation
Decreased urine output, elevated serum creatinine level	Vessels open, RI > 0.9, renal pelvis not dilated	Suspected rejection, US-guided biopsy, further management depending on histology
Decreased urine output, elevated serum creatinine level	Dilated renal pelvis and ureter:	
	(a) Free fluid → suspected lymphocele	(a) Aspiration/possibly pigtail catheterization, most often surgery with fenestration of lymphocele necessary
	(b) No free fluid → suspected ureteral stenosis	(b) Possibly surgery
Hematuria	Bladder with hyperechoic mass–suspected tamponade; bladder empty–suspected hemorrhage from pelvocaliceal system or ureter	Irrigation, observation, possibly reoperation
Decreased urine output	Free fluid	Suspected urine leak, aspiration, potassium/creatinine level, possibly renal scintigraphy, possibly reoperation
Late postoperative phase		
Elevated serum creatinine level	No suspicious findings, vessels open, significant increase in RI	Suspected toxicity of calcineurin inhibitors (CNI), change of immunosuppressive regimen
Elevated serum creatinine level	Turbulent arterial flow signal at anastomosis, accelerated flow, aliasing	Suspected arterial stenosis, DSA to clarify possible intervention
Elevated serum creatinine level (possible swelling of ipsilateral lower limb)	Liquid mass at transplant bed	Suspected lymphocele (DD: hematoma, urinoma), possibly aspiration, surgery with fenestration of lymphocele

Liver Transplantation

Basic Facts

- In 2005, 976 livers were transplanted in Germany, of which 88 were from living-related donors (Deutsche Stiftung Organtransplantation [German Foundation of Organ Transplantation: www.dso.de]), the latter rate being on the rise in some centers; one-year patient survival rate is 80–90%.
- The liver is viewed from below and between the ribs; Doppler analysis of the hepatic portal is best carried out from a right intercostal view.
- **Caveat:**
  • Whole liver transplant (orthotopic position) or reduced-size graft (part of a donor liver),
  • Split liver transplant (SLT) (liver divided and transplanted into two recipients)
  • Auxiliary transplant (transplantation of whole/partial liver without [or possibly just partial] removal of recipient's own liver; rather rare indication, usually only in fulminant liver failure or metabolic disorder
- *Location and number of vascular anastomoses:* In orthotopic LTx, usually end-to-end anastomoses of the suprahepatic and infrahepatic inferior vena cava and portal vein of the donor and recipient are performed (except in piggy-back transplants, where the recipient vena cava is left undisturbed and only the hepatic veins are anastomosed). Arterial anastomoses are more varied: Besides the common anatomical variants of the arterial tree (accessory hepatic arteries originating from the superior mesenteric or left gastric artery), pathological changes (e.g., stenosis of the celiac trunk) may also influence the choice of anastomosis (surgical report, consult surgeon!).
- Donor and recipient common bile duct are usually anastomosed in end-to-end fashion (or donor duct with Roux-en-Y loop of upper jejunum) (Fig. 16.**8**).
- After routine cholecystectomy the gall bladder is always missing–long cystic duct remnant can, however, dilate and mimic the presence of the gallbladder.
- Rate of arterial complications is 12% (higher in pediatric patients); portal vein thrombosis 7%.
- Rate of biliary complications post-LTx is about 10%: arterial malperfusion (bile duct supply exclusively via the hepatic artery!), rejection, or technical problems (biliary stricture or leak).
- *Pre*-LTx: (Doppler) Sonographic assessment for: hepatic parenchyma (tumor?); vascular anatomy; particularly flow direction in portal vein (orthograde, retrograde, or total occlusion; in case of retrograde flow always consider possible portocaval shunts. **Caveat**: Portal vein thrombosis may impact on surgical approach); status of suprahepatic vena cava in Budd–Chiari syndrome; shunt function (e.g., after TIPSS).

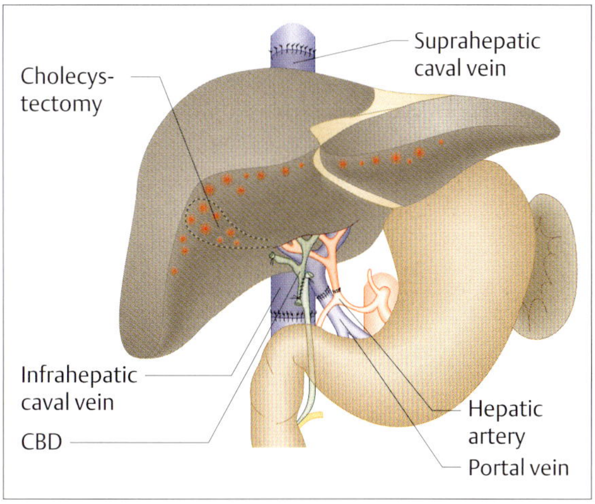

Fig. 16.**8** Liver transplantation: typical anastomoses.

- *Post*-LTx: Immediate postoperative Doppler analysis for vascular baseline status. *Recommendation:* Daily follow-up throughout the first week, then twice a week, and later at each outpatient follow-up, if possible. Doppler imaging plays a central role whenever hepatic function becomes impaired, particularly so during the early post-operative phase.
- Look for arterial signal not only at the hepatic portal but also within the liver (in both lobes!) (Fig. 16.**9**, 16.**10**), particularly if there are accessory hepatic arteries. Note: Even on Doppler investigation, the hepatic artery cannot always be outlined as a vascular structure.
- The arterial flow waveform may initially demonstrate little or no diastolic flow (due to high vascular resistance).
- Portal venous blood flow is hepatopetal, with little variation on respiration. Shortly after LTx, it is often higher than in normal livers (up to 40–60 cm/s).
- Spectral analysis of hepatic veins demonstrates characteristic bidirectional triphasic flow (due to reflux from the right atrium into the vena cava during systole).
- In addition to the resistive index RI, described in the preceding section on kidney transplantation, the damping index (DI) can be determined: DI = minimum flow velocity/peak flow velocity → evaluation of hepatic perfusion.
- Assessment for rejection with FNA/biopsy, as well as interventional drainage (for hematoma or bilioma), always under US guidance, ideally with Doppler imaging for identification of vessels: → breath holding, sonographic check for possible hemorrhage immediately post intervention and 4–6 h later; always check CBC!

- In **workup for rejection**, two paracentesis sites are possible: intercostal or subcostal in the medioclavicular line; **Caveat**: Intercostal FNA: pneumothorax, risk of hemorrhage from marked collaterals between the ribs and on diaphragm. For topographic reasons, subcostal FNA does not encompass the whole transplant. The preferred site in our institution is primarily intercostal FNA.
- *Additional workup:* US guided FNA/biopsy, contrast-enhanced spiral CT, MRI, angiography, ERCP, cholescintigraphy.
- *Specifics in special LTx techniques:*
  - "Reduced-size graft" LTx: Left lateral segments (particularly in children) and left lobe → right upper quadrant filled with loops of bowel, resection surface and Roux-en-Y loop of biliary anastomosis are at right edge of transplant.
  - Right lobe → no bowel shift, resection surface and Roux-en-Y loop are at left edge of transplant.
  - Auxiliary LTx: Most often left hepatic lobe → vascular anastomoses varied, frequently with left recipient vessels, Roux-en-Y loop. **Caveat:** Auxiliary LTx carries higher risk of vascular complications. Important consideration: evaluation of recipient hepatic function over time (homogeneous parenchyma? necrosis?).

Sonographic Criteria of Assessment

- Evaluation of homogeneity of parenchymal echotexture, of bile duct diameter, and of hepatic perfusion.
- Portal triads are often pronounced (usually without pathological significance, normalization within a few weeks); biliary tree is also pronounced postoperatively.
- Strength of sonography: localized parenchymal changes. Weakness of sonography: diffuse changes (domain of FNA!).
- Parenchymal condensation in fatty changes → often sequela of ischemia/reperfusion injury.
- Hypoechoic intrahepatic areas: hematoma, necrosis (gridlike structure), abscess, biloma.
- Hypoechoic perihepatic areas: ascites, hematoma, abscess, seroma, bile leak, or lymphocele (Figs. 16.**13**–16.**16**).
- In arterial stenosis: turbulent arterial flow signal and accelerated flow (aliasing) at the porta hepatica (Fig. 16.**17**).
- Complete absence of Doppler signals in the early postoperative phase is an indication for emergency angiography and/or laparotomy (preferably before clinical manifestation). Severe parenchymal damage (e.g., major reperfusion injury) may occasionally present with RI > 1.0, but this does not indicate a higher incidence of arterial thrombosis.
- Parenchymal damage (acute rejection or severe reperfusion injury) will attenuate the hepatic vein signal (damping) (Fig. 16.**18**).
- Secondary attenuation of the hepatic vein signal, possibly in combination with increasing RI in the hepatic artery, raises suspicion of rejection, but in our own experience FNA or biopsy is always mandatory for confirmation.
- **Caveat:** Oscillating arterial flow or lack of diastolic flow is not an indicator of impaired venous run-off.
- In ascites: Determine flow direction and velocity in portal vein (always rule out portal vein thrombosis). In poor portal vein flow (thrombosis) there is often unusually easy detection of arterial signals, particularly of the intrahepatic arteries (Fig. 16.**19**).

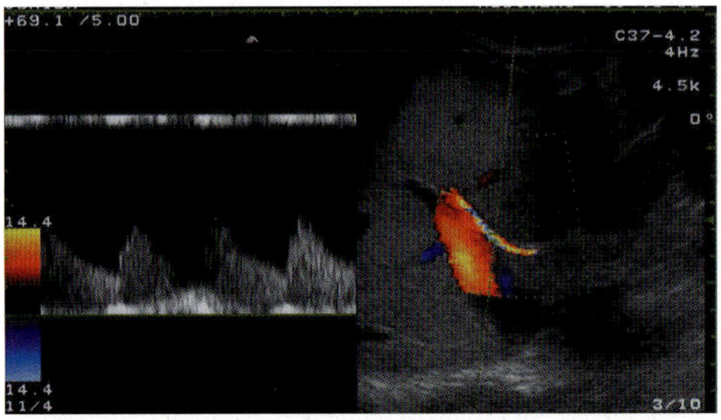

Fig. 16.**9a** Normal arterial signal alongside the portal vein in a liver transplant–the artery appears as a vascular structure.

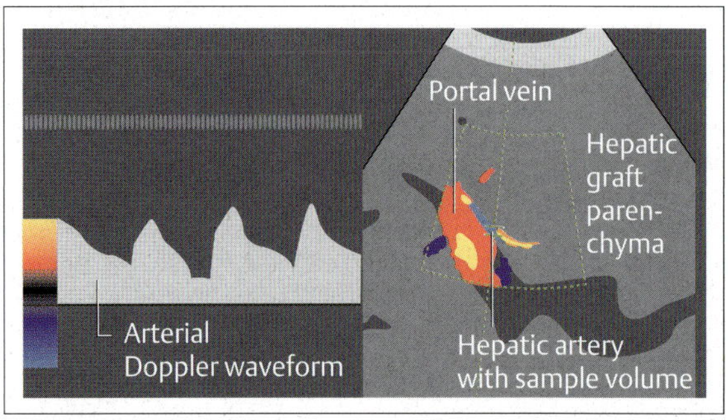

Fig. 16.**9b** Line drawing.

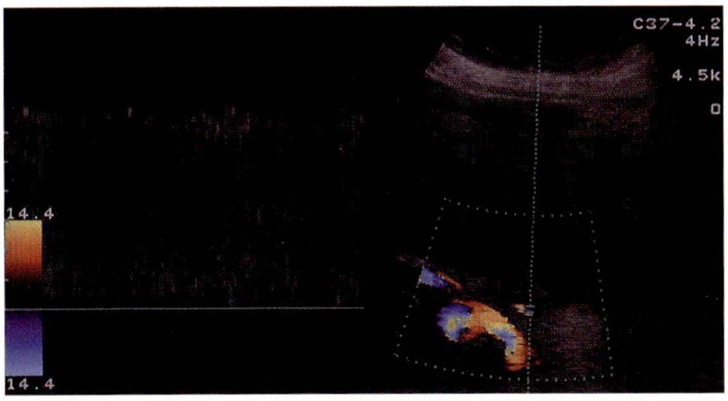

Fig. 16.**10 a** Normal arterial signal alongside the portal vein in a liver transplant–the artery cannot be delineated as a vascular structure.

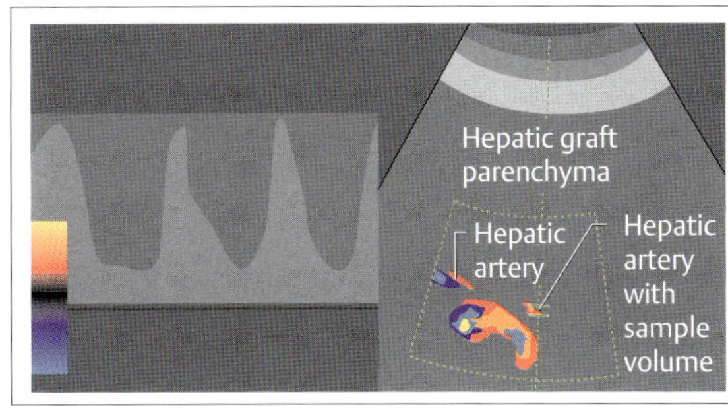

Fig. 16.**10 b** Line drawing.

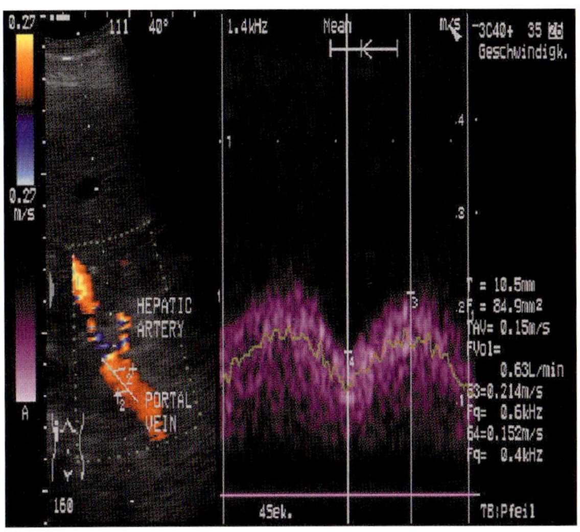

Fig. 16.**11 a** Normal portal vein signal in a liver transplant–flow rate 0.63 l/min.

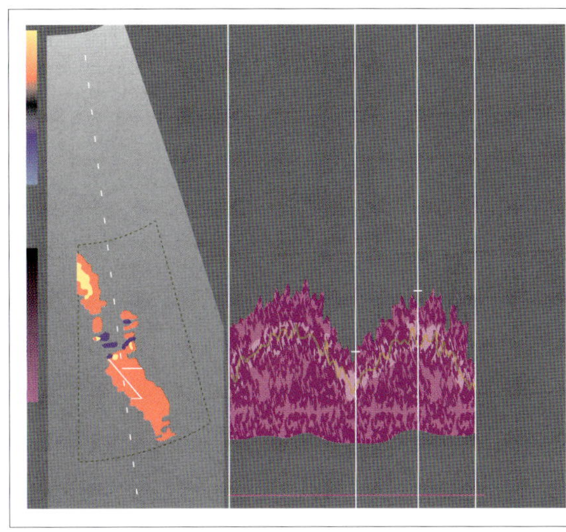

Fig. 16.**11 b** Line drawing.

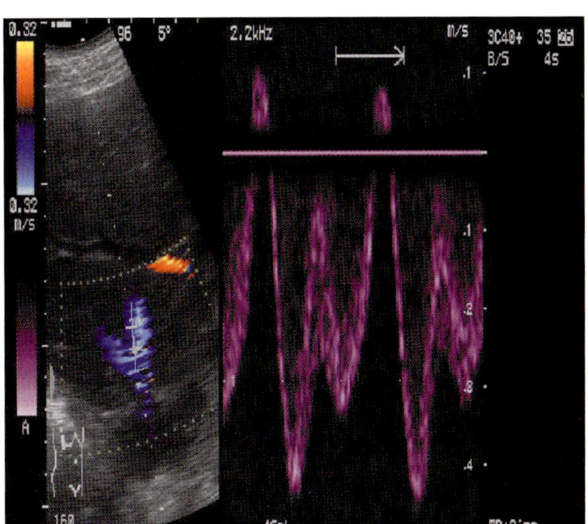

Fig. 16.**12 a** Normal triphasic Doppler waveform of the hepatic veins in a liver transplant.

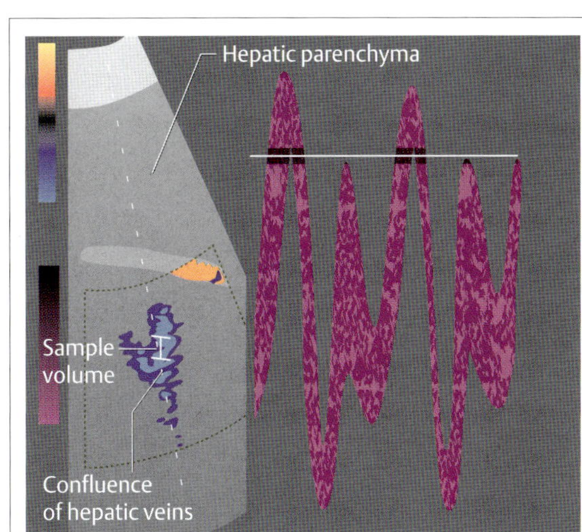

Fig. 16.**12 b** Line drawing.

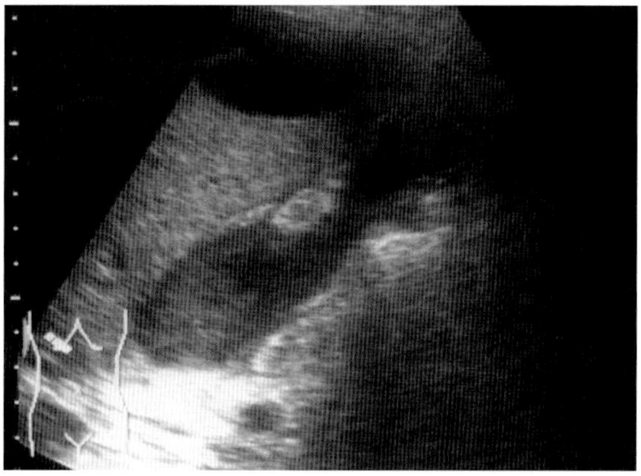

Fig. 16.**13 a** Hypoechoic (liquid) mass at the edge of the liver–FNA confirmed the suspected bilioma.

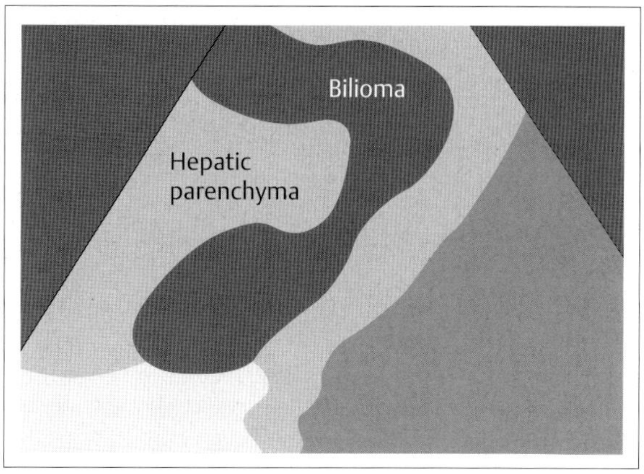

Fig. 16.**13 b** Line drawing.

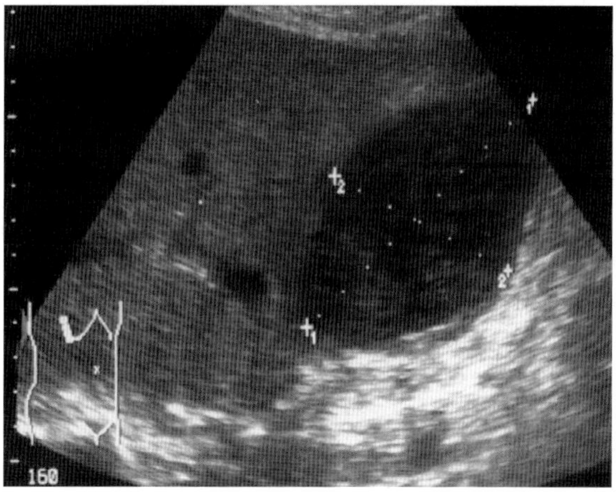

Fig. 16.**14 a** Hypoechoic (liquid) mass at the edge of the liver–FNA confirmed the clinically suspected abscess.

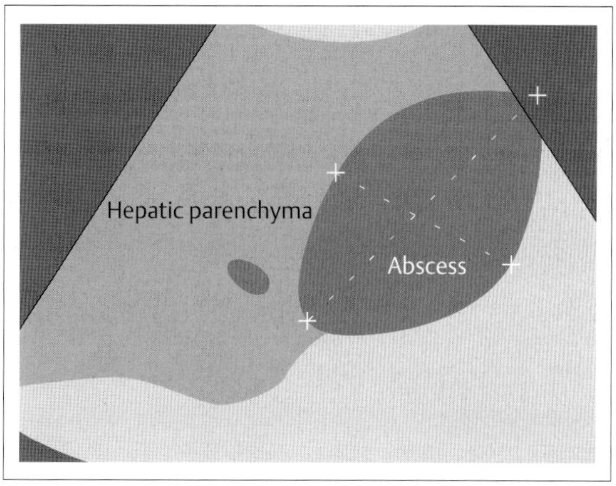

Fig. 16.**14 b** Line drawing.

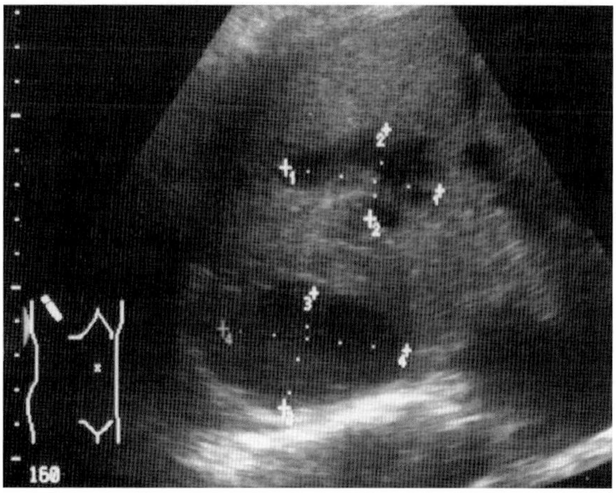

Fig. 16.**15 a** Hypoechoic (liquid) intrahepatic mass, confirmed as liquefaction necrosis.

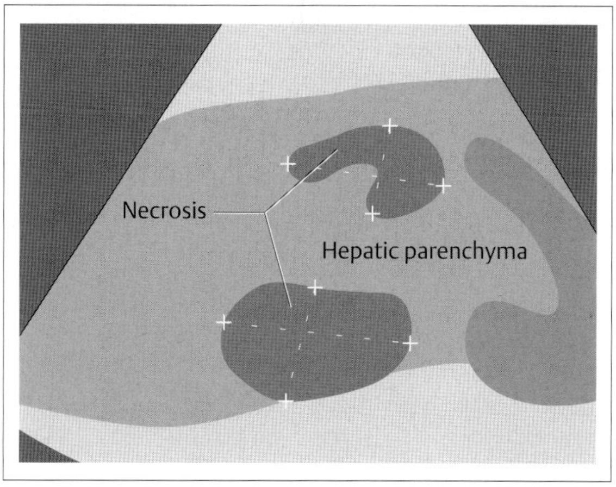

Fig. 16.**15 b** Line drawing.

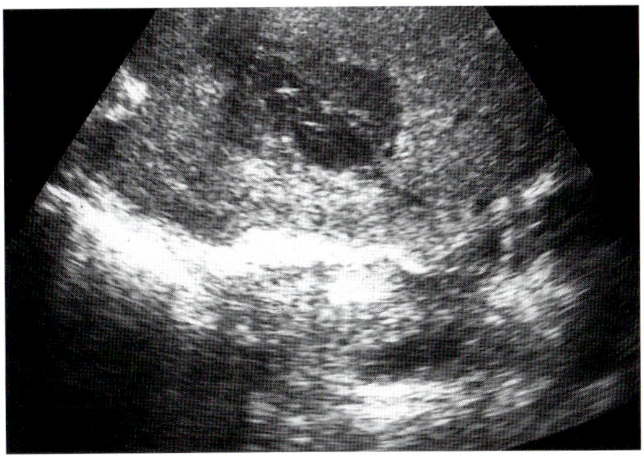

Fig. 16.**16 a** Hypoechoic (liquid) intrahepatic mass; organized hematoma on biopsy.

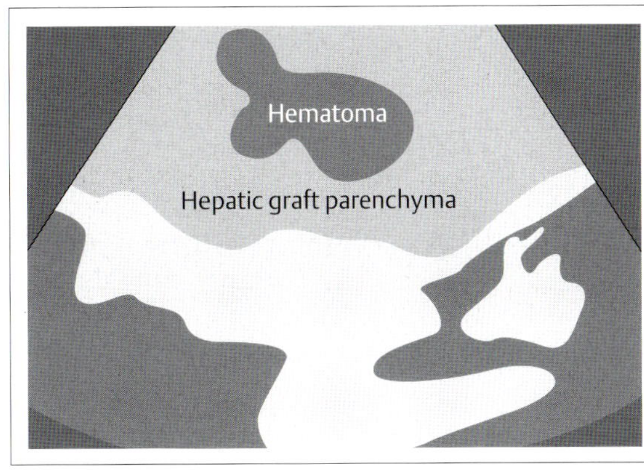

Fig. 16.**16 b** Line drawing.

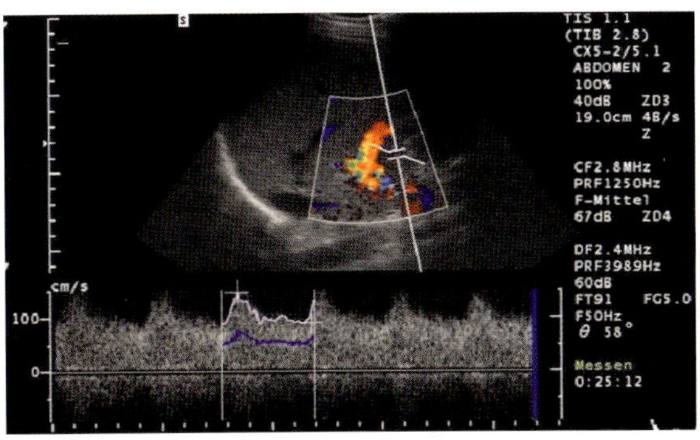

Fig. 16.**17 a** Suspected stenosis of the donor hepatic artery with accelerated prestenotic flow.

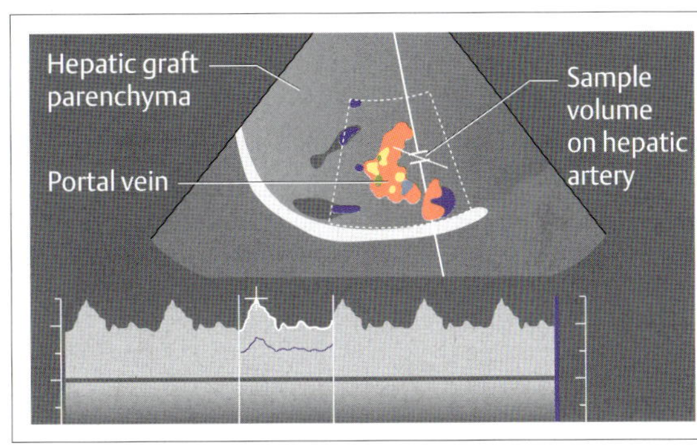

Fig. 16.**17 b** Line drawing.

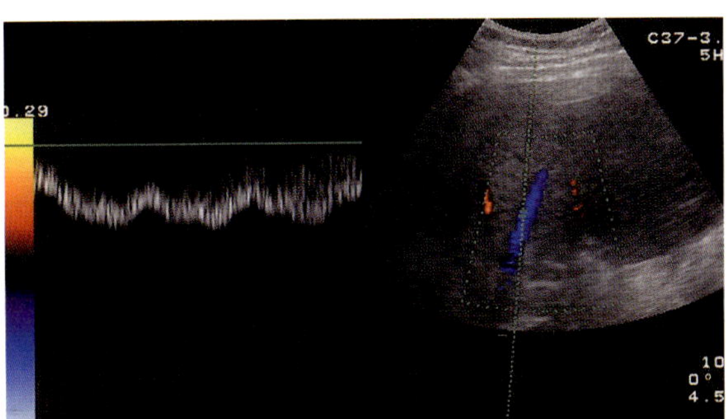

Fig. 16.**18 a** Attenuated signal of the hepatic vein on day 1 post-LTx–marked edematous swelling of the liver due to ischemia/reperfusion injury.

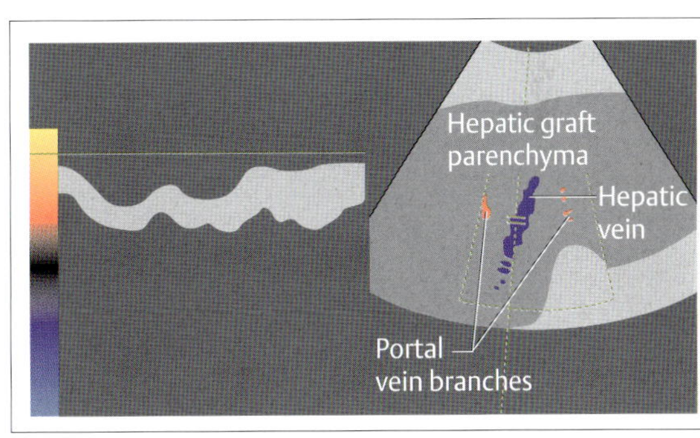

Fig. 16.**18 b** Line drawing.

Consequences for Surgical Treatment

Diagnosis	Characteristic Findings	Management
Early postoperative phase		
Marked transaminase elevation (> 1000 U/l), coagulation factor substitution, absence of bile production, elevated serum lactate level	Vessels open, condensed parenchyma, attenuated hepatic vein signal, intrahepatic biliary tree not distended	Differential diagnosis: Reperfusion injury or initially nonfunctional graft, watchful waiting for the indication of retransplantation
Masked elevation of transaminase levels including GLDH	No arterial signal visible	If initially present, suggestive of arterial occlusion; consider DSA or immediate reoperation
Drop in Hb	Free fluid around liver and elsewhere in abdomen	Suggestive of hemorrhage; FNA for DD of ascites; possibly reoperation if hemorrhagic
Secondary elevation of transaminase levels	Liver with hypoechoic area (gridlike texture), artery open	Suggestive of liver necrosis; CT; reoperation rarely required
Elevated transaminase levels, increased ascites, serum lactate level may be elevated	No portal vein signal, easy demonstration of intrahepatic arterial signals	Suggestive of portal vein thrombosis, possibly reoperation
Elevated body temperature, elevated transaminase levels	Vessels open, condensed parenchyma, attenuated hepatic vein signal	Suspected rejection: FNA or biopsy
Treatment of rejection	If responding, the attenuated and possibly monophasic hepatic vein signal becomes increasingly bidirectional	Possibly FNA/biopsy for follow-up
Elevated body temperature, AP, GGT, and bilirubin elevated (cholestasis)	Intrahepatic biliary tree prominent or distended	Suspected cholangitis, antibiotics. Consider: stenotic bile duct anastomosis; possibly ERCP to decide on stent/reoperation
Elevated bilirubin, liver enzyme levels normal or barely elevated	Intrahepatic biliary tree normal or slightly prominent, artery open, accelerated hilar flow (aliasing)	Suggestive of bile duct ischemia in arterial stenosis; DSA; possibly reoperation
Late postoperative phase		
Routine outpatient follow-up, normal blood chemistry	Artery open, accelerated hilar flow (aliasing), turbulence	Suspected arterial stenosis, follow-up, DSA to clarify possible intervention
Recurrent elevated temperature, elevated AP, GGT, and bilirubin levels (cholestasis), jaundice	(a) Biliary tree distended (b) Condensed parenchymal texture, biliary tree not distended but rarefied on the whole	(a) suspected chronic recurrent cholangitis, possibly ERCP to rule out bile duct stenosis (b) Consider vanishing bile duct syndrome: biopsy if chronic rejection is suspected

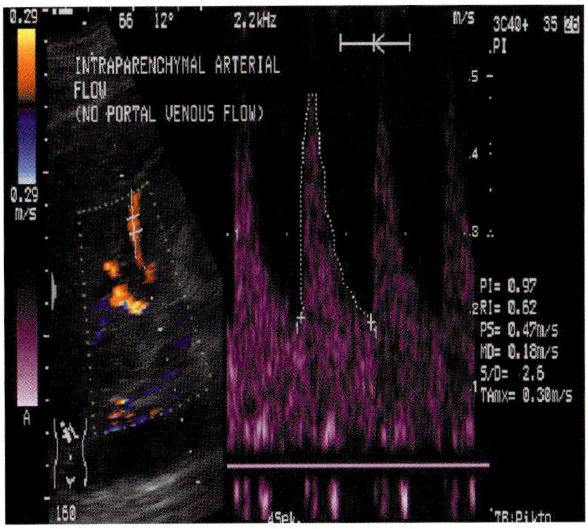

Fig. 16.**19a** Unusually prominent intrahepatic arterial Doppler signal and lack of portal vein signal secondary to portal vein thrombosis.

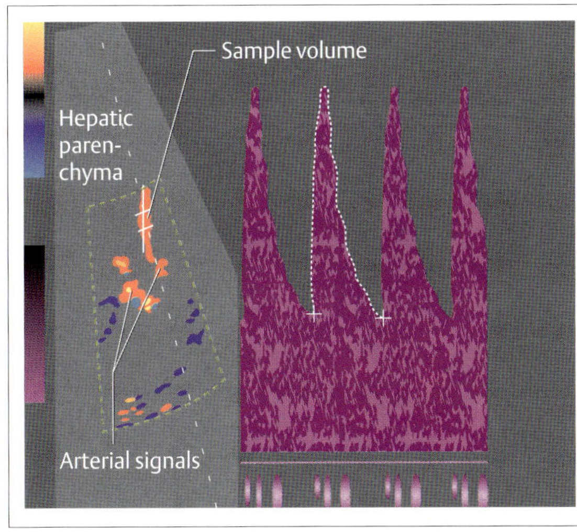

Fig. 16.**19b** Line drawing.

Pancreas Transplantation

Basic Facts

- In 2005, 165 pancreatic transplantations were performed in Germany, mostly combined with a renal graft (Deutsche Stiftung Organtransplantation [German Foundation of Organ Transplantation: www.dso.de]).
- Indication: insulin-dependent diabetes mellitus. Since the underlying disease frequently results in ESRD, simultaneous grafting of pancreas and kidney from the same donor has proved more favorable immunologically than pancreas transplantation alone.
- Monitoring for rejection is often easier in the kidney, as rejection affects both organs in > 80% of cases; diagnosis is simple if serum creatinine is elevated, clinical signs of rejection occur earlier in the kidney, and diagnostic workup for renal rejection is easier via low-risk biopsy.
- *Surgical technique:* Previously, for exocrine pancreatic drainage the donor duodenum was anastomosed to the urinary bladder (Fig. 16.**20b**), with monitoring of urine amylase (drop) as a marker of renal function (rejection). A drawback is significant bicarbonate loss.
  - Today, for exocrine drainage the donor duodenum is anastomosed to a Roux-en-Y loop of jejunum (Fig. 16.**20a**) or even directly to the second jejunal loop.
  - Arterial and venous anastomoses are mostly to the iliac vessels (Fig. 16.**20a**), the venous limb is possibly also anastomosed to the superior mesenteric vein. Often complex vascular reconstruction is required: request precise information from the surgeon.
- If drainage is into the urinary bladder, the bladder should be full for ultrasound in order to distend the duodenal segment and displace the bowel loops cephalad.
- Particularly in long-term follow-up, delineation of the pancreas graft from the surrounding loops of bowel may be difficult–look for peristalsis.
- Vessels can usually be pursued well into the organ periphery.
- *Recommendation:* Immediate postoperative Doppler analysis for baseline status of vessels and blood flow.
- Even if rejection is suspected, biopsy of the pancreas is not recommended due to possible bleeding, pancreatitis, and pancreatic fistula formation.
- In exocrine pancreatic drainage via the urinary bladder, organ function may be monitored via the urine amylase level.
- Vascular problems mainly involve the donor vein → thrombosis.
- *Additional workup:* amylase (serum and possibly urine), blood sugar and required insulin substitution, procalcitonin, spiral CT; MRI is increasingly becoming the standard imaging modality for follow-up of organ perfusion; possibly DSA.

Sonographic Criteria of Assessment

- Transplant more likely to be hyperechoic (Fig. 16.**21**–16.**23**).
- Transplant pancreatitis echomorphology is similar to that of general pancreatitis (edema, swelling, altered echotexture, less distinct margin).
- Organ texture: homogeneous bloating of edematous swollen organ, hypoechoic areas in early necrosis.
- Consideration of peripancreatic processes: free fluid indicating hemorrhage or pancreatitis, liquid mass signaling pseudocyst, hematoma, seroma, abscess, lymphocele
- Resistive index (RI): RI > 0.75 is suggestive of rejection; RI < 0.7 suggests acute pancreatitis or toxicity of immunosuppressive drugs.

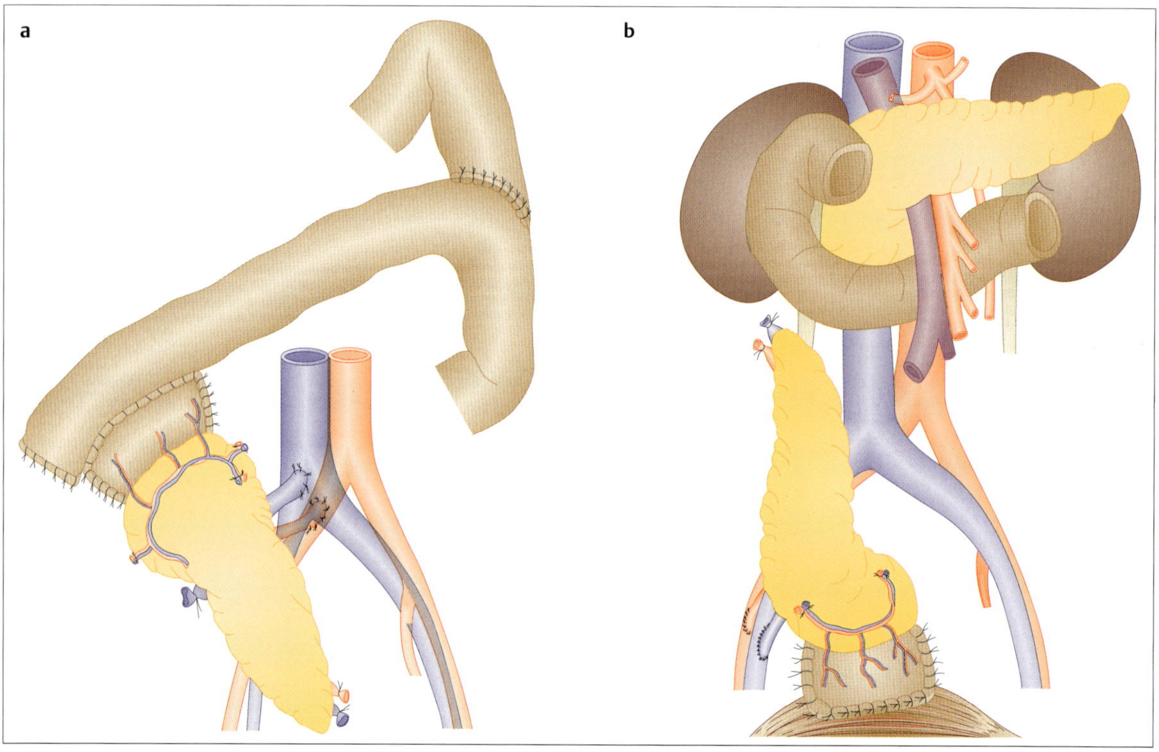

Fig. 16.**20 a** Pancreas transplantation: exocrine drainage into Roux-en-Y loop of jejunum.

Fig. 16.**20 b** Exocrine drainage into urinary bladder.

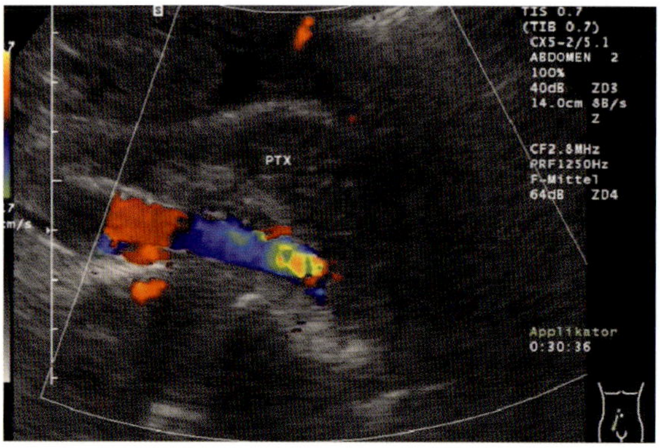

Fig. 16.**21 a** Pancreas transplant (PTX) in right iliac fossa.

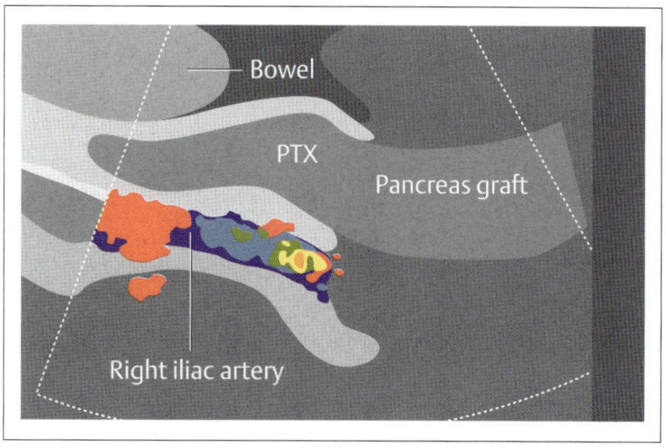

Fig. 16.**21 b** Line drawing.

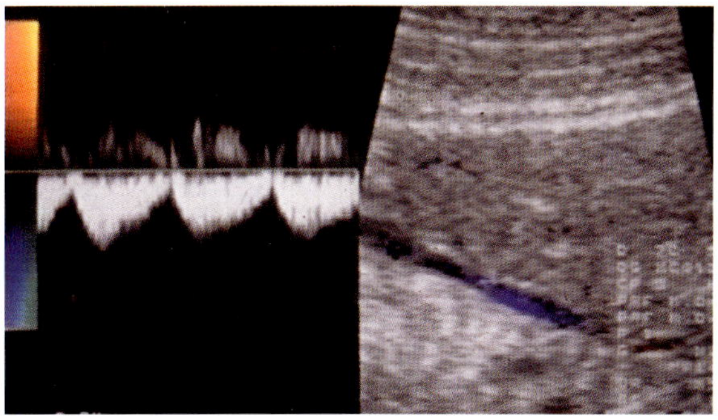

Fig. 16.22a Normal venous flow signal after pancreas transplantation.

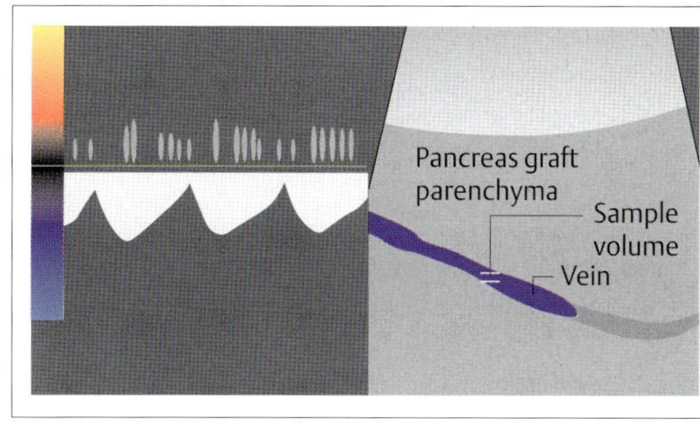

Fig. 16.22b Line drawing.

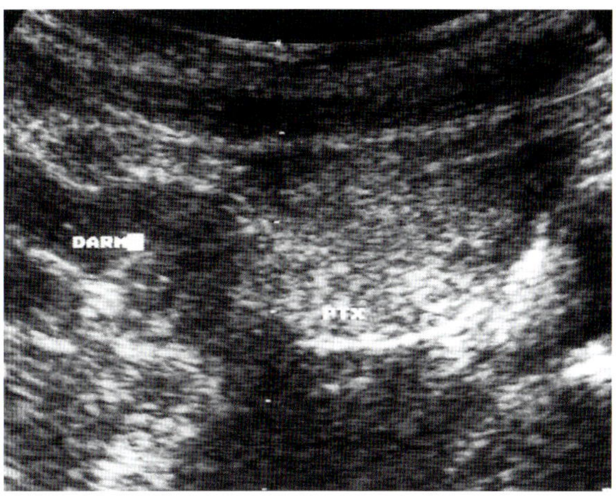

Fig. 16.23a Well-functioning pancreas transplant (PTX) with jejunal anastomosis eight years post transplantation, difficult to delineate from the surrounding loops of small bowel (DARM).

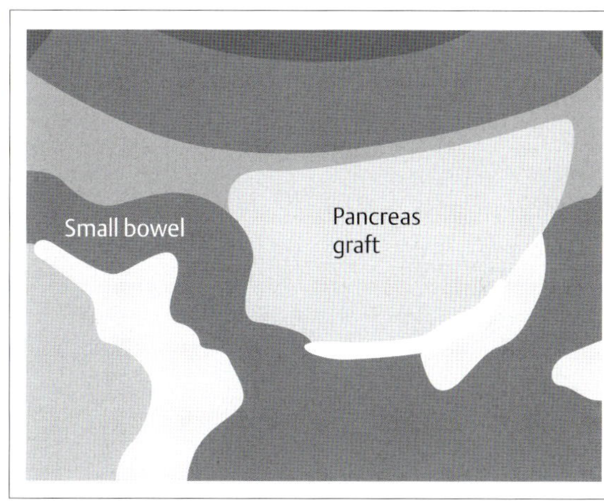

Fig. 16.23b Line drawing.

Bibliography

Ball CG, Kirkpatrick AW, Yilmaz S, Monroy M, Nicolaou S, Salazar A. Renal allograft compartment syndrome: an underappreciated postoperative transplantation. Am J Surg. 2006; 191: 619–24.

Berrocal T, Parron M, Alvarez-Luque A, Prieto C, Santamaria ML. Pediatric liver transplantation: a pictorial essay of early and late complications. Radiographics 2006; 26: 1187–209.

Breitenseher M, Helbich T, Kainberger F, et al. Farbdopplersonographie von Nierentransplantaten. Ermöglicht der Resistive Index die Diagnose der chronischen Funktionsstörung? Ultraschall Med. 1994; 15: 24–8.

Casalino DD, Winsberg F. Doppler ultrasonography in liver transplantation. In: Gandolfi L, Fukuda M, eds. Current Trends in Digestive Ultrasonography. Front. Gastrointest. Res. Basel: Karger; 1997: 305–22.

Chang JM, Lee JM, Suh KS, et al. Biliary complications in living donor liver transplantation: imaging findings and the role of interventional procedures. Cardiovasc Intervent Radiol. 2005; 28: 756–7.

Coulden RA, Britton PD, Farman P, Noble-Jamison G, Wight DGD. Preliminary report: hepatic vein Doppler in the early diagnosis of acute liver transplant rejection. Lancet. 1990; 336: 273–5.

Duda SH, Erley CM, Huppert PE, Lauchart W, Risler T, Claussen CD. Posttransplant renal artery stenosis–outpatient intraarterial DSA versus color aided duplex Doppler sonography. Eur J Radiol. 1993; 16: 95–101.

Fobbe F. Transplantatniere. In: Wolf KJ, Fobbe F, eds. Farbkodierte Duplexsonographie: Grundlagen und klinische Anwendung. Stuttgart: Thieme; 1993: 186–94.

Friedewald SM, Molmenti EP, Friedewald JJ, Dejong MR, Hamper UM. Vascular and nonvascular complications of renal transplants: sonographic evaluation and correlation with other imaging modalities, surgery, and pathology. J Clin Ultrasound 2005; 33: 127–39.

Galanski M, Ringe B. Radiologische Diagnostik vor und nach Lebertransplantation. Radiologe. 1992; 241-7.

Goel MC, LaPerna L, Whitelaw S, Modlin CS, Flechner SM, Goldfarb DA. Current management of transplant renal artery stenosis: clinical utility of duplex Doppler sonography. Urology 2005; 66: 59–64.

Harms J, Chavan A, Ringe B, Galanski M, Pichlmayr R. Vascular complications in adult patients after orthotopic liver transplantation: role of color duplex sonography in the diagnosis and management of vascular complications. Bildgebung. 1994; 61: 14–9.

Consequences for Surgical Treatment

Diagnosis Early postoperative phase	Characteristic Findings	Management
Drop in Hb	Free perigraft fluid	Suggestive of hemorrhage, possibly reoperation
Fever, elevated serum amylase and lipase levels	Newly arising free perigraft fluid, liquid mass	Suggestive of pancreatitis (anastomotic leak?); in peripancreatic abscess possibly drainage, reoperation
Fever, maybe abdominal symptoms	(a) Edematous swelling of graft, no venous signal (b) Graft with hypoechoic areas, venous signal present	(a) Suggestive of donor vein thrombosis, immediate reoperation (b) Suggestive of pancreatic necrosis, possibly reoperation
Exocrine drainage into urinary bladder, hematuria	Urinary bladder with liquid mass of heterogeneous echogenicity	Intravesical hemorrhage, irrigation; check of graft and vessels always mandatory
Exocrine drainage into urinary bladder, urine amylase level dropping	Graft only edematous, vessels open, RI > 0.75	Suggestive of rejection, start antirejection treatment protocol
Suspected rejection	If responsive to antirejection treatment, RI will decrease over time	
Shock symptoms	Free intra-abdominal fluid	Suspected erosion of iliac artery → immediate reoperation

Hellinger A, Roll C, Stracke A, Erhard J, Eigler FW. Impact of colour Doppler sonography on detection of thrombosis of the hepatic artery and the portal vein after liver transplantation. Langenbecks Arch Chir. 1996; 381: 182–5.
Kaneko T, Sugimoto H, Hirota M, Kure S, Kiuchi T, Nakao A. Intrahepatic venous anastomosis formation of the right liver in living donor liver transplantation: evaluations by Doppler ultrasonography and pulse-inversion ultrasonography with Levovist. Surgery 2005; 138: 21–7.
Kock T, Slooff MJH, Thijn CJP, et al. Routine Doppler ultrasound for detection of clinically unsuspected vascular complications in the early postoperative phase after orthotopic liver transplantation. Transplant Int. 1998; 11: 272–6.
Lang H, Lück R, Weimann A, et al. Experience with color-coded duplex sonography after combined kidney/pancreas transplantation–preliminary results. Bildgebung. 1996; 63: 90–3.
Morton MJ, James EM, Wiesner RH, Krom RAF. Applications of duplex ultrasonography in the liver transplant patient. Mayo Clin Proc. 1990; 65: 360–72.
Nolten A, Sproat IA. Hepatic artery thrombosis after liver transplantation: temporal accuracy of diagnosis with Duplex US and the syndrome of impending thrombosis. Radiology 1996; 198: 553–9.
Preidler KW, Szolar D, Schreyer H, Ebner F, Kern R, Holzer H, Horina JH. Differentiation of delayed kidney graft function with gadolinium-DPTA-enhanced magnetic resonance imaging and Doppler ultrasound. Invest Radiol. 1996; 31: 364–71.
Rob PM, Jansen O, Richter V, Erbsloh-Moller B, Marienhoff N, Wiedemann G. Diagnosis of renal transplant failure by real-time and duplex Doppler sonography. Clin Invest. 1993; 71: 531–6.
Schwarz A, Gwinner W, Hiss M, Radermacher J, Mengel M, Haller H. Safety and adequacy of renal transplant protocol biopsies. Am J Transplant. 2005; 5: 1992–8.
Schwenger V, Korosoglou G, Hinkel UP, et al. Real-time contrast-enhanced sonography of renal transplant recipients predicts chronic allograft nephropathy. Am J Transplant. 2006; 6: 609–15.
Tublin ME, Dodd GD 3rd. Sonography of renal transplantation. Radiol Clin North Am. 1995; 33: 447–59.
Patel B, Wolverson MK, Mahanta B. Pancreatic transplant rejection: assessment with duplex ultrasound. Radiology 1989; 173: 131–5.
Pozniak MA. Ultrasound evaluation of the transplant liver, kidney and pancreas. In: McGahan JP, Goldberg BB, eds. Diagnostic Ultrasound: A Logical Approach. Philadelphia: Lippincott-Raven, 1998; 561–98.
Propeck PA, Scanlan KA. Reversed or absent hepatic arterial diastolic flow in liver transplants shown by Duplex sonography: a poor predictor of hepatic artery thrombosis. Am J Radiol. 1992; 159: 1199–201.
Rifkin MD, Needleman L, Pasto ME, et al. Evaluation of renal transplant rejection by duplex Doppler examination: value of resistive index. Am J Radiol. 1987; 148: 759–62.
Rode A, Ducerf C, Adham M, et al. Influence of systemic echodoppler artery survey on hepatic artery thrombosis after liver transplantation in adults. Transplant Int. 1998; 11(Suppl. 1): S292–5.

Acknowledgment

The authors would like to thank the following colleagues for their courteous support in compiling the images: Marco Dömland MD, Department of General and Transplant Surgery, Essen University Medical Center, and Jürgen Müller MD, Department of Diagnostic Radiology, both of the University of Leipzig.

17 Color-Flow Doppler Imaging of the Intra-abdominal Arteries

E. Wrenger

Technical Principles of Color-Flow Doppler Imaging (CFDI)

Color-Flow

- Brief pulses of ultrasound reflected from acoustic interfaces in the body are analyzed on their return at the transducer with regard to (a) time interval from transmission to reception, (b) amplitude, and (c) Doppler frequency shift relative to the transmission frequency. B-mode images are constructed from the time interval and amplitude information.
- If the reflecting interface (e.g., RBC agglomerates) is moving away with respect to the ultrasound beam emitted from the transducer, the frequency of the echo pulses received at the transducer will be lower than the transmission frequency. If the ultrasound waves are reflected by red blood cells moving toward the transducer, the frequency of the echo received will be higher than the transmission frequency (Doppler effect). The moving areas in the image are displayed in color, and by convention targets moving toward the transducer are displayed in red, while targets moving away will be colored blue. Slow-moving blood is depicted by saturated colors, while fast blood flow is displayed by brighter, less saturated colors.
- "Aliasing" is an artifact arising from ambiguity in the measurement of high Doppler frequency shifts. In color-flow Doppler display, aliasing results in a wraparound of the frequency color map from one flow direction to the opposite direction, passing through a transition of unsaturated color. If the pulse repetition frequency is set correctly, aliasing alone may signal an arterial stenosis (e.g., renal artery).
- Color-flow Doppler display is primarily used for locating and differentiating the various intra-abdominal vessels.

Duplex Imaging

- Duplex scanners combine real-time imaging with Doppler capability, with either the imaging transducer or a separate transducer used to collect continuous or pulsed wave Doppler signals, either simultaneously with imaging or sequentially. This allows precise measurement of the Doppler shift at any given point of the sonogram.
- Once the angle between the ultrasound beam and the vessel examined (Doppler angle) is known, the flow velocity can be computed and is displayed by the ultrasound unit in meters per second.
- The flow velocity is depicted in the so-called Doppler flow profile.

Flow Resistance Indices

- In solid abdominal and retroperitoneal organs (e.g., the kidneys), arterial blood usually flows in antegrade direction throughout the entire cardiac cycle (Fig. 17.**1**). Two indices that provide information on the prevailing arterial flow resistance are derived from relationships between peak systolic velocity (V_{max}), end-diastolic flow velocity (V_{ed}), and mean flow velocity (V_{mean}) according to the following equations:

Resistive index: $RI = (V_{max} - V_{ed})/V_{max}$
Pulsatility index: $PI = (V_{max} - _{ed})/V_{mean}$

- In general, large index values reflect high peripheral arterial flow resistance. Compared with absolute measurements of velocity, the indices do not depend on the Doppler angle (the angle is canceled out in the equation).

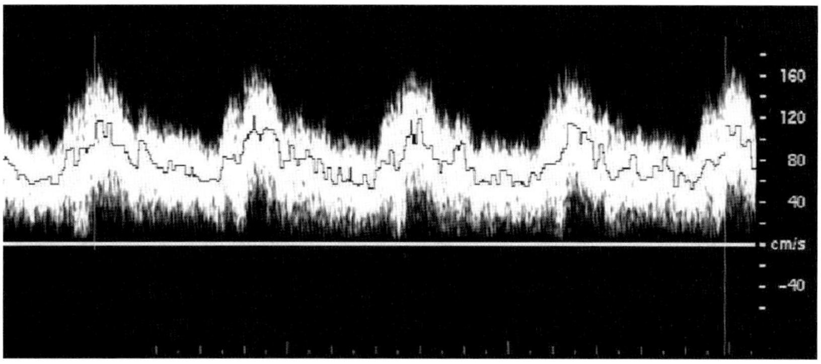

Fig. 17.**1** Characteristic holodiastolic antegrade arterial flow in solid organs of the abdomen (in this case the renal artery).

Aorta

Basic Facts

Indications for Sonography

- Evaluation for abdominal aortic aneurysm (AAA):
  - Pulsatile abdominal mass
  - Acute abdomen
  - Shock of undetermined etiology, suggestive of ruptured AAA
  - Follow-up after surgical or interventional therapy
  - Screening for AAA in patients with other aneurysms
  - Workup for source of peripheral arterial embolism
- Classification:
  - True aneurysm with dilatation of all layers of the aortic wall: saccular aneurysms affecting predominantly the anterior wall, or fusiform aneurysms characterized by circular dilatation in all directions.
  - Pseudoaneurysm subsequent to puncture does not involve the layers of the aortic wall and corresponds to a paravascular hematoma.
  - Dissecting aortic aneurysm with aortic dilatation due to a tear in the intima and media, which appear as a floating membrane within the lumen of the aorta. Blood courses a variable distance in the wall and reenters the true lumen of the aorta farther distal to the original intimal defect.
- Evaluation of arterial stenoses superior to the inguinal ligament
- Evaluation for aortic dissection:
  - Aortic dissection need not be accompanied by aneurysmal dilatation of the vessel (cf. dissecting aneurysm).
  - Defining the extent of abdominal involvement in thoracic aortic dissection.
  - Clarification from which lumen the mesenteric and/or renal arteries branch off.
- Examination technique:
  - Median transverse epigastric view with 3.5 MHz curved array probe which is slowly tilted and swept caudad. Mandatory measurement of the anteroposterior aortic diameter is routinely performed in the infrarenal segment. The ultrasound probe is then turned 90° for the longitudinal view in which the Doppler-angle corrected flow velocity is measured.
  - When imaging the aorta in the longitudinal view, peak systolic velocity should be measured without aliasing; usually, this calls for adjustment of the velocity color map.
  - Systematic morphological assessment includes the course (kinking), caliber, wall deposits (plaques, thrombi), intraluminal structures (dissection membrane), and para-aortic structures (lymph nodes, hematomas).
  - Normally, the aorta displays a biphasic or triphasic flow profile on duplex scanning, with a signal-free systolic window and a color change from systole to diastole. Superior to the origin of the renal arteries there may be antegrade end-diastolic flow. Farther caudad, owing to the high peripheral resistance the end-diastolic Doppler flow profile coincides with or runs below the baseline. Normal value: $V_{max} = 0.6–1.4$ m/s.
- *Additional workup:* CT, spiral CT, MRI, DSA.

Sonographic Criteria of Assessment

- In B-mode imaging, aortic aneurysms (Fig. 17.**2**) and their surroundings are assessed for:
  - Longitudinal length and anteroposterior diameter.
  - Thrombosis? Width of thrombus.
  - Floating intraluminal structures: Nonsessile plaques, membranes.
  - Thickness of the aneurysmal wall and estimation of risk of rupture.
  - Spontaneous echo contrast.
  - Suspected (contained) rupture in case of free fluid, anechoic halo around the aneurysm, retroperitoneal hematoma.
  - In aneurysms, CFDI may yield additional information: easier delineation of the perfused residual lumen in the presence of hypoechoic thrombotic wall deposits (Fig. 17.**3**), reliable differentiation of heterogeneous mural thrombi from dissection membranes by color-flow in the false lumen (even if flow is low), relation of renal arteries to aneurysm.
- **Aortic dissection on B-mode imaging:**
  - As it is very thin (< 1 mm) and of low echogenicity (gain set to High), the dissection membrane is difficult to visualize.
  - Transverse section is mandatory for diagnostic confirmation of dissection (many artifacts are possible on longitudinal view).
  - Attempted delineation of distal end.
- In aortic dissection, CFDI may yield additional information:
  - In most cases, the false lumen is larger and flow there is characterized by slow retrograde perfusion with a monophasic signal (antegrade and faster flow in the true lumen).
  - Clarification from which lumen the mesenteric and/or renal arteries branch off.
  - Interconnection between both lumina.

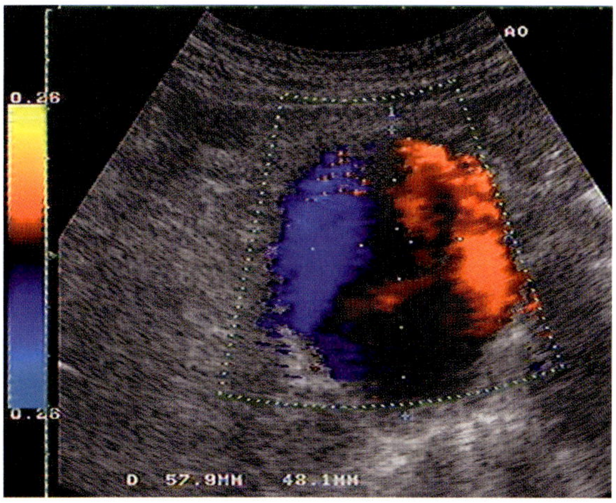

Fig. 17.**2 a** Transverse umbilical view of an infrarenal aortic aneurysm with a maximum anteroposterior diameter of 5.8 cm. The entire lumen remains perfused and exhibits turbulent flow.

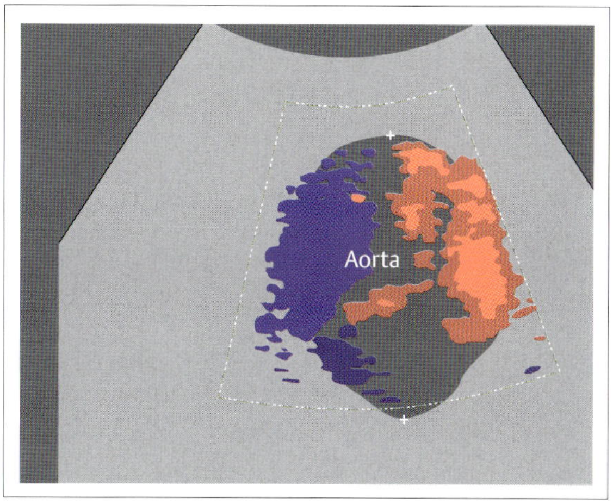

Fig. 17.**2 b** Line drawing.

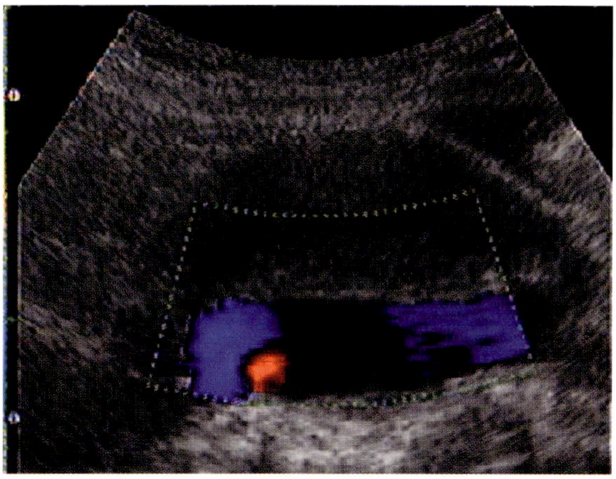

Fig. 17.**3 a** Longitudinal view of an infrarenal aortic aneurysm with marked mural thrombus. The colored area represents the perfused part of the lumen.

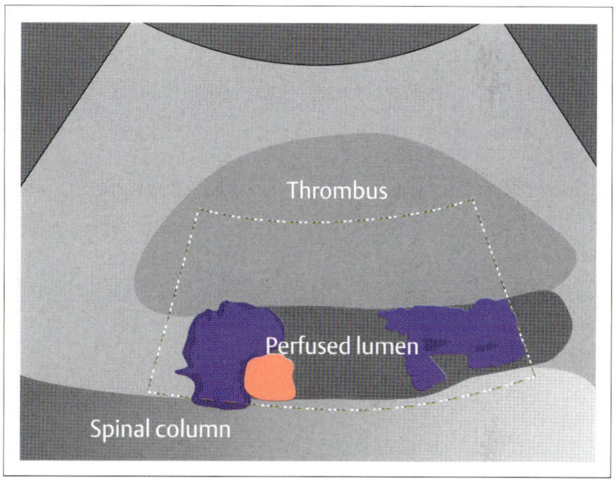

Fig. 17.**3 b** Line drawing.

Consequences for Surgical Treatment

Diagnosis	Characteristic Findings	Management
AAA, diameter: 3–5 cm	Dilatation with/without mural thrombus	Strict treatment of hypertension, follow-up after 3–6 months
AAA, diameter: 5–8 cm	Dilatation with/without mural thrombus; possibly thin mural lining	Risk of rupture < 15% in 5 years Additional workup: CT and MRI Usually vascular surgery Endovascular treatment by aortic stenting, if distance to renal branches > 2 cm (Bürger, 1998, Sternberg et al., 1998, van der Vliet and Boll, 1997)
AAA, diameter: > 8 cm	As above	Risk of rupture > 75% in 5 years, as above
Contained perforation	Hypoechoic material, usually posterior to the aneurysm	Urgent surgery
Frank perforation, usually with symptoms of fulminant shock	Free intra-abdominal fluid	Resuscitation, emergency surgery
Aortic dissection	Two perfused lumina with/without aneurysmal dilatation	Assessment of cephalad spread by TEE, CT, or MRI Assessment of caudal spread into the iliofemoral vessels Close follow-up, e.g., every 3 months, particularly of the thoracic aorta Surgery indicated in peripheral ischemia (Bürger, 1998; Donaldson et al., 1997; Sternberg et al., 1998; van der Vliet and Boll, 1997)

Celiac Trunk and Mesenteric Arteries

Basic Facts

- Indications for study:
  - Evaluation for mesenteric arterial insufficiency
  - Relation of celiac trunk and mesenteric arteries to any aortic aneurysm or aortic dissection
  - Workup of acute abdomen (acute arterial intestinal ischemia)
  - Evaluation for celiac artery compression (median arcuate ligament syndrome or Dunbar syndrome)
- Examination with epigastric transverse and longitudinal views.
- Blood flow in the celiac trunk does not vary with digestive activity; normal values: V_{max} systolic = 1.0–2.3 m/s; V_{ed} = 0.3–0.6 m/s.
- Flow in the superior mesenteric artery (SMA) clearly varies with digestive activity; no end-diastolic flow in fasting, while the postprandial decrease in resistance results in antegrade end-diastolic flow; normal values: V_{max} systolic (fasting) = 1.0–1.8 m/s; V_{max} systolic (postprandial) = up to 2.6 m/s; V_{ed} end-diastolic (postprandial) = up to 0.5 m/s; resistive index (fasting) = 0.8–0.9; resistive index (postprandial) < 0.7.
- The inferior mesenteric artery can only be demonstrated in slender patients and hardly ever permits sufficient access for conclusive evaluation.
- Provocation test in abdominal angina and suspected hemodynamic significance of a stenosis, particularly in the SMA: meal of 4000 kJ, after 45 minutes V_{max} increases to 1.5–2 times baseline and V_{ed} to 2.5–3 times the baseline levels.
- *Additional workup:* DSA or standard angiography.

Sonographic Criteria of Assessment

- Detection of localized aneurysms on CFDI.
- Detection of dissection–posttraumatic or as part of aortic dissection.
- Aliasing on CFDI suggestive of stenosis.
- In the SMA, V_{max} (fasting) > 2.2 m/s highly suspicious for a hemodynamically significant stenosis (Fig. 17.**4**).
- Provocation test:
  - In mild to moderate stenosis, disproportionate rapid rise of flow velocity to three or four times the fasting baseline level.
  - In more severe stenosis, only a slight rise in postprandial velocity is possible.

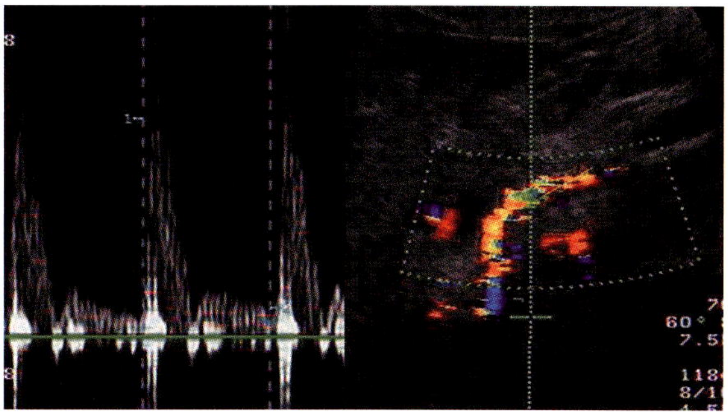

Fig. 17.**4a** Longitudinal epigastric view of a normal superior mesenteric artery with a V_{max} of 1.65 m/s.

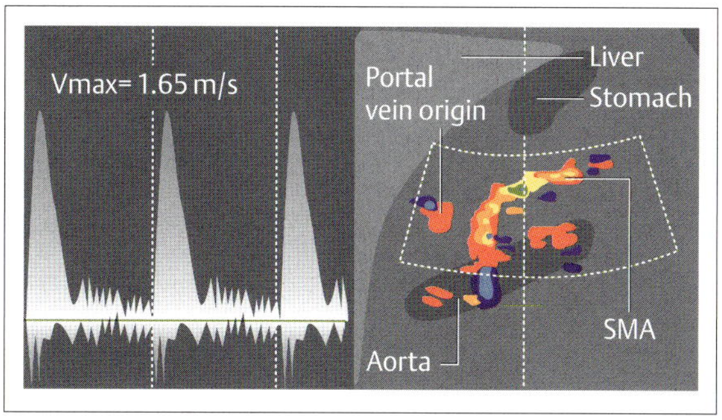

Fig. 17.**4b** Line drawing.

Consequences for Surgical Treatment

Diagnosis	Characteristic Findings	Management
Calcified plaques	No sign of hemodynamically significant stenosis	No proven treatment
Stenosis (particularly of superior mesenteric artery)	Abdominal angina and increased flow velocity in fasting, possibly pathological provocation test	Additional workup including DSA; surgery is the treatment of choice (Bürger, 1998) (thrombendarterectomy or vein/prosthetic graft) aiming for prevention of postprandial pain and weight increase in malabsorption syndrome

Native Kidneys and Renal Arteries

Basic Facts

- CFDI is used for screening in suspected renovascular hypertension (1–2% of all hypertension).
- Renovascular hypertension is primarily caused by atheromatous changes (in older patients) followed by fibromuscular dysplasia (mostly in younger women). Less common causes include renal artery aneurysm, embolic/thrombotic occlusion, AV fistulas, and dissection of various origin.
- Clinically suspected in cases of brittle hypertension (despite more than four medications), hypertension onset at < 25 or > 50 years, sudden deterioration of previous hypertension, arterial bruit, severe hypertension with unilaterally small kidney on sonography, and lack of nocturnal fall in blood pressure.
- Not all renal artery stenosis results in renovascular hypertension, since only hemodynamically significant narrowing will stimulate the renin–angiotensin system.
- Vascular supply of the kidney by more than one renal artery (15–20% of cases) poses problems in examination and interpretation; branches to the lower pole may even originate at the iliac arteries.
- Examination of fasting patient with 2.0–3.5 MHz probe.
- Renal arteries are delineated in 60–90% of examined subjects depending on the ultrasound unit and the investigator's skills (in obese patients, the distance of the renal artery from the skin of the abdomen may reach 15–20 cm).
- The renal artery is assessed on transverse abdominal view, and the kidney on oblique lateral view (possibly in corresponding lateral decubitus position).
- As the arteries become less elastic with age, the resistive index (RI) will increase (Table 17.**1**).
- When combining the direct and indirect criteria for stenosis (see below), sensitivity and specificity for diagnosing hemodynamically significant stenosis reaches > 90%, provided imaging quality suffices (Krumme et al., 1996).
- Intrarenal RI > 0.80 (usually measured on the nonstenosed side) indicates renal damage caused by nephrosclerosis; these patients may not benefit from PTA in terms of better control of blood pressure or amelioration of renal function (Radermacher et al., 2001).
- *Additional workup:* Spiral CT, MR angiography, angiography (DSA), always with option of PTA.

Sonographic Criteria of Assessment

- After their aortic origin, both renal arteries briefly course anteriorly (red) before they turn and run deep posteriorly (blue); angle-corrected measurement of flow velocity (Fig. 17.**5**).
- Optimum view and measurement of both kidneys is obtained with B-mode imaging.
- The Doppler sample volume is positioned on 3–6 interlobular arteries at the transition zone between parenchyma and renal pelvis for recording of the Doppler flow profile and computing the resistance indices (especially the resistive index) (Fig. 17.**6**).
- **Direct criteria of stenosis:**
  - V_{max} > 2 m/s (Fig. 17.**7**) or V_{max} of renal artery more than 3.5 times the aortic flow velocity.
- **Indirect criteria of stenosis (in stenosis > 70%):**
  - Difference in intrarenal RI > 0.05 on contralateral reference signals unilateral prerenal stenosis on the side with the lower RI (Fig. 17.**8**).
  - Unphysiologically low RI in both kidneys points to impaired bilateral run-in.
  - Massive differences within one kidney indicate polar or segmental artery stenosis.
- **Limitations of color-flow Doppler imaging:**
  - Color flow Doppler imaging is not a morphological modality for precisely quantifying the degree of stenosis!
  - In localized lack of perfusion, renal vein thrombosis, and tumors of the native kidney, CFDI can only complement the findings of conventional ultrasound.

Table 17.**1** Intrarenal resistive index as a function of age

Age	Resistive Index (RI)
≤ 30 years	0.52–0.62
31–50 years	0.55–0.68
51–60 years	0.60–0.73
61–70 years	0.65–0.82

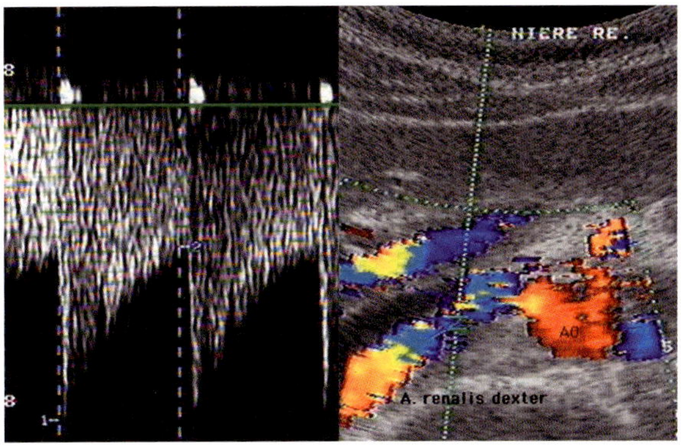

Fig. 17.5 a B-mode imaging of the right renal artery and measurement of the angle-corrected flow velocities (normal findings).

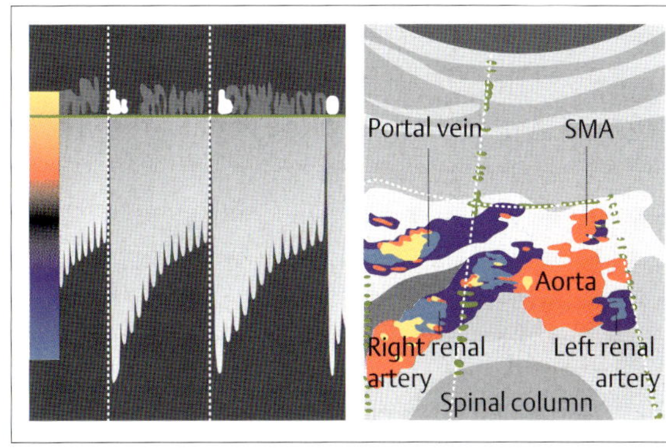

Fig. 17.5 b Line drawing.

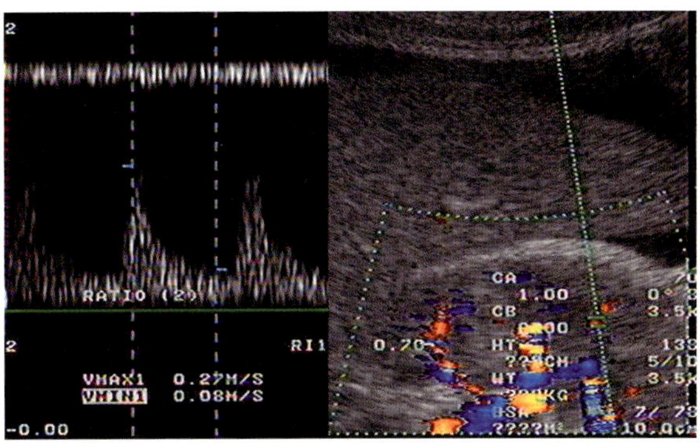

Fig. 17.6 a Doppler sample volume positioned on an interlobular artery of the right kidney with computation of the resistive index (normal findings).

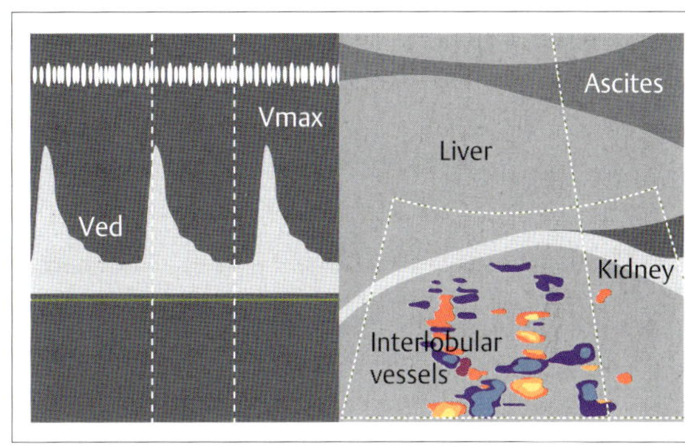

Fig. 17.6 b Line drawing.

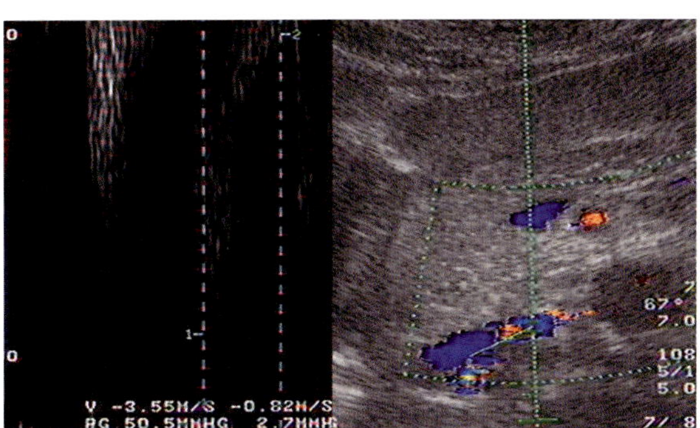

Fig. 17.7 a Right renal artery stenosis with a peak systolic velocity of 3.55 m/s.

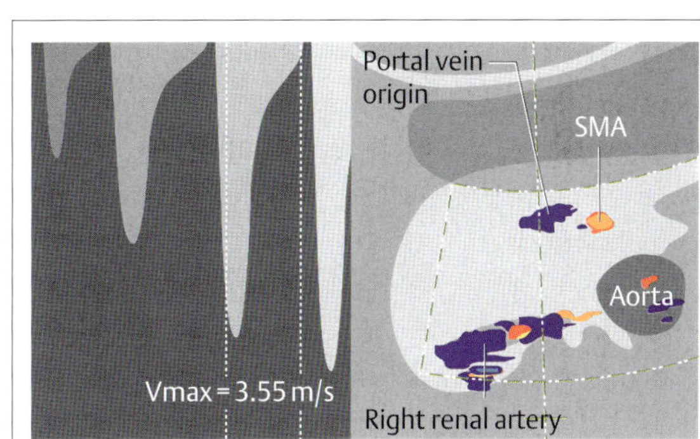

Fig. 17.7 b Line drawing.

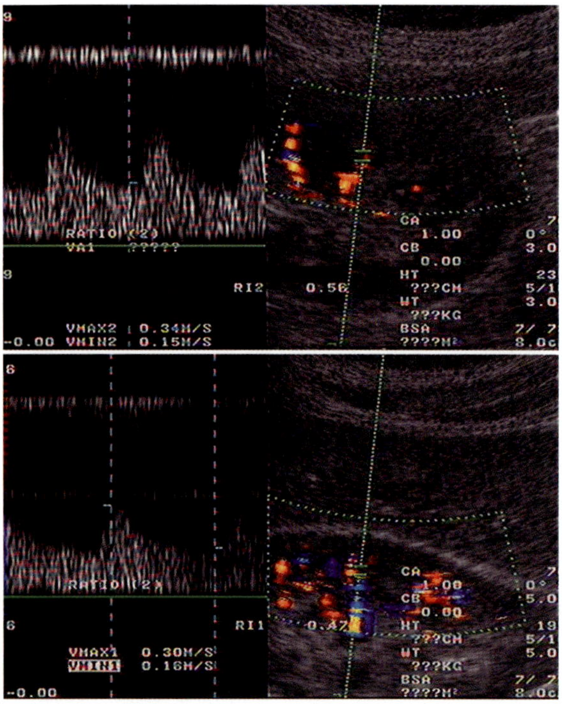

Fig. 17.**8 a** Comparison of the intrarenal resistive index of the left (RI = 0.56; upper panel) and right kidney (RI = 0.47; lower panel) in stenosis of the right renal artery.

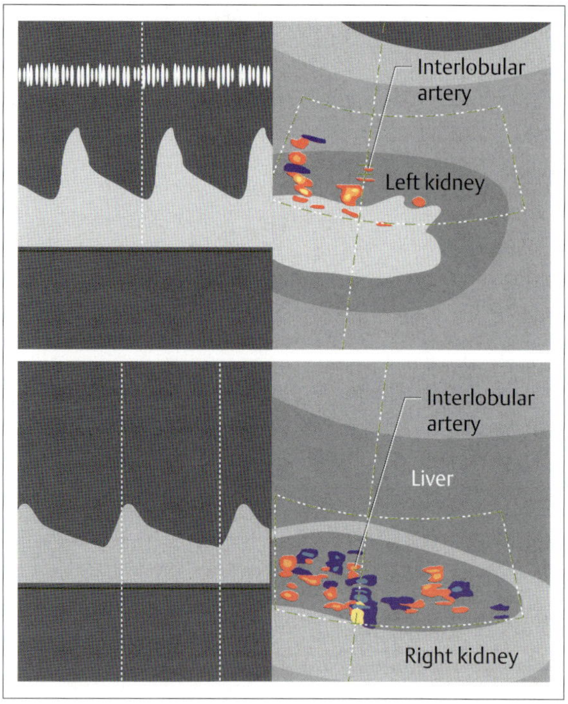

Fig. 17.**8 b** Line drawings.

Consequences for Surgical Treatment

Diagnosis	Characteristic Findings	Management
Calcified plaques in renal arteries	No sign of hemodynamically significant stenosis	No proven treatment
Ostial stenosis	Hemodynamically significant stenosis mostly in older patients	Usually atheromatous stenoses: DSA plus PTA (possibly including stenting); depending on surgical risk, also aortorenal bypass as primary measure with better outcome (Erdoes et al., 1996)
Nonostial stenosis	Hemodynamically significant stenosis mostly in younger patients (predominantly female)	Usually fibromuscular dysplasia: primarily DSA with PTA indicated (stenting usually not necessary)
Bilateral stenoses or stenosis in solitary kidney	Hemodynamic significance and renal insufficiency	Primarily aortorenal bypass in order to preserve renal function, also provides better outcome (Erdoes et al., 1996), or PTA plus stenting

Bibliography

Bürger T. Gefäßchirurgie. In: Lippert H, ed. Praxis der Chirurgie. Stuttgart, New York: Thieme; 1998: 811–36.

Donaldson MC, Belkin M, Whittemore AD. Mesenteric revascularization during aneurysmectomy. Surg Clin North Am. 1997; 77: 443–59.

Erdoes LS, Berman SS, Hunter GC, Mills JL. Comparative analysis of percutaneous transluminal angioplasty and operation for renal revascularization. Am J Kidney Dis. 1996; 27: 496–503.

Krumme B, Blum U, Schwertfeger E, et al. Diagnosis of renovascular disease by intra- and extrarenal Doppler scanning. Kidney Int. 1996; 50: 1288–92.

Radermacher J, Chavan A, Bleck J, et al. Use of Doppler ultrasonography to predict the outcome of therapy for renal-artery stenosis. N Engl J Med. 2001; 344: 410–7.

Sternbergh WC, Gonze MD, Garrard CL, Money SR. Abdominal and thoracoabdominal aortic aneurysm. Surg Clin North Am. 1998; 78: 827–43.

Van der Vliet JA, Boll AP. Abdominal aortic aneurysm. Lancet. 1997; 349: 863–6.

18 Sonography in Pediatric Surgery

H. Krause, V. Aumann

Indications for Sonography

This chapter discusses the characteristic sonographic manifestations of selected pediatric disorders that may require surgical therapy. As this textbook on sonography in surgery could not possibly present all disorders relevant in pediatrics and pediatric surgery, the authors had to limit their focus on the particular aspects central to all studies in pediatric sonography. Just as the physical examination of infants requires special sensitivity, care, and much patience on the part of medical practitioners, so practitioners must familiarize themselves with an expanding spectrum of sonographic findings, because almost all of the pathologies presented here are restricted to the pediatric age group. Apart from incidence and prevalence, the necessary technical equipment and potential consequences also played a role in the authors' selection process. As a result, listed here are the core characteristics of some childhood diseases that any practicing surgeon may encounter and that usually can be diagnosed with a "standard" ultrasound unit. Not only will the role of sonography as a decision-making tool for potential surgical intervention be considered, but just as importantly its value in determining when treatment should remain conservative.

Infantile Hypertrophic Pyloric Stenosis

Basic Facts

- Manifestation of infantile hypertrophic pyloric stenosis (IHPS) is during the first few weeks of life; incidence is 2–4 per 1000 live births; familial clustering is still controversial.
- It is more predominant in males than females (male-to-female ratio 5 : 1)
- A characteristic is progressive nonbilious vomiting or regurgitation after feeding, possibly becoming projectile since marked hypertrophy and spasticity of the pylorus lead to a narrowed pyloric opening, thus blocking passage.
- Hypokalemic-hypochloremic metabolic alkalosis, severe dehydration, and failure to thrive.
- Diagnosis is confirmed by sonography.
- The diameter of the normal pylorus is 12 mm; a diameter of 12–15 mm is regarded as borderline. Pyloric diameter ≥ 15 mm, pyloric canal length ≥ 16 mm, and pyloric muscle thickness ≥ 4 mm are definitely pathological.
- *Additional workup:* radiographic upper GI series in selected cases.

Sonographic Criteria of Assessment

- Depending on the degree of gastric filling, an annular structure with typical gut signature inferior to the liver; in IHPS, a "doughnut" with hypoechoic thickened muscle mass just superficial to the hyperechoic mucosal layer of the pyloric canal (Figs. 18.**1** and 18.**2**).

Consequences for Surgical Treatment

Diagnosis	Characteristic Findings	Management
Changing symptoms in suspected IHPS	Borderline sonographic findings	Conservative attempts with numerous small feedings and spasmolytic (anticholinergic) medication
Marked symptoms in suspected IHPS	Characteristic sonographic findings	Pyloromyotomy according to Weber, Ramstedt, and Fredet

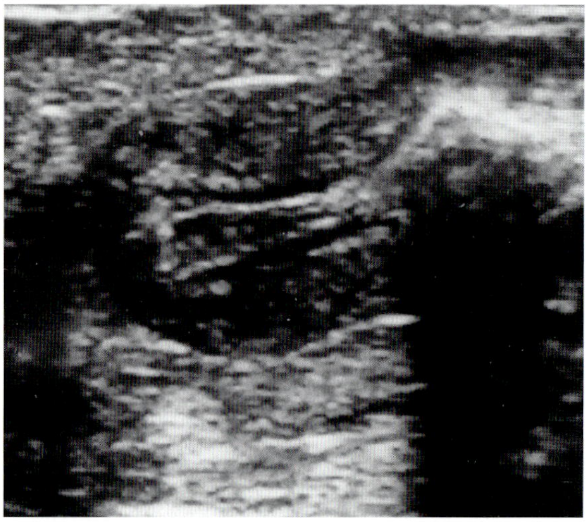

Fig. 18.**1 a** Longitudinal view of the pylorus.

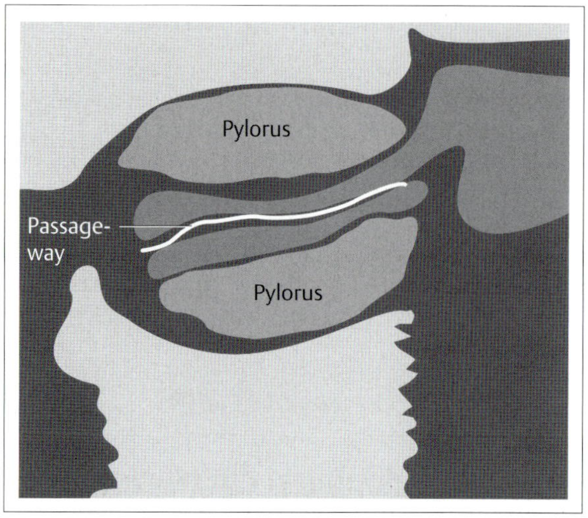

Fig. 18.**1 b** Line drawing.

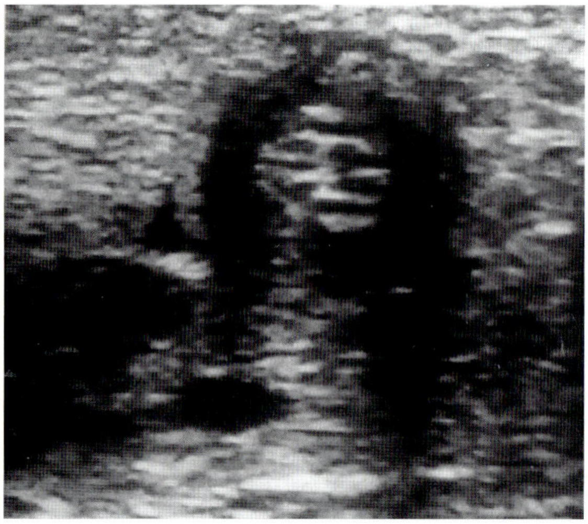

Fig. 18.**2 a** Transverse view of the pylorus. Depending on the degree of gastric filling, there will be an annular structure with typical gut signature inferior to the liver. This sonogram of IHPS depicts a pathognomonic "doughnut" with hypoechoic thickened muscle mass just superficial to the hyperechoic mucosal layer of the pyloric canal with its anechoic fluid-filled crevices.

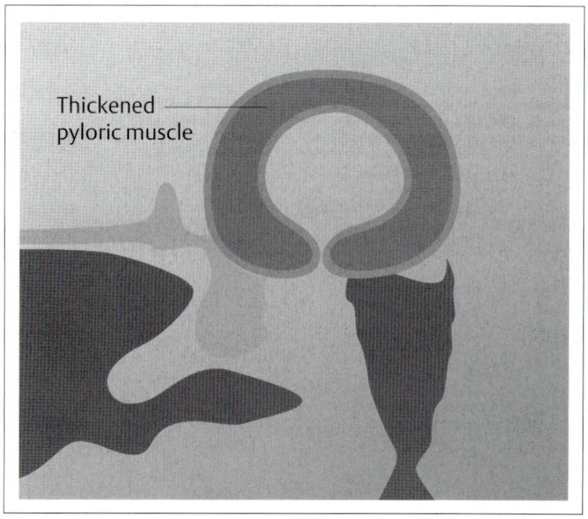

Fig. 18.**2 b** Line drawing.

Intussusception

Basic Facts

- The most common cause of small-bowel obstruction in well-nourished children between the ages of 6 months and 4 years. Male-to-female ration 3 : 1–2, for terminology, see Table 18.**1**.
- Etiology is unknown; there is evident correlation with the presence of enlarged Peyer's patches, Meckel's diverticulum, and intestinal polyps.

Table 18.**1** Terminology of intussusception

Ileoileal intussusception	Small bowel telescoped into small bowel
Ileocecal intussusception	Small bowel telescoped into cecum
Ileocolic intussusception	Small bowel telescoped into colon
Colocolic intussusception	Colon telescoped into colon

- Clinical presentation is characterized by intermittent short attacks of sudden-onset colicky abdominal pain. In the later course there are vomiting and lethargy, with "currant jelly" (bloody) stools being a late symptom. Palpable abdominal mass in some cases.
- Diagnosis is confirmed by sonography.
- *Additional workup:* In case of characteristic symptoms but lack of the pathognomonic target sign, diagnostic and therapeutic contrast reduction (**no barium**) if the history is less than 24 hours and there is no passage of bloody stools. **Caveat:** There is increased risk of perforation in this case.

Sonographic Criteria of Assessment

- The characteristic "target sign" is frequently seen in the right upper quadrant, with numerous concentric rings of alternating hypoechoic and hyperechoic echotexture (Fig. 18.**3**).

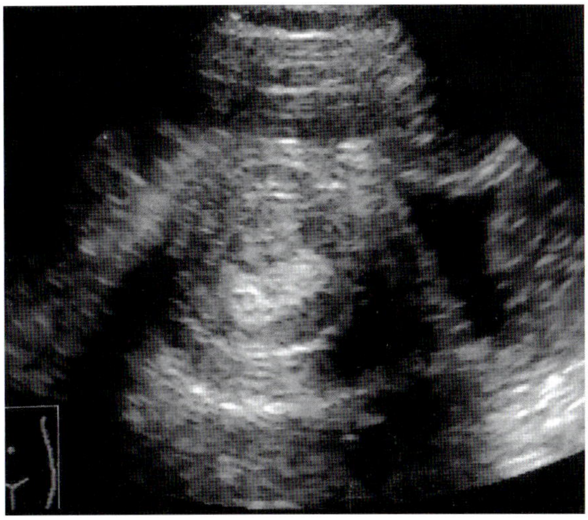

Fig. 18.**3 a** Characteristic target sign in ileocolic intussusception; depending on localization and duration, a "target sign" (frequently in the right upper quadrant) with numerous concentric rings resulting from the interfaces between telescoped bowel walls can be demonstrated.

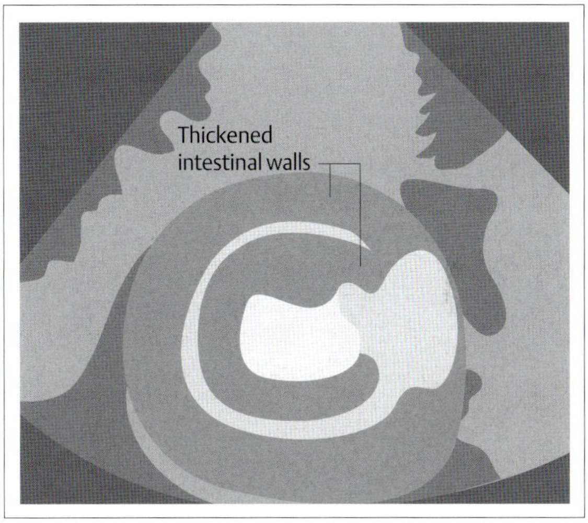

Fig. 18.**3 b** Line drawing.

Consequences for Surgical Treatment

Diagnosis	Characteristic Findings	Management
Intussusception diagnosed by experienced investigator and standby surgical team	Positive target sign	US-guided attempt at hydrostatic (saline) or pneumatic reduction
Intussusception diagnosed by experienced investigator and standby surgical team	No definite sonographic confirmation, no passage of "currant jelly" stools, no ileus	Contrast enema and possible attempt at reduction under fluoroscopy
Intussusception	Unsuccessful hydrostatic/ pneumatic reduction, passage of "currant jelly" stools, or signs of ileus	Indication for laparotomy with attempt at manual reduction by gentle retrograde milking of the intussusceptum (Hutchinson maneuver). Irreversibly damaged bowel must be resected

Henoch–Schönlein Purpura

Basic Facts

- This disease is discussed here because clinical signs and symptoms as well as sonographic findings may resemble those of intestinal intussusception, and, conversely, it may act as lead point in intussusception.
- It is probably caused by an allergic vasculitis of small vessels in a variety of body systems (primarily involving the skin, joints, and kidneys), frequently involving the GI tract with the main symptom of abdominal pain.
- The clinical picture is characterized by colicky abdominal pain and subsequently vomiting and passage of bloody stools or melena.
- Diagnostic workup relies on sonography and search for the characteristic skin rash.
- *Additional workup:* Fever, arthralgia, and later renal involvement (about 40%) help settle the diagnosis.

Sonographic Criteria of Assessment

- Hyperechoic **thickened (edematous) bowel wall** with hardly any evidence of gut signature. Blood flow within the thickened wall is almost impossible to demonstrate. Frequently there is free fluid within the intraperitoneal cavity (Fig. 18.**4**).

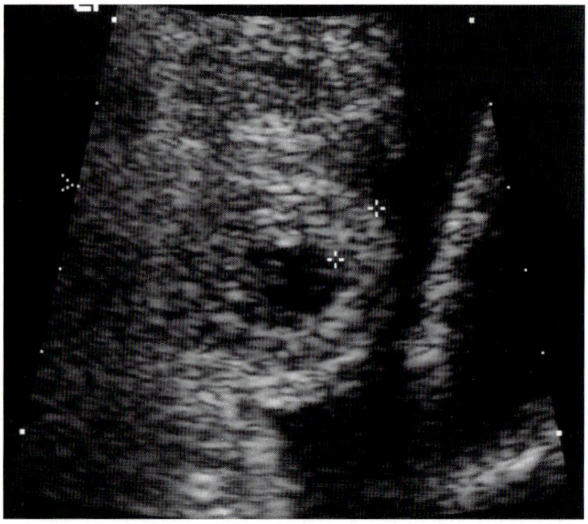

Fig. 18.**4a** Characteristic edematous wall thickening of the small bowel with free fluid.

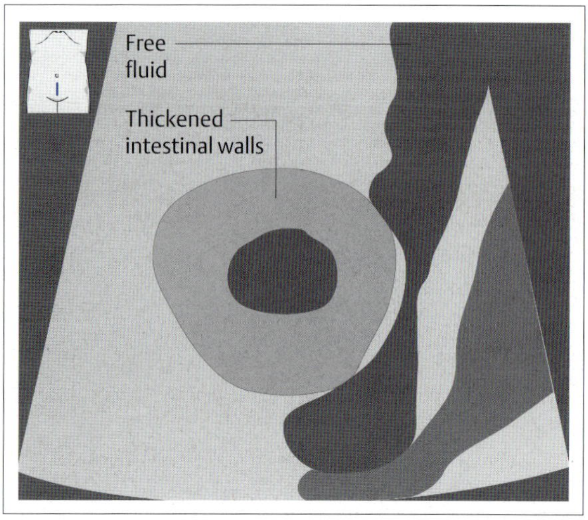

Fig. 18.**4b** Line drawing.

Consequences for Surgical Treatment

Diagnosis	Characteristic Findings	Management
Confirmation of suspected Henoch–Schönlein purpura	Thickened intestinal wall without characteristic gut signature on sonography	Strictly conservative
Abdominal symptoms not resolving with conservative treatment	Presence of a target sign	Sonographic follow-up ruling out intussusception

Alimentary Tract Duplications

Basic Facts

- Duplications may be found anywhere along the alimentary tract, always on the mesenteric side of the bowel.
- Errors in embryology of the primordial gut are hypothesized as a possible cause. The small bowel is involved in more than half of gastrointestinal duplications. The vascular supply of these structures is mostly from the adjacent intestinal segment.
- The form is varied, from diverticulum to cyst and tubular structure. As congenital malformations, the first signs and symptoms are already present during infancy.
- *Note:* Alimentary tract duplications are often associated with other malformations.
- Clinical presentation varies depending on size, location, and communication with the intestinal lumen. Nonspecific abdominal pain, failure to thrive, and even complete intestinal obstruction may be the initial symptoms.

Sonographic Criteria of Assessment

- Depending on site, duplications present as fluid-filled monocystic or polycystic masses. Mass with smooth outline; contents of cyst either hypoechoic or homogeneously hyperechoic. The margin usually has the characteristic gut signature. Mural blood flow is demonstrated in most cases (Figs. 18.**5** and 18.**6**).

- Diagnostic workup relies on sonography and contrast meal.
- Planning for surgery and informed consent of parents is based on sonographic delineation of size (if possible).
- *Additional workup:* CT/MRI is helpful in selected cases.

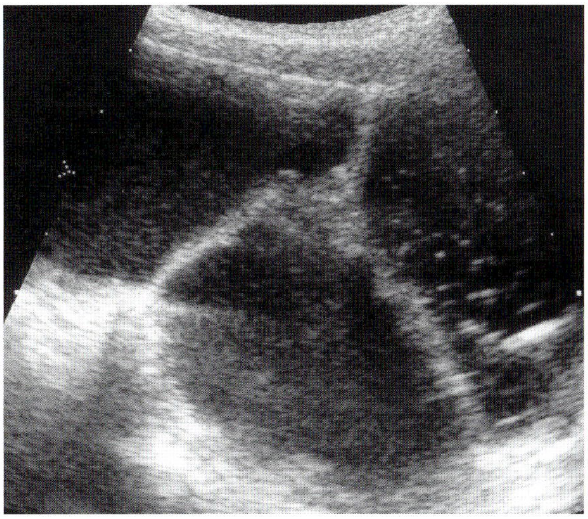

Fig. 18.**5 a** Longitudinal view of a smooth cystic mass.

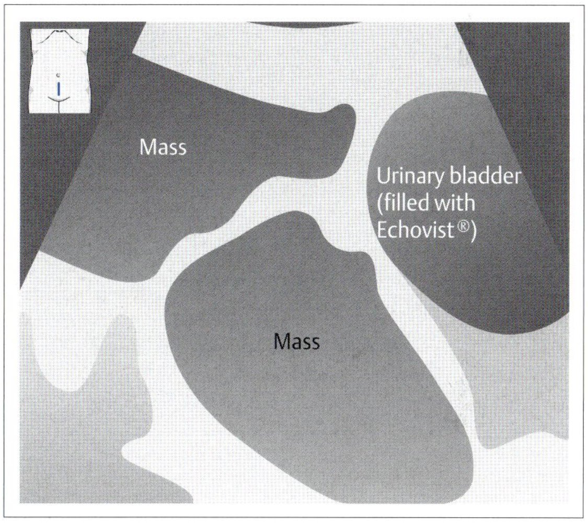

Fig. 18.**5 b** Line drawing.

Consequences for Surgical Treatment

Diagnosis	Characteristic Findings	Management
Short intestinal duplication	Circumscribed changes	Excision of the mucosa-bearing malformation by en-bloc resection with the adjacent normal bowel segment and restoration of continuity with end-to-end anastomosis
Long intestinal duplication	Large, ill-defined changes often combined with cystic components	Excision of the mucosa-bearing parts by subtle mucosectomy

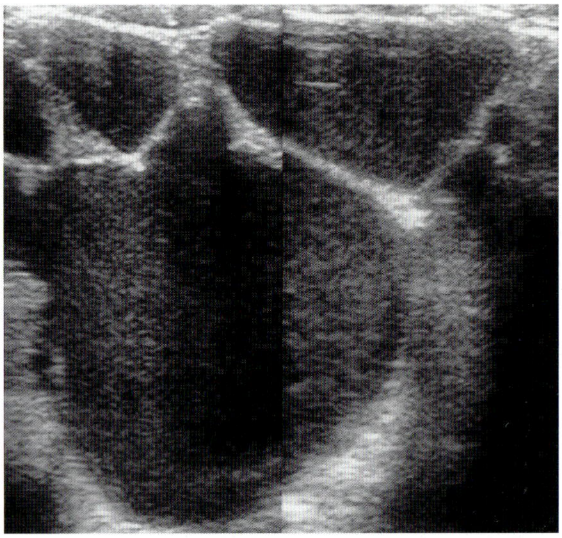

Fig. 18.**6a** Transverse view of a cystic mass in the lower abdomen. The margin displays the characteristic gut signature and there is mural blood flow.

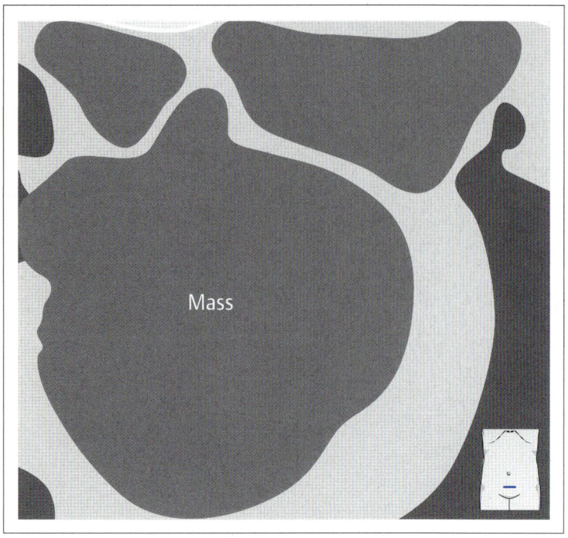

Fig. 18.**6b** Line drawing.

Undescended Testis/Cryptorchidism

Basic Facts

- Testicular descent is along the processus vaginalis peritonei via the inguinal canal into the scrotum between the 25th and 32nd weeks of gestation.
- Undescended testes are seen in 3–5% of full-term newborns and in approximately 33% of premature male infants weighing less than 2550 grams.
- In bilateral cryptorchidism associated with abnormal external genitalia, chromosomal sex determination is recommended.
- Always establish diagnosis, determine etiology, and institute treatment before the third year of life, since after the second year parenchymal testicular damage with subsequent subfertility or infertility is highly likely. A higher rate of testicular torsion remains controversial.
- Strictly speaking, cryptorchidism (a *state*) results from the *process* of "incomplete testicular descent" (maldescensus testis). Semantic confusion is common, both terms often being used synonymously (see Table 18.**2** for terminology).
- There is a rather frequent association with inguinal hernia (about 75%). The clinical picture of undescended testis is characterized by mobile swelling. Diagnosis is confirmed by sonography.
- *Additional workup:* indication for laparoscopy (MRI/scintigraphy in selected cases) if there is no sonographic confirmation

Sonographic Criteria of Assessment

- Delineation of a **normal testis** of splenic echogenicity and echotexture, smooth, rather homogeneous, and little blood flow. Epididymis somewhat hypoechoic to testis and located superior to it (Fig. 18.**7**).
- **Inguinal testis** still demonstrating normal testicular echotexture, but significantly smaller and with internal speckling (Fig. 18.**8**).

Table 18.**2** Terminology of Undescended Testis/Cryptorchidism

Anorchidism	Congenital absence of testis
Cryptorchidism	Hidden testis; term usually reserved for abdominal testis
Undescended testis	Incomplete descent, i.e., the testis has not completed its path from the abdomen through the inguinal canal into the scrotum
Highly retractile testis	Testis can be "milked" into the scrotum but will quickly retract into the inguinal canal
Retractile testis	In warm temperatures and in the absence of stimuli, the testis remains in the scrotum, moving up to the external inguinal ring due to a hyperactive cremaster reflex or reaction to cold

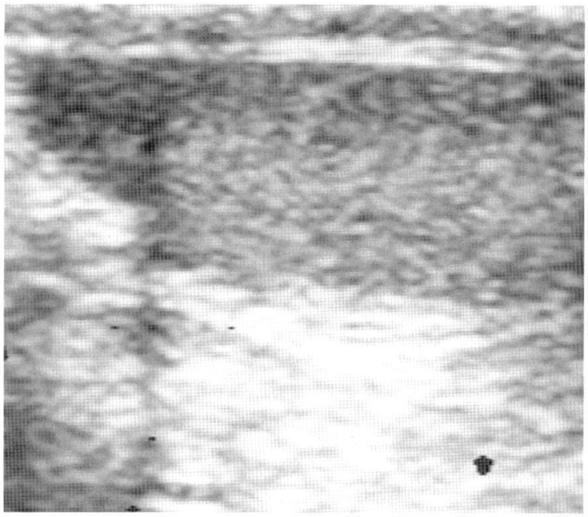

Fig. 18.**7 a** Normal testis of splenic echogenicity and echotexture, smooth, rather homogeneous, and little blood flow; the epididymis superior to the testis is somewhat less echogenic.

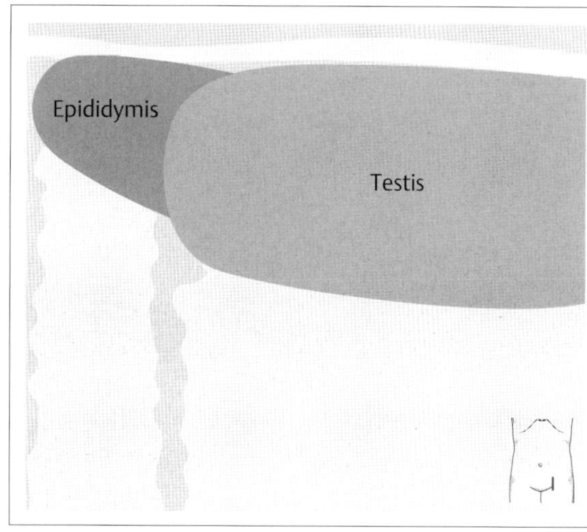

Fig. 18.**7 b** Line drawing.

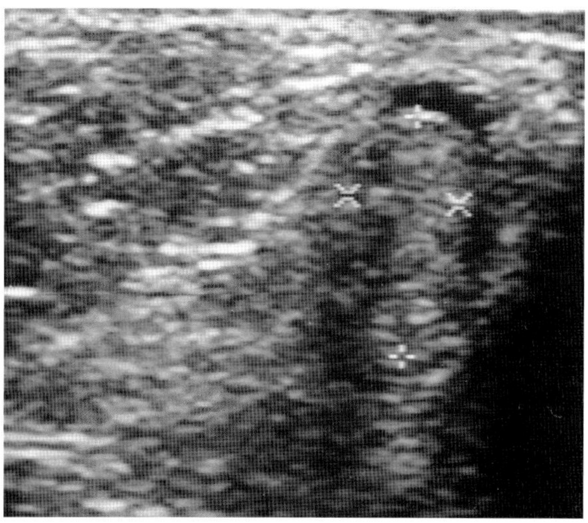

Fig. 18.**8 a** Inguinal testis still demonstrating normal testicular echotexture, but significantly smaller and with prominent hyperechoic parenchymal areas.

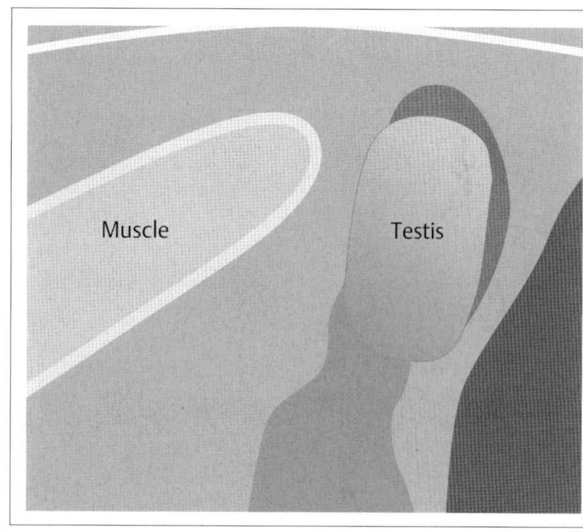

Fig. 18.**8 b** Line drawing.

Consequences for Surgical Treatment

Diagnosis	Characteristic Findings	Management
Inguinal/highly retractile testis	Characteristic parenchymal echotexture (splenic) at the inguinal canal, palpable swelling	Conservative hormone treatment with HCG or GnRH is possible in almost inguinal testes. If accompanied by inguinal hernia, curative effect is **unlikely**
Inguinal testis (after hormone treatment or in boys > 2 years)	Mostly unchanged echogenicity and texture (as above), sometimes smaller than contralateral reference	Orchiopexy and search for incidental hernia. Recurrence is often due to initially overlooked and thus untreated hernia
Retractile testis	Characteristic parenchymal echotexture (splenic); before examination the testis is usually palpable in scrotum	Close follow-up
Intra-abdominal testis	No testicular structure in scrotum or inguinal area	Laparoscopy; if a dysplastic gonad is found, removal vs. orchiopexy, possibly staged

Inguinal Hernia

Basic Facts

- Congenital inguinal hernias almost always the result of a patent processus vaginalis (indirect hernia)
- Incidence for full-term newborns about 5%, with a male-to-female ratio of 9 : 1. Incidence much higher in premature infants
- Hernias in boys more commonly right sided (later testicular descent)
- Incarceration in boys involves the intestines and in girls primarily the ovaries
- Diagnosis confirmed by sonography
- *Additional workup:* None. History provided by the child's caretakers of utmost importance

Sonographic Criteria of Assessment

- In the inguinal region, a gap in the abdominal wall muscles is visualized at the edge of which the ovary, characterized by its typical cystic structure, can frequently be delineated. In boys, the hernial contents often are bowel loops (sometimes protruding as far as the scrotum) (Fig. 18.**9**).

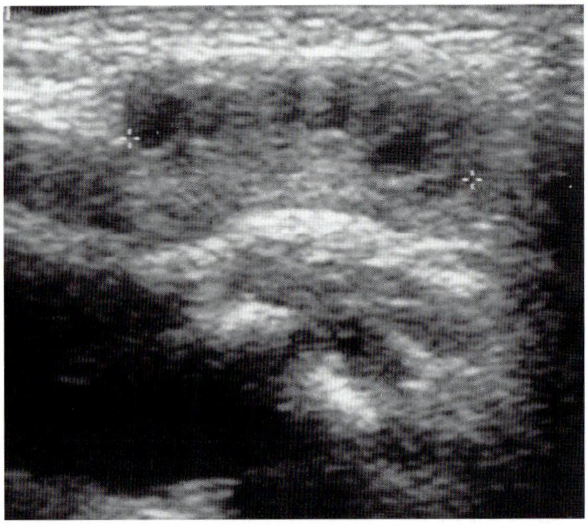

Fig. 18.**9 a** Inguinal hernia in a girl, with irreducible swelling (ovary) in inguinal canal. A gap in the abdominal wall muscles is visualized at the edge of which the ovary, characterized by its typical cystic structure, is delineated.

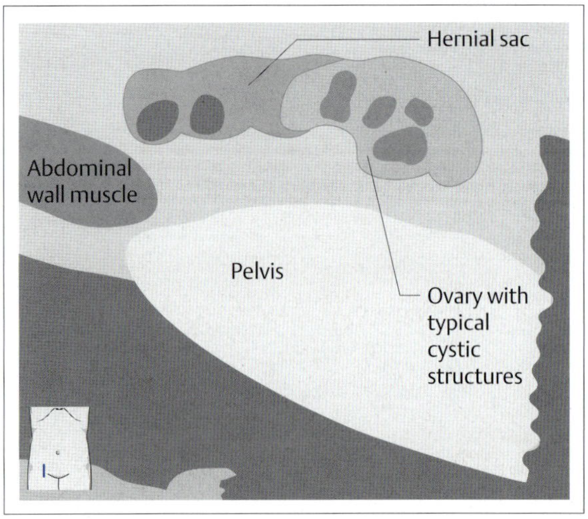

Fig. 18.**9 b** Line drawing.

Consequences for Surgical Treatment

Diagnosis	Characteristic Findings	Management
Inguinal hernia	History, sonographic confirmation not always successful	Indication for (elective) surgery. One such typical operation is herniotomy according to Ferguson
Irreducible hernia in boys	Usually demonstration of distended bowel loops	Emergency herniotomy (risk of intestinal ischemia)
Irreducible hernia in girls with confirmed herniation of the ovary	Demonstration of cystic structure	Urgent surgery, otherwise risk of tubal obliteration

Dermoid and Epidermoid Cysts

Basic Facts

- Subcutaneous cystic indolent benign tumor, most often encased in a fibrous capsule (see Table 18.**3** for terminology).
- Favored sites: periorbital region and scalp; less frequently the jugular, sternal, and scrotal areas.
- Diagnosis is confirmed by sonography. Blood supply and any intracranial communication must be assessed preoperatively. Differential diagnosis includes Langerhans cell histiocytosis and meningocele, and in the neck branchial and thyroglossal cysts. Definite diagnosis requires histopathological work-up. Surgical excision is therefore indicated for assessment of possible malignancy.
- *Additional workup:* In deeper-reaching lesions, CT or MRI may be indicated.

Sonographic Criteria of Assessment

- Smooth (punched out) bone defect, completely filled by moderately hypoechoic mass also demonstrating smooth margins (Fig. 18.**10**).

Table 18.**3** Terminology of dermoid and epidermoid cysts

Dermoid cyst	Ectopic epithelium invested with stratified squamous epithelium, possibly containing appendages of the skin (e.g., hair)
Epidermoid cyst	Ectopic epithelium invested with stratified squamous epithelium, lacking any appendages of the skin

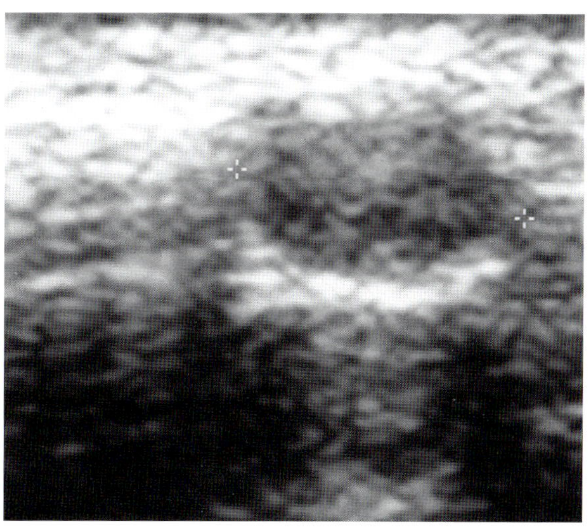

Fig. 18.**10 a** Typical localization of an (epi-)dermoid cyst above the left eyebrow, presenting as tense elastic indolent tumor. The sonogram demonstrates a smooth (punched out) bone defect, completely filled by moderately hypoechoic mass also with smooth margins.

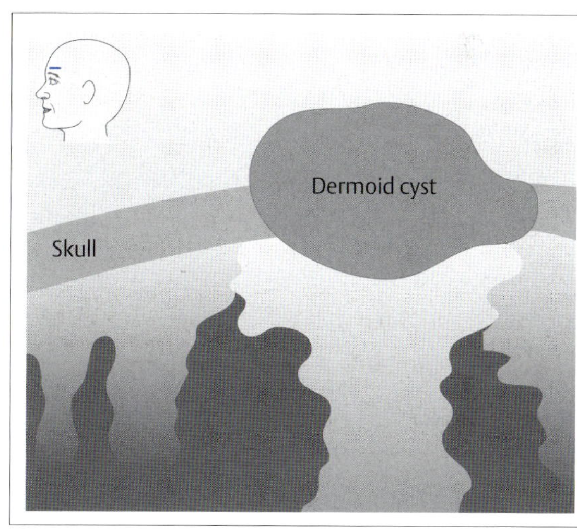

Fig. 18.**10 b** Line drawing.

Consequences for Surgical Treatment

Diagnosis	Characteristic Findings	Management
Suspected (epi-)dermoid cyst	Smooth hypoechoic mass mostly in the face/head	On perforation, pasty yellowish-white material is seen. In case of partial excision, sonographic follow-up is indicated as recurrent cysts may arise from leftover remnants of the wall

Lymphangioma

Basic Facts

- Lymphangiomas represent congenital malformations of the lymphatic system: elastic, partly mobile, ill-defined indolent tumors found at numerous sites (frequently neck, shoulder girdle, and lateral thoracic or abdominal wall). The different types are presented in Table 18.**4**.
- Spontaneous regression, as sometimes seen in hemangiomas, is unlikely

Sonographic Criteria of Assessment

- Multilocular cystic mass (often with communicating compartments) with hypoechoic or anechoic contents and a thin hyperechoic margin (Fig. 18.**11**).
- No flow signals on CFDI. **Caveat:** Contents shifting due to probe movement may mimic flow (Fig. 18.**12**).

Table 18.**4** Terminology of Lymphangioma

Lymphangioma simplex	Proliferation of the lymphatic capillaries
Cavernous lymphangioma	Dilatation of the lymphatics
Cystic lymphangioma	Cysts with endothelial lining
Hematolymphangioma	Mixed entity of hemangioma and lymphangioma

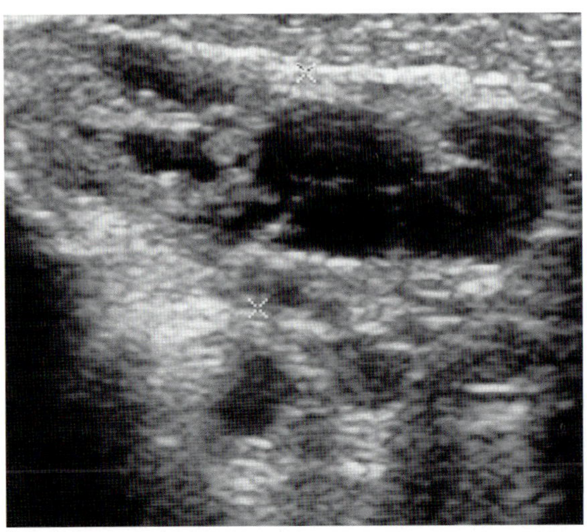

Fig. 18.**11 a** Lymphangioma of the right neck. Multilocular cystic mass (often with communicating compartments) with hypoechoic or anechoic contents and a thin hyperechoic margin.

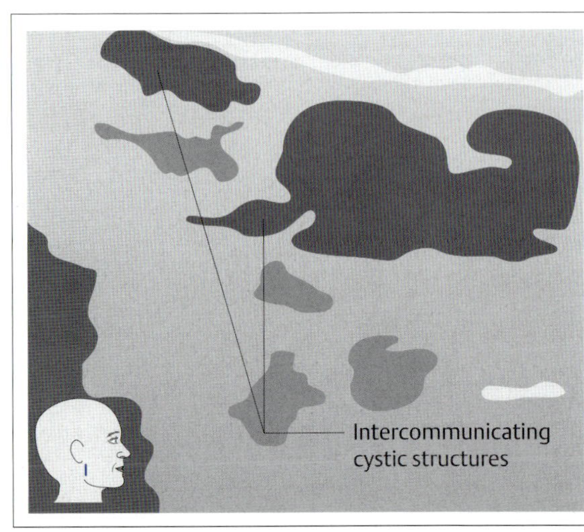

Fig. 18.**11 b** Line drawing.

Consequences for Surgical Treatment

Diagnosis	Characteristic Findings	Management
Lymphangioma immediately adjacent to major vessels/nerves	Cystic mass with hypoechoic contents and hyperechoic margin and no flow signals on CFDI	Radical wide excision (often difficult dissection), possibly unsatisfactory cosmesis
Lymphangioma not immediately adjacent to major vessels/nerves	Cystic mass with hypoechoic contents and hyperechoic margin and no flow signals on CFDI	Laser coagulation (e.g., Nd-YAG) for localized devitalization via a bare-fiber inserted transcutaneously (small skin incision!) through a cannula. US and local (pilot laser) monitoring during the procedure are possible

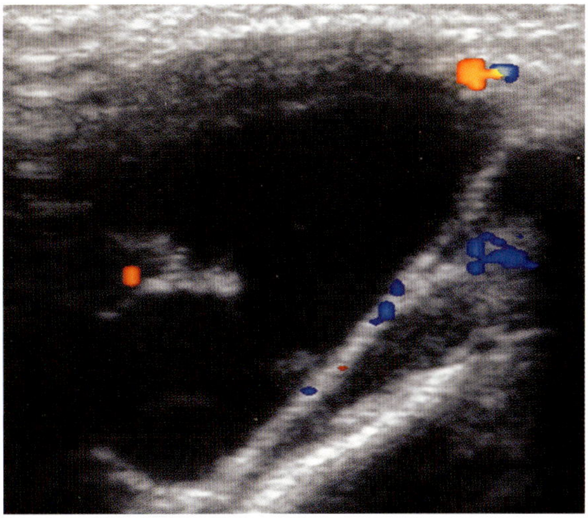

Fig. 18.**12a** No flow signals on CFDI. **Caveat:** Contents shifting due to probe movement may mimic flow.

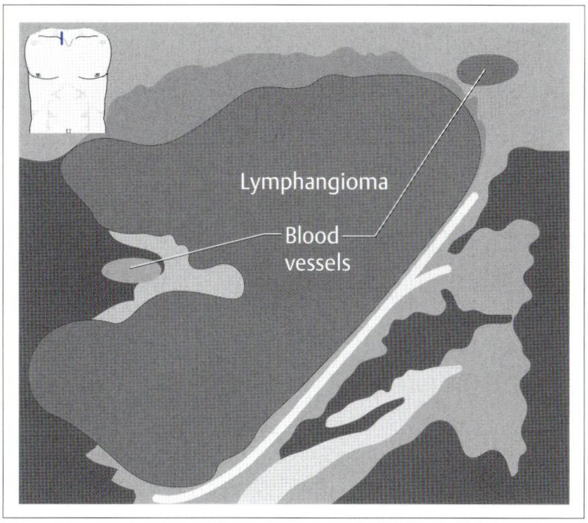

Fig. 18.**12b** Line drawing.

Hemangioma of the Skin

Basic Facts

- Hemangiomas commonly either present at birth or arise and proliferate during the first months of life. It is important to differentiate them from telangiectasia. Male-to-female ratio is 1 : 2; favored sites are the head and trunk. Up to 80% regress within the first 2–5 years of life (see Table 18.**5** for terminology).
- Telangiectasia: nevus flammeus/telangiectaticus, nuchal nevus, vascular spider, port wine stain.
- **Caveat:** In case of other abnormalities (paraclinical changes, contralateral difference, etc.) differential diagnosis must include Klippel–Trénaunay syndrome, Louis–Bar syndrome, and Kasabach–Merritt syndrome.
- Diagnosis is confirmed by sonography (CFDI).
- *Additional workup:* Monstrous lesions are best assessed by angio-MRI/DSA.

Sonographic Criteria of Assessment

- Relatively hyperechoic lesion with heterogeneous internal echotexture, defined from its surroundings; CFDI revealing massive high-velocity blood flow. **Caveat:** In substantial venous run-off, very slow peripheral flow is possible (Fig. 18.**13**).

Table 18.**5** Terminology of Hemangioma

Cutaneous hemangioma	Greatest extension in the cutaneous plane, protuberant, sharply delimited soft-tissue mass with frequently progressive growth in the first months of life, but a high tendency to involution
Cavernous hemangioma	Maximum extension subcutaneously, with spontaneous growth phases and a low tendency to involution

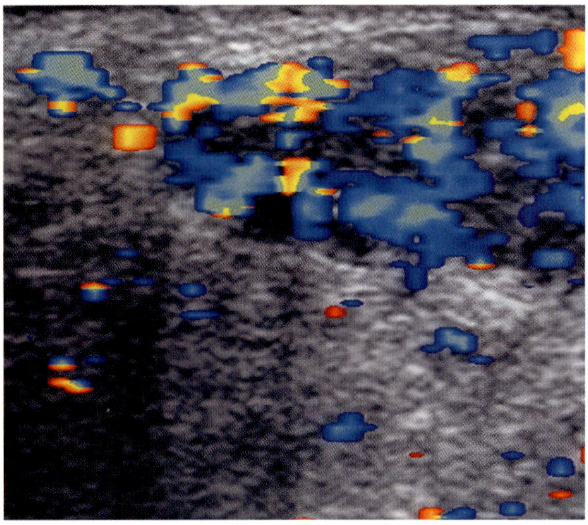

Fig. 18.**13 a** Cavernous hemangioma of the right chest. Relatively hyperechoic lesion with heterogeneous internal echotexture, defined from its surroundings; CFDI reveals massive high-velocity blood flow. **Caveat:** In substantial venous run-off, very slow peripheral flow may also be possible.

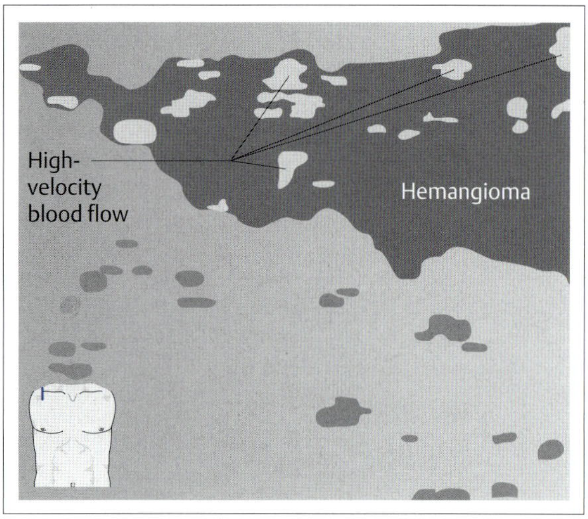

Fig. 18.**13 b** Line drawing.

Consequences for Surgical Treatment

Diagnosis	Characteristic Findings	Management
Inconspicuous cutaneous hemangioma without growth tendency, no functional impairment	Usually circumscribed areas with heterogeneous hyperechoic internal texture and marked flow signals on CFDI	Conservative; spontaneous involution is highly likely
Cutaneous or cavernous hemangioma with rapid growth, conspicuous location, recurrent bleeding, ulceration, or functional impairment	Circumscribed areas of different size with heterogeneous hyperechoic internal texture and marked flow signals on CFDI. If a marked venous component is present, flow velocity on CFDI is much lower	Corticosteroids and irradiation are obsolete. Open surgery (as in lymphangioma) is technically difficult and often with poor cosmesis. Currently, laser coagulation (e.g., Nd-YAG) appears to be the best treatment option. Cavernous hemangioma is devitalized under pilot laser and US guidance via bare-fiber introduced into the convoluted vessels through a cannula. Cutaneous hemangioma can be laser-treated quite well via an ice cube or cooled glass spatula. Alternatively, small hemangioma may also be treated by cryotherapy

Nephroblastoma (Wilms Tumor)

Basic Facts

- Nephroblastomas stem from maldevelopment of the metanephrogenic blastoma.
- Wilms tumor is the most common intra-abdominal malignant tumor to occur in the child (1 : 9000), in Germany accounting for about 6.5% of all newly diagnosed malignancies in childhood.
- Peak incidence is at the 3rd year of life, and approximately 80% of all Wilms tumors are diagnosed by the age of 5 years. Increased incidence in Beckwith–Wiedemann syndrome (synonym: EMG syndrome [exomphalos, macroglossia, gigantism]) points to a genetic contribution.
- Not linked to sex.
- Diagnostic workup relies on a multitude of investigations, but any child with recurrent abdominal pain, hematuria, or equivocal findings on abdominal palpation should undergo sonographic screening as this modality is simple, painless, fast, and inexpensive. If performed promptly, it may result in a decisive time gain, increasing the chances of cure for the child.

Sonographic Criteria of Assessment

- Usually **well-delineated** (pseudo-encapsulated) **tumor** within the renal bed. In the early phase the tumor appears **homogeneous** (some larger nephroblastomas display necrosis) and in most cases is of **hepatic texture** and echogenicity. Calcifications are usually absent, while residual kidney parenchyma can be demonstrated in almost all cases. CFDI shows diminished perfusion compared with the normal renal tissue (Fig. 18.**14**).

- Two different strategies in the treatment of the Wilms tumor are most commonly used:
  - Surgery is tailored to the individual response to preoperative downstaging (SIOP–Societé International d'Oncologie Pédiatrique, Europe).
  - Definitive surgery to obtain exact histological results – (NWTS–National Wilms Tumor Study, USA).
- Depending on the stage, follow-up treatment may not become necessary.

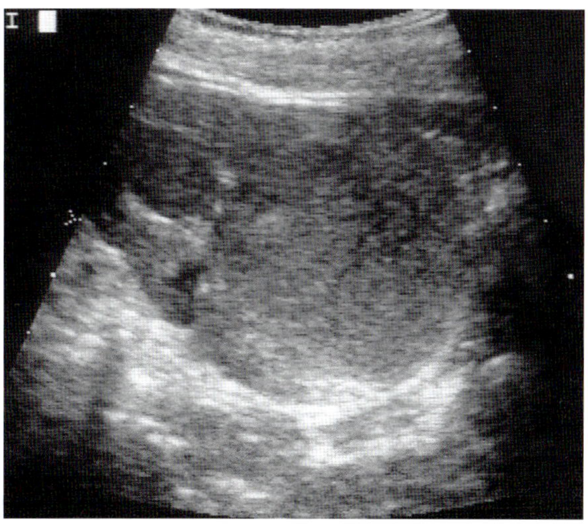

Fig. 18.**14a** Usually well-delineated (pseudo-encapsulated) tumor within the renal bed. In the early phase the tumor appears homogeneous (some larger nephroblastomas display necrosis) and in most cases is of hepatic texture and echogenicity. Calcifications are usually absent, while residual kidney parenchyma can be demonstrated in almost all cases. CFDI shows diminished perfusion compared with the normal renal tissue. This sonogram depicts residual renal parenchyma cephalad and caudad, while the anterior border of the kidney has already been breached.

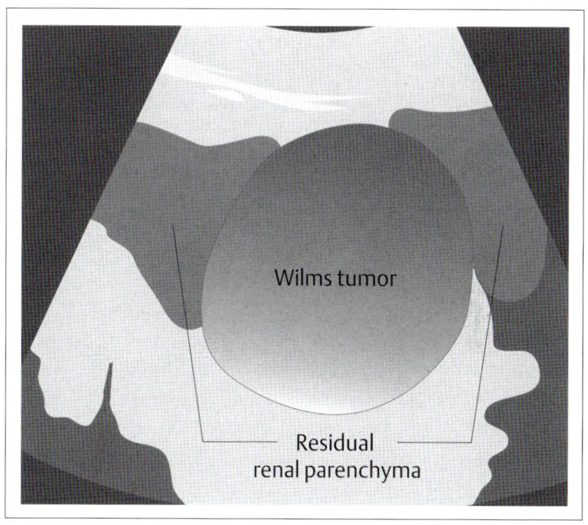

Fig. 18.**14b** Line drawing.

Consequences for Surgical Treatment

Finding (according to National Wilms Tumor Study)	Characteristic Findings	Management (according to SIOP: preoperative chemotherapy mandatory)
Stage I	Limited to one side and one kidney	Individual treatment protocol aiming for total resection No follow-up treatment
Stage II	Limited to one side but with invasion of adjacent tissue	Individual treatment protocol aiming for total resection No follow-up treatment
Stage III	Limited to one side, but peritoneal or lymph node metastasis (or intraoperative rupture)	Individual treatment protocol aiming for total resection of the tumor plus postoperative (radio-)chemotherapy
Stage IV	Hematogenous spread	Individual treatment protocol aiming for total resection of the tumor plus postoperative (radio-)chemotherapy
Stage V	Bilateral renal involvement	Individual treatment protocol (possibly resection of the larger tumor and subtotal excision of the contralateral malignancy)

Neuroblastoma

Basic Facts

- Neuroblastomas stem from maldevelopment of the neural crest. More than 50% are located in the retroperitoneum, 30% of which arise in the adrenals. In Germany, neuroblastomas represent 7.8% of all newly diagnosed childhood malignancies.
- Spontaneous involution in infancy is possible; age peak is at 2 years of life.
- Screening modalities are currently under development.
- Diagnostic workup involves numerous modalities. Even more so than in nephroblastoma, any child with recurrent abdominal pain, hematuria, equivocal findings on abdominal palpation, or equivocal anemia and frequent fatigue should undergo sonographic screening, as this can improve prognosis dramatically. If performed promptly, it may result in a decisive time gain, increasing the chances of cure for the child.

Sonographic Criteria of Assessment

- Most neuroblastomas are **ill-defined tumors** of heterogeneous internal texture, often displaying necrosis and characteristic calcifications. The kidney is displaced. CFDI shows diminished perfusion compared with the normal renal tissue. Occasionally, hepatic metastases will already be present (Fig. 18.**15**).
- Differential diagnosis must rule out adrenal hemorrhage. Characteristically, the latter caps the kidney as a somewhat hypoechoic mass without flow signals on CFDI (Fig. 18.**16**).

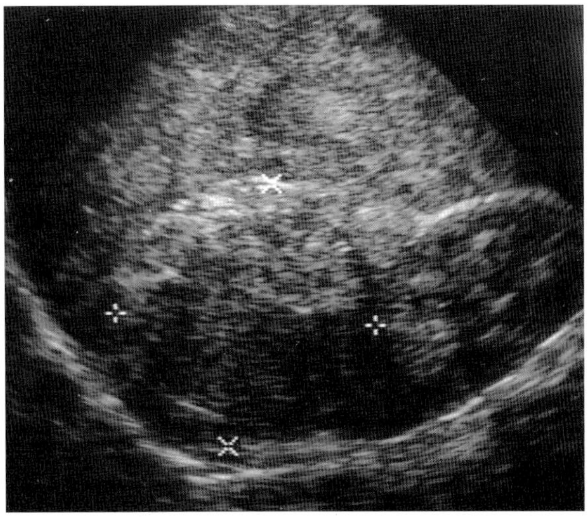

Fig. 18.**15 a** Neuroblastoma is usually an ill-defined tumor of heterogeneous internal texture, often displaying necrosis and characteristic calcifications. The kidney is displaced. CFDI shows increased perfusion compared with the normal renal flow profile. Hepatic metastases are already present in the sonogram. The kidney has been displaced caudad.

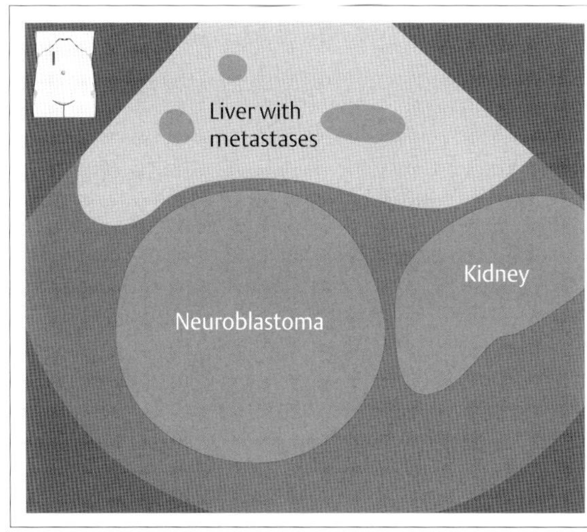

Fig. 18.**15 b** Line drawing.

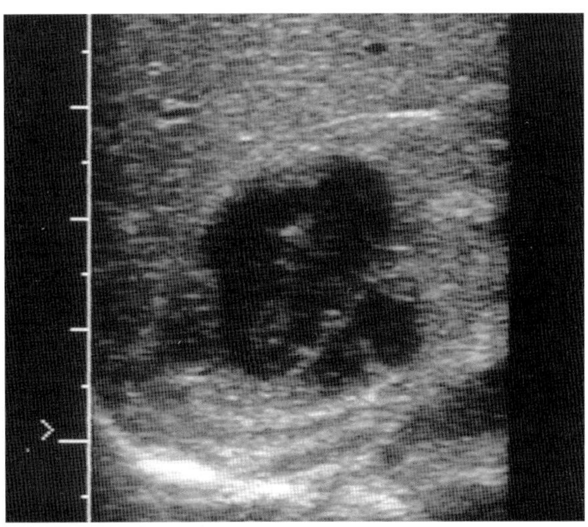

Fig. 18.**16 a** Differential diagnosis must rule out adrenal hemorrhage. Here, the kidney is capped by a somewhat hypoechoic mass without flow signals on CFDI.

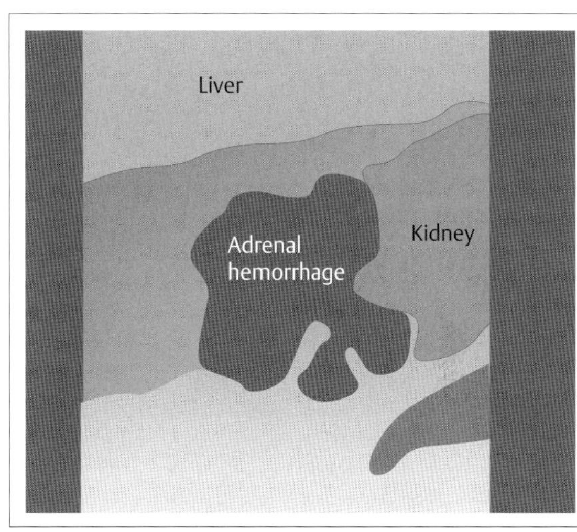

Fig. 18.**16 b** Line drawing.

Consequences for Surgical Treatment

Finding (according to Evans)	Characteristic Findings	Management (in stage II and higher, preoperative chemotherapy is mandatory)
Stage I	Limited to organ of origin (rare)	Total resection
Stage II	Invasion of surroundings without crossing the midline. Homolateral regional lymph node involvement is possible	Individual treatment protocol aiming for total resection of the tumor plus postoperative RT/CT
Stage III	Invasion of surroundings crossing the midline, and regional lymph node involvement on both sides of the midline is possible	Individual treatment protocol aiming for total resection of the tumor plus postoperative RT/CT
Stage IV	Stage III plus hematogenous spread	Individual treatment protocol aiming for total resection of the tumor plus postoperative RT/CT
Stage IV/S	Stage I or II plus distant spread without osseous involvement	Individual treatment protocol aiming for total resection of the tumor plus postoperative RT/CT

Teratoma

Basic Facts

- This tumor stems from maldevelopment of germ cells comprising all three germinal layers. About 50% are located around the sacrum (sacrococcygeal teratoma) and manifest rather quickly, while the remainder favor the ovaries, testes, retroperitoneum, and mediastinum. In principle, any site may be involved.
- Although "classic" sacrococcygeal teratoma is benign at birth, the rate of malignancy increases rapidly after the first few months of life.
- In other types of teratoma, definite assessment is possible only after preoperative diagnostic workup (tumor markers) and histopathological evaluation.

Sonographic Criteria of Assessment

- Rather **heterogeneous** tumor with cystic as well as solid areas (Fig. 18.**17**).

Consequences for Surgical Treatment

Finding	Characteristics	Management
Teratoma	Varied sites and heterogeneous sonogram	Individual timing of surgery, aiming for total resection depending on localization, age, and preoperative staging. In probably benign and well-localized tumors, rapid resection should be attempted. In probable malignancies and unfavorable sites, preoperative chemotherapy is an option
Sacrococcygeal teratoma	Typical site in newborn	Early surgery with coccygectomy

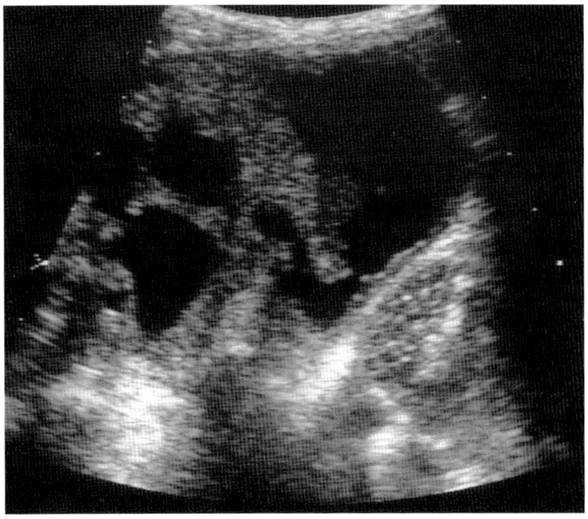

Fig. 18.**17 a** Teratoma arising from the left ovary. The large tumor is rather heterogeneous with cystic as well as solid areas.

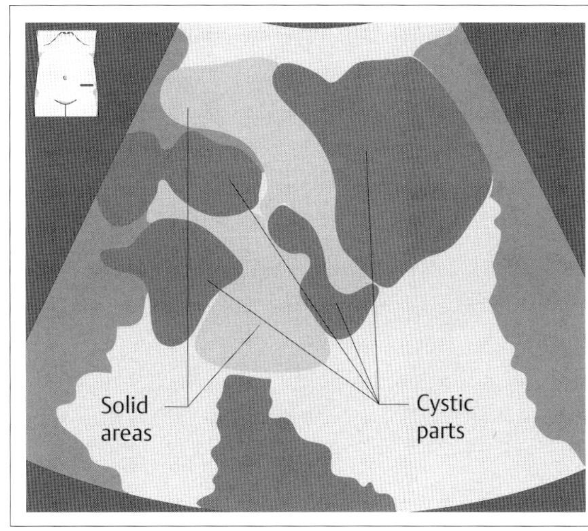

Fig. 18.**17 b** Line drawing.

19 Contrast-Enhanced Sonography

H. P. Weskott

■ Introduction and Technical Background

Sonography is often the first-line imaging modality in patients with suspected abdominal pathology. New gray-scale imaging techniques, such as tissue harmonic imaging and compound scanning, and transducer technology such as matrix array probes have greatly improved image quality. The advantages of real-time gray-scale sonography are well known and accepted, but compared to imaging modes with routine use of contrast media, such as CT and MRI, there are some important shortcomings, including a significantly lower detection rate for liver lesions (Kinkel et al., 2002; Noone et al., 2004) the specific diagnosis of which often remains doubtful. With the advent of dedicated contrast media, sonography can combine the imaging of tissue with that of macrovasculature and microvasculature in organs. Ultrasound contrast agents (UCAs) may act by their presence in the vascular system, from where they are ultimately metabolized (blood pool agents) or by their selective uptake in tissue after a vascular phase.

Between 1996 and 2001, two UCAs were approved in Europe for examination of abdominal vessels and organs: Levovist™ (SH U 508A, Schering, Berlin, Germany) and Sonovue™ (BR 01, Bracco, Milan, Italy). Definity™ is approved in Canada, Brazil, Israel, and Mexico; Sonovue in China. An overview of trade-marketed UCAs is presented in Table 19.**1**.

The strongly reflecting UCA microbubbles introduced into the vascular system seek to increase the backscatter of the tissue that bears them (macrovasculature and microvasculature). The bubbles comprise air or other gas encapsulated in a hard shell (Levovist) or a soft shell (Sonovue, Definity). The bubble size ranges between 3 and 7 µm and, unlike CT and MRI contrast agents, UCAs do not leave the vascular bed and therefore act as blood pool tracers. They survive passage through the capillary network without being destroyed and can thus enhance vessels and organs such as the abdominal organs or the brain. UCAs do not appear in the biliary system or the urinary tract. The microbubbles are eliminated in the lungs, while the shell and stabilizing agents are metabolized in the liver. As they do not affect kidney function, renal insufficiency is not a contraindication for their use. UCAs are not approved for use during pregnancy and childhood.

Due to their soft, more flexible shells, second-generation microbubble UCAs are more stable within the acoustic field, as long as the acoustic pressure is low (applying a low mechanical index = "low-MI imaging"). Another acoustic advantage is their ability to oscillate within the acoustic field; the microbubbles emit harmonic frequencies and the reflected second harmonics still have sufficiently high acoustic power to allow for their detection. In order to display only the signals originating from the contrast bubbles, a special imaging technique (phase-inversion imaging) is used. In most cases, this technique eliminates the gray-scale tissue background image. The bubbles break at higher acoustic pressure, producing much more intense backscatter signals (Burns et al., 2000; Correas et al., 2001).

Table 19.**1** Ultrasound contrast agents approved in the EU and Canada

Contrast Agent; Company	Reflector	Shell	Concentration (Single bolus volume)	Stability after Reconstitution	Approval in the EU
Levovist™; Schering[a]	Air	Galactose/ palmitic acid	200–400 mg/ml [6–20 ml]	15 min	1995
Sonovue™; Bracco[b]	Gas: sulfur hexafluoride	Phospholipid	[1–5 ml]	6 h	2001
Definity™; Bristol-Myers Squibb[c]	Gas: octafluoropropane	Phospholipid	10 µl/kg	12 h (agent has to be activated)	**Not EU approved.** Approved in Canada 2001

[a] Schering Company, Berlin, Germany; [b] Bracco Company, Milan, Italy; [c] BMS Medical Imaging: New York, NY, USA.

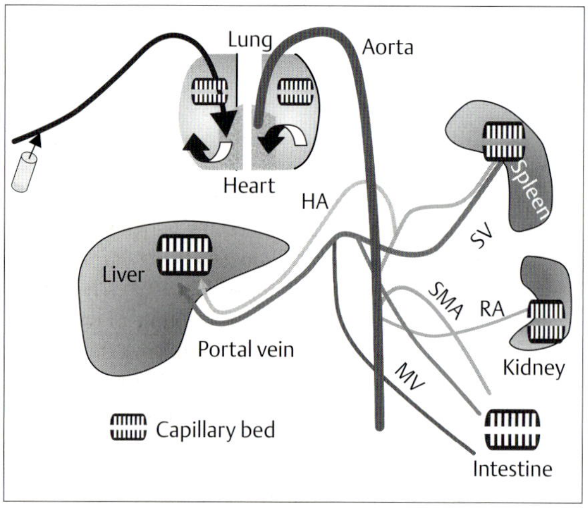

Fig. 19.**1** Schematic contrast pathways after intravenous injection.
HA hepatic artery
RA renal artery
SV splenic vein
MV mesenteric veins
SMA superior mesenteric artery

Practical Considerations

- UCAs are given as an intravenous bolus via the antecubital vein. A size < 21G needle is recommended. The UCA is administered as a rapid bolus injection followed by a 5–10 ml saline flush. A stopwatch should be started at the time of UCA injection. It is mandatory for all contrast examinations to use dedicated contrast software designed for the specific agent being employed.
- When using low-MI contrast-specific imaging modes, it is crucial to provide a balance between sufficient tissue cancellation and adequate depth penetration. A pathway and distribution scheme for intravenously administered US contrast agents is illustrated in Figure 19.**1**.
- Special settings offered on most scanners have to be used when working with Levovist. Since the bubbles can be destroyed when hit by sound waves, a dedicated one-sweep examination technique should be used. These sweeps are performed during the different contrast phases.
- Sonography with Sonovue or Definity is performed just like basic gray-scale examinations in real mode at a low acoustic power output level (low-MI imaging). The contrast behavior of organ tissue and focal lesions should be evaluated and compared. In liver studies, continuous scanning for 60–90 seconds is recommended to fully assess the arterial and portal phases. In a basic liver examination the entire liver should be scanned, especially during the portal and late phases. The different phases of liver enhancement are characterized in Table 19.**2**.
- The time of onset of the three vascular phases in a given patient is influenced by the individual global hemodynamic situation.

Table 19.**2** Vascular phases in contrast-enhanced ultrasonography of the liver (from the EFSUMB Study Group [Albrecht et al., 2004])

Phase	**Visualization Post-Injection Time (s) Start**	**End**
Arterial	10–20	25–35
Portal venous	30–45	120
Late	> 120	Bubble disappearance (approx. 240–360)

Detection of Focal Liver Lesions

Basics

- Compared to contrast-enhanced CT, MRI, or PET (Kinkel et al., 2002; Noone et al., 2004), non-enhanced B-mode sonography has a lower sensitivity in the detection of focal liver lesions. In patients with favorable scanning conditions, however, the use of UCAs increases the detection rate in the number of focal liver lesions by about at least 30% (Harvey et al., 2000; Beissert et al., 2000; Bernatik et al., 2001; Solbiati et al., 2001; Albrecht et al., 2003; Quaia et al., 2004). The European guidelines for the use of ultrasound contrast agents recommend their use in all patients with malignancy whenever liver metastases have to be confirmed or ruled out (Albrecht et al., 2004).
- Focal liver infections or abscesses, especially in the immune-compromised patient, mostly after high dose chemotherapy, benefit from UCAs in the detection of multiple small infectious lesions during the portal or late phases.
- UCAs can be used to guide liver biopsies, especially when the lesion cannot be imaged well in non-enhanced sonography.
- Malignant liver lesions can be detected as hyperenhancing lesions during the early arterial phase (best in hypervascular lesions) or as hypoenhancing or contrast cleared lesions during late phases (Fig 19.**2**). The hyperenhancing phase may last for only a couple of seconds.
- Benign lesions can be detected best during the arterial phase; during the late phase they mostly show isoenhancement and thus cannot be differentiated from surrounding normal liver. FNH, HCC, and hypervascularized liver lesions fill up with contrast prior to the liver, so the early arterial phase is helpful for detection, while the late phase helps to differentiate hypervascularized benign from malignant lesions (Table 19.**3**).
- During the late phase CEUS can be used for needle guidance in difficult or nondetected lesions on baseline US study. It has been shown that ablation therapy can be successfully monitored by contrast-enhanced US (Solbiati et al., 2003).

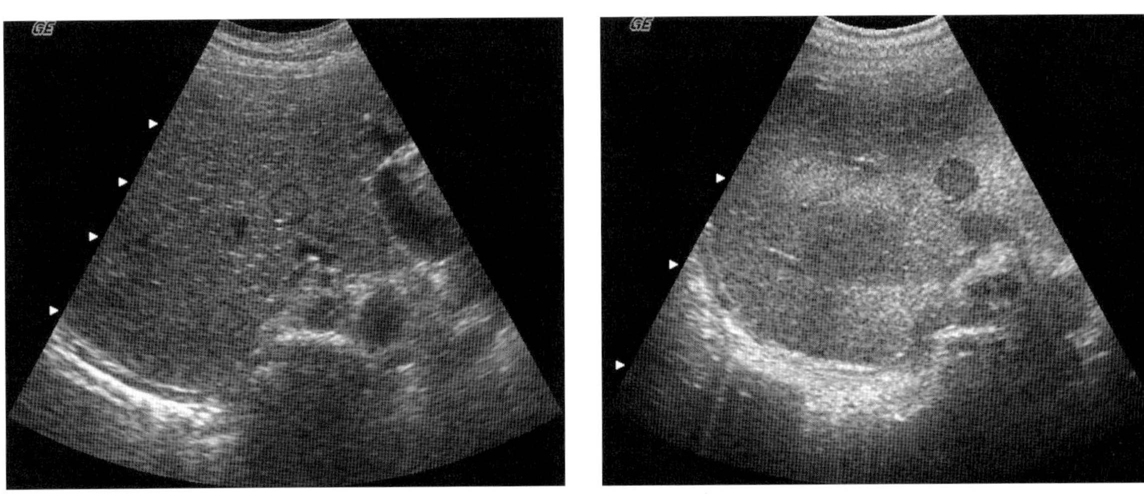

Fig. 19.**2** Liver metastasis in breast cancer, difficult to detect on a plain B-mode scan (**left**), but easily visualized in a contrast-enhanced study during the portal venous phase (**right**).

Table 19.**3** Best contrast phases for detection the most common liver lesions

	Arterial Phase	Portal Venous Phase	Late Phase
Hemangioma	+++	+	–
FNH	+++	+	–
HCC	+++	+	+
CCC	++	+	++
Hypervascularized metastases	+++	++	+++
Hypovascularized metastases	+	++	+++

Characteristics of Focal Liver Lesions

- Compared to nonenhanced sonography, UCAs markedly improve identification of focal hepatic lesions and may, in patients with favorable scanning conditions, compete with CT and MRI (Beissert et al., 2000; Vilgrain et al., 2000; Hohmann et al., 2003; Quaia et al., 2003; Strobel et al., 2003; Nicolau and Bru, 2004). This chapter discusses the most common focal liver lesions and lists their characteristic contrast-enhanced ultrasound (CEUS) findings.
- In order to **correctly** characterize different tumor types all contrast phases should be analyzed. The late phase behavior is best for differentiation between benign and malignant lesions. The arterial phase is best in differentiating between benign lesions and between hyper- and hypovascular lesions (Table 19.**4**).

Table 19.**4** Best contrast phases to characterize the most common liver lesions

	Arterial Phase	Portal Venous Phase	Late Phase
Hemangioma	+++	+++	+++
FNH	+++	+++	+++
HCC	+++	+	+
CCC	++	+	++
Hypervascularized metastases	+++	++	–
Hypovascularized metastases	+++	++	+++

Hemangioma

Basics

- Hemangiomas are the most common benign solid liver lesions.
- The reported incidence of hepatic hemangiomas is approximately 2%, with a prevalence at autopsy as high as 7.4%.
- There is a female preponderance of 4–6 : 1.
- Histology: vascular channels and calcifications may be present; thrombosis is a frequent finding.

Sonographic Features

In a gray-scale imaging, 70% have a "characteristic" appearance: Hyperechoic, well-defined tumor, enhancement often visible (Fig. 19.**3 b**). With increasing size, hypoechoic areas arise and an echogenic rim may be present. Color-flow Doppler imaging reveals little to no flow in most hemangiomas. The majority of hemangiomas are located in the periphery, adjacent to venous branches. Atypical hemangiomas occur in about 30%, often appearing as hypoechoic lesions in fatty liver disease, some with an echogenic rim. Hemangiomas may have an arterial supply, a portal venous supply, or a mix of both. Intratumoral arteriosystemic shunts may exist. Contrast behavior reflects the vascular patterns described (Vilgrain et al., 2000; Wilson et al., 2000; Kim et al., 2002; Albrecht 2001; Quaia et al., 2002, 2003; Isozaki et al., 2003). Arterialized hemangiomas take up contrast very quickly during the arterial phase; these mostly small hemangiomas (< 3 cm) are completely filled after 20–30 seconds. Due to shunting, vascular channels can fill completely during the arterial phase ("high-flow hemangiomas"). Typical features of a hemangioma are peripheral globular enhancement ("eclipse sign" Fig. 19.**3 a**) and a centripetal filling of the lesion (see Table 19.**5**). On dynamic bolus CT, globular enhancement is considered a highly sensitive (88%) and specific (84–100%) feature (Quinn and Benjamin, 1992; Leslie et al., 1995). UCA enhancement patterns have a specificity and accuracy of 99.4% and 97.8%, respectively (Isozaki et al., 2003). Completely thrombosed hemangiomas remain nonenhanced at all times.

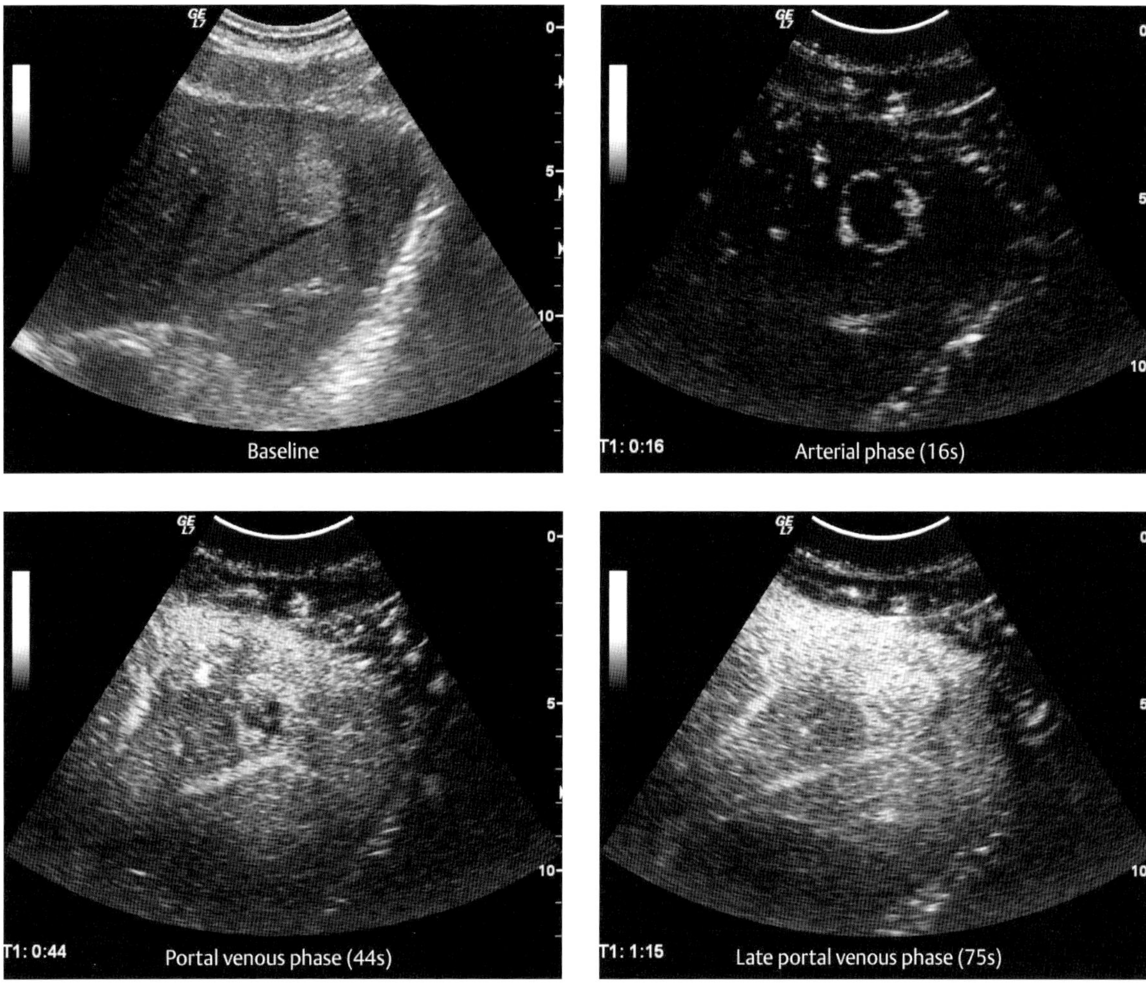

Fig. 19.3 a Typical hemangioma (in a 63-year-old man). "Eclipse sign" during the early arterial phase.

Table 19.5 Most common CEUS findings in hemangiomas

	Arterial Phase	Portal Venous Phase	Late Phase
Characteristic features	Peripheral nodular enhancement	Progressive centripetal enhancement	Complete enhancement
Optional/other features	Complete enhancement	Peripheral nodular enhancement	Nonenhanced areas
	No intratumoral vessels	Complete enhancement	

Focal Nodular Hyperplasia

Basics

- Focal nodular hyperplasia (FNH) is a benign hepatic tumor without malignant potential, predominantly found in younger females.
- It most likely represents a local hyperplastic response of hepatocytes to a congenital vascular anomaly.
- Most lesions have central scars that contain thick-walled vessels providing excellent arterial blood supply; hemorrhage, necrosis, and infarction are, therefore, extremely unusual.
- Histology: hepatocytes, reticuloendothelial system (RES) of varying proportions, bile ducts, fibrous tissue.
- Most patients with FNH are asymptomatic and the lesions are incidental findings. If imaging techniques fail to identify the lesion, biopsy is recommended.
- In case of tumor related symptoms, resection should be considered.
- Discontinuation of oral contraceptive use is recommended for women.

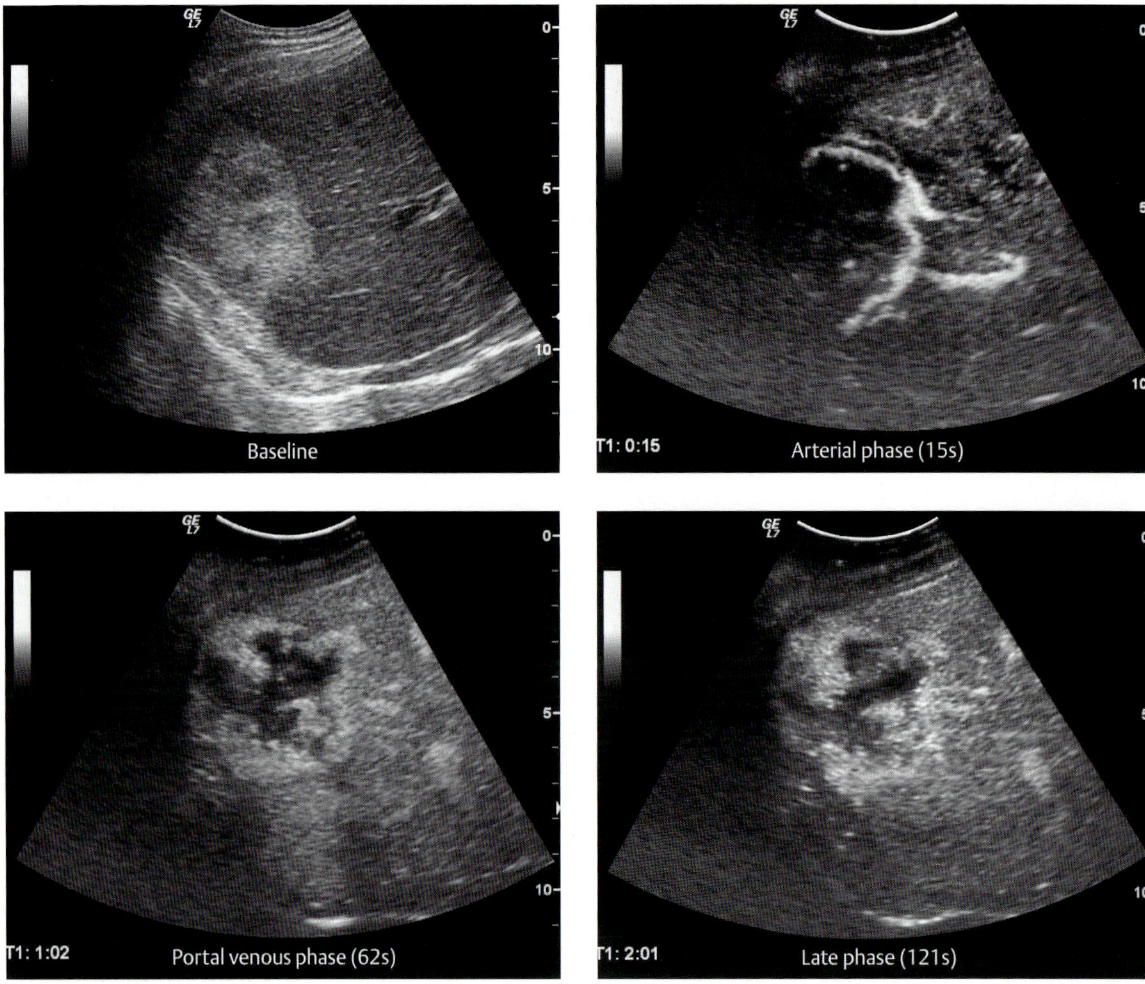

Fig. 19.**3 b** Typical hemangioma (in a 51-year-old woman).

Sonographic Features

FNH gray-scale image depends on coexisting fatty liver changes. Central scar. Blood vessels: dense network of arteries feeding the tumor from the center (spoke-and-wheel sign) or the periphery. Due to the low peripheral resistance, the resistance index (RI) of the feeding artery is also low. Uggowitzer et al. (1999) found the RI of the feeding artery to be lower than that of the hepatic artery (mean 0.51 ± 0.09 vs. 0.65 ± 0.06). FNHs have a portal venous supply and arteriosystemic shunts. Degeneration leads to tumor shrinkage, and the portal venous branches often thrombose. In contrast studies, FNHs display a rapid early uptake of contrast agent (Fig. 19.**4 a**). Maximum enhancement occurs during the arterial and early portal phases. Decrease of enhancement depends on the portal venous supply. Therefore, a long and intense enhancement can be seen, as well decreasing enhancement during the portal venous phase (Bartolotta et al., 2003; Strobel et al., 2003).

In order to better differentiate benign lesions, the contrast behavior during the arterial phase is most important as all benign tumors show an iso- (some a hyper-) enhancement during late phase (Table 19.**6**).

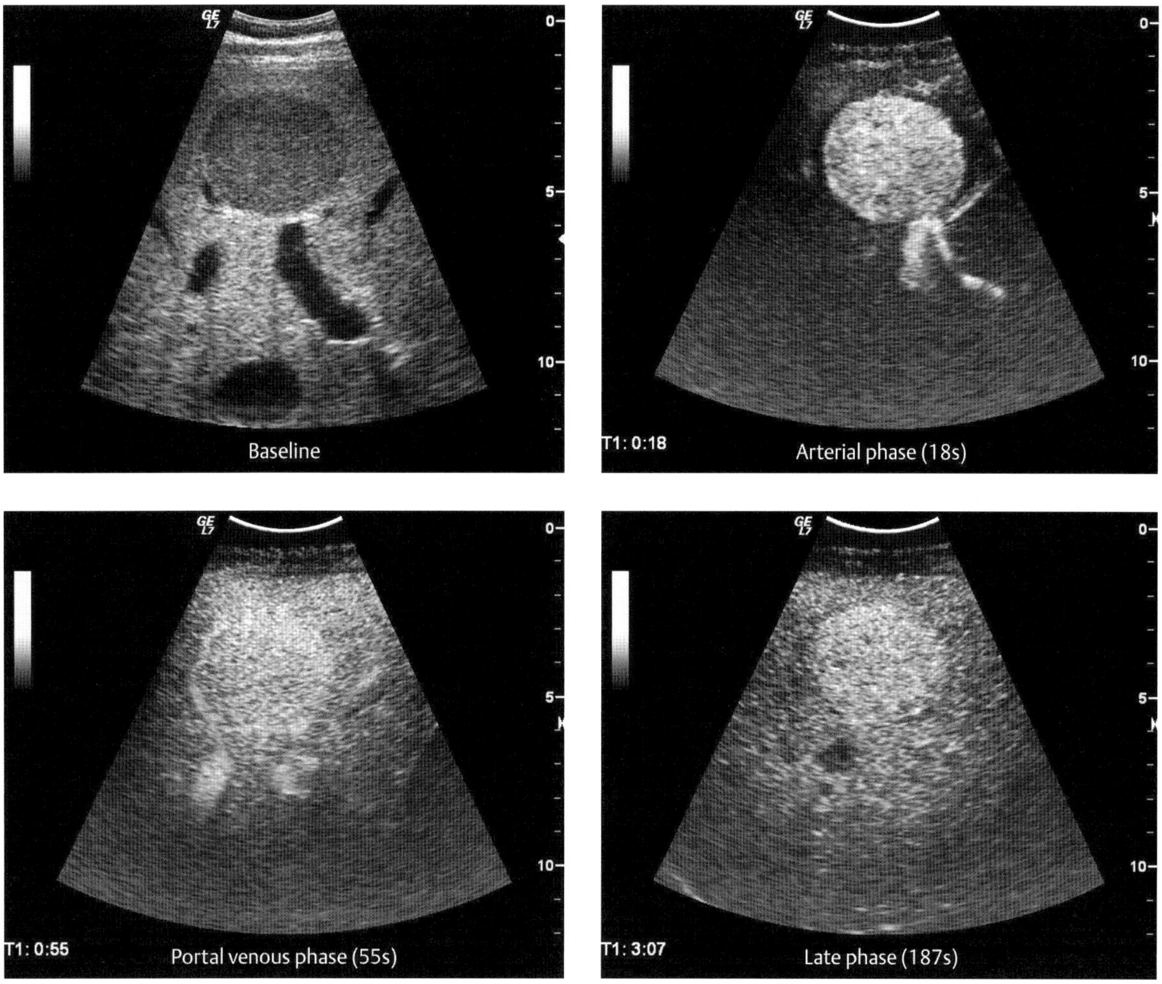

Fig. 19.**4 a** Typical contrast enhancement in focal nodular hyperplasia (FNH) during the arterial phase (in a 30-year-old woman). Very early enhancement of arteries radiating to the center (7 seconds); one second later, the FNH is completely filled, draining liver veins, hyperenhancing compared to liver tissue during all phases.

Table 19.**6** Most Common CEUS Findings in FNH

	Arterial Phase	Portal Venous Phase	Late Phase
Characteristic features	Early complete enhancement	Hyperenhancing	Iso-/hyperenhancing
Optional/other features	Feeding artery	Central scar	
	Radiating arteries		
	Centrifugal filling pattern		

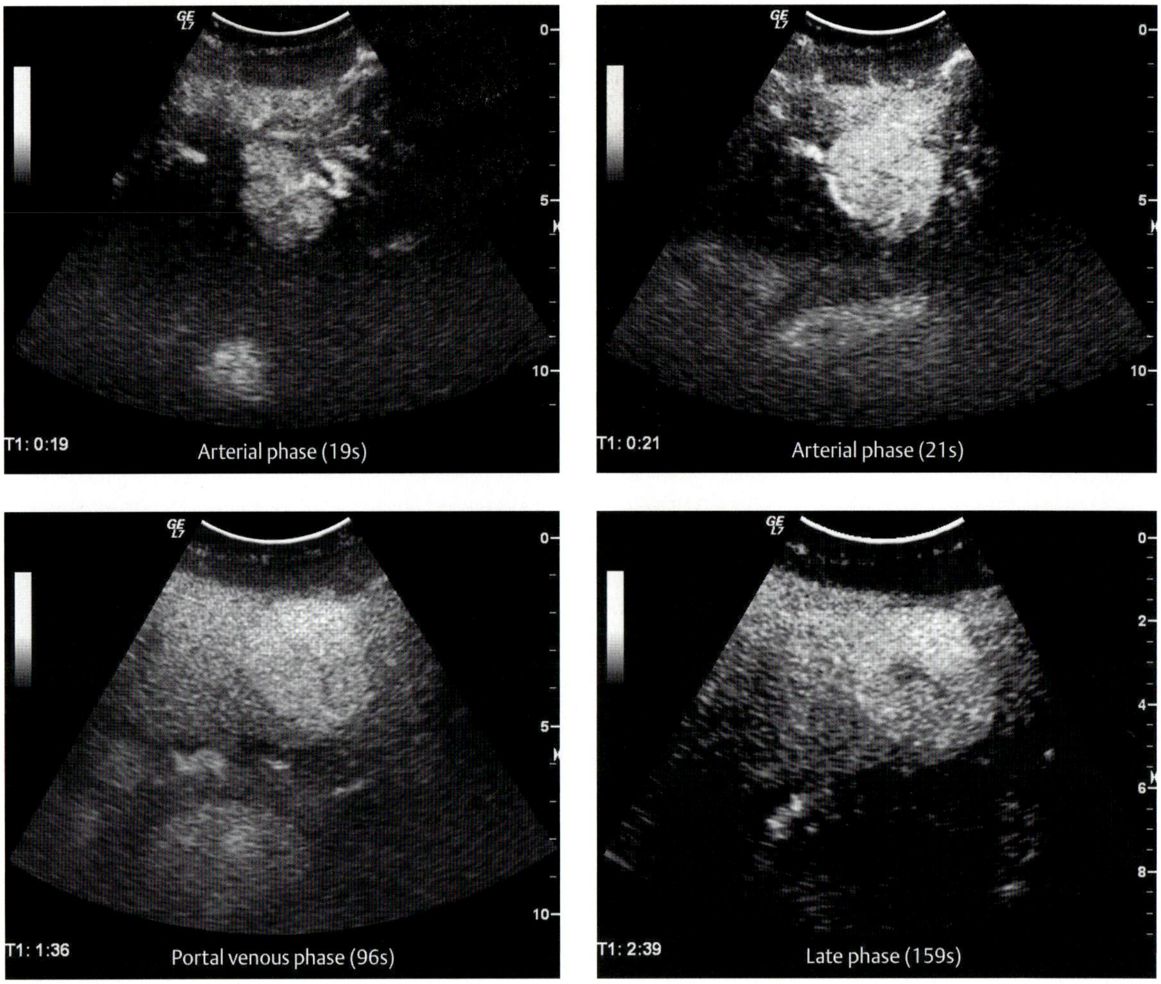

Fig. 19.**4** b FNH in the left hepatic lobe (in a 28-year-old woman), with a central scar and feeder artery. Hyperenhancing during all phases.

Fatty Liver Disease

Basics

- In most cases, fatty liver disease arises from metabolic disorders, such as obesity, alcohol abuse, diabetes, or toxicity (for example, chemotherapy).
- Nonalcoholic steatohepatitis (NASH) is increasingly being recognized as an important and common condition, affecting approximately 13–15% of the general population (Tchelepi et al., 2002; Mofrad and Sanyal, 2003).
- Focal sparing can be seen, most likely as a result of higher regional liver perfusion, most commonly posterior to the gallbladder, in segment IV at the hepatic hilum, and in the caudate lobe.

Sonographic Features

Fatty infiltration (area of hyperechogenicity) is often patchy or focal. A circumscribed hypoechoic area in a fatty liver may mimic a focal liver lesion. UCAs can help to easily rule out a focal liver lesion, since these areas display the same contrast behavior as the surrounding hepatic tissue (Table 19.**7**).

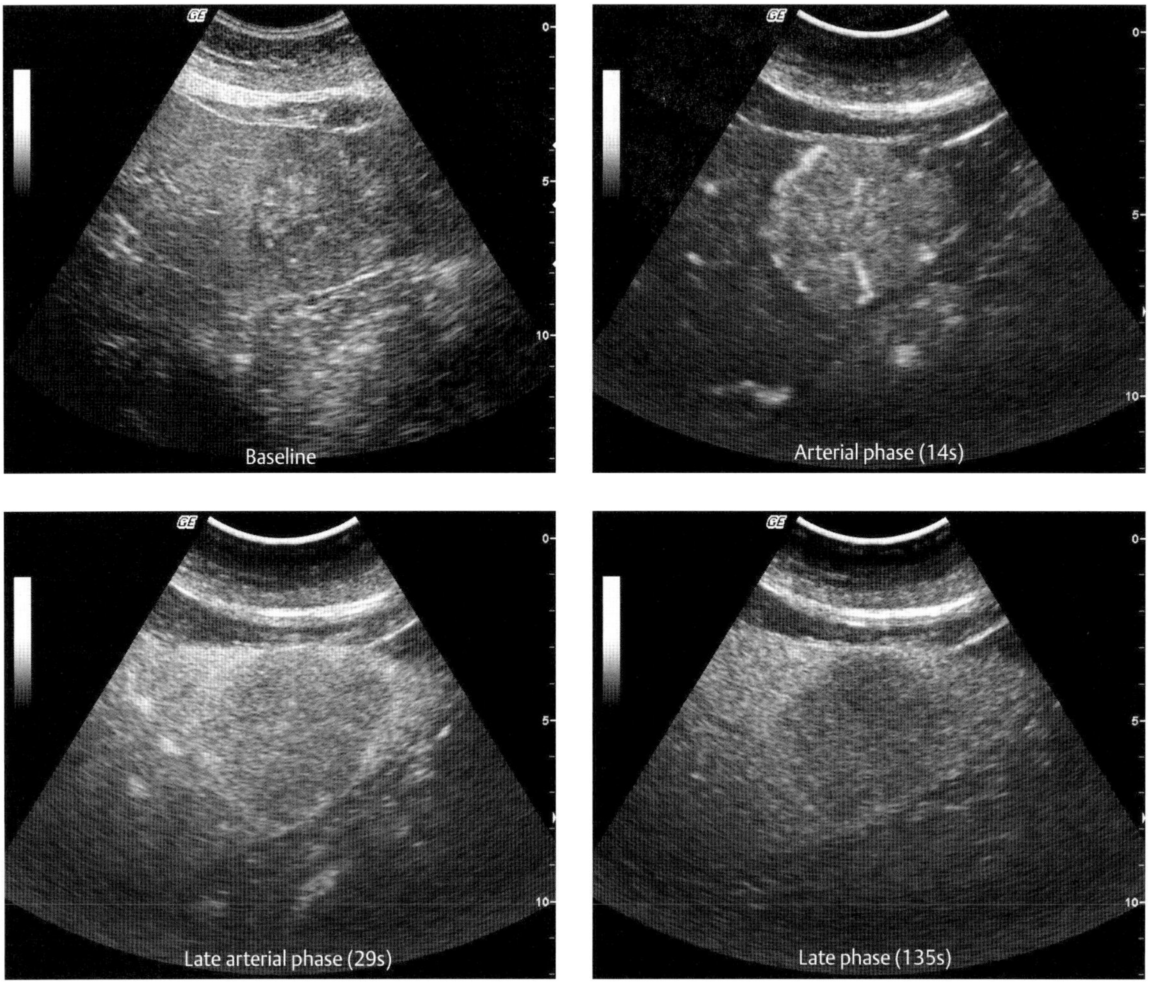

Fig. 19.**4c** Atypical FNH (in a 51-year-old woman). Note the beginning of washout during the early portal phase. FNH was proved by surgical specimen (HIDA scintigraphy characterized the lesion as malignant).

Table 19.**7** Most common CEUS findings in livers with uneven distribution of fatty liver tissue

	Arterial Phase	**Portal Venous Phase**	**Late Phase**
Focal fatty sparing (no fat)/ Focal fatty change (focal fatty infiltration)			
Typical features	Isoenhancement	Isoenhancing	Isoenhancing

Pyogenic Abscess

Basics

- Liver abscess may result from infection of the biliary tract, sepsis, and septic emboli from various sources, such as intestinal infections, endocarditis, or pyelonephritis.
- Contiguous spread from cholecystitis and the perihepatic space may also result in pyogenic abscesses.
- Other sources may be perforated bowel, postoperative infections, or trauma to the liver.
- Additional nonbacterial causes include amebiasis due to infection with *Entamoeba histolytica* (a protozoan)
- Abscesses may also stem from fistula formation between localized intra-abdominal infections.

Sonographic Features

Bacterial abscess is characterized by increased perfusion around it, often leading to hyperperfusion of this liver segment. During the arterial phase, enhancement of the rim (Fig. 19.**5**) and of some local arteries adjacent to the abscess becomes evident (Table 19.**8**). The destruction of liver tissue may leave some viable septations displaying enhancement (Catalano et al., 2004). The acuity of the inflammatory process defines the degree of vascular reaction around the abscess, which decreases under interventional or antibiotic therapy.

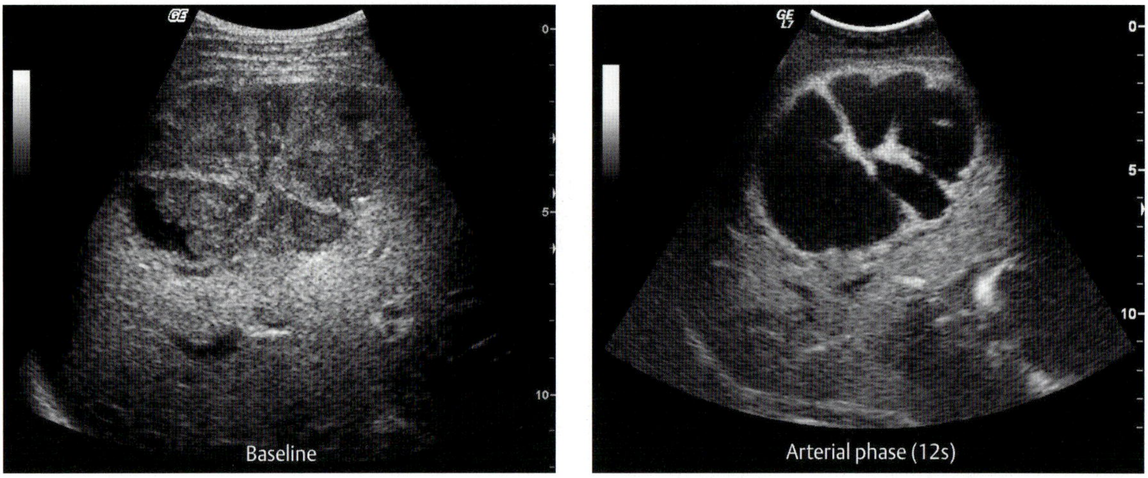

Fig. 19.**5** Pyogenic liver abscess; 12 seconds after bolus injection, a hyperenhancing rim and enhanced septations can be seen.

Table 19.**8** Most common CEUS findings in liver abscess

	Arterial Phase	Portal Venous Phase	Late Phase
Characteristic features	Hyperenhancing rim	Nonenhancing areas	Iso-/hypoenhancing rim
	Nonenhancing areas	Enhancing septa	Nonenhancing areas
Optional/other features	Arteries within the margin	Hypoenhancing rim	
	Hyperenhanced liver segment	Hyperenhanced liver segment	

Liver Metastases

Basics

- The liver is the organ second most commonly involved by metastatic disease, after the lymph nodes.
- While liver tissue is characterized by a dual blood supply (portal vein plus hepatic artery, see Fig. 19.**1**), liver metastases are supplied solely by arteries. This explains the early contrast enhancement during the arterial phase and the quick wash-out during the portal phase, when the normal liver tissue exhibits the most intense enhancement (Fig. 19.**6**).

Sonographic Features

Liver metastases may be classified as hypervascularized (such as in renal cell carcinoma, breast cancer, or neuroendocrine tumors) (Fig. 19.**8**) or hypovascularized (Fig. 19.**7**). Hypervascularization refers to the level of enhancement during the arterial phase and the number of larger-sized detectable arteries. The vasculature of the lesion can be visualized best during the arterial phase and in the postarterial phase, as malignant lesions lack a portal supply (Table 19.**9**). The UCA enhancement pattern of liver metastases has specificity and accuracy of 94.3% and 93.4%, respectively (Isozaki et al., 2003).

In summary, solid lesions that are nonenhancing in the late phase are most likely malignant (except, for example, completely thrombosed hemangiomas and mycotic focal liver inflammations). Lesions with almost no change in late phase enhancement most likely have a benign character.

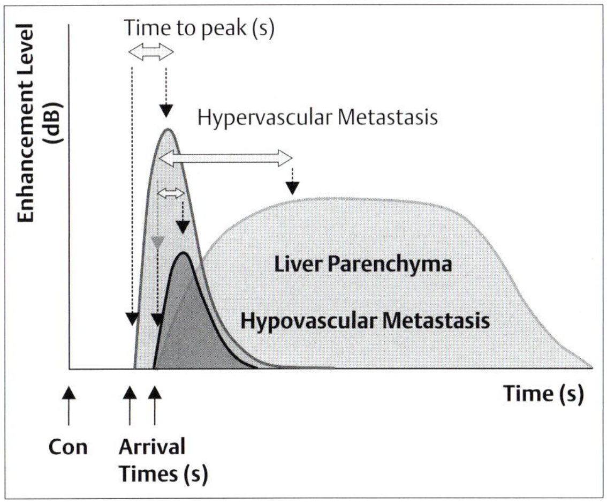

Fig. 19.**6** Schematic contrast kinetics in liver metastasis compared to normal liver tissue enhancement.
CA: Contrast agent

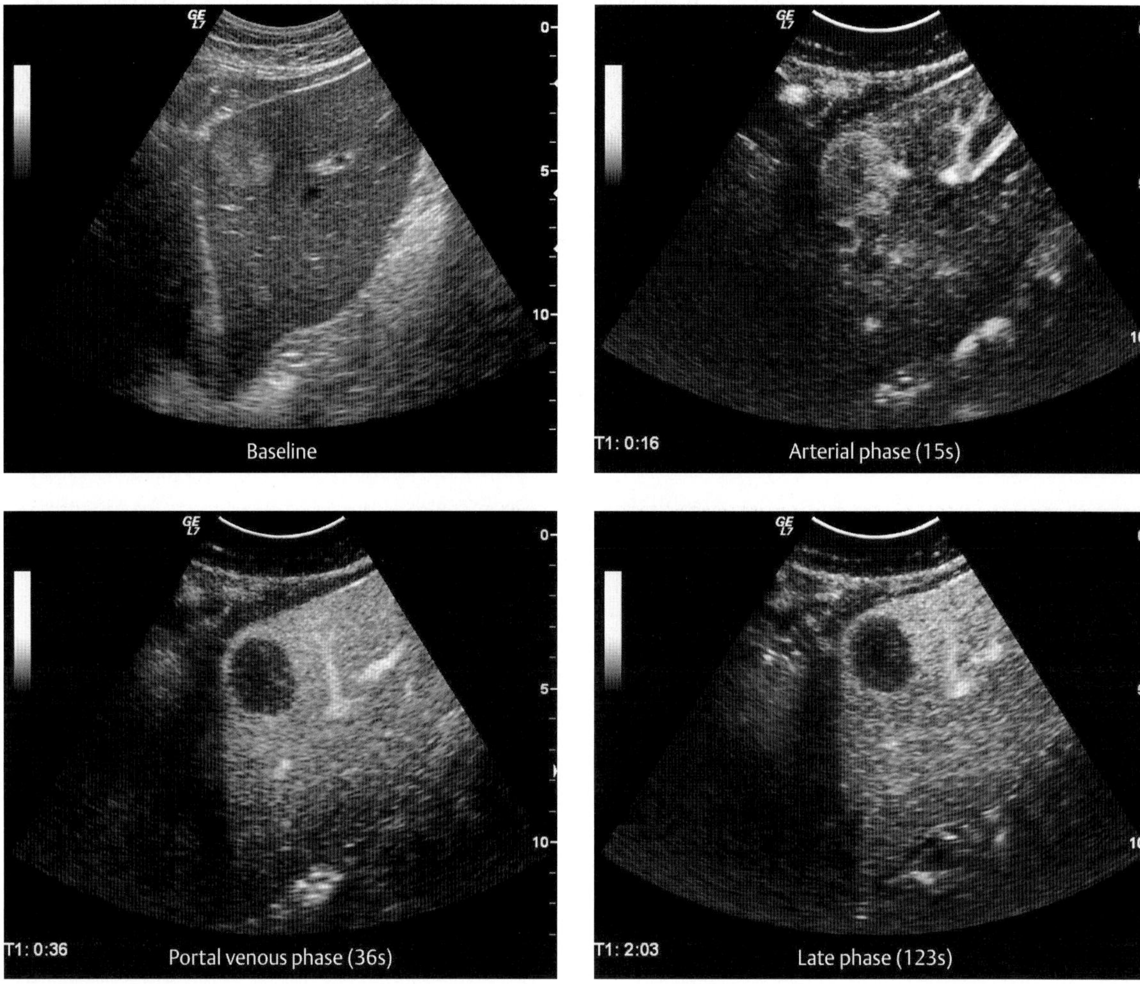

Fig. 19.7 Hypovascular liver metastases (urothelial carcinoma, 65-year-old man).

Table 19.9 Most common CEUS findings in liver metastases

	Arterial Phase	Portal Venous Phase	Late Phase
Hypovascular metastases			
Characteristic features	Rim enhancement, tiny tumor vessels	Hypoenhancing/nonenhancing area	Nonenhancing lesion
Optional/other features	Nonenhancing areas	Nonenhancing areas	("= black hole")
	Mostly weak, nearly complete enhancement		
Hypervascular metastases			
Characteristic features	Strong, nearly complete enhancement, large feeding arteries. Enhancement prior to liver tissue	Hypoenhancing	Regional hypoenhancing areas
Optional/other features	Nonenhancing/low-enhancing areas	Nonenhancing areas	Nonenhancing lesion

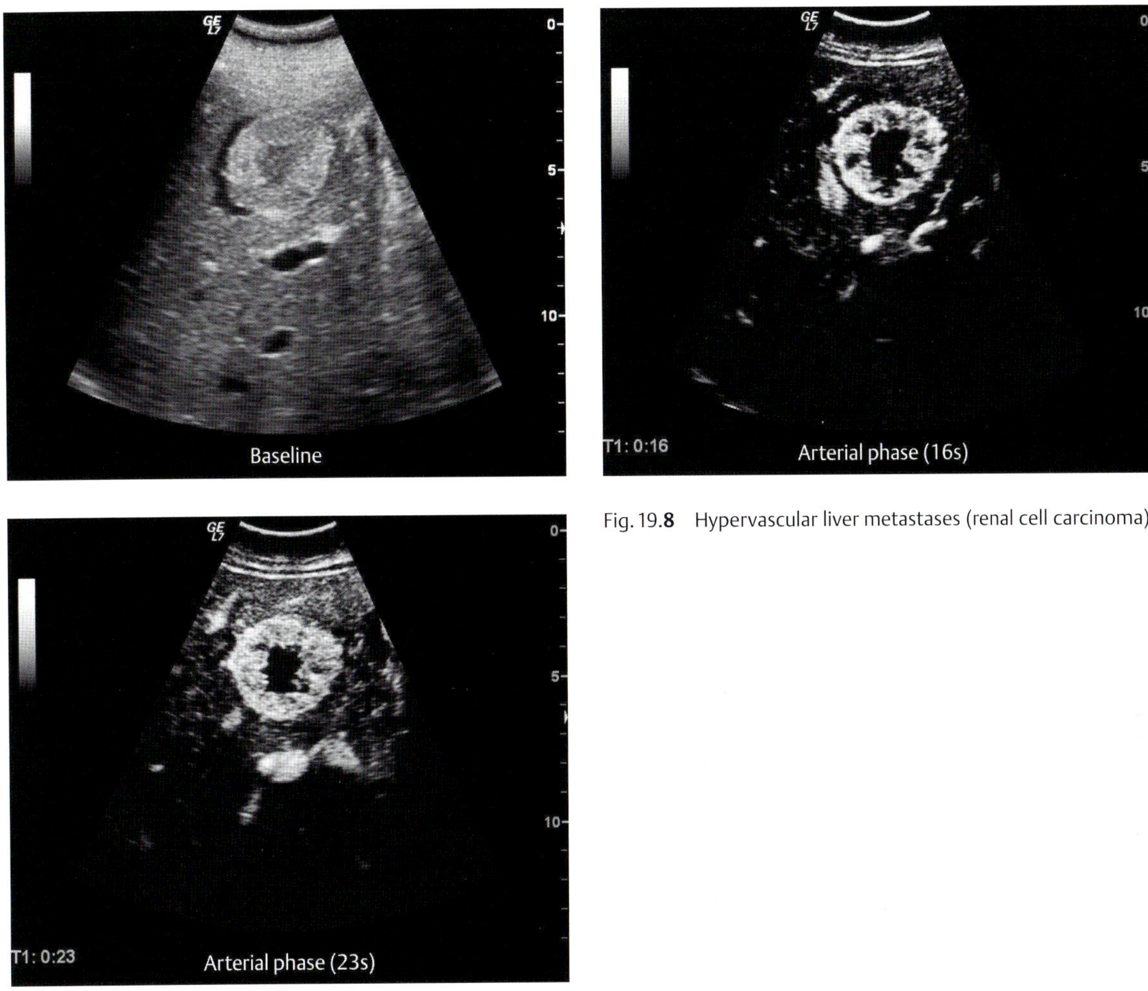

Fig. 19.**8** Hypervascular liver metastases (renal cell carcinoma).

Hepatocellular Carcinoma

Basics

- Hepatocellular carcinoma (HCC) is the fifth most common cancer in the world.
- While HCCs also comprise bile ducts, blood vessels, and fat-storing cells, liver cells (hepatocytes) make up 80% of an HCC lesion.
- The majority of HCCs develop in a cirrhotic liver.
- Apart from establishing the diagnosis, the most important indication for UCAs is the search for tumor thrombosis and follow-up sonography after local ablation therapy.

Sonographic Features

Local hemodynamics in a cirrhotic liver are characterized by an increase in arterial blood flow and a relative decrease in the portal blood supply. Therefore, tumors in a cirrhotic liver are embedded in a hyperarterialized organ. Most HCCs are characterized by a rich network of feeder arteries originating at the periphery of the tumor (basket sign). Intratumoral arteries of different sizes, mostly of chaotic architecture, can be visualized (Fig. 19.**9**). They strongly enhance during the early arterial phase and often demonstrate long-lasting enhancement. In tumor thrombosis, the portal vein thrombus exhibits enhancement during the early arterial phase (Table 19.**10**).

UCA enhancement patterns of HCC have a specificity and accuracy of 94.0% and 94.5%, respectively (Isozaki et al., 2003).

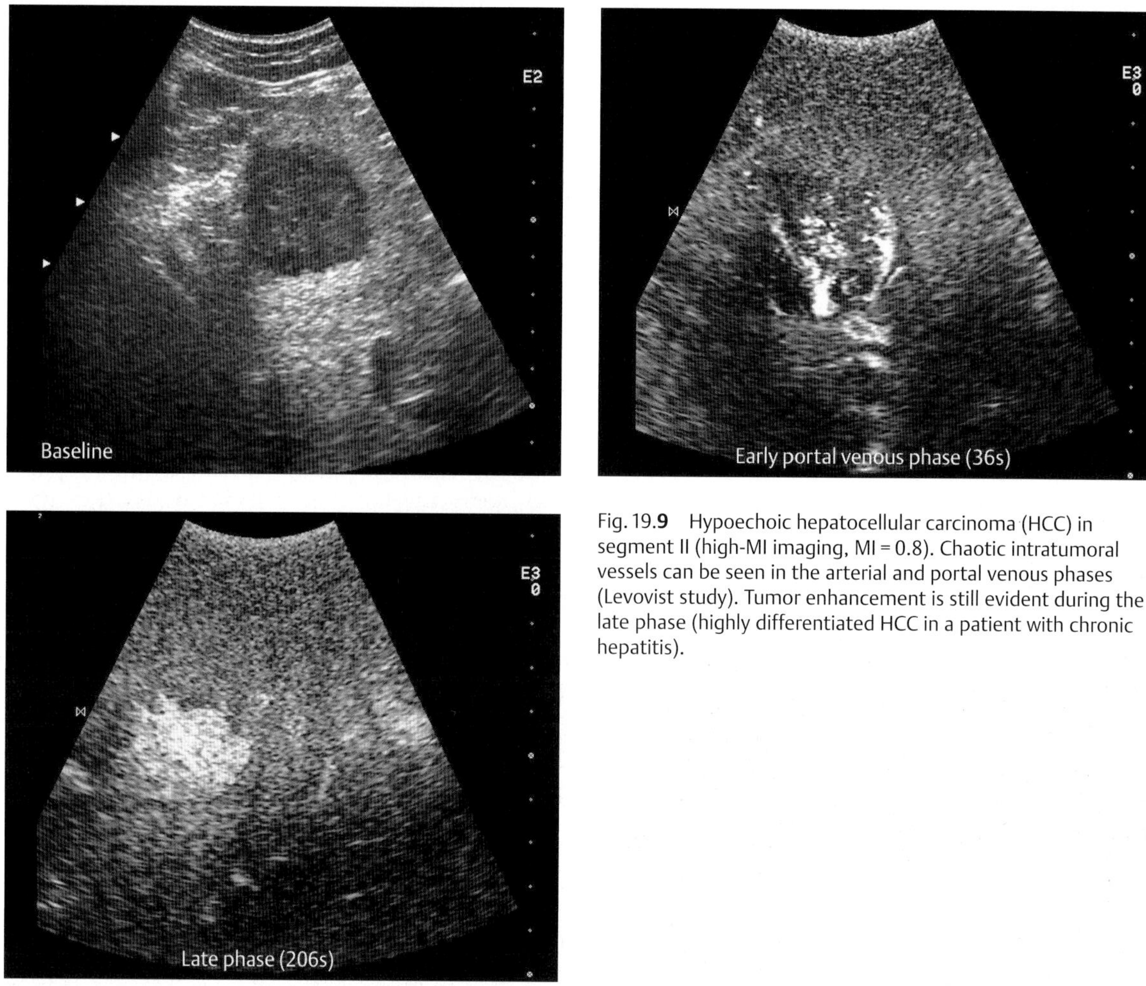

Fig. 19.**9** Hypoechoic hepatocellular carcinoma (HCC) in segment II (high-MI imaging, MI = 0.8). Chaotic intratumoral vessels can be seen in the arterial and portal venous phases (Levovist study). Tumor enhancement is still evident during the late phase (highly differentiated HCC in a patient with chronic hepatitis).

Table 19.**10** Most common CEUS findings in regenerative nodules and HCC

	Arterial Phase	Portal Venous Phase	Late Phase
Regenerative nodules			
Characteristic features	Iso-/hyperenhancing	Isoenhancing	Isoenhancing
HCC			
Characteristic features	Early complete or most complete enhancement	Iso/hypoenhancing	Hypoenhancing
Optional/other features	Intratumoral chaotic vessels	Nonenhancing areas	Nonenhancing areas
	Portal venous thrombus enhancement	Hypoenhancing portal venous thrombus	Nonenhancing portal venous thrombus

Infarction

Basics

- Infarction of abdominal organs may stem from numerous underlying diseases.
- Vascular disease, embolism from the left atrium (atrial fibrillation) and ventricle, endocarditis, and sepsis arising from other organs are the most frequent causes.

Sonographic Features

Liver infarction, particularly after liver surgery (transplantation, resection; Fig. 19.**10**), can easily be visualized as a sharply delineated nonenhancing (occluded liver artery and portal vein) or late-enhancing hypoperfused segmental area due to a low residual flow mainly from branches of the liver artery (Table 19.**11**).

The size of nonenhancing areas in the spleen depends on the number and size of occluded arteries. Multiple defects may be seen in embolic infarction. Splenic infarction may have a nonenhancing triangular shape or a large nonperfused splenic segment (Fig. 19.**11**).

In case of superinfection, the resulting abscess will have a hyperechoic rim while the infarct itself will show only minor enhancement.

In acute renal infarction (Fig. 19.**12**), a well-defined section of the kidney is excluded from blood flow; while an old infarct may still show some individual vessels, it will not display any parenchymal enhancement. Capsular arteries may contribute somewhat to the oxygen supply of the renal cortex.

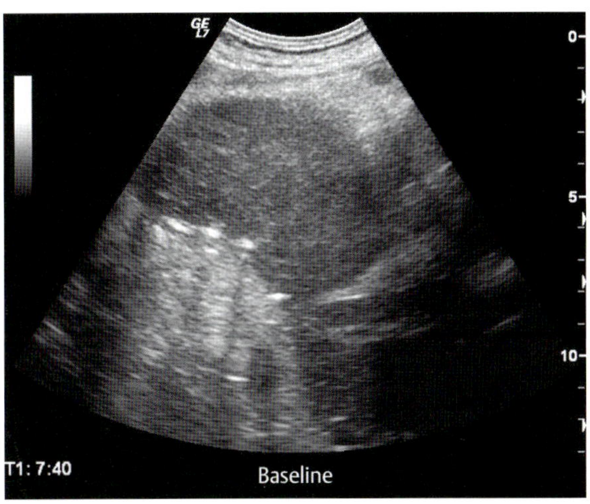

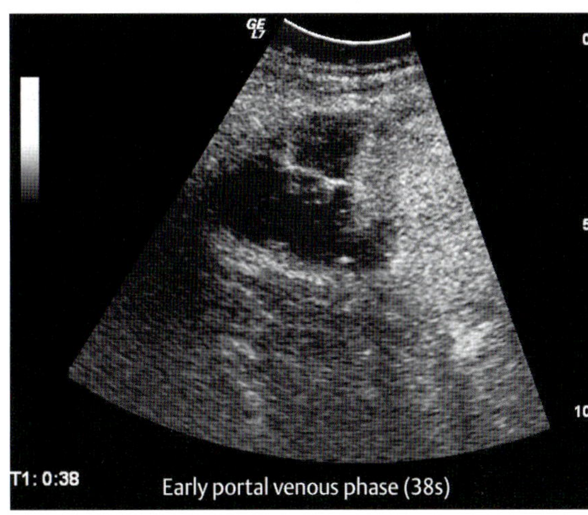

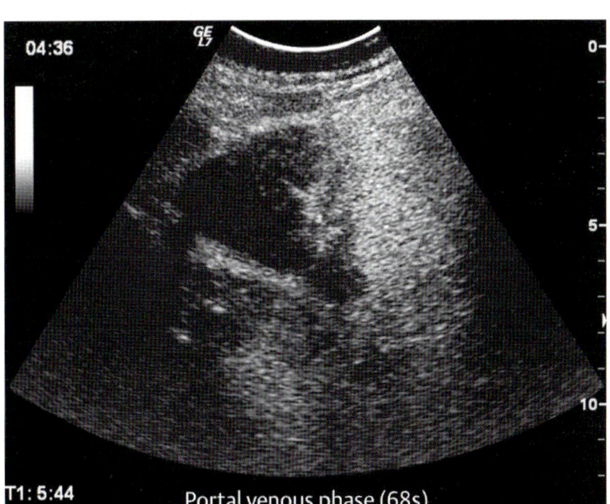

Fig. 19.**10** Liver infarction after atypical hemihepatectomy, not detectable in gray-scale imaging.

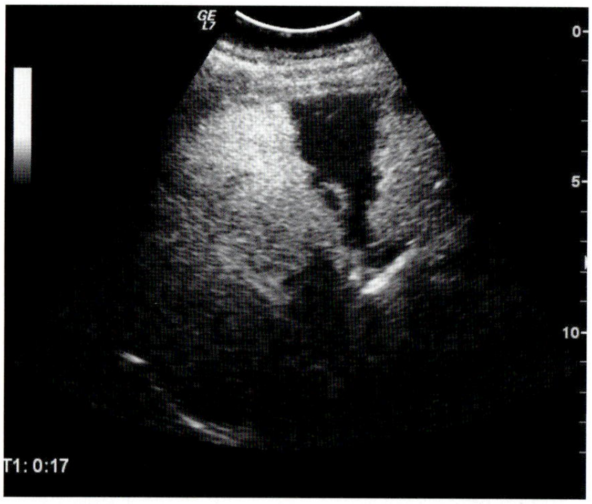

Fig. 19.**11** Acute splenic infarction in a patient with leukemia (17 seconds post contrast injection).

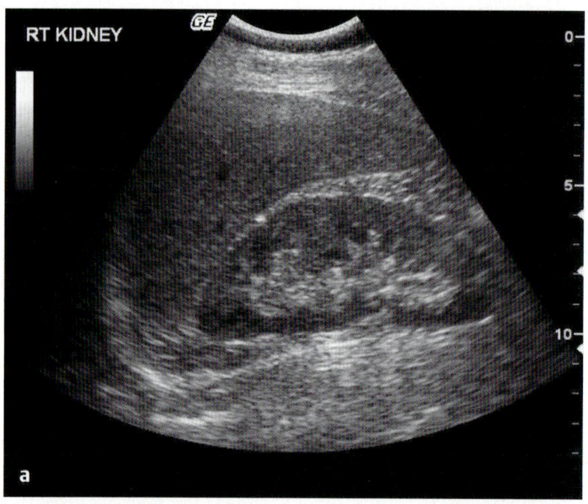

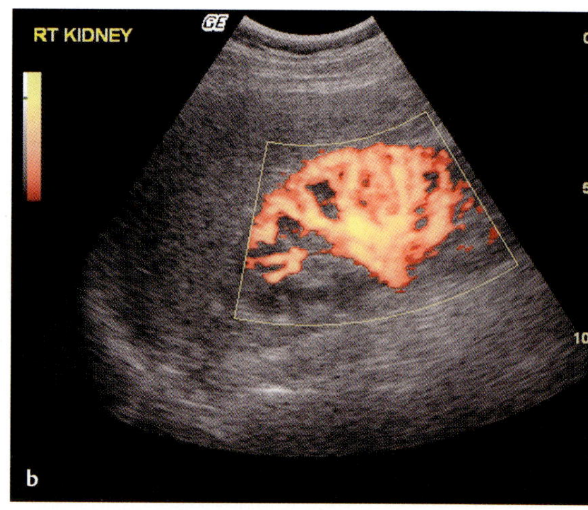

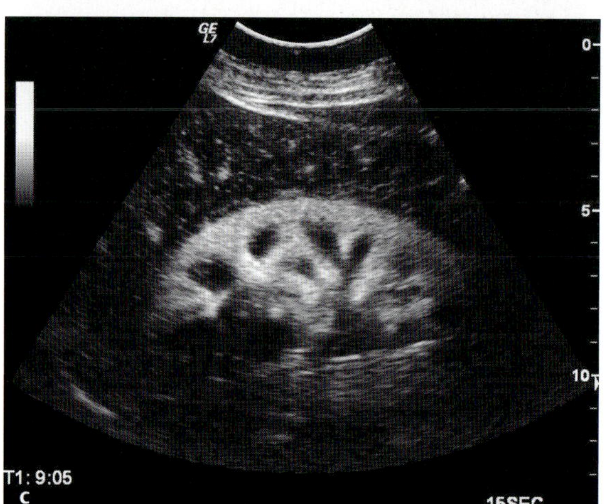

Fig. 19.**12 a–c** Renal infarction. Enhancement defect in the medial portion of the left upper renal pole (15 seconds after injection of 2.4 ml Sonovue).
a B-mode image.
b Power Doppler image.
c Contrast image 15 s post bolus injection.

Table 19.**11** Most common CEUS findings in infarction

	Arterial Phase	Portal Venous Phase	Late Phase
Characteristic features	Segmental nonenhancing area	Segmental nonenhancing area	Segmental nonenhancing area

Bibliography

Albrecht T, Blomley MJ. Characteristics of hepatic hemangiomas at contrast-enhanced harmonic US. Radiology. 2001; 220: 269–70.

Albrecht T, Blomley MJ, Burns PN, et al. Improved detection of hepatic metastases with pulse-inversion US during the liver-specific phase of SHU 508A: multicenter study. Radiology. 2003; 227(2): 361–70.

Albrecht T, Blomley M, Bolondi L, et al. EFSUMB Study Group. Guidelines for the use of contrast agents in ultrasound. January 2004. Ultraschall Med. 2004; 25(4): 249–56.

Bartolotta TV, Midiri M, Scialpi M, et al. Focal nodular hyperplasia in normal and fatty liver: a qualitative and quantitative evaluation with contrast-enhanced ultrasound. Radiol Med (Torino). 2003; 106(4): 320–8.

Beissert M, Jenett M, Keberle M, et al. Comparison of contrast harmonic imaging in B-mode with stimulated acoustic emission, conventional B-mode US and spiral CT in the detection of focal liver lesions. Rofo Fortschr Geb Rontgenstr Neuen Bildgeb Verfahr. 2000; 172(4): 361–6.

Bernatik T, Strobel D, Hahn EG, Becker D. Detection of liver metastases: comparison of contrast-enhanced wide-band harmonic imaging with conventional ultrasonography. J Ultrasound Med. 2001; 20(5): 509–15.

Burns PN, Wilson SR, Simpson DH. Pulse inversion imaging of liver blood flow: improved method for characterizing focal masses with microbubble contrast. Invest Radiol. 2000; 35: 58–71.

Catalano O, Sandomenico F, Raso MM, Siani A. Low mechanical index contrast-enhanced sonographic findings of pyogenic hepatic abscesses. AJR Am J Roentgenol. 2004; 182(2): 447–50.

Correas JM, Bridal L, Lesavre A, et al. Ultrasound contrast agents: properties, principles of action, tolerance, and artifacts. Eur Radiol. 2001; 11(8): 1316–28.

Harvey CJ, Blomley MJ, Eckersley RJ, et al. Pulse-inversion mode imaging of liver specific microbubbles: improved detection of subcentimetre metastases. Lancet. 2000; 355(9206): 807–8.

Hohmann J, Skrok J, Puls R, Albrecht T. Characterization of focal liver lesions with contrast-enhanced low MI real time ultrasound and SonoVue. Rofo Fortschr Geb Rontgenstr Neuen Bildgeb Verfahr. 2003; 175(6): 835–43.

Isozaki T, Numata K, Kiba T, et al. Differential diagnosis of hepatic tumors by using contrast enhancement patterns at US. Radiology. 2003; 229(3): 798–805.

Kim JH, Kim TK, Kim BS, et al. Enhancement of hepatic hemangiomas with Levovist on coded harmonic angiographic ultrasonography. J Ultrasound Med. 2002; 21(2): 141–8.

Kinkel K, Lu Y, Both M, et al. Detection of hepatic metastases from cancers of the gastrointestinal tract by using noninvasive imaging methods (US, CT, MR imaging, PET): a meta-analysis. Radiology. 2002; 224(3): 748–56.

Leslie DF, Johnson CD, Johnson CM, et al: Distinction between cavernous hemangiomas of the liver and hepatic metastases on CT: value of contrast enhancement patterns. AJR Am J Roentgenol. 1995; 164(3): 625–9.

Mofrad PS, Sanyal AJ. Nonalcoholic fatty liver disease. Med Gen Med. 2003; 5(2): 14.

Nicolau C, Bru C. Focal liver lesions: Evaluation with contrast-enhanced ultrasonography. Abdom Imaging. 2004; 29(3): 348–59.

Noone TC, Semelka RC, Chaney DM, Reinhold C. Abdominal imaging studies: comparison of diagnostic accuracies resulting from ultrasound, computed tomography, and magnetic resonance imaging in the same individual. Magn Reson Imaging. 2004; 22(1): 19–24.

Quaia E, Bertolotto M, Dalla Palma L. Characterization of liver hemangiomas with pulse inversion harmonic imaging. Eur Radiol. 2002; 12(3): 537–44.

Quaia E, Bertolotto M, Calderan L, et al. US characterization of focal hepatic lesions with intermittent high-acoustic-power mode and contrast material. Acad Radiol. 2003; 10(7): 739–50.

Quaia E, Calliada F, Bertolotto M, et al. Characterization of focal liver lesions with contrast-specific US modes and a sulfur hexafluoride-filled microbubble contrast agent: diagnostic performance and confidence. Radiology. 2004; 232(2): 420–30.

Quinn SF, Benjamin GG. Hepatic cavernous hemangiomas: simple diagnostic sign with dynamic bolus CT. Radiology. 1992; 182(2): 545–8.

Solbiati L, Tonolini M, Cova L, Goldberg N. The role of contrast-enhanced ultrasound in the detection of focal liver lesions. Eur Radiol. 2001; 11(Suppl. 3): E15–26.

Solbiati L, Ierace T, Tonolini M, Cova L. Guidance and control of percutaneous treatments with contrast-enhanced ultrasound. Eur Radiol. 2003; 13(Suppl. 3): N87–90.

Strobel D, Raeker S, Martus P, et al. Phase inversion harmonic imaging versus contrast-enhanced power Doppler sonography for the characterization of focal liver lesions. Int J Colorectal Dis. 2003; 18(1): 63–72.

Tchelepi H, Ralls PW, Radin R, Grant E. Sonography of diffuse liver disease. J Ultrasound Med. 2002; 21(9): 1023–32.

Uggowitzer MM, Kugler C, Mischinger HJ, et al. Echo-enhanced Doppler sonography of focal nodular hyperplasia of the liver. J Ultrasound Med. 1999; 18(7): 445–51.

Vilgrain V, Boulos L, Vullierme MP, et al. Imaging of atypical hemangiomas of the liver with pathologic correlations. Radiographics. 2000; 20: 379–97.

Wilson SR, Burns PN, Muradali D, et al. Harmonic hepatic US with microbubble contrast agent: initial experience showing improved characterization of hemangioma, hepatocellular carcinoma, and metastasis. Radiology. 2000; 215(1): 153–61.

20 New Technologies in Ultrasonic Imaging

J. C. Schlegel

Introduction

The number of innovations in diagnostic ultrasound has increased significantly in recent years. This development was mainly initiated by the on-going digitalization of ultrasound devices. While only some years ago ultrasound systems were based on analog circuitry, signal processing components of today's devices are mainly digital. This technology is now able to process many times the information of analog systems in real time. Especially the introduction of digital beamformers as well as the development of fast and powerful application-specific integrated circuits (ASICs) has triggered this quantum leap in ultrasound imaging technology.

Digital beamformers have also led to a substantial increase in beam shaping precision and therefore to significantly improved resolution and uniformity of ultrasonic images. Digital technology has introduced the capability of simultaneous processing of multiple scan lines and advanced signal and image processing technologies such as tissue harmonic imaging, real-time compounding or panoramic imaging. Because of their outstanding versatility, a number of these technologies became standard features in high-end scanners within a very short time and are currently being integrated into smaller systems.

Another effect of the digitalization of ultrasound devices is the increasing miniaturization of components, leading to the development of increasingly powerful portable ultrasound systems. Much as laptops have changed our way of working, it is expected that portable ultrasound devices will change the role of ultrasound as a diagnostic tool. Especially the ubiquitous availability will expand its versatility and diagnostic potential considerably.

Due to the continuously increasing capabilities of ultrasound devices, examinations have also become more and more complex. Accordingly, ergonomics, ease of use, and workflow optimization are currently topics drawing special attention. Major new developments in this area include automated image optimization and measurements as well as tools for workflow guidance to support the management of examinations. Moreover, fully digital handling of image and patient data as well as reporting are gaining ever more attention as important tools for quality assurance and clinical workflow optimization.

This chapter provides an overview of the newly developed key technologies and their clinical applications.

Image Quality Improvements

The propagation of sound waves in the human body is a very complex process. This results in a number of limitations of ultrasonic imaging with respect to sensitivity, resolution, and detail definition. The powerful architecture of state-of-the-art ultrasound devices enables the application of increasingly complex and sophisticated signal processing algorithms to process a number of scan lines or images simultaneously before actual display on the monitor. This has led to a number of important new techniques for image quality improvement and artifact reduction in ultrasonic imaging.

Tissue Harmonic Imaging

Harmonic imaging was initially developed to detect ultrasonic contrast agents. It was believed that ultrasonic waves would propagate linearly in tissue, while contrast-agent bubbles would vibrate under the influence of sound waves and thus produce strong nonlinear backscatter signals at higher harmonic frequencies. Nonlinear backscatter signals coming from tissue were initially treated as artifacts. However, soon they turned out to be an excellent source for B-mode imaging.

Apparently tissue harmonic signals have a number of very interesting characteristics. Because their center frequency is doubled and their beam width is reduced, the spatial resolution of tissue harmonic signals is significantly higher than that of fundamental frequencies. Moreover, the low side lobe level of tissue harmonic signals results in substantially improved contrast resolution. And because tissue harmonic signals are generated inside the body, they travel only half the distance compared to the transmitted waves and pass the upper fatty layer—a major source of signal distortion—only once before reception. Thus tissue harmonic signals are less attenuated and less distorted, resulting in enhanced image quality and better penetration compared to a setup transmitting and receiving at the harmonic frequency.

Figure 20.**1** demonstrates these effects in an example of a breast cyst. On the right side the fundamental image is shown. While the penetration in the tissue harmonic image of the same cyst as displayed on the left is slightly de-

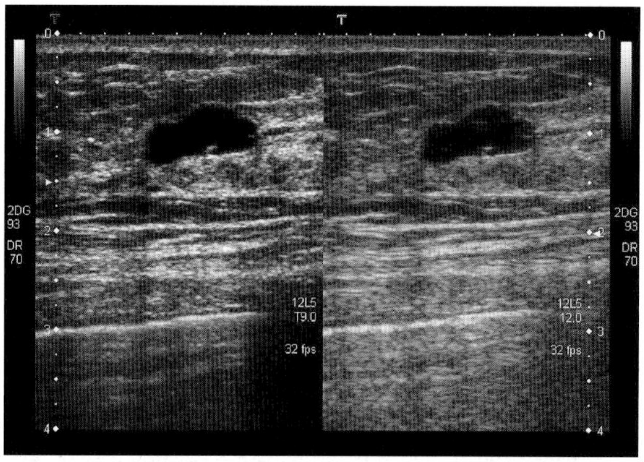

Fig. 20.1 Comparison of fundamental (right) and tissue harmonic (left) images of a breast cyst showing advantages of THI such as improved spatial resolution and gray scale contrast. (Image courtesy of Dr. L. Steyaert, AZ Sint Jan, Brugge, Belgium.)

creased, spatial and contrast resolution are significantly improved.

The principle of tissue harmonics generation is simple. Sound is a longitudinal mechanical wave, which means that the positive half-cycle of a traveling wave compresses the tissue whereas the negative half-cycle expands it. Because the speed of sound in a medium depends on the density of the medium, sound waves travel faster in compressed and slower in expanded tissues. This periodic change leads to a deformation of the initially perfectly sinusoidal sound wave, which then contains, as well as the fundamental frequency, components at higher harmonic frequencies.

Obviously it is necessary for the sound wave to travel a certain distance before its deformation reaches a detectable level. Higher frequencies, on the other hand, are much more attenuated than lower frequencies. Thus tissue harmonic imaging works most effectively at mid-range depths.

To create a tissue harmonic image it is necessary to separate harmonic from fundamental signals in the echo. The simplest way of doing this is to filter the fundamental components out of the received signals by means of a high-pass filter. The major disadvantage of this method is that the frequency spectra of fundamental and second harmonic signals overlap, which makes it quite difficult to cancel fundamental components completely. Another problem is that filtering limits the bandwidth of the received signals, which has a deleterious effect on the axial resolution in the ultrasonic image.

Pulse inversion is the most common method for separating tissue harmonic from fundamental components. A pair of inverted pulses is sent consecutively into the same tissue. Summing up both received echoes cancels linear components completely, because they are perfectly mirror-inverted. Second-harmonic components of both echoes have different characteristics and are therefore maintained in the summation process. The downside of this method is that the frame rate is halved, because two pulses are required to generate one line.

Only a fraction of the incident sound energy is shifted to harmonic frequencies. Therefore, tissue harmonic signals are generally weaker than fundamental signals. To detect and display tissue harmonic signals adequately, transducers and system electronics with enhanced sensitivity and bandwidth and a minimum noise level are required. Due to the strongly increased attenuation of sound waves at higher frequencies, this is especially important for applications such as vascular, small parts, or intra-operative imaging.

Because of its usefulness, tissue harmonic imaging became a routine function in ultrasound imaging in an amazingly short time. Nearly all ultrasound systems offered today have tissue harmonic imaging available as an option or as a standard feature, at least on low-frequency transducers such as standard cardiac sector and abdominal convex types.

Real-Time Compounding

Visibility, echo pattern (also referred to as „speckles"), and detail definition of small objects are strongly dependent on transducer frequency and angle of insonation. Speckles, which are actually not a reproduction of the tissue structure but interference patterns, limit contrast resolution and thus the detail definition of ultrasonic images. Also borders, such as vessel walls, are known to be depicted best if hit by the incoming sound wave at an angle of 90°.

Compounding makes use of these effects by acquiring independent, noncoherent ultrasonic images or scan lines of the same object. There are several ways of doing this. Independent ultrasound images can be acquired, for example, at multiple points of observation, scan angles, frequencies, or times. Before display on the monitor, these data are superimposed, which results in images with significantly increased quality and detail resolution. At the same time artifacts are suppressed.

Real-time compounding performs this process in the ultrasound system during live scanning and is therefore especially useful for applications such as abdominal or small parts imaging, where high spatial and contrast resolution are required to identify small lesions reliably.

Spatial compounding has been commercialized under a variety of names. Its basic principle is to acquire scan lines or images of the same object from different viewing angles, which is similar to the steering function of linear probes. After images from all views have been acquired sequentially, they are superimposed to form a new ultrasonic image with improved uniformity and contrast resolution. Moreover, the delineation of structures and boundaries is enhanced and shadowing artifacts are reduced. Live scanning at a high frame rate is maintained by consecutive updating of individual views followed by the formation of a new compound image. Increasing the number of superimposed views will lead to an enhanced effect. The penalty of adding

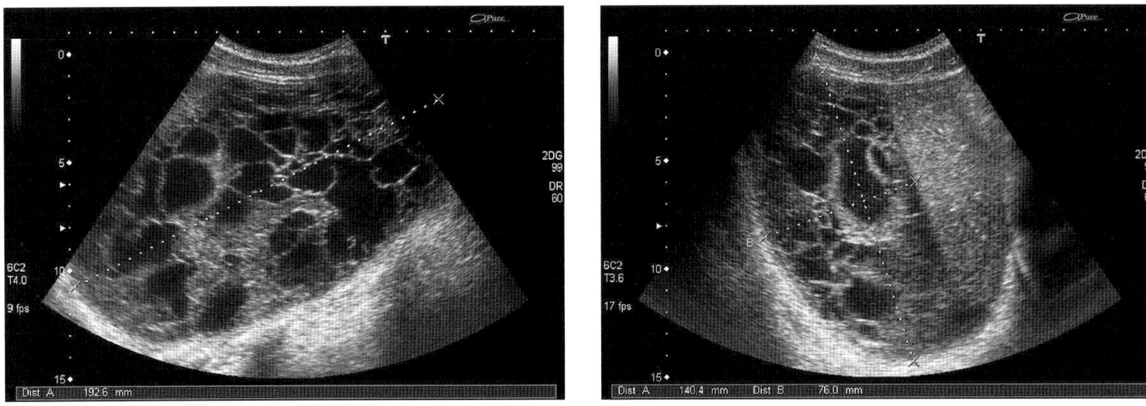

Fig. 20.**2** Real-time compound images of a liver hematoma demonstrating typical effects such as enhanced contrast resolution, improved continuity of structures, and a homogeneous presentation of liver tissue with reduced speckles. (Images courtesy of Dr. L. Steyaert, AZ Sint Jan, Brugge, Belgium.)

more views to a compound image is that it takes an increasingly long time to collect all the data from different angles. Consequently this technique becomes more and more susceptible to motion, which can, for example, be caused by the patient's breathing or by transducer movement. This will then result in a significant deterioration of images.

In frequency compounding, ultrasonic data from different frequency bands are acquired simultaneously. While lower frequencies are less attenuated and thus afford good penetration and sensitivity, higher frequencies are used to maximize the spatial resolution. State-of-the-art transducers allow transmission and reception of signals of within a remarkably wide range of frequencies. Thus images of the same region of interest can be acquired at different frequencies at the same time. Although they depict exactly the same object, ultrasonic data received at different frequencies contain different echo patterns. Compounding such data sets will result in enhanced spatial and contrast resolution as well as in optimized sensitivity and penetration. Because in frequency compounding all data can be acquired simultaneously, this method does not suffer from reduced frame rate or increased persistence.

The most recent techniques perform a combination of both spatial and frequency compounding, and are thus able to combine the advantages of both methods. Figure 20.**2** shows an example of such real-time compound imaging in a giant liver hematoma. The display of liver tissue is very homogeneous due to the effect of speckle reduction. Moreover, because of the high contrast resolution, the texture of the hematoma can be depicted clearly. Even small structures are displayed with high spatial resolution and improved continuity.

High-Resolution Color Doppler Imaging

Color Doppler imaging was introduced commercially in 1986 and gained broad clinical acceptance very rapidly. Its performance and diagnostic value, however, have increased dramatically since then. Next to the refinement of detection and signal processing algorithms, this development was initiated by a strong increase in hardware and software performance. Particularly the introduction of digital beamformer technology has again enabled the implementation of many advanced techniques and thus helped to overcome a number of previous limitations, e.g., in frame rate, artifact suppression, and spatial resolution.

Parallel Signal Processing

Ultrasound waves travel at quite low velocity and therefore the time required to create an image is relatively long. This is especially problematic in color Doppler imaging, where multiple pulses are required to create a scan line. The introduction of parallel signal processing has enabled reception and processing of multiple scan lines simultaneously, which improves the frame rate of B-mode and especially of color Doppler imaging significantly.

In parallel processing, a pulse with relatively wide beam profile is transmitted into the tissue. A digital beamformer is used to receive and store the returning echo signals of each transducer element. Using different focusing patterns, the digital beamformer is then able to calculate a number of neighboring scan lines within the transmitted beam profile. The current state of the art is the ability to create up to four scan lines simultaneously in color Doppler as well as in B-mode. As a result, the frame rate is improved by a factor of up to 4 compared to conventional imaging.

This technique is therefore of special interest for cardiac imaging. Due to the rapid motion of the heart, the ability to detect and depict fast events with high temporal and spatial resolution is of vital importance for a comprehensive and secure diagnosis and therapy planning such as cardiac valve

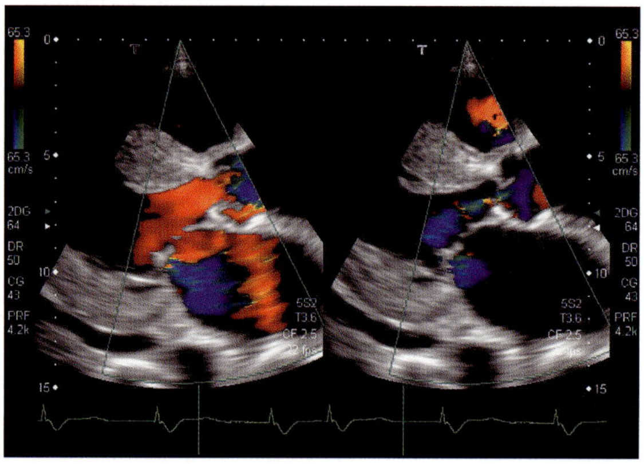

Fig. 20.**3** Parasternal long-axis view of the left heart showing both aortic (right) and mitral (left) insufficiencies in color Doppler with high spatial and temporal resolution. (Images courtesy of Dr. Nesser, Krankenhaus der Elisabethinen, Linz, Austria.)

surgery. Figure 20.**3** shows regurgitant jets of both mitral (left) and aortic (right) valves, in a parasternal long-axis view. Although the color ROI is relatively wide, the frame rate is still high. Because the duration of each frame is significantly below 50 ms, even fast cardiac events can be detected. Moreover, the high temporal and spatial resolution of the ultrasonic image enables the precise depiction of both valve morphology and jet areas.

Although the need for very high frame rates is less important in radiology, parallel signal processing for color Doppler imaging plays an important role here also. The ability to generate many more scan lines per second considerably increases the amount of data available for velocity estimation. The result is first of all an improved signal-to-noise ratio with enhanced sensitivity and improved artifact suppression. Furthermore, it is now possible to maintain reasonable frame rates even when using multiple focal points or wide color ROIs, or when working in triplex mode.

Wideband Doppler Techniques

While spatial and contrast resolution are the most important criteria for B-mode, sensitivity plays a major role in color Doppler imaging in general. Echo signals from blood are more than two orders of magnitude weaker than tissue signals. To achieve a high sensitivity and to determine blood flow velocities accurately, Doppler techniques usually make use of long transmit pulses. The bandwidth of these signals is small, however, which results in a generally poor spatial resolution of color Doppler compared with gray-scale imaging.

New transducer materials, a significantly reduced intrinsic noise level, a high number of physical beamformer channels, and the capability of ultrasound systems to perform increasingly complex signal processing algorithms in real time have led to increased sensitivity and artifact suppression. It therefore became possible to increase the bandwidth and thus the spatial resolution of Doppler signal processing significantly.

The results are a substantially refined display of vascular structures and improved ability to resolve individual vessels. Fig. 20.**4** demonstrates the effect on two similar color Doppler images showing kidney perfusion. While Fig. 20.**4 b** shows an image using conventional power Doppler, Fig. 20.**4 a** demonstrates the same kidney using a wideband Doppler imaging method. Obviously both methods are able to detect and display kidney perfusion. Using conventional power Doppler, however, it is impossible to identify small vessels. A wideband Doppler such as advanced dynamic flow (ADF), on the other hand, has a much better spatial resolution and is therefore able to resolve individual vessels up to the cortical region. Doppler processing enables also the determination of the direction of flow, resulting in a similar directional color coding to that familiar from conventional color Doppler imaging. Wideband Doppler techniques are also very useful for improving the visualization of flow patterns around vascular obstructions such as plaques and for displaying submillimeter vessels such as can be found in small organs.

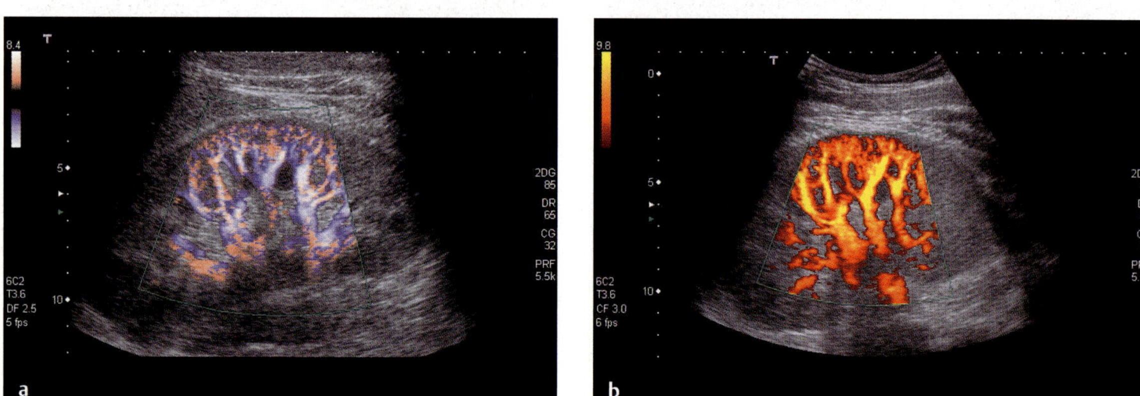

Fig. 20.**4 a, b** Wideband Doppler techniques such as Advanced Dynamic Flow (**a**) offer superior spatial resolution compared to conventional color or power Doppler imaging (**b**).

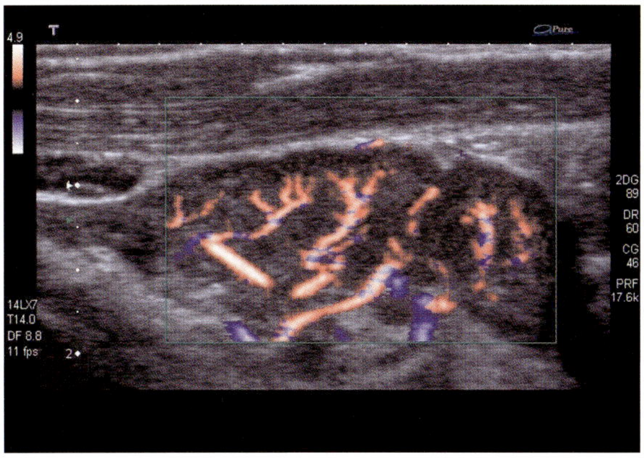

Fig. 20.**5** Enhanced vascularization of a hypervascular lymph node as depicted with a high-frequency 1.5D linear transducer and ADF.

Advances in Transducer Technology

While the development of ultrasound system design was enormous in the last decade, the number of fundamental changes in electronic transducer design was relatively low. Major new developments such as high-frequency transducers and two-dimensional transducer arrays have nevertheless expanded the image quality and application range of diagnostic ultrasound significantly.

High-Frequency Transducers

One of the fundamental characteristics of ultrasonic imaging is the tradeoff between resolution and penetration, which both depend on the transducer frequency. The majority of applications require some substantial penetration and therefore a relatively low frequency. The introduction of more effective ceramic materials and the improved bandwidth of ultrasound scanners have enabled the development of transducers with frequencies of up to 15 MHz or more.

These high-frequency transducers are able to resolve very small objects like tendons or submillimeter lesions with high detail definition. Thus, they are especially important for imaging of small organs such as the thyroid and breast, and also for all kinds of musculoskeletal applications. In combination with wideband Doppler techniques they enable the depiction of submillimeter vessels such as are found in small organs. Figure 20.**5** demonstrates this by showing the enhanced vascularization in a hypervascular lymph node.

Other devices working at even higher frequencies of up to several hundred Megahertz have been developed for special applications such as imaging of skin tumors. High-frequency transducers are also used for the imaging of small animals like mice; this has recently become a very important tool for cancer and gene therapy research.

1.5D Matrix Transducers

Conventional transducers enable to focus the ultrasonic beam in the imaging plane very precisely. However, in the elevation direction, perpendicular to the imaging plane, the beam shape is set by an acoustic lens with fixed focusing properties and one predetermined focal point. Thus, the slice thickness of the ultrasonic image varies over depth as demonstrated in Fig. 20.**6a**. This is especially problematic in the far field, where slice thickness artifacts can degrade image quality and noise level.

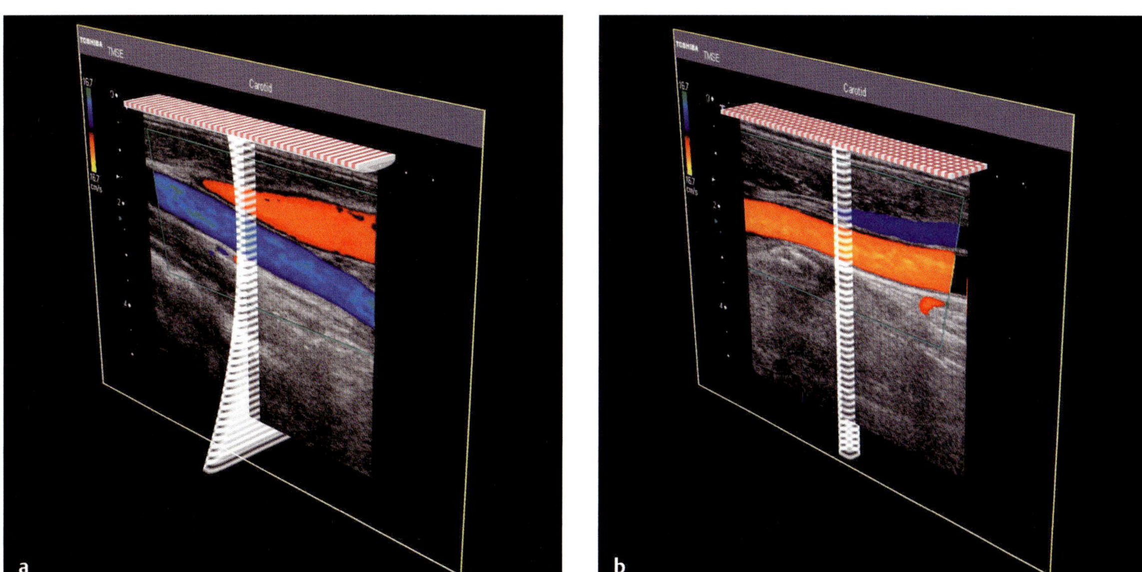

Fig. 20.**6a, b** The varying slice thickness of conventional one-dimensional transducers (**a**) leads, especially in the far field, to imaging artifacts. Two-dimensional slicing of the transducer allows control of the ultrasonic beam dynamically in both lateral and elevation directions to create a uniform slice thickness (**b**).

Two-dimensional slicing of the transducer elements allows control of the ultrasonic beam shape dynamically in both lateral and elevation directions (see Fig. 20.**6b**). A small number of slices in the elevation direction leads already to a substantial improvement in image quality and artifact suppression. Because the number of slices in the elevation direction is much lower than in the imaging plane, these transducers are also referred to as 1.5-dimensional or 1.5D transducers.

Because 1.5D transducers are capable of controlling the ultrasonic beam electronically in both dimensions, a continuous thin beam at all depths and in all dimensions and improved artifact suppression can be achieved. The results are improved image uniformity, increased spatial resolution, and enhanced image contrast and less clutter. Consequently, even small lesions can be visualized more accurately from shallow regions to the far field.

Beyond 2D Imaging

Diagnostic ultrasound is a real-time, nonirradiating technique that can be applied at any time and in any place. But while other modalities such as CT or MRI deliver 3D datasets that allow the user to create arbitrary cross-sections through the whole human body, ultrasound devices usually deliver only two-dimensional images with a limited field of view. During scanning this is not a problem in most cases, because by moving the transducer over the area of interest the investigator can easily obtain an overview and put the currently displayed image into relation with its surroundings.

Problems occur if the region of interest exceeds the field of view of the transducer or if the structure of interest is very complex, like the feeding vessels of a tumor, and thus cannot be captured in a single 2D image. In many cases the limited field of view also makes it impossible to display the region of interest and typical surrounding landmarks clearly in one image for documentation purposes. This is especially problematic for the surgeon, who usually has to rely on stored or printed images.

A number of techniques have been developed to overcome these problems. Next to continuous efforts to enlarge the field of view of the transducers themselves, 3D/4D and panoramic imaging are the most important.

Panoramic Imaging

Panoramic images are created by slowly drawing the transducer along a cut plane of interest across the human body. While this is being done, individual ultrasonic images are collected in the system and stitched together to give one resulting image with extended field of view. State-of-the-art techniques are able to create images with a total width of more that half a meter in real time. Two examples are shown in Figs. 20.**7** and 20.**8**. Figure 20.**9** demonstrates the different fields of view and the relationship of conventional 2D (left) and panoramic (right) images in an example showing the right carotid artery. The box displayed in the panoramic image equals the size of a conventional 2D image.

Most of today's panoramic imaging techniques do not require a positioning device attached to the transducer. By means of pattern recognition these techniques are able to generate a panoramic image from a series of regular 2D images. If the transducer is moved slowly enough to maintain the correlation between consecutive images, the accuracy of the resulting panoramic image is fairly high. Even back-and-forth movements will be mapped correctly. Advanced devices are able to generate and display the panoramic image in real time on the monitor of the ultrasound scanner; others will create it off-line after acquisition of the 2D images.

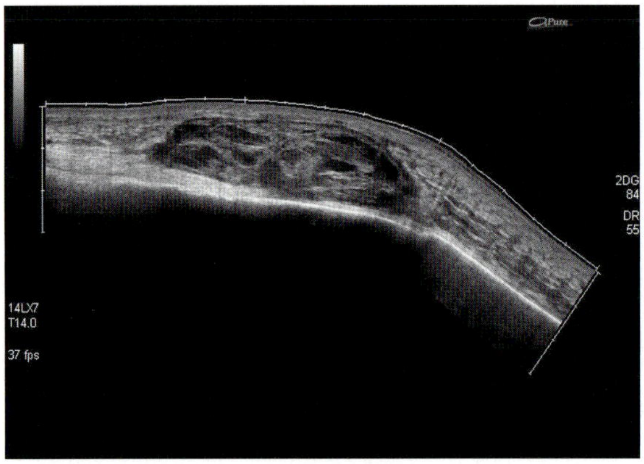

Fig. 20.**7** Panoramic view of lower limb with hematoma.

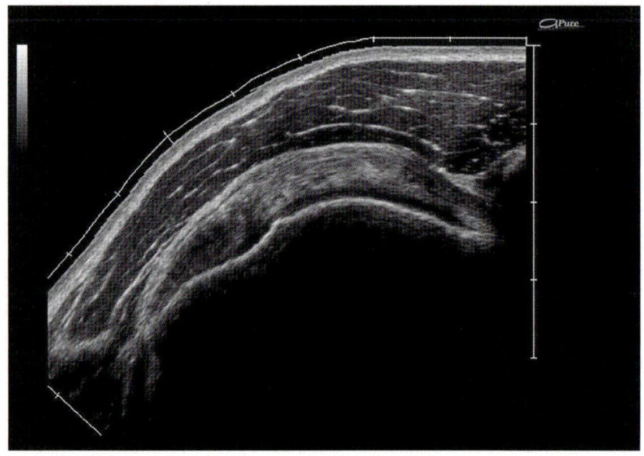

Fig. 20.**8** Panoramic view of a shoulder.

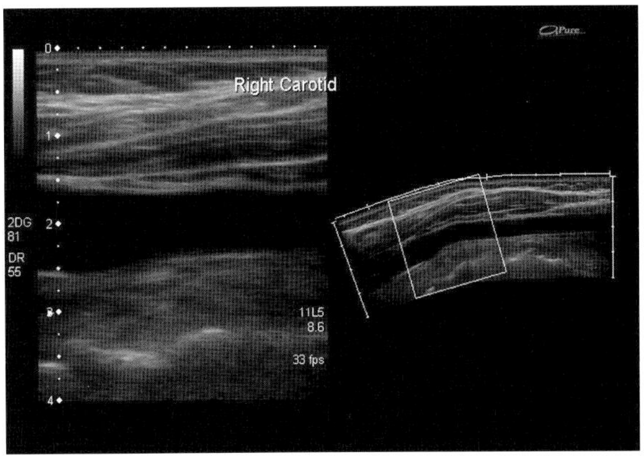

Fig. 20.**9** Comparison of the fields of view of conventional 2D (left) and panoramic (right) images in a normal right carotid artery. The box displayed in the panoramic image equals the size of the 2D image.

Panoramic imaging is available in a number of commercially obtainable systems for gray-scale imaging and power Doppler mode. Gray-scale panoramic imaging is used in many applications to visualize structural information in the enhanced field of view. Power Doppler mode can help to identify vascular occlusions or to improve the visualization of complex vascular structures, including surrounding tissues and landmarks for a better understanding of each particular pathology.

3D/4D Imaging

Diagnostic ultrasound delivers two-dimensional images of 3D objects. Therefore, the investigator has to move and tilt the transducer while examining the patient in order to obtain an overview of the region of interest. Depending on their skills, investigators will be able to transform the series of two-dimensional images seen on the monitor into volumetric information in their mind and thus be able to appreciate complex structures and their relationship with surrounding tissues. However, the result is not reproducible nor can it be stored, printed, or shared with others.

By moving the cut-plane of a transducer over the region of interest it is possible to acquire a set of neighboring images in a reasonably short time. If this movement is carried out in a well-defined manner, exact 3D datasets of the region of interest can be obtained, and in fact most manufacturers of diagnostic ultrasound equipment offer such a function or as add-ons to their systems.

There are a number of approaches for acquiring 3D datasets. Freehand techniques have the advantage of working with standard transducers and skilled users are able to produce reasonably good results. To increase the accuracy and to enable reliable distance measurements within the 3D dataset, some freehand products make use of positioning devices that can be attached to any transducer. As a result, freehand techniques deliver static 3D volume data of high resolution and accuracy.

Today's standard is to use special arrays that are swept mechanically inside the transducer housing in much the same way that mechanical transducers used to work. These ultrasound probes are able to produce accurate volume data sets within a split second. This results in a quasi real-time display and the continuous acquisition of 3D datasets enables the display of moving 3D images, sometimes also referred to as 4D imaging (three spatial dimensions and time as the fourth dimension).

The number of volumes per second created by such mechanical arrays is rather low and thus not suitable for depicting fast-moving structures such as heart valves. Using two-dimensional (2D) electronic arrays improves the volume imaging speed enormously, but currently available array technology suffers from limited spatial resolution. This is not a big problem for cardiac applications, where frame rate is most important and contrast between cavum and myocardium is high. Radiological or obstetric applications, where spatial and contrast resolution are of vital importance, so far rely on mechanically swept one-dimensional arrays.

There are also several ways to display 3D datasets. Surface rendering is most probably the best-known method. It is very useful for depicting the inside or outside surfaces of objects filled with or surrounded by echo-weak fluids, such as fetuses, bladders, gallbladders, or heart chambers and valves. This mode is commonly also used to display 3D power Doppler data. Volume rendering enables visualizing of 2D images on the surface of a data cube. By moving the surfaces of the data cube through an acquired data set, any combination of scan planes can be displayed. Multiplanar reslicing (MPR) is a method to display arbitrary two-dimensional cut-planes of a given 3D dataset. This can either be single planes or multiple views at the same time.

Figure 20.**10** shows an example of a 3D image of the carotid bifurcation. 3D volume data were acquired for both B-mode and power Doppler. This image shows the surface reconstruction of power Doppler data in a 3D mode. For a better overview the gray-scale data are displayed in an independent volume-rendered mode as 2D cut-plane. The cut-plane can be freely positioned and the dataset freely rotated to obtain the best diagnostic view.

Figure 20.**11** shows an example of MPR in a liver data set. While in the lower right a 3D reconstruction is displayed, the other views show simultaneously three perpendicular 2D slicings of the dataset. In this way MPR permits views in any cut-plane through the 3D dataset easily and with high spatial resolution.

Although the clinical usefulness and diagnostic relevance of 3D/4D scanning is still under investigation, it is widely accepted that procedures such as surgical planning, the understanding of anatomical relationships, or the accuracy of volume measurements can strongly benefit from 3D/4D scanning and that it will become an important tool in advanced ultrasound diagnostics in the future.

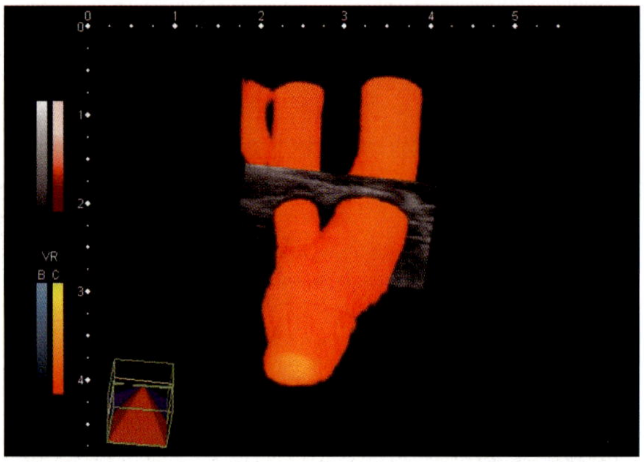

Fig. 20.**10** Three-dimensional display of the carotid bifurcation with surface-rendered power Doppler and volume-rendered gray-scale image.

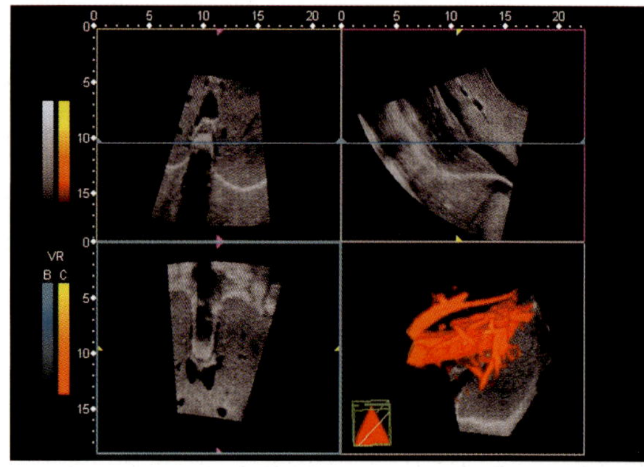

Fig. 20.**11** Multi-planar reslicing of a 3D volume dataset of a normal liver. In the lower right a 3D reconstruction is displayed; the other views show simultaneously three perpendicular 2D slicings of the dataset.

Ultrasonic Contrast Imaging

Contrast agents have been used as a standard tool to visualize vascular structures and blood flow in most imaging modalities for a long time. In diagnostic ultrasonography, however, this has not been the case. One of the reasons is most certainly the significant gap in echogenicity between tissue and blood, which makes it easy to depict vessels using a standard ultrasound scanner. Moreover, spectral and color Doppler allow us not only to detect blood flow very sensitively, but also to quantify its velocity and direction in the main branches.

To display and quantify perfusion and perfusion dynamics, however, ultrasonic imaging requires the support of a contrast agent as well. Today there is an ever-growing number of reports describing an enormous variety of detection techniques as well as their clinical application and usefulness. And although contrast agents are not yet approved for some applications and in a number of counties, today contrast echography is rapidly moving from the research field into routine clinical use.

Ultrasonic Contrast Agents

The first report describing an ultrasonic contrast agent dates back to 1968, when Gramiak and Shah detected echoes in the heart chambers, which are normally echo-poor, after injecting agitated saline. Agitation of the fluid generated small air bubbles and, because the mechanical impedance of gases and liquids differs strongly, the reflectivity of these gas bubbles is enormous, resulting in a strong echo signal. This method turned out to be useful in diagnosing septal shunt defects, which were previously only detected incidentally using ultrasound.

However, these gas bubbles were not stable and because of their size they were not able to pass through the lungs, which made catheterization of the patients necessary. Today's commercially available contrast agents are coated gas bubbles of much smaller size and more stable and they can be applied intravenously. Initially they were intended for detection of shunts and to enhance blood flow detectability in regions difficult to access, e.g. to improve the visualization of flow around plaques for a better assessment of the degree of stenosis.

Detection of Ultrasonic Contrast Agents

In fact it is much more interesting to trace contrast agents in areas that cannot be accessed with conventional Doppler techniques, such as in the microvasculature of organs. Besides the need for increased sensitivity, the major challenge in the development of suitable contrast imaging techniques for this purpose is to separate bubble echoes from overlying tissue signals effectively. In addition to their high echogenicity it turned out to be useful that microbubbles resonate or even disintegrate under the influence of ultrasound. The alternating pressure of the incident sound waves causes the bubbles to expand and to shrink. Because this is an asymmetric process, a portion of the backscattered sound energy is shifted to higher harmonic frequencies, which are nonlinear bubble echoes not present in the transmitted waveform.

Because of the high echogenicity of the microbubbles, blood flow can be detected even if the vessel diameter is smaller than the resolution of the ultrasonic image or if blood flow velocities are very close to or equal to zero, as in the microvasculature. Therefore, ultrasonic contrast imaging enables us to visualize and to quantify blood flow in the vascular phase as well as blood volume in the perfusion phase of an organ.

The amplitude of the harmonic signals depends on the strength of insonation, which can be characterized by the mechanical index (MI). At low MI, contrast agent bubbles contract and expand under the influence of the incident mechanical sound wave. With increasing MI, the probability of introducing cracks in the bubble shells grows. This results in fragmentation of bubbles and in rapid dissolution of the free gas.

A large number of contrast imaging techniques have been developed and commercialized under a virtually endless variety of names. However, there are just a few basic principles and all of these techniques employ at least one of them. From an application standpoint, all contrast imaging methods can be separated into two groups. The first group is based on the destruction of microbubbles at high MI, the other on the nonlinear response from resonating microbubbles at low MI.

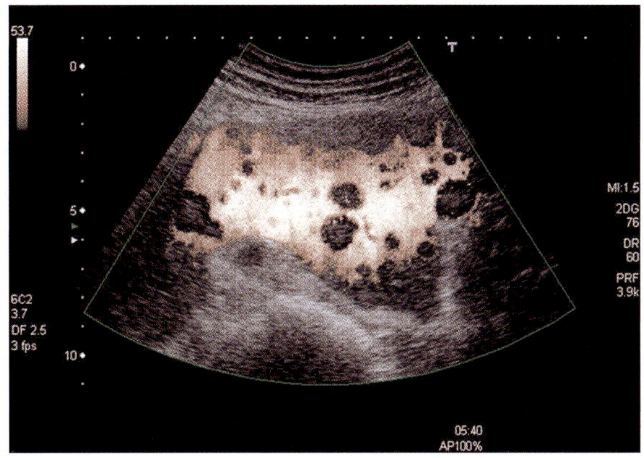

Fig. 20.**12** Late-phase imaging of a liver at high MI clearly identifies multiple liver metastases. (Image courtesy of Dr. Dittmar, Leverkusen, Germany.)

Destructive Contrast Imaging Techniques

High-MI techniques are based on the destruction of microbubbles to detect their presence in the area of interest. This effect produces a strongly nonlinear response over a wide range of frequencies. In fact these nonlinear bubble echoes can be seen as pseudo-Doppler signals spread over a wide range of velocities (= Doppler frequencies). Therefore, Doppler signal processing or similar correlation techniques can be used to detect the nonlinear echoes coming from the disintegrating bubbles. This can be done at either fundamental or harmonic frequencies or at both.

The destruction of bubbles, on the other hand, is also a major drawback of these methods, because most of the microbubbles are destroyed after making only one image. Depending on the supplying vessels, it may take up to several seconds to refill the insonated area with contrast agent. Thus, high-MI techniques can only be applied as intermittent scanning methods, leading to long, difficult clinical procedures.

Since the introduction of real-time imaging methods and contrast agents operating effectively at low MI, the clinical importance of high-MI techniques has declined substantially. Nevertheless, because of the very strong nonlinear response of the disintegrating microbubbles, they are still the most sensitive detection methods. Especially for perfusion imaging in the late phase of contrast agent wash-in, high-MI techniques are still valuable diagnostic tools. Wideband Doppler techniques allow the acquisition of perfusion images of outstanding sensitivity and spatial resolution. Thus, perfusion defects can be visualized very sensitively, which is essential for detection of lesions. Figure 20.**12** shows an example of multiple liver metastases as depicted using high MI after bolus injection of the contrast agent.

Real-Time Contrast Imaging Techniques

The destruction of microbubbles has to be avoided for visualization of ultrasonic contrast agents in real time. This requires a method that can separate bubble echoes effectively from all other echo components even at a very low MI. Filtering is a very simple method of separating harmonic from fundamental components. However, it is not very effective and limits the bandwidth of the nonlinear signals, resulting in decreased resolution.

The most commonly used technique today is pulse inversion, which makes use of the fact that bubbles respond differently to positive and negative incident pressure as described above. Two identical but phase-inverted waveforms are sent in the same direction into the tissue. Linear tissue echoes are canceled when the two received waveforms are added, because they are mirror-inverted. Bubble echoes of the two inverted pulses have different characteristics and their summation reveals the even harmonic components of the backscattered signals. Because a very low MI can be used here to detect the contrast agent, almost no tissue harmonic signals are generated, which is of vital importance for the tissue-contrast separation.

Amplitude modulation is another detection technique. It uses two similar pulses to be sent into the tissue, with the second pulse having double the amplitude of the first. While the linear components of the second echo are exactly doubled in amplitude compared to the first, nonlinear components coming from bubble echoes show a more complex behavior. Multiplying the amplitude of the first echo by a factor of 2 and subtracting the echoes results in the cancellation of linear components and in the preservation of nonlinear components.

Apart from these basic techniques, many derivatives as well as a number of combinations of these techniques exist.

Although the above-mentioned techniques are very sensitive, the presentation of contrast agents is limited in regions with very low bubble concentration. This is especially

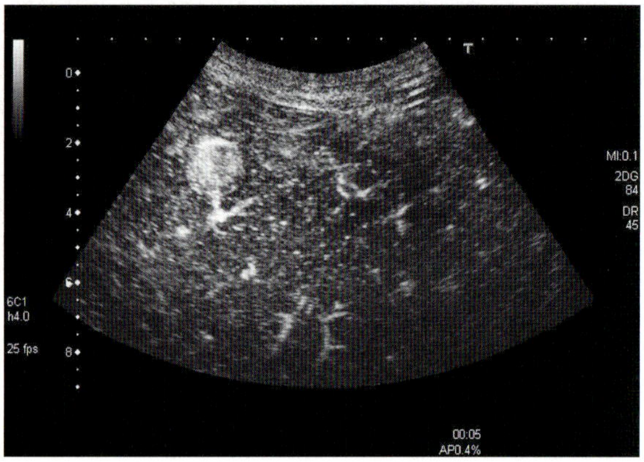

Fig. 20.**13** Enhanced vascularization and rapid filling of an HCC as revealed by real-time contrast harmonic imaging using low MI Pulse Subtraction. (Image courtesy of Professor D. Cosgrove, Hammersmith Hospital, London, UK.)

the case in slowly perfused organs like the breast or in the microvasculature of organs. Continuous imaging using low MI allows us to track the path of individual microbubbles over time. Microflow imaging captures and displays these traces, resulting in a significantly refined display of contrast agent, especially in the microvasculature (Fig. 20.**14**).

By imaging the propagation of microbubbles in the vascular system, wash-in/wash-out dynamics as well as arteriovenous transient times can be assessed. Time–intensity curves are a simple but efficient tool to visualize and quantify these transient events. Figure 20.**15** shows an example of HCC with very rapid contrast agent uptake in the HCC (red curve) compared to the liver parenchyma (green curve).

With the use of these tools, ultrasonic imaging is now able to detect, characterize, and classify lesions with high sensitivity and specificity in many kinds of tissues such as liver, breast, testis, myocardium, and others.

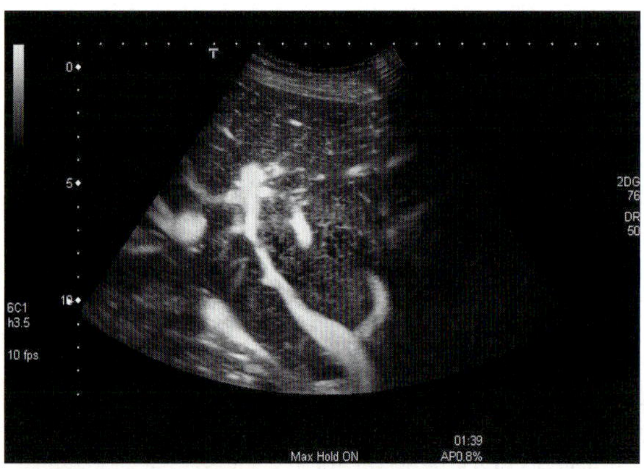

Fig. 20.**14** MFI is used to trace microbubbles in this contrast-enhanced image of a lymphoma in the splenic hilus resulting in a significantly refined display, especially of the microvasculature. (Image courtesy of Dr. C.F. Dietrich, Caritas Krankenhaus, Bad Mergentheim, Germany.)

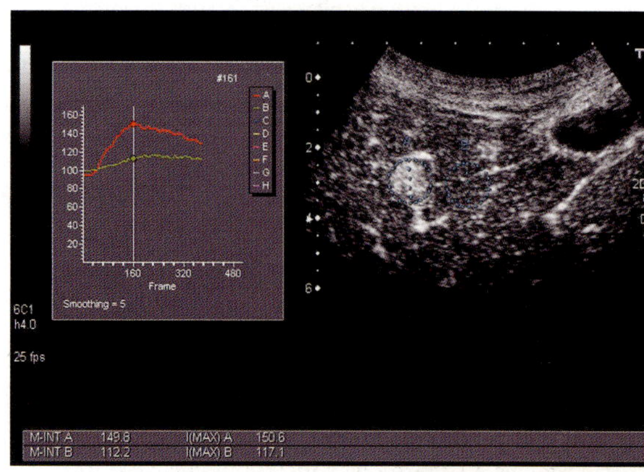

Fig. 20.**15** Time–intensity curves allow quantification of the dynamics of contrast agent wash-in as demonstrated in this low-MI pulse subtraction study of an HCC. Due to the arterial supply, contrast agent uptake in the HCC (red curve) occurs much faster than in the parenchyma (green curve). (Image courtesy of Professor D. Cosgrove, Hammersmith Hospital London, UK.)

Clinical Workflow Support and Automation

Image quality is of course the key to rapid and secure diagnosis. In ultrasound, unlike in other diagnostic imaging techniques, examination results and image quality vary substantially from patient to patient. Because it is impossible to scan patients with a fixed set of system settings, the operator has to optimize a number of scanning parameters for each patient and each view. The increasing diagnostic capabilities and accuracy of ultrasound scanners have in general made their operation more complex and thus made them more difficult to use.

To facilitate ultrasound examinations, a number of functions to assist automated or semi-automated image quality adjustment and measurements have been developed. These features can help to simplify examinations, to save time, and to increase the overall quality of examination results. A positive side-effect of these technologies is also that they support non-experts and beginners in making a reliable high quality diagnosis.

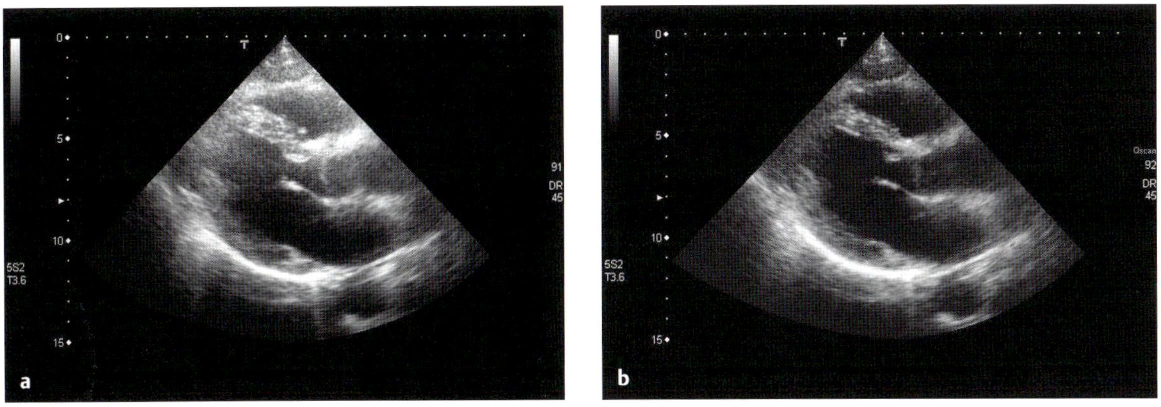

Fig. 20.**16 a, b** Parasternal long-axis view of the heart before (**a**) and after (**b**) automatic image optimization.

Automatic Image Optimization

Although today virtually all ultrasound scanners are able to display 256 different gray levels, the adapted human eye can only distinguish up to 60 shades of gray. The simplest way to increase the contrast resolution for the human eye is to colorize the ultrasonic images. To visualize subtle differences in echogenicity, however, it is always required to optimize brightness and contrast of the ultrasonic images and to distribute echo levels over the full range of the 256 gray levels. Scanners are equipped with a number of dials and sliders for adjustment, but it requires some experience and can be quite time-consuming to optimize all system settings.

To simplify this process, many of today's high-end scanners offer an automatic image quality adjustment function that performs all these tasks instantaneously simply with the push of a button. Figure 20.**16 a** demonstrates the effect on a nonoptimized parasternal long-axis view of the heart. After automatic optimization (Fig. 20.**16 b**), the image contrast is visibly increased and the noise level is reduced significantly.

Similar techniques also exist for the automatic optimization of spectral Doppler traces. Automatic adjustment of pulse repetition frequency, zero shift, and gain helps to avoid aliasing and to optimize the quality and display size of Doppler curves, which is important for accurate Doppler measurements.

Automatic Measurements

Another group of workflow-supporting features is that of automated measurements. In particular, tracings can be quite cumbersome and difficult to perform with high accuracy. Tracings are usually carried out on objects with well-defined borders such as cavities, vessels, or spectral Doppler curves. Since the ability of software algorithms to detect such well-defined borders automatically is quite good, a number of methods with surprisingly high accuracy are available in commercial systems.

The most common and useful feature implemented in a number of ultrasound systems is the automatic tracing of spectral Doppler curves. In addition to the exact tracing of the Doppler spectrum, many of these software packages are also able to detect systolic and end-diastolic velocities as well as to calculate all kinds of ratios and indices automatically. Figure 20.**17** shows an example of such tracing performed on a vertebral artery. While some packages perform these tasks in real time, others work offline after freeze.

Another common application for automatic measurements is the tracing of the left ventricle over the cardiac cycle and the automatic calculation of performance parameters such as the ejection fraction.

The accuracy of automatic tracing depends strongly on the quality of the underlying images. Automatic image optimization tools are thus very useful for delivering optimum imaging results for automatic measurements with the best possible accuracy. Both kinds of functions can also facilitate

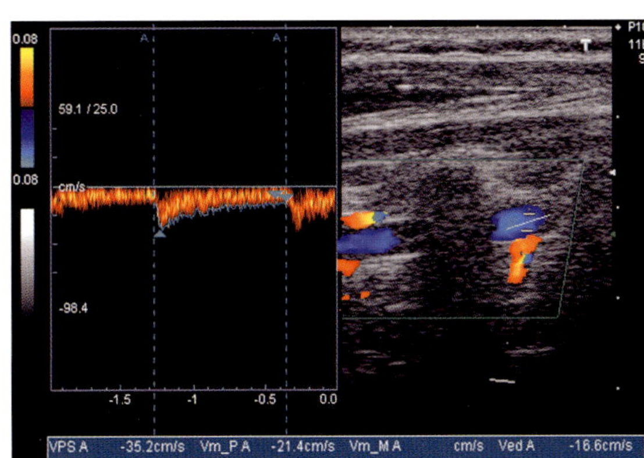

Fig. 20.**17** Automatic Doppler tracing and measurements on Doppler spectrum of the vertebral artery.

the examination and shorten the examination time significantly. It can therefore be expected that in future an increasing number of such workflow automation tools will become available.

Digital Documentation and Archiving

In recent years DICOM (Digital Imaging and COmmunication in Medicine) has become a keyword for digital image storage and transfer. Most diagnostic ultrasound systems offered today already support DICOM functions to some extent, and more and more hospitals are in the process of building up an infrastructure for fully digital management of patient records and diagnostic imaging. The basic idea behind the DICOM standard is to transfer, store, print, or review diagnostic images or clips digitally. This has a number of benefits, e. g., there is no image degradation, measurements can be taken any time after the examination, and data from previous examinations of each patient are available at any time in any place in the hospital. Moreover, images can be shared instantaneously with colleagues over the internal network or via the Internet.

But DICOM can do even more. Almost the entire workflow of an imaging department can be performed based on the DICOM standard. This includes electronic transfer of patient data into the diagnostic device, generation and transfer of reports and measurements taken during an examination to a central archive, or sending the details of a performed examination automatically to the Hospital Information System (HIS) for further patient management, accounting or statistical purposes.

Because DICOM is an open standard and applicable to all medical imaging modalities such as CT, MRI, or diagnostic ultrasound, data from different manufacturers and imaging modalities can be collected and shared. Thus, it is easy to compare or superimpose the results of different diagnostic procedures or to review previous examinations of a patient.

Index

D

V

W

Z